STANDARDS, RECOMMENDED PRACTICES, AND GUIDELINES

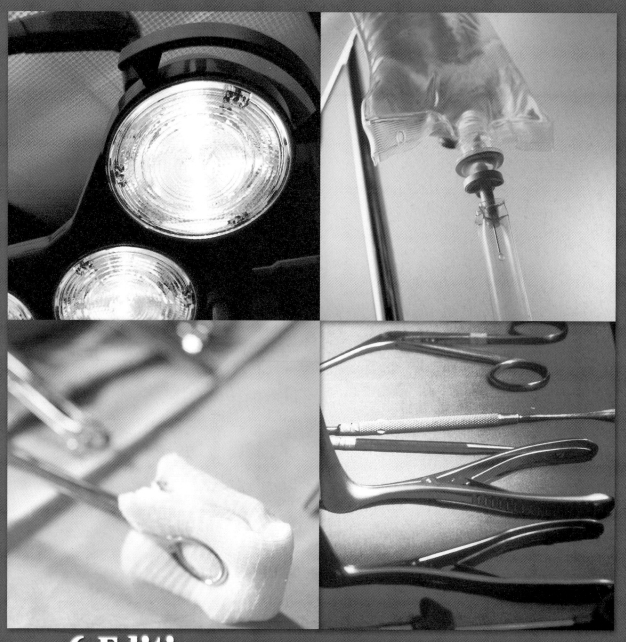

2006 Edition
With Official AORN Statements

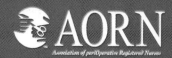

AORN

Association of periOperative Registered Nurses

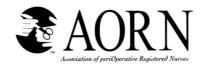

Association of periOperative Registered Nurses

2170 South Parker Road
Suite 300
Denver, CO 80231-5711
(800) 755-2676

Standards, Recommended Practices, and Guidelines

Copyright © 2006
AORN, Inc.

Clinical Editor: Ramona Conner, RN, MSN, CNOR
Senior Editor: Deb Reno
Cover Design: Masako James
Production Manager: Terry Isaacs

ISBN 1-888460-50-4

Printed in USA

Table of Contents

* *Indicates items newly revised in 2005 or published here for the first time.*

Table of Contents

* Indicates items newly revised in 2005 or published here for the first time.

Introduction to 2006 Edition

Historically, AORN has demonstrated an ongoing commitment to the surgical patient, the perioperative nurse, and the nursing profession. AORN was the first specialty nursing organization to develop process, structure, and outcome standards. This publication represents a compilation of the AORN-approved model, standards, statements, and recommended practices and reflects the perioperative nurse's scope of responsibility. Additionally, the publication contains AORN's mission and philosophy, bylaws, and position statements.

AORN offers a unified network of interrelated principles that systematically guide activities while allowing for flexibility, individuality, and change. The standards and recommended practices are broad in scope and are attainable, definitive, and relevant for the perioperative setting. They represent a comprehensive approach to meeting surgical patients' health needs in the practice setting.

Section 1: Perioperative Nursing Practice

AORN is dedicated to enhancing the professionalism of perioperative nurses, promoting standards of perioperative nursing practice to better serve the needs of society, and providing a forum for interaction and exchange of ideas related to perioperative health care. In support of this mission, this section includes AORN's competency statements, position statements, and guidelines for perioperative practice.

This year, the competency statements for perioperative nurses, perioperative advanced practice nurses, and perioperative care coordinators have been extensively revised and reformatted to incorporate the standardized terminology of the Perioperative Nursing Data Set. In addition, AORN's official position statements now include the new statements on correct site surgery, fire prevention, care of the patient with an implanted electronic device, and the revised statement on entry into practice, as ratified by the House of Delegates in April 2005.

AORN's new guidance statements on human and avian influenza, environmental responsibility, the role of the health care representative in the perioperative setting, and creating a patient safety culture appear in this edition for the first time. Also featured are revised guidance statements on the reuse of single-use devices and safe medication practices. AORN guidelines on bariatric surgery, latex safety, malignant hyperthermia, and the ethical responsibilities of perioperative nurses also are included in this section.

Section 2: Standards of Nursing Practice

The "Statement on perioperative patient care quality" recognizes the active participation of the perioperative nurse in shaping the practice environment. Clinical and organizational indicators of quality are identified through structure, process, and outcome standards.

The "Standards of perioperative administrative practice" were developed to guide professionals in administrative roles. They suggest criteria for the creation and maintenance of an environment in which nursing knowledge and skills can be used effectively. Professional nursing encompasses the responsibility to lead and manage others.

The "Standards of perioperative clinical practice" are process standards, based on the nursing process, that provide a basic model by which the quality of perioperative nursing practice can be evaluated. The standards are intended to assist perioperative nurses to expand their knowledge, increase their sensitivity to human needs, and maintain accountability to the consumer. The standards suggest criteria for continuous and systematic data collection, making a nursing diagnosis, identifying nursing actions, and evaluating observable outcomes. The perioperative nurse's special contribution lies in providing integrated, continuous care.

The "Standards of perioperative professional practice" describe the role activities that the nurse is expected to engage in (ie, providing quality care, pursuing education, practicing collegiality, ethical conduct, performance appraisal, collaboration, research, and resource utilization). These standards reflect a competent level of behavior and describe the roles expected of all perioperative nurses.

The "Quality and performance improvement standards for perioperative nursing" are intended to assist the perioperative nurse in monitoring and evaluating the quality of patient care. The standards were developed using the quality assessment and improvement standards of the Joint Commission on Accreditation of Healthcare Organizations. The standards suggest criteria for continuous monitoring and evaluation as a foundation for selecting methods for quality improvement.

The "Perioperative patient outcomes" reflect the ongoing development of the Perioperative Nursing Data Set (PNDS). These outcomes, interpretive statements, and accompanying outcome indicators provide a framework for measuring patient responses. They are designed to assist in evaluating the degree to which patient outcomes were attained, to support current nursing practice, or to provide a rationale for change.

Finally, the newly revised "AORN standards for RN first assistant education programs " have been updated and reformatted to reflect their continuity with the underlying standards of perioperative practice.

Section 3: Recommended Practices

AORN's "Recommended practices for perioperative nursing" (RPs) are written by selected members of the Association and liaisons from the Centers for Disease Control and Prevention, the Association for Professionals in Infection Control and Epidemiology, the American Society of Healthcare Central Service Professionals, the International Association of Healthcare Central Service Materiel Management, the American College of Surgeons, and the American Society of Anesthesiologists. Each recommended practice is reviewed and revised as appropriate at regular periodic intervals.

These recommended practices are based on principles of microbiology, scientific literature, research, and the opinions of experts and are periodically updated to reflect research data and advanced technology. They represent AORN's official position on questions of aseptic and technical practices by perioperative nurses. While policies and procedures will reflect variations in practice settings, individual commitment and professional conscience must guide the perioperative nurse in the use of these recommended practices.

Section 4: Additional Resources

Additional resources include the "Glossary of times used for scheduling and monitoring of diagnostic and therapeutic procedures" developed by the Association of Anesthesia Clinical Directors (AACD) and an index of important terms and concepts found throughout the text.

AORN Vision, Mission, Philosophy, and Values

AORN Vision and Mission

Preamble

Understanding that the term *perioperative* may not be well known outside the surgical arena, AORN defines the term *perioperative nursing* as the practice of nursing directed toward patients undergoing operative and other invasive procedures. AORN recognizes the *perioperative nurse* as one who provides, manages, teaches, and/or studies the care of patients undergoing operative or other invasive procedures.

Vision statement

AORN is the global leader in promoting excellence in perioperative nursing practice.

Mission statement

AORN supports registered nurses in achieving optimal outcomes for patients undergoing operative and other invasive procedures.

Philosophy

AORN is a voluntary organization of professional registered nurses concerned with perioperative patient care.

The Association believes that:

- Nursing is a social institution that provides essential and significant health care services to meet evolving societal needs. The perioperative nurse uses knowledge, judgment, and skills based on the principles of physical, biological, physiological, behavioral, social, and nursing science.
- Nurses must be ethical, responsible, and accountable for quality patient care. The nurse engaged in perioperative nursing practice provides or facilitates care to surgical or other perioperative patients.
- Research should be the foundation for perioperative nursing practice.
- Learning is a lifelong process, and perioperative nurses must assume responsibility for their ongoing education. The Association is committed to enabling perioperative nurses to meet that responsibility.
- Standards of nursing practice, interdisciplinary collaboration, and appropriate resource utilization enhance perioperative nursing practice.

- Its activities should be structured to anticipate and meet society's perioperative health care needs.

Values Statement

AORN is committed to excellence in support of its mission. Therefore, the Association values:

1. Educational services that are:
   - Cost effective
   - Accessible
   - Ongoing
   - Driven by member needs
   - Current/timely
   - Approved for contact hours
   - Convenient

2. Representation that is:
   - Effective
   - Comprehensive
   - Visible
   - Current/timely
   - Present in diverse health care arenas
   - Cost effective
   - Collaborative

3. Standards that are:
   - Research based
   - Current/timely
   - Comprehensive
   - Applicable
   - Achievable

Strategic Initiatives

1. AORN will partner with other perioperative associations and industry to achieve our goals.

2. AORN will be an indispensable resource for the perioperative nursing profession.

3. AORN will be the recognized leader of the perioperative nursing profession.

4. AORN will have strong, mutually supportive connections with its grassroots members.

Article I

The name of this professional organization is AORN, Inc (Association of periOperative Registered Nurses), hereinafter referred to as the "Association."

Article II

PURPOSES

The purposes of this Association are:

A. To unite registered professional operating room nurses for the purpose of maintaining an Association dedicated to the constant endeavor of promoting the highest professional standards of perioperative nursing practice for the optimum care of the patient before, during, and after surgery;

B. To provide opportunity for continuous learning through diversified educational activities;

C. To study, discuss, research, and exchange information in the field of perioperative nursing;

D. To hold meetings at intervals for the purposes of this Association;

E. To cooperate lawfully with other professional associations, health care facilities, universities, industries, technical societies, research organizations, and governmental agencies in matters affecting the foregoing purposes of the Association;

F. To otherwise lawfully adopt policies and conduct programs for the improvement of perioperative nursing practice, provided that the policies and programs are consistent with the requirements that the Association is not organized for profit and no part of its earnings inure to individuals.

Article III

MEMBERSHIP AND DUES

Section 1: Membership in the Association is contingent on compliance with requirements as specified in these bylaws.

Section 2: Membership is unrestricted by consideration of nationality, race, creed, lifestyle, color, sex, or age.

Section 3: Categories of membership in this Association are chapter member, member at large, retired, student, and associate.

A. CHAPTER MEMBER: A registered professional nurse who supports the mission of AORN living in an area where a chapter exists.

B. MEMBER AT LARGE: A registered professional nurse who supports the mission of AORN and does not have access to e-Chapter or consistent access to a local chapter.

C. RETIRED: A retired registered professional nurse who supports the mission of AORN.
   1. Qualifies to be a member at large.
   2. If a chapter membership is selected, applicable chapter dues may be assessed.

D. STUDENT: An individual pursuing education leading to eligibility to sit for the registered nurse licensing examination.
   1. Qualifies to be a member at large.
   2. If a chapter membership is selected, applicable chapter dues may be assessed.
   3. May not hold elective office.
   4. May not serve as a delegate to the AORN House of Delegates.

E. ASSOCIATE: An individual who supports the mission of AORN and who is primarily engaged in one of the following professions: health care industry representative, central service professional, physician, health care administrator, perioperative and facility material management, informatics personnel, or pharmacist.
   1. Qualifies to be an associate at large.
   2. If a chapter membership is selected, applicable chapter dues may be assessed.
   3. May not hold elective office.
   4. May not serve as a delegate to the AORN House of Delegates.
   5. This is a nonvoting category.

Section 4: Termination

A. The Board of Directors may terminate a membership for failure to meet membership requirements, provided the member was offered an opportunity to have an unprejudiced hearing, if requested, at which the member was permitted to defend against the termination.

B. If terminated, a member may be allowed to rejoin by the Board of Directors after demonstrating eligibility for membership.

Section 5: Dues

A. Annual membership dues in this Association are determined by the Board of Directors and subject to ratification by the House of Delegates.

B. Dues shall be paid according to established policy.

C. Delinquency: Any member whose dues are not received by the last working day of the member's renewal month is automatically terminated as a member, and all privileges of the Association are withdrawn.

Article IV

OFFICERS

The officers of this Association are President, President-elect, Vice President, Secretary, and Treasurer.

A. President:

Serves as the official representative of the Association and presides at all meetings of the House of Delegates, the Board of Directors, and the Executive Committee.

B. President-elect:

Observes and assists the President in preparation for assuming the duties and responsibilities of that office.

C. Vice President:

Performs the duties of the President in the absence or inability of the President to act.

D. Secretary:

Assures records are maintained of the proceedings of all business meetings of the House of Delegates and the Board of Directors.

E. Treasurer:

Monitors the fiscal affairs of the Association and provides reports and interpretation to the House of Delegates and the Board of Directors.

Article V

NOMINATING COMMITTEE – NOMINATIONS
ELIGIBILITY – ELECTIONS
TERMS – VACANCIES – REMOVAL

Section 1:   Nominating Committee

A. The Nominating Committee consists of five (5) members. Three (3) members are elected in the even-numbered years and two (2) in the odd-numbered years, each serving for a term of two (2) years.

B. The immediate past President will automatically become a nonvoting member of the committee for a term of one (1) year following the term of office as President.

Section 2:   Nominations

A. The Nominating Committee prepares and presents a slate of candidates to serve in elected capacity.

B. Nominations may be made from the floor of the House of Delegates, provided that eligibility has been verified and written consent to serve if elected was obtained from the nominee and is submitted at the time of the nomination.

Section 3:   Eligibility

A. To be eligible for elective office as a member of the Board of Directors or as a member of the Nominating Committee, a nominee must currently provide or have previously provided perioperative nursing care that addresses(ed) the needs of patients preoperatively, intraoperatively, and postoperatively.

B. To be eligible for elective office as a member of the Board of Directors or a member of the Nominating Committee, a nominee must have been a member of the Association continuously for two (2) years immediately prior to being nominated and may not be an employee of AORN Headquarters.

C. To be eligible for the office of President-elect or Vice President, a nominee must have served at least one (1) year as a member of the Board of Directors.

D. The members of the Nominating Committee may not be listed as candidates for election on a slate that they have prepared.

Section 4:   Elections

A. The Officers, Board of Directors, and Nominating Committee shall be elected by written ballot at the annual Congress, and plurality elects. In case of a tie, choice is by lot.

B. Any member holding an elective office may not be a candidate for another office unless the current term of the member expires at the impending annual election.

Section 5:   Term of office

A. A President-elect is elected each year and serves in that capacity for one (1) year, and then as President for one (1) year.

B. The Vice President and Secretary shall be elected in the even-numbered years for a term of two (2) years and shall serve until their successors have assumed office.

C. The Treasurer shall be elected in the odd-numbered years for a term of two (2) years and shall serve until a successor has assumed office.

D. Three (3) members of the Board of Directors shall be elected in the even-numbered years for a term of two (2) years and shall serve until their successors have assumed office.

E. Four (4) members of the Board of Directors shall be elected in odd-numbered years for a term of (2) years and shall serve until their successors have assumed office.

F. No officer or member of the Board of Directors shall serve more than two (2) consecutive terms in the same office.

Section 6: Vacancies

A. President: The Vice President immediately assumes office.

B. President-elect and Vice President: A vacancy in the office of President-elect or Vice President is filled by a vote of the Board of Directors from a slate submitted by the Nominating Committee, and eligibility requires the nominee to have served at least one (1) year as a member of the Board of Directors.

C. The Board of Directors fills all other vacancies.

D. Any member filling a vacancy for an unexpired term of one (1) year or more is deemed to have served one term.

Section 7: Removal

Any elected official, regardless of the manner of election or appointment, may be removed by the House of Delegates upon two-thirds (2/3) affirmative vote whenever, in its judgment, the best interests of the Association would be served thereby, provided the elected official, upon request, was offered an opportunity to have an unprejudiced hearing at which the elected official was permitted to defend against the termination.

Article VI

MEETINGS

A. House of Delegates

1. The annual meeting is designated as the annual Congress, and the time and place is determined by the Board of Directors.

2. The voting body of the annual Congress is the House of Delegates constituted as follows:

   a) The maximum size of the House of Delegates is 1,500 voting members, excluding the delegates described in paragraphs b) and c).

   b) All officers and members of the Board of Directors are delegates and entitled to all the privileges of a delegate at the time they assume office. (May not serve as a chapter delegate.)

   c) The three (3) most recent and eligible past Presidents attending the annual Congress are delegates. (May not serve as a chapter delegate.)

   d) The delegate count shall be allocated annually to chapters and MAL category members based upon the ratio of total chapter membership to total Association membership as of June 30, with each chapter and the MAL category having a minimum of one (1) delegate and one (1) alternate delegate.

   e) Each selected delegate shall serve for a term commencing at the beginning of the first annual Congress that follows the election of the delegate and ending immediately prior to the beginning of the next annual Congress.

3. The House of Delegates convenes at least twice during each annual Congress.

4. Special meetings of the House of Delegates may be called during the annual Congress by the national President, or upon request of one-third (1/3) of the total number of members of the House of Delegates, or by written request of five (5) members of the Board of Directors.

5. Special meetings of the House of Delegates may be held between annual Congresses on the written request of five (5) members of the Board of Directors. A delegate may vote at a special meeting by proxy granted to the Secretary of the Association or such other person or persons as the notice of the meeting may specify.

6. Delegates shall not vote by proxy at meetings of the House of Delegates held during the annual Congress.

7. The presence of twenty percent (20%) of the registered delegates constitutes a quorum for all meetings of the House of Delegates.

Article VII

BOARD OF DIRECTORS

The Board of Directors consists of the officers and seven (7) elected members. It has power, authority, and responsibility to manage the affairs of the Association, except modifying action of the House of Delegates.

Section 1: Meetings
A. Meets at least three (3) times per year; once immediately before, once immediately following the annual Congress, and once in the interim between Congresses.
B. Special meetings of the Board of Directors may be called by the President or upon written request of three members of the Board of Directors.
C. Five (5) members of the Board, two of whom are officers, constitutes a quorum.

Section 2: Executive Committee
A. Consists of at least three (3) members: the President, the President-elect, and the Vice President.
B. Assists the President in expediting the business of the Association between meetings of the Board of Directors. A majority constitutes a quorum.

Article VIII

ORGANIZATIONAL UNITS

Section 1: Committees and Task Forces
In order to facilitate the Association's mission and strategic plan as well as the needs of the profession, the Board of Directors shall at least annually create such committees and ad hoc task forces as it deems desirable. The President-elect shall appoint the members of all such committees and ad hoc task forces. Each committee or task force shall consist of a chair and at least two (2) additional members. Each committee or task force shall have only such powers as are specifically delegated to it by the Board of Directors. A majority of the members of the committee or task force shall constitute a quorum.

Section 2: Organizational Units
To achieve the mission and purposes of AORN, the Board of Directors may establish organizational units to serve special interests of the membership.

Section 3: State Councils
State Councils composed of registered nurses may be recognized as AORN affiliates by the Board of Directors.

Article IX

EXECUTIVE DIRECTOR AND HEADQUARTERS

A. The Executive Director is the salaried employee of the Association accountable to the Board of Directors and given the authority to administer the Association according to policies established by the House of Delegates and the Board of Directors.
B. The Executive Director shall employ, direct, promote, and terminate Headquarters staff of the Association.

Article X

OFFICIAL PUBLICATION

The official publication of the Association is the *AORN Journal.*

Article XI

PARLIAMENTARY AUTHORITY

Robert's Rules of Order Newly Revised is the parliamentary authority of this Association.

Article XII

AMENDMENTS

A. Amendments to the bylaws may be made at the annual Congress by a two-thirds (2/3) vote of the delegates present and voting, provided that the proposed amendments have been submitted to all members at least forty-five (45) days prior to the annual Congress.
B. Amendments to the bylaws may be made at the annual Congress by a four-fifths (4/5) vote of the delegates present and voting, provided the amendments are submitted at one meeting and voted upon at the next meeting.

Revised March 2004.

Perioperative Patient Focused Model

Introduction

AORN has demonstrated an ongoing commitment to the surgical patient through its concern for the quality of operating room nursing practice. To provide quality patient care, AORN has developed standards of practice.

The first official statement defining nursing care in the operating room, "Definition and objective for clinical practice of professional operating room nursing," was published in 1969.[1] This statement was intended to serve as an ultimate guideline for nurse practitioners in nursing education and nursing service. It provided direction to nurses at that time.

AORN continued to establish its commitment to the surgical patient by the approval of the following resolutions. At the 1973 AORN Congress, the House of Delegates adopted a resolution, "The necessity for the registered nurse in the operating room."[2] In 1975, the AORN House of Delegates approved the statement, "Mandate for the registered nurse as circulator in the operating room."[3]

In the fall of 1976, a proposal to define the role of nurses in the operating room, Project 25, was approved by the AORN Board of Directors. The report of the Project 25 Task Force was accepted by the House of Delegates at the 25th AORN Congress in New Orleans in 1978. Within the report is the definition of the perioperative role and nursing activities performed during the preoperative, intraoperative, and postoperative phases of the patient's surgical intervention.[4]

In 1984–1985, the Nursing Practices Committee was charged with the responsibility of reviewing and revising the 1978 definition of nursing in the operating room. The 1978 definition was determined to be too restrictive in that it addressed the individual practitioner rather than the scope of nursing practice in the operating room. The term *perioperative nursing practice* was determined to be more descriptive than the term *perioperative role*.

In 1990, as part of the Project 2000 activities to position AORN for the future, the Board of Directors charged the Project Team to Redefine/Reconceptualize Perioperative Nursing to scrutinize the 1985 definition of nursing practice in the operating room. This definition addressed the registered nurse in the operating room responsible for providing nursing care to surgical patients.[5] Then as now, many noninvasive procedures were being performed outside the traditional operating room,[6] and many were

questioning who exactly is the "surgical" patient. The Project Team was charged to recommend a new definition of and conceptual framework for perioperative nursing, carefully analyzing who the recipients of perioperative nursing care are and what services they require. Their conclusions and recommendations were presented to the AORN House of Delegates and adopted in 1994.[7]

The Perioperative Patient Focused Model

In 1998, the AORN Board of Directors appointed a special Project Team on a Perioperative Model and charged its members to evaluate existing nursing theoretical models and recommend one of the models to the Board as applicable for incorporating the professional practice of perioperative nursing. If an existing model could not be identified as satisfying perioperative practice and the underpinning concepts of patient care, the team was charged with developing a theoretical model for perioperative nursing.[8]

The selection process. After conducting a literature search, the team generated an initial list of possible theories and models. The Project Team examined and evaluated 15 selected theories and models. Team members agreed that the most basic and essential characteristics of a theory were that it had to be

- logical;
- relatively simple, yet generalizable to various perioperative practice settings and patient populations;
- able to be used by practicing perioperative nurses to guide and improve practice; and
- researchable, so that hypotheses could be tested leading to contributions to the general body of knowledge within the specialty of perioperative nursing.

Each theory or model was evaluated for internal criticism (ie, the construction of the theory or model) and external criticism (ie, the theory or model and its relationship to people, nursing, and health). External criticism regarding the relationship between perioperative nursing and perioperative patient care also was specified. Based on the ratings and on the summary and recommendation of the team member who reviewed the theorist or model, the Project Team chose the conceptual model developed by AORN's Data Elements Coordinating Committee (Figure 1). In addition to the scoring and commentary by the team reviewer, other salient and compelling reasons guided this choice.

Figure 1

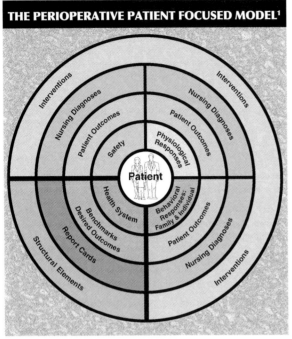

THE PERIOPERATIVE PATIENT FOCUSED MODEL[1]

NOTE
1. S Beyea, ed, Perioperative Nursing Data Set, *second ed* (Denver: AORN, 2002) 25 and inside front cover.

Patient focused. The model is patient focused. The patient is at the center of the model, which clearly and emphatically represents perioperative patient care. Regardless of practice setting, geographic location, or nature of the patient population, there is nothing more important to the practicing perioperative nurse than his or her patient. This model makes this concept of patient care "visible" in and between all other variables in the surgical setting.

The Perioperative Patient Focused Model consists of four domains: patient safety, physiologic responses, behavioral responses, and the health system. Nursing diagnoses, nursing interventions, and patient outcomes comprise the patient safety, physiologic response, and behavioral response domains. These foci represent the phenomena of concern to perioperative nurses and the needs of surgical patients and their families. These components of the model are in continuous interaction with the health system encircling the focus of perioperative nursing practice: the patient. The fourth domain, the health system, is composed of the structural data elements and focuses on clinical processes and outcomes.[9]

The model focuses on outcomes. This is important, as nursing theories and models should embrace and represent all elements of the nursing process, including outcomes. AORN's model represents the outcomes focus of perioperative nurses by placing outcomes immediately adjacent to the patient care domains. The Project Team members believed that perioperative nurses have a unique knowledge base that supports high-quality patient outcomes in surgical settings. An individualized patient assessment guides the identification of nursing diagnoses and selection of nursing interventions for each patient.

Conclusion. Components of the Perioperative Patient Focused Model, such as safety, physiologic responses, and behavioral responses of patients, reflect the nature of the surgical experience for the patient and guiding precepts for providing care by perioperative nurses. The Perioperative Patient Focused Model is logical, and the concepts and principles are supported in practice environments. Although this model and the theoretical concepts that underpin it are descriptive in nature and in early stages of development, it holds much promise for research.

The model represents the "real world" for practicing perioperative nurses and has utility for practicing nurses, educators, and researchers. A simultaneous simplicity and elegance is reflected in this model. The interrelationships of the domains and concepts provide a picture of the building blocks of perioperative nursing practice in a way that instructs and educates the student, guides nursing practice, and offers infinite opportunities for testing and further validation through research.

The model as a whole illustrates the dynamic nature of the perioperative patient experience and the nursing presence throughout that process. Working in a collaborative manner with other members of the health care team and the patient, the nurse establishes outcomes, identifies nursing diagnoses, and provides nursing care. The nurse intervenes within the context of the health care system to assist the patient to achieve the highest attainable health outcomes (ie, physiological, behavioral, and safety) throughout the perioperative experience.[10]

Goal of perioperative nursing practice

The goal of perioperative nursing practice is to assist patients and their families to achieve a level of wellness equal to or greater than that which they had prior to the procedure.

Philosophy of perioperative nursing practice

Nursing is a social institution providing an essential and significant component of the health care services needed by people. As such, nursing must be concerned with meeting evolving societal needs in relation to the nature and delivery of such services. Nursing is a science and derives a large portion of its knowledge base from the natural, behavioral, and social sciences and the humanities. Nursing integrates and applies these principles through use of the nursing process directed to and from the focal point of all nursing activities—the patient.

The practice of nursing is directed toward the patient who, as a biopsychosocial being, is a product of and responds to internal and external phenomena. Nursing responds by helping to alter these phenomena to promote and maintain health, to help cure disease, to assist adaptation to chronic disease, or to support the achievement of a peaceful, dignified death. Nursing is a caring art based on the creative application of knowledge, skills, and interpersonal competencies to provide quality, individualized patient care.

The patient who experiences the prospect or performance of an operative or other invasive procedure is the focus of perioperative nursing. Perioperative nursing practice addresses resulting patient needs amenable to nursing intervention. While basic life-sustaining needs may be of the highest priority, the perioperative nurse is concerned with all physiological, psychological, sociocultural, and spiritual dimensions of the patient's human responses.

Through the use of the nursing process, perioperative nurses provide care designed to meet individual patient needs and the needs of their families. *Families* may be defined as the person or persons that the patient defines as his or her family or significant other. Perioperative nursing occurs within a social setting characterized by rapidly changing technological, economic, and cultural forces that require continuous adaptation by professional practitioners. The complexity of knowledge and skill required compels nurses to be well educated and to continue their education beyond generic nursing programs.

Perioperative nursing practice includes providing direct care, coordinating comprehensive care, educating recipients of perioperative nursing, and generating perioperative nursing knowledge in a variety of settings. The perioperative nurse uses substantial knowledge, judgment, and skill based on the principles of biological, physiological, behavioral, social, and nursing sciences. Knowledge and skills acquired by the nurse are used to implement the nursing process and the "Standards of [perioperative] nursing practice."[11] In this context, the perioperative nurse works with the patient to make decisions regarding the patient's needs and to assist and support the patient.

The perioperative nurse also works in collaboration with other health professionals to meet patients' needs. The perioperative nurse has primary responsibility and accountability for the nursing care of patients who are experiencing operative and other invasive procedures.

Definition of perioperative nurse

Perioperative nurse is defined as the registered nurse who, using the nursing process, develops a plan of nursing care and then coordinates and delivers care to patients undergoing operative or other invasive procedures. Perioperative nurses have the requisite skills and knowledge to assess, diagnose, plan, intervene, and evaluate the outcomes of interventions. The perioperative nurse addresses the physiological, psychological, sociocultural, and spiritual responses of surgical patients.

Scope of perioperative nursing practice

Perioperative nurses provide care across the surgical continuum, beginning when the patient is first told of the need for an operative or invasive procedure and ending when the patient returns to his or her usual roles and responsibilities. The perioperative registered nurse provides care in a variety of clinical settings including acute care and ambulatory facilities as well as office-based settings and home care. The perioperative nurse's focus of concern is the patient and his or her family members, significant others, and friends.

Perioperative professional nurses identify patients' needs, set goals with patients, and implement nursing interventions and activities to achieve optimal patient outcomes. Each patient is viewed as a unique individual, and care is planned and provided to meet each patient's specific needs. The perioperative nurse is concerned with the patient's safety as well as physiological and behavioral responses throughout the surgical experience.

The perioperative nurse may function in one or more roles as a clinical practitioner, manager, educator, and researcher. Perioperative nursing practice is defined both as a caring art and as a science incorporating the critical thinking skills that are derived from knowledge of natural, behavioral, and social sciences and the humanities. Nursing integrates and applies this knowledge through use of the nursing process.

Glossary

Invasive procedures: Those in which the body is entered (eg, by use of a scalpel, tube, device, ionizing or nonionizing radiation, or any other invasion) and in which protective reflexes or self-care abilities are potentially compromised.

Perioperative: Surrounding the operative and other invasive experience (ie, before, during, and after).

Perioperative nursing care: The nursing activities that address the needs of patients, their families, and significant others that occur preoperatively, intraoperatively, and postoperatively.

Perioperative nursing services: Services extended to a variety of other groups to enhance the care ultimately provided to the patient. These groups include, but are not limited to, hospitals, clinics, schools and colleges of nursing, physicians, other nurses, insurers, and medical device and pharmaceutical manufacturers.

NOTES
1. "Definition and objective for clinical practice of professional operating room nursing," *AORN Journal* 10 (November 1969) 43-48.

2. "Delegates approve statements on RN and nursing students in OR, institutional licensure, abortion," *AORN Journal* 17 (April 1973) 187-191.

3. "Delegates approve statements, resolutions at 22nd Congress," *AORN Journal* 21 (May 1975) 1067-1082.

4. "Operating room nursing: Perioperative role," *AORN Journal* 27 (May 1978) 1156-1175.

5. "Project 2000 final report: A work plan for the future," *AORN Journal* 57 (January 1993) 54-77.

6. *Ibid.*

7. "Bylaws amendments, member at large delegates, redefinition of perioperative nursing top business issues this year," *AORN Journal* 59 (June 1994) 1167-1191.

8. J Rothrock, D Smith, "Select the Perioperative Patient Focused Model," *AORN Journal* 71 (May 2000) 1030-1037.

9. S Beyea, ed, *Perioperative Nursing Data Set,* second ed (Denver: AORN, 2002) 25.

10. Rothrock, Smith, "Select the Perioperative Patient Focused Model," 1030-1037.

11. "Standards of nursing practice," in AORN *Standards and Recommended Practices* (Denver: Association of Operating Room Nurses, Inc, 1993) 57-90.

Original statement submitted February 1978 and adopted February 14, 1978, by the House of Delegates, New Orleans, Louisiana.
Revised November 1984.
Revised March 1988 by the House of Delegates, Dallas, Texas.
Revised March 1994 by the House of Delegates, New Orleans, Louisiana.

This document was compiled in December 2001 based on "A model for perioperative nursing practice" (in Standards, Recommended Practices, and Guidelines *[Denver: AORN, 2001] 15-17) and the "Perioperative Patient Focused Model" (in* Perioperative Nursing Data Set, *second ed, S Beyea, ed [Denver: AORN, 2002]).*

PERIOPERATIVE NURSING PRACTICE

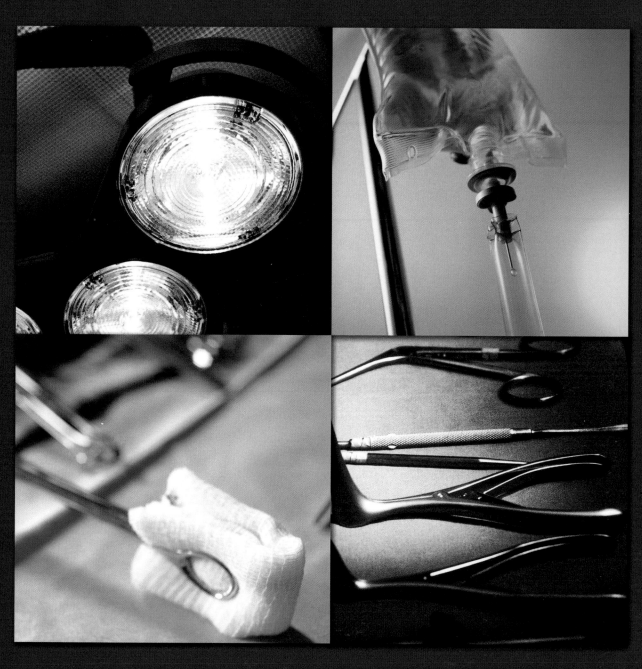

Section One

T he following definitions were developed by the AORN Center for Nursing Practice and were approved by the Board of Directors in November 2004. These definitions are intended to assist perioperative nurses in distinguishing among the different types of documents and statements developed by AORN and published in this section of *Standards, Recommended Practices, and Guidelines*.

Please note that all documents are subject to review or revision at any time during the review cycle if new information, technology, legislation, regulation, or other relevant developments require a more timely update of the document.

* Documents are listed in order of rigor.

Document name*	Suggested definition	Author	Review/revision process	Approval authority
Standard	Authoritative statements that describe the responsibilities for which perioperative nurses are accountable. Standards reflect the values and priorities of the profession. They are a means to direct and evaluate professional nursing practice.	Board appointed (Nursing Practice Committee)	Undefined, suggest 5-year review cycle	Board
Recommended practice	Achievable recommendations representing what is believed to be an optimal level of perioperative nursing practice. Recommended practices are broad statements to be used to guide policy and procedure development in specific work environments. Although they are considered to represent the optimal level of practice, variations in practice settings and clinical situations may limit the degree to which each recommendation can be implemented.	Board appointed (Recommended Practices Committee)	3 years	Board
Guideline	Addresses a specific medical diagnosis or clinical condition and is based on empirical data. A guideline should assist practitioners in clinical decision making, be used to assess and assure the quality of care, and to guide clinical practice (eg, malignant hyperthermia, latex allergy).	Board appointed	Undefined, suggest 5-year review cycle	Board
Guidance statement	Provides suggested strategies to assist practitioners in developing facility-specific processes related to clinical and administrative issues (eg, medication guidance statement, staffing guidance statement).	Board appointed	Undefined, suggest 5-year review cycle	Board

Document name*	Suggested definition	Author	Review/revision process	Approval authority
Competency statements	Represents expected, measurable, perioperative nursing behaviors. Defines the knowledge, skills, and abilities necessary to fulfill the professional role functions of a perioperative registered nurse.	Board appointed (Nursing Practices Committee)	Variable, determined by Board	Board
Position statement	Articulates AORN's official position or belief about certain perioperative nursing-related topics.	Board appointed	Variable, determined by Board sunset policy	Board and House of Delegates

Competency Statements in Perioperative Nursing

These statements of competency for perioperative nursing have been established as part of AORN's continuing commitment in providing care to surgical patients. The Association believes that validating competency is a necessary outgrowth of its beliefs about nursing and patient care. The philosophy of perioperative nursing developed by AORN states that "nursing is a caring art based on the creative application of knowledge, skills, and interpersonal competencies," adding that "the ultimate goal of such nursing is the provision of quality individualized patient care."[1,2]

In 2005, the National Committee on Education was charged by the AORN Board of Directors to incorporate the Perioperative Nursing Data Set (PNDS) into these competency statements. This supports the goal of the AORN Board to increase awareness, generate interest, and support use of the PNDS by perioperative nurses. The members of the National Committee on Education are nurses who either currently function in the role of perioperative educators, or who have in the past. They each have between 15 and 35 years of experience. The majority of members are educationally prepared at the bachelor's or master's level. The committee took the current perioperative competencies and, with the help of PNDS experts, translated them into the four domains with the corresponding measurable criteria and recommendations for validation. The literature search that was completed by the prior committee was not repeated. The competency statements were sent for review to the Advanced Practice Issues Task Force, the Nursing Practices Committee, and governing council members for the Nurse Educator/Clinical Nurse Specialist specialty assembly. They were then reviewed internally by the Nursing Practice and Editorial departments at AORN.

The PNDS is "a dictionary that applies to surgical patients' preadmission preparation, preoperative assessment, intraoperative nursing care, postoperative recovery, discharge teaching, and at-home postoperative convalescence. The PNDS is a consistent, comprehensive set of terms for describing patient safety interventions, physiological effects, and behavioral responses before, during, and after surgery."[3] Incorporating the PNDS into the AORN competency statements required restructuring the framework to reflect the PNDS domains rather than the nursing process.

AORN continues to define *competency* as the knowledge, skills, and abilities necessary to fulfill the professional role functions of a registered nurse in the operating room.[4] Competencies are the behavioral, observable evidence of clinical knowledge. Competency assessment is an objective measurement of an individual's performance of essential job responsibilities. Competency assessment can occur

- at the end of an orientation program,
- before independent practice in a specialty,
- to address the requirements of the Joint Commission on Accreditation of Healthcare Organizations related to nurse preparedness to manage low volume, high risk issues,[5] and
- to address institutional initiatives.

Identifying competency is essential to providing an understanding of the fundamental knowledge and skills necessary to fulfill the functions/activities of a registered nurse in the practice setting. The competencies have been developed to address all settings and all patient types. Individual facilities should select those that are appropriate for their setting and patient populations.

Background

In the fall of 1976, a proposal to define the role of nurses in the operating room, Project 25, was approved by the AORN Board of Directors. The report of the Project 25 Task Force, which included the definition of perioperative nursing, was accepted by the House of Delegates at the 25th AORN Congress in New Orleans in 1978.[1] The definition of *perioperative nursing practice* is:

The registered nurse specializing in perioperative nursing practice performs nursing activities in the preoperative, intraoperative, and postoperative phases of the patient's surgical experience. Registered nurses enter perioperative nursing practice at a beginning level depending on their expertise and competency to practice. As they gain knowledge and skills, they progress on a continuum to an advanced level of practice.[6]

In 1982, through the Ad Hoc Committee on Basic Competencies, 25 statements were developed as basic competencies for perioperative nursing. These statements were intended as guidelines for what a nurse who has been employed in the perioperative setting for six months to one year can be reasonably expected to achieve. Originally, basic competency was defined as:

the knowledge, skills, and abilities necessary to fulfill, at a minimum level, the professional role functions (as defined in the Standards of Perioperative Nursing Practice) of the registered nurse in the operating room. Basic competency is expected to be attained within a specific time span (six to twelve months). The knowledge, skills, and abilities are common to all nursing practice and are used in providing care to the surgical patient and his family/significant others regardless of the practice setting.[7]

In 1984, the Nursing Practices Committee was charged with the responsibility of reviewing and revising the 1978 statement. While exploring the original document, the committee felt that any reference to a level of competency within a given time frame should be deleted from the competency statements. Consequently, competency was redefined as "the knowledge, skills, and abilities necessary to fulfill the professional role functions of a registered nurse in the operating room."[4]

Using the nursing process as the framework, the existing statements were revised to fit that model. In some instances, statements could be combined so that the result was 18 competency statements. The committee, working as a panel of experts and aided by previous works of the Association and their own experience, developed a list of expected behaviors or nursing actions that could be used to measure the achievement of each competency statement.

An awareness of the need for a comprehensive database describing perioperative nursing began in 1988 with the AORN Critical Issues Committee. A four-year evaluation clearly demonstrated the need to identify the relationship of nursing interventions to patient outcomes and the need for a database capable of providing evidence of the value of the perioperative nurse during the patient's surgical experience. The AORN Board established the Task Force on Perioperative Data Elements in November 1993 to begin the process of defining the "data elements" of the database.[8]

From 1995 to 1998, that work was carried on by the Data Elements Coordinating Committee, and in February 1999 the PNDS received recognition from the Amerian Nurses Association (ANA) Committee on Nursing Practice Information Infrastructure as a data set useful in the practice of nursing.[8] The first edition of *Perioperative Nursing Data Set: The Perioperative Nursing Vocabulary,* was published in 2000, followed by the second edition in 2002.

Suggestions for implementation

Incorporating the PNDS into the competency statements has not changed their potential use as delineated by the work of the original committee, but only enhances that use. The PNDS provides a consistent organizing framework for

♦ policies and procedures,
♦ job descriptions,
♦ performance improvement activities,
♦ performance appraisals,
♦ orientation,
♦ staff development,
♦ peer review, and
♦ clinical ladders.[9]

Competency statements based on the PNDS also can be used in the generic curriculum to provide faculty with a structure for course outline and a specific means of measuring the performance of students in perioperative nursing.[4] Additionally, the statements can become a valuable tool in quality assurance activities demonstrating accountability in the care of the surgical patient.[9]

By using the PNDS as the overall framework for defining clinical competency, perioperative nurses may better describe and validate their practice. Prospective nursing students and RNs who are interested in perioperative nursing will be better informed regarding the specific functions/actions of that specialty practice. Federal agencies, as well as other medical and nursing organizations, can be provided with definite statements about the use of the nursing process in perioperative nursing.[2,10] These competency statements reaffirm AORN's position that only registered nurses can be responsible for nursing care during surgery.

How to use these statements

The competency statements that follow are intended to serve as guidelines to what a nurse who has been employed in the perioperative setting for six months to one year can reasonably be expected to achieve. These competency statements are formatted in the following manner:

♦ Competencies are divided by Domains (Column 1);
♦ Outcomes are identified for each domain (Column 1);

◆ Interventions are defined for each outcome (Column 2); and

◆ Observable behaviors for validation of competency are listed (Column 3).

Facilities can use the observable behaviors to develop their own templates, checklists, and/or validation tools to document or verify competency. The value of PNDS in competency assessment is that the standardized language accurately describes the clinical perioperative practice that takes place every day in a variety of settings. As a vocabulary that is recognized, computerized, and comprehensive, the PNDS offers nurses the opportunity to verify their professional knowledge and skills, demonstrate their competency to practice, and validate their contribution to patient outcomes.[3]

NOTES

1. "Operating room nursing: Perioperative role," *AORN Journal* 27 (May 1978) 1156-1175.

2. "A model for perioperative nursing practice," in *Standards, Recommended Practices, and Guidelines* (Denver: AORN, Inc, 2005) 15.

3. S Kleinbeck, *PNDS @ Work: Clinical Competencies and Job Descriptions* (Denver: AORN, Inc, 2005).

4. "Competency statements in perioperative nursing," in *Standards, Recommended Practices, and Guidelines* (Denver: AORN, Inc, 2005) 33.

5. S Beyea, ed, *Perioperative Nursing Data Set: The Perioperative Nursing Vocabulary,* second ed (Denver: AORN, Inc, 2002) 38.

6. "A model for perioperative nursing practice," *AORN Journal* 41 (January 1985) 188.

7. *Developing Basic Competencies for Perioperative Nursing* (Denver: Association of Operating Room Nurses, 1982) 2.

8. S Beyea, ed, "In search of perioperative data elements," in *Perioperative Nursing Data Set: The Perioperative Nursing Vocabulary,* second ed (Denver: AORN, Inc, 2002) 13-27.

9. S Beyea, ed, "The value of a clinical information infrastructure," in *Perioperative Nursing Data Set: The Perioperative Nursing Vocabulary,* second ed (Denver: AORN, Inc, 2002) 3-11.

10. S Kleinbeck, *PNDS @ Work: Policies, Procedures, and Pathways* (Denver: AORN, Inc, 2005) 16-18.

Editor's note: To help perioperative nurses incorporate the PNDS standardized vocabulary into facility competency statements, job descriptions, patient records, and policies and procedures, AORN publishes the *PNDS @ Work* series, written by S V M Kleinbeck (Denver: AORN, Inc, 2004–2005). Titles in the series include the following:

Building a Perioperative Patient Record
ISBN 1-888460-27-X

Policies, Procedures, and Pathways
ISBN 1-888460-36-9

Encouraging Perioperative Clinical Experiences
ISBN 1-888460-38-5

Staff Nurse Development
ISBN 1-888460-41-5

Clinical Competencies and Job Descriptions
ISBN 1-888460-42-3

Please contact AORN for more information.

Perioperative Nurse Competency Statements

These statements identify the basic competencies required for perioperative nurses. They are guidelines for what a nurse who has been employed in the perioperative setting for six months to one year can be reasonably expected to achieve. These competencies utilize PNDS terminology and include measurable criteria and recommendations for validation of the stated competency.

Patient Outcome	PNDS Interventions as Measurable Criteria	Recommendations for Validation of Competency
	**Domain 1: SAFETY O2 – O9**	
	*Competency Statement:* **The perioperative registered nurse demonstrates the ability to establish an environment of safety for the surgical patient.**	
O2 The patient is free from signs and symptoms of injury caused by extraneous objects.	**(I138) Implements protective measures prior to operative or invasive procedure.** The patient, equipment, and environment are prepared to ensure safety during the operative or other invasive procedure. ♦ Reviews preoperative checklist ♦ Confirms preoperative assessment of physical status ♦ Confirms required diagnostic testing prior to procedure ♦ Assures that variances from preoperative testing have been addressed ♦ Introduces self to patient and explains role ♦ Identifies and addresses barriers to communication (eg, interpreter services etc) ♦ Verifies NPO status ♦ Verifies medications taken immediately prior to admission ♦ Reviews surgical consent form for completeness and accuracy including addressing discrepancies ♦ Confirms room readiness (ie, suction and lights) ♦ Removes environmental hazards (eg, removes unnecessary equipment, provides appropriate waste receptacles)	♦ Direct observation of patient assessment ♦ Verification of communication with patient's health care team members Other: _____
	(I26) Confirms identity before the operative or invasive procedure. Verifies verbally and visually the identity of the individual undergoing the operative or invasive procedure. ***Alert and oriented patient*** ♦ Greets patient using full name. ♦ Introduces self. ♦ Asks patient to state name and operative procedure. ♦ Verifies name and hospital number on transfer documentation with patient's identification bracelet, the patient's chart, and the consent. ♦ Communicates discrepancies to attending physician and validates resolution. ***Child*** ♦ Follows steps above, engaging parent or guardian with the child in the process. ♦ Observes interaction with unit nursing staff to identify patient in absence of parent or legal guardian. ***Comatose and disoriented patient*** ♦ Verifies patient's identification bracelet and patient's chart. ♦ Asks family member, if present, to identify patient. ♦ Observes interaction with unit nursing staff to identify patient in absence of parent or legal guardian.	♦ Direct observation ♦ Review of patient health record ♦ Verification of communication with patient/child/family members Other: _____

Patient Outcome	PNDS Interventions as Measurable Criteria	Recommendations for Validation of Competency
	Domain 1: SAFETY O2 – O9 *(continued)*	
	Competency Statement: **The perioperative registered nurse demonstrates the ability to establish an environment of safety for the surgical patient.**	
(continued) **O2 The patient is free from signs and symptoms of injury caused by extraneous objects.**	**(I143) Verifies operative procedure, surgical site, and laterality.** Verifies patient's/family member's understanding by listening to their explanations of procedure to be performed, site, and laterality. ♦ Reviews surgery schedule ♦ Reviews surgical consent form for completeness, accuracy, and congruency with patient's statements ♦ Determines that physician's notations on health record are consistent with surgical consent ♦ Visually inspects patient identification band to verify correct name and number ♦ Encourages patient/family member to verbalize identity ♦ Encourages patient/family member to describe understanding of intended procedure, site, and laterality ♦ Encourages patient/family member to indicate site and laterality ♦ Informs surgeon and/or administrative authority of any discrepancy ♦ Follows facility policies regarding verification of site and laterality ♦ Evaluates patient's responses	♦ Direct observation of patient interaction ♦ Verification of communication with physician ♦ Review of patient's health record Other: _____
	(I11) Applies safety devices. Prepares, applies, attaches, uses, and removes devices (eg, restraints, padding, support devices) and takes action to minimizes risks. ♦ Examines the surgical environment for equipment or conditions that pose a safety risk and takes corrective action. ♦ Selects safety devices based on patient's needs and the planned operative or invasive procedure. ♦ Applies safety devices to patient according to the plan of care, applicable practice guidelines, facility policies, and manufacturers' documented instructions. ♦ Ensures that safety devices are readily available, clean, free of sharp edges, padded as appropriate, and in working order prior to use.	♦ Direct observation ♦ Review of patient's medical record ♦ Evidence of education ♦ Documentation of annual equipment review Other: _____
	(I76) Implements protective measures to prevent skin or tissue injury due to thermal sources. Prevents skin and tissue trauma secondary to thermal sources including hot instruments, solutions, casting materials, thermal regulation devices, and light sources. ♦ Assesses patient's risk for skin injury related to thermal hazards ♦ Identifies nursing diagnoses that describe the patient's degree of risk for skin injury related to thermal hazards	♦ Direct observation ♦ Review of patient's medical record ♦ Evidence of education ♦ Documentation of annual equipment review Other: _____

Patient Outcome	PNDS Interventions as Measurable Criteria	Recommendations for Validation of Competency
	**Domain 1: SAFETY O2 – O9** *(continued)*	

Competency Statement: **The perioperative registered nurse demonstrates the ability to establish an environment of safety for the surgical patient.**

Patient Outcome	PNDS Interventions as Measurable Criteria	Recommendations for Validation of Competency

(continued)
O2 The patient is free from signs and symptoms of injury caused by extraneous objects.
	(continued)
	♦ Inspects skin periodically during and after using thermoregulation devices
	♦ Plans interventions to protect and maintain skin integrity
	♦ Monitors temperature when using thermoregulation devices
	♦ Protects patient from injury related to application of plaster
	♦ Monitors active electrode of electrosurgical unit during procedure
	  – Places active electrode in clean, dry, nonconductive, highly visible area during procedure
	  – Prevents active electrode from contacting metal clamps
	  – Prevents active electrode from lying on patient during the procedure
	♦ Ensures alarms are active and functioning
	♦ Monitors function of dispersive electrode of electrosurgical unit during procedure
	  – Places dispersive electrode as close as possible to the surgical site
	  – Sets dysfunction alarm to audible status
	♦ Evaluates temperature safety of irrigating/infusion solutions immediately prior to administration
	♦ Protects skin and internal organs from heat transfer by endoscopes or other hot instruments	

	(I77) Implements protective measures to prevent skin/tissue injury due to mechanical sources.
	Prevents skin and tissue trauma secondary to mechanical sources including the use of devices such as positioning equipment, tourniquets, sequential compression devices, clippers, tape, and the OR bed.
	♦ Assesses patient's risk for skin injury related to mechanical hazards.
	♦ Assesses skin for injury from invasive devices (eg, tubes, drains, indwelling catheters, cables).
	♦ Identifies the nursing diagnoses that describe the patient's degree of risk for skin injury related to mechanical hazards.
	♦ Plans interventions to protect and maintain skin integrity.
	♦ Selects safest method of hair removal (if indicated) that preserves skin integrity.
	  – Reassesses skin immediately after hair removal, observing for redness, clipper nicks, or skin abrasions.
	  – Evaluates skin postoperatively for redness, clipper nicks, or skin abrasions.
	♦ Provides cast care to patients with fresh plaster cast to prevent injury to skin.
	♦ Cleans and dries skin around incision site before applying dressing.
		♦ Direct observation
		♦ Review of patient's medical record
		♦ Evidence of education
		♦ Documentation of annual equipment review
		Other: _____

Patient Outcome	PNDS Interventions as Measurable Criteria	Recommendations for Validation of Competency
	Domain 1: SAFETY O2 – O9 *(continued)*	
	Competency Statement: **The perioperative registered nurse demonstrates the ability to establish an environment of safety for the surgical patient.**	

(continued) **O2 The patient is free from signs and symptoms of injury caused by extraneous objects.**	*(continued)*
	♦ Secures dressing with tape without stretching the skin
	♦ Inspects, tests, and uses powered surgical instruments according to manufacturers' documented instructions
	♦ Uses tourniquet according to procedural need
	  – Avoids allowing prep solution to seep under cuff. Removes cuff, dries extremity, and replaces cuff with dry cuff if solution has wet cuff
	  – Inspects skin after cuff removal for signs of bruising, blistering, pinching, and/or necrosis	

	(I93) Performs required counts.
	Ensures that the patient is free from injury related to retained sponges, instruments, and sharps.
	
	Sponges
	♦ Counts sponges before the procedure to establish a baseline, at the time of permanent relief of either the scrub person or the circulating nurse, before closure of a cavity within a cavity, before would closure begins, and at skin closure or end of procedure
	  – Counts audibly and concurrently with team counterpart (ie, scrub person or circulating nurse)
	  – Separates sponges when counting
	  – Uses only x-ray-detectable sponges during the procedure
	  – Keeps sponges, linen, and trash in the OR during entire procedure
	  – Reports count results to surgeon
	  – Documents count on patient record according to policy
	
	Sharps
	♦ Counts sharps before the procedure to establish a baseline, at the time of permanent relief of either the scrub person or the circulating nurse, before closure of a cavity within a cavity, before would closure begins, and at skin closure or end of procedure
	  – Counts audibly and concurrently with team counterpart (ie, scrub person or circulating nurse)
	  – Counts needles according to number indicated on package
	  – Verifies number of needles with circulating nurse when package is opened
	  – Retains sharps in OR during procedure
	  – Reports count results to surgeon
	  – Documents count on patient record according to policy
		♦ Direct observation
		♦ Review of patient's medical record
		♦ Evidence of education
		Other: _____

Patient Outcome	PNDS Interventions as Measurable Criteria	Recommendations for Validation of Competency
	Domain 1: SAFETY O2 – O9 *(continued)*	
	Competency Statement: **The perioperative registered nurse demonstrates the ability to establish an environment of safety for the surgical patient.**	
(continued) **O2 The patient is free from signs and symptoms of injury caused by extraneous objects.**	*(continued)* **Instruments** ♦ Counts instruments before the procedure to establish a baseline, at the time of permanent relief of either the scrub person or the circulating nurse, and before would closure begins – Counts audibly and concurrently with team counterpart (ie, scrub person or circulating nurse) – Isolates and accounts for all removable instrument parts and all pieces of broken instruments – Reports count results to surgeon – Documents count on patient record according to policy **Unresolved counts** ♦ Notifies surgeon of unresolved counts ♦ Resolves count according to facility policy ♦ Implements documentation procedures according to facility policy	
	(I84) Manages specimen handling and disposition. Collects, identifies, labels, processes, stores, preserves, and transports specimens. ♦ Establishes chain of custody for cultures and tissue specimens ♦ Provides supplies and equipment needed for collection of cultures and specimens ♦ Labels culture and tissue specimen containers ♦ Completes laboratory slips ♦ Documents collection of cultures and specimens on the patient's operative record ♦ Obtains and processes frozen sections for pathology examination as quickly as possible ♦ Prepares surgical specimens for disposition according to hospital policy ♦ Directs transfer of cultures and specimens to laboratory ♦ Communicates intraoperative pathology reports to physician	♦ Direct observation ♦ Review of patient's medical record ♦ Evidence of education ♦ Communication with health care team members Other: _____
	(I122) Uses supplies and equipment within safe parameters. Ensures that use of supplies, equipment, and instruments does not compromise patient safety. ♦ Obtains necessary supplies and equipment for procedure ♦ Consults manufacturers' documented instructions for use of supplies, equipment, and instruments ♦ Operates equipment according to manufacturers' documented instructions ♦ Verifies safety/biotechnology inspections are current on all equipment	♦ Direct observation ♦ Review of patient's medical record ♦ Evidence of education ♦ Documentation of annual equipment review Other: _____

Patient Outcome	PNDS Interventions as Measurable Criteria	Recommendations for Validation of Competency
	**Domain 1: SAFETY O2 – O9** *(continued)*	
	*Competency Statement:* **The perioperative registered nurse demonstrates the ability to establish an environment of safety for the surgical patient.**	
(continued) **O2 The patient is free from signs and symptoms of injury caused by extraneous objects.**	*(continued)* ♦ Isolates malfunctioning equipment and defective supplies ♦ Checks for manufacturer outdates before using packaged items ♦ Provides care using the principles of aseptic technique and transmission-based precautions ♦ Opens supply packages according to manufacturers' documented instructions, principles of aseptic technique, and facility policy and procedure ♦ Discards contaminated packages	
	(I112) Records devices implanted during the operative or invasive procedure. Verifies and records the placement of implants, manufacturer, lot number, type, size, and other identifying information in compliance with federal regulations for tracking implantable devices. ♦ Complies with federal regulations for tracking implantable devices ♦ Completes required internal and external paperwork ♦ Notifies appropriate personnel, facility, or manufacturer of implant defects or failure ♦ Provides patient with implant identification documentation/card	♦ Direct observation ♦ Review of patient's medical record ♦ Evidence of education Other: _____
	(I95) Performs venipuncture. Obtains diagnostic blood samples. ♦ Collects appropriate supplies for procedure ♦ Verifies order for venipuncture ♦ Reviews chart for allergies, laboratory results, and patient history ♦ Assesses barriers to communication ♦ Assesses patient's ability to understand information ♦ Provides information about procedure to be completed and offers emotional support ♦ Reviews with patient presence of allergies, clotting problems, or medications that may affect clotting ♦ Maintains aseptic technique throughout procedure ♦ Applies tourniquet above insertion site ♦ Cleanses area with appropriate solution per facility policy or protocol ♦ Inserts needle per appropriate policy or protocol ♦ Observes for blood in flash chamber/blood collection tube ♦ Evaluates patient's response to procedure	♦ Direct observation ♦ Review of patient's medical record ♦ Verification of communication with patient/child/family members Other _____

Patient Outcome	PNDS Interventions as Measurable Criteria	Recommendations for Validation of Competency
center	**Domain 1: SAFETY O2 – O9** *(continued)*	

Competency Statement: The perioperative registered nurse demonstrates the ability to establish an environment of safety for the surgical patient.

Patient Outcome	PNDS Interventions as Measurable Criteria	Recommendations for Validation of Competency
(continued) **O2 The patient is free from signs and symptoms of injury caused by extraneous objects.**	**(I128) Maintains continuous surveillance.** Acquires, interprets, and synthesizes patient data so as to detect and prevent potential adverse clinical events. ◆ Continually monitors physiological and psychological indicators to detect discrete changes in overall condition. ◆ Utilizes critical thinking skills. ◆ Recognizes patients at high risk for complications. ◆ Communicates information about patient's risk status to appropriate member(s) of health care team. ◆ Monitors and controls clinical environment for safety or infection risks and other potential hazards. ◆ Prioritizes nursing actions based on clinical situation and patient's condition. ◆ Institutes appropriate care utilizing clinical practice guidelines. ◆ Notes type and amounts of effluent from drainage tube and notifies appropriate member of health care team regarding significant changes. ◆ Troubleshoots surgical equipment and clinical systems.	◆ Direct observation ◆ Review of patient's medical record ◆ Evidence of education ◆ Documentation of annual equipment review Other: _____
	(I152) Evaluates for signs and symptoms of physical injury to skin and tissue. Observes for signs and symptoms of physical injury to skin or tissue acquired from extraneous objects. ◆ Verifies preoperative nursing assessment. ◆ Assesses skin postoperatively for clipper nicks or skin abrasions. ◆ Inspects entire area prepped with antimicrobial solution for signs of redness, rash, abrasion, or blisters. ◆ Inspects skin for signs of bruising, pinching, and necrosis after removal of tourniquet cuff. ◆ Observes extremities for ability to move fingers/toes after removal of tourniquet. ◆ Assesses peripheral sensation after removal of tourniquet. ◆ Evaluates skin integrity after electrocautery use, paying close attention to any imprint on the dispersive pad itself, areas under dispersive electrode, skin under the electrocardiogram (ECG) leads, and at temperature probe entry sites. ◆ Assess circulation, sensation, and motion of extremities.	◆ Direct observation ◆ Review of patient's medical record ◆ Evidence of education ◆ Documentation of annual equipment review Other: _____
O3 The patient is free from signs and symptoms of chemical injury.	**(I75) Implements protective measures to prevent skin and tissue injury due to chemical sources.** Prevents skin and tissue trauma secondary to chemical agents, including antimicrobial agents, chemical disinfectants, liquid sterilants, irrigation solutions, ethylene oxide, methylmethacrylate, and tissue preservatives. ◆ Assess the patient's risk for skin injury related to chemical hazards during the perioperative period.	◆ Direct observation ◆ Review of patient's medical record ◆ Evidence of education ◆ Documentation of annual equipment review Other _____

Patient Outcome	PNDS Interventions as Measurable Criteria	Recommendations for Validation of Competency
**Domain 1: SAFETY O2 – O9** *(continued)*		
*Competency Statement:* **The perioperative registered nurse demonstrates the ability to establish an environment of safety for the surgical patient.**		

(continued)
O3 The patient is free from signs and symptoms of chemical injury.
	(continued)
	♦ Identifies nursing diagnoses that describe the patient's degree of risk for skin injury related to chemical hazards.
	♦ Plans interventions to protect and maintain skin integrity.
	♦ Follows manufacturer's documented instructions regarding skin testing and use of chemical depilatories when removing hair.
	♦ Prepares skin with antimicrobial agents before surgical intervention in a manner that preserves skin integrity
	  – Selects antimicrobial agents based on patient's allergies and sensitivities, incision locations, and skin conditions.
	  – Places sterile towels under the patient before skin preparation to prevent antimicrobial solutions from saturating bed linens. Removes before draping patient.
	  – Allow antimicrobial solutions drying time.
	  – Documents type of prep solution used and site prepped.
	  – Observes skin for any allergic-type responses to prep solutions.
	♦ Allows flammable solutions (eg, alcohol, acetone, fat solvents) to dry and fumes to evaporate before draping or activating electrosurgical or laser equipment.
	♦ Observes patient's skin integrity immediately postoperatively for redness, rash, abrasion, or blisters.
	♦ Uses sterile water to thoroughly rinse items disinfected with chemical germicides prior to use in an invasive procedure.
	♦ Prevents burns to patient's skin/tissue by completing full aeration cycle for gas-sterilized items/supplies before use.
	♦ Protects patient from skin/tissue burn by completely rinsing high-level disinfectants solutions form the surface of equipment or devices.
	♦ Prevents undiluted sterilant from touching patient by completing entire sterilization cycle when using low-temperature liquid chemical sterilization methods.
	♦ Cleans and dries skin around incision before applying dressing to prevent applying tape over dried preparation solutions.
	♦ Evaluates skin/tissue for chemical injury.	

	(I123) Verifies allergies. Identifies allergies, idiosyncrasies, and sensitivities to medications, latex, chemical agents, foods, and/or adhesives. ♦ Queries patient about allergies or hypersensitivity reaction to adhesives, egg products, latex, or iodine products. ♦ Queries patient about medications and foreign proteins that cause anaphylaxis (eg, antibiotics, opiates, insulin, vasopressin, protamine, allergen extracts, muscle relaxants, vaccines, local anesthetics, whole blood, cryoprecipitate, immune globulin, iodinated contrast media).	♦ Direct observation ♦ Review of patient's medical record ♦ Identification of patient allergies in patient care record and use of facility allergy alert system (eg, arm band) ♦ Verification of communication with health care team members. Other: _____

Patient Outcome	PNDS Interventions as Measurable Criteria	Recommendations for Validation of Competency
	**Domain 1: SAFETY O2 – O9** *(continued)*	
	*Competency Statement:* **The perioperative registered nurse demonstrates the ability to establish an environment of safety for the surgical patient.**	
(continued) **O3 The patient is free from signs and symptoms of chemical injury.**	*(continued)* ♦ Determines type of food, nutritional supplement, or substance and type of reaction experienced, if any, as reported by the patient. ♦ Records and communicates to the anesthesia care provider a patient history of anaphylaxis, asthma, or other respiratory difficulties related to the presence of allergens, toxins, or antigens.	
	(I139) Implements latex precautions as needed. Protects patient with risks for or latex-sensitivity from exposure to natural rubber. ♦ Stores essential non-natural-rubber supplies in a quick access location. ♦ Assesses/monitors for latex allergy response. ♦ Initiates approved latex precautions protocol as needed. ♦ Evaluates effectiveness of precautions taken.	♦ Direct observation ♦ Review of patient's medical record ♦ Evidence of education ♦ Documentation of annual equipment review Other: _____
	(I36) Evaluates for signs and symptoms of chemical injury. Observes for allergic reactions, burns, rashes, blistering, respiratory distress, or other signs and symptoms of chemical injury. ♦ Assesses skin for any allergic type responses to prep solutions. ♦ Inspects entire area prepped with solution(s) for signs of redness, rash, abrasion, or burns. ♦ Assesses dependent areas of skin for injury due to pooling of prep or irrigation solution. ♦ Assesses respiratory status for signs and symptoms such as dyspnea, shortness of breath, labored respirations, wheezing, or stridor.	♦ Direct observation ♦ Review of patient's medical record ♦ Verification of communication with health care team members. Other: _____
O4 The patient is free from signs and symptoms of electrical injury.	**(I72) Implements protective measures to prevent injury due to electrical sources.** Prevent injury secondary to dispersive electrode placement, active electrode handling, electrosurgical unit use, or stray radiofrequency current. ♦ Implements general electrosurgery safety precautions. ♦ Implements dispersive patient electrode safety precautions. ♦ Implements active electrode safety precautions. ♦ Inspects insulation of active electrodes for cracks, breaks, and holes before use in minimally invasive surgery. ♦ Avoids using a hybrid cannula system (metal and plastic components) during minimally invasive surgery. ♦ Avoids coiling, bundling, or clamping active and patient dispersive electrodes. ♦ Avoids wrapping active electrode cords around a metal instrument. ♦ Removes all metal patient jewelry to prevent current diversion and to avoid contact with other metals.	♦ Direct observation ♦ Review of patient's medical record ♦ Evidence of education ♦ Documentation of annual equipment review Other: _____

Patient Outcome	PNDS Interventions as Measurable Criteria	Recommendations for Validation of Competency
	**Domain 1: SAFETY O2 – O9** *(continued)*	

Competency Statement: **The perioperative registered nurse demonstrates the ability to establish an environment of safety for the surgical patient.**

Patient Outcome	PNDS Interventions as Measurable Criteria	Recommendations for Validation of Competency
(continued) **O4 The patient is free from signs and symptoms of electrical injury.**	*(continued)* ♦ Reviews chart to determine special considerations (eg, pacemaker, automated implanted cardioverter-defibrillator [AICD]). ♦ Applies safety devices to patient according to manufacturers' documented instructions, plan of care, and applicable facility practice guidelines. ♦ Removes safety devices from patient when indicated. ♦ Inspects insulation on reusable and disposable electrodes. ♦ Encourages lowest possible power settings and verbally confirms settings with surgeon. ♦ Secures ESU cords to avoid displacement of pad. ♦ Records placement of dispersive electrode, identification number of unit, and settings used.	
	(I37) Evaluates for signs and symptoms of electrical injury. Observes for redness, blistering, or burn to the skin. ♦ Examines patient dispersive electrode site for any skin changes. ♦ Evaluates skin integrity, paying close attention to any imprint on the dispersive pad itself, areas under dispersive electrode, skin under the ECG leads, and at temperature probe entry sites. ♦ Assesses skin at bony prominences or pressure sites for reddened or raised areas.	♦ Direct observation ♦ Review of patient's medical record ♦ Verification of communication with health care team members Other: _____
O5 The patient is free from signs and symptoms of injury related to positioning.	**(I64) Identifies physical alterations that require additional precautions for procedure-specific positioning.** Determines those at risk for positioning injury and implements appropriate precautions. ♦ Identifies individuals at risk for positioning injury (eg, those with implanted devices or amputations, the elderly, infants, the morbidly obese, and those who have limited mobility or incontinence). ♦ Reviews chart for information on patient's weight, preexisting medical conditions, and laboratory results. ♦ Interviews patient for history of implanted devices. ♦ Examines patient skin condition, level of comfort, perception of pain, presence of peripheral pulses, and mobility impairments. ♦ Assesses external devices (eg, drains, catheters, and orthopedic immobilizers). ♦ Applies antiembolism stockings in a manner to minimize friction injuries. ♦ Implements measures to prevent inadvertent hypothermia. ♦ Maintains safe transport environment through use of elevated bed rails, safety straps applied, and additional devices secured (eg, oxygen tanks, IV poles, Foley catheters, chest tubes). ♦ Supervises placement of equipment and/or surgical instruments on patient. ♦ Monitors patient for external pressures applied by members of health care team.	♦ Direct observation ♦ Review of patient's medical record ♦ Evidence of education ♦ Documentation of annual equipment review Other: _____

Patient Outcome	PNDS Interventions as Measurable Criteria	Recommendations for Validation of Competency
	Domain 1: SAFETY O2 – O9 *(continued)*	
	Competency Statement: **The perioperative registered nurse demonstrates the ability to establish an environment of safety for the surgical patient.**	
(continued) **O5 The patient is free from signs and symptoms of injury related to positioning.**	**(I127) Verifies presence of prosthetics or corrective devices.** Identifies presence of or use of prosthetics or corrective devices and modifies nursing care as indicated for planned procedure. ♦ Determines presence of metal and synthetic prostheses and implants, pacemakers, automated implanted cardioverter-defibrillators, hearing augmentation devices, intraocular lenses, or plastic/fluid implants (eg, penile implants, testicular implants, breast implants) and notifies appropriate members of health care team. ♦ Individualizes plan of care to accommodate prosthetic or corrective devices.	♦ Direct observation ♦ Review of patient's medical record ♦ Evidence of education ♦ Documentation of annual equipment review Other: _____
	(I96) Positions the patient. Determines the need for, prepares, applies, and removes devices designed to enhance operative exposure, prevent neuromuscular injury, maintain skin and tissue integrity, and maintain body alignment and optimal physiological functioning. ♦ Selects positioning devices based on patient's identified needs and the planned operative or invasive procedure. ♦ Positions patient on stretcher with side rails up and wheels locked when: 　– Awaiting admission to OR. 　– Procedure is completed on the stretcher. ♦ Determines that devices are readily available, clean, free of sharp edges, padded as appropriate, and in working order before placing patient on the OR bed. ♦ Modifies OR bed as necessary before attaching positioning devices. ♦ Reviews chart for information on patient's weight, preexisting medical conditions, previous surgeries, and laboratory results. ♦ Assesses functional limitations while patient is awake and responsive. ♦ Assesses patient for presence of skin conditions, level of comfort, perception of pain, presence of peripheral pulses, and mobility impairments while awake. ♦ Adapts positioning plan to accommodate limitations. ♦ Maintains body alignment. ♦ Maintains proper alignment of legs (uncrossed). ♦ Uses positioning devices to protect, support, and maintain patient position. ♦ Attaches padded arm boards to bed at less than 90-degree angle. ♦ Places patient's arms on boards with palms up and fingers extended or secures arms at patient's side in neutral position. ♦ Places fingers in position clear of table breaks or other hazards.	♦ Direct observation ♦ Review of patient's medical record ♦ Evidence of education ♦ Documentation of annual equipment review Other: _____

Patient Outcome	PNDS Interventions as Measurable Criteria	Recommendations for Validation of Competency
	**Domain 1: SAFETY O2 – O9** *(continued)*	
	*Competency Statement:* **The perioperative registered nurse demonstrates the ability to establish an environment of safety for the surgical patient.**	
(continued) **O5 The patient is free from signs and symptoms of injury related to positioning.**	*(continued)* ♦ Applies safety belt loosely so blood flow is not compromised. ♦ Protects body parts from contact with metal portions of OR bed. ♦ Protects patency of tubes, drains, and catheters. ♦ Prevents limbs from dropping below bed level to prevent compression of peripheral nerves. ♦ Rechecks body alignment, extremities, safety strap, and all padding if repositioning occurs. ♦ Removes positioning devices cautiously after surgery while maintaining body alignment and homeostatic status.	
	(I38) Evaluates for signs and symptoms of injury as a result of positioning. Observes for signs and symptoms of injury to integumentary, neuromuscular, and cardiopulmonary systems as a result of the patient's position during the procedure. ♦ Examines patient to assess peripheral pulses and/or neuromuscular impairments. ♦ Examines sites related to positional devices for signs and symptoms of skin/tissue injury. ♦ Examines pressure areas for signs of skin injury. ♦ Assesses and monitors vital signs.	♦ Direct observation ♦ Review of patient's medical record ♦ Verification of communication with health care team members Other _____
O6 The patient is free from signs and symptoms of laser injury.	**(I73) Implements protective measures to prevent injury due to laser sources.** Provides safety equipment and protective measures during the procedure using laser sources. ♦ Verifies that surgeon is credentialed to perform laser surgery ♦ Assesses patient for mobility and comfort ♦ Controls access to laser treatment area and laser equipment ♦ Removes patient's makeup from surgical site ♦ Coordinates distribution of appropriate laser safety eyewear that is labeled with appropriate optical density and wave length for the laser in use for staff (eg, glasses, goggles, and microscope or ophthalmoscope shutters) and the patient (eg, wet eye pads, laser protective eyewear, and laser-specific eye shields). ♦ Protects skin and non-targeted tissues from unintended laser beam exposure ♦ Reduces exposure to smoke plume generated during laser surgery (eg, wall suction unit with in-line filter or appropriate smoke evacuator unit and high-filtration surgical masks) ♦ Implements fire protection measures ♦ Inspects equipment, including laser, for electrical hazards	♦ Direct observation ♦ Review of patient's medical record ♦ Evidence of education ♦ Documentation of annual equipment review Other: _____

Patient Outcome	PNDS Interventions as Measurable Criteria	Recommendations for Validation of Competency
	**Domain 1: SAFETY O2 – O9** *(continued)*	
	*Competency Statement:* **The perioperative registered nurse demonstrates the ability to establish an environment of safety for the surgical patient.**	
(continued) **O6 The patient is free from signs and symptoms of laser injury.**	**(I40) Evaluates for signs and symptoms of laser injury.** Observes for injury unrelated to the intended therapeutic effects of the laser therapy. ♦ Inspects and assesses skin and adjacent tissue for discoloration, reddened, raised, or painful areas around surgical site ♦ Instructs patient to report any complaints of visual problems postoperatively ♦ Assesses for complaints of vision difficulty	♦ Direct observation ♦ Review of patient's medical record ♦ Verification of communication with health care team members Other: _____
O7 The patient is free from signs and symptoms of radiation injury.	**(I142) Assesses history of previous radiation exposure.** Assesses patient's history of radiation exposure for therapeutic and diagnostic purposes. ♦ Ensures that premenopausal women are aware of radiation risks associated with pregnancy ♦ Delays, if possible, surgical procedure for 24 hours after radioactive diagnostic studies ♦ Recognizes risk of compromised would healing in patients who have received radiation in large doses preoperatively	♦ Direct observation ♦ Review of patient's medical record ♦ Verification of communication with health care team members Other: _____
	(I74) Implements protective measures to prevent injury due to radiation sources. Provides safety equipment and protective measures such as gonadal protection for diagnostic and therapeutic uses of radiation. ♦ Assembles proper protective equipment ♦ Limits exposure to radiation to therapeutic levels (eg, fluoroscope is off when not in use, radioactive elements remain in lead-lined containers until ready for implantation) ♦ Provides shields to protect body areas from scatter radiation or focused beam whenever possible (fetus/gonadal shields, thyroid/sternal shields, lead aprons, lead gloves) ♦ Implements appropriate procedures for handling of radiated tissue specimens ♦ Implements measures to protect the patient from direct and scatter radiation ♦ Manages body fluids and tissue removed from patients who have undergone recent diagnostic studies using radioactive materials according to the recommendations of the radiation safety department ♦ Documents protective measures	♦ Direct observation ♦ Review of patient's medical record ♦ Evidence of education ♦ Documentation of annual equipment review Other: _____
	(I43) Evaluates for signs of radiation injury to skin and tissue. Observes for signs and symptoms of injury to skin and tissue unrelated to the intended diagnostic or therapeutic effects of radiation. ♦ Follows facility policies, procedures, guidelines, or protocols for skin assessment ♦ Monitors patient for skin changes (eg, redness, abrasions, bruising, blistering, or edema) ♦ Reports variances from expected to appropriate members of health care team	♦ Direct observation ♦ Review of patient's medical record ♦ Verification of communication with health care team members Other: _____

Patient Outcome	PNDS Interventions as Measurable Criteria	Recommendations for Validation of Competency
\multicolumn{3}{c}{**Domain 1: SAFETY O2 – O9** *(continued)*}		

Domain 1: SAFETY O2 – O9 *(continued)*

Competency Statement: **The perioperative registered nurse demonstrates the ability to establish an environment of safety for the surgical patient.**

Patient Outcome	PNDS Interventions as Measurable Criteria	Recommendations for Validation of Competency
O8 The patient is free from signs and symptoms of injury related to transfer/transport.	**(I118) Transports according to individual needs.** Ensures transfer without tissue injury; altered body temperature; ineffective breathing patterns; altered tissue perfusion; and undue discomfort, pain, or fear. ♦ Correctly identifies patient ♦ Assesses mobility limitations ♦ Explains what patient can expect prior to implementing transfer/transport ♦ Adapts plan of care to address mobility impairments ♦ Performs or directs patient transfer ♦ Positions patient to maintain respiration and circulation ♦ Maintains body alignment during transfer ♦ Applies safety devices ♦ Implements measures to prevent inadvertent hypothermia ♦ Ensures adequate number and properly trained personnel for safe transfer ♦ Plans for special needs during transport and transfer	♦ Direct observation ♦ Review of patient's medical record ♦ Evidence of education ♦ Documentation of annual equipment review Other: _____
	(I42) Evaluates for signs and symptoms of skin and tissue injury as a result of transfer or transport. Observes for signs and symptoms of injury to skin and tissue related to transfer or transport. ♦ Assesses patient for correct anatomical alignment by checking position of arms, legs, torso, and head and neck ♦ Assesses pain/discomfort level using an approved pain scale ♦ Visually inspects skin for areas of redness, bruising, abrasion, compression, and/or pressure related to transport	♦ Direct observation ♦ Review of patient's medical record ♦ Verification of communication with health care team members Other: _____
O9 The patient receives appropriate medication(s), safely administered during the perioperative period.	**(I123) Verifies allergies.** Identifies allergies, idiosyncrasies, and sensitivities to medications, latex, chemical agents, foods, and/or adhesives. ♦ Queries patient about allergies or hypersensitivity reaction to adhesives, egg products, latex, or iodine products ♦ Queries patient about medications and foreign proteins that cause anaphylaxis (eg, antibiotics, opiates, insulin, vasopressin, protamine, allergen extracts, muscle relaxants, vaccines, local anesthetics, whole blood, cryoprecipitate, immune globulin, iodinated contrast media) ♦ Determines type of food, nutritional supplements or substance and type of reaction experienced, if any, as reported by the patient ♦ Records and communicates to the anesthesia care provider a patient history of anaphylaxis, asthma, or other respiratory difficulties related to the presence of allergens, toxins or antigens	♦ Direct observation ♦ Review of patient's medical record ♦ Verification of communication with health care team members Other: _____

Patient Outcome	PNDS Interventions as Measurable Criteria	Recommendations for Validation of Competency
	Domain 1: SAFETY O2 – O9 *(continued)*	
	Competency Statement: **The perioperative registered nurse demonstrates the ability to establish an environment of safety for the surgical patient.**	

(continued) **O9 The patient receives appropriate medication(s), safely administered during the perioperative period.**	**(I8) Administers prescribed medications and solutions.** The correct prescribed medication or solution is administered to the right patient, at the right time, in the right dose, via the right route.
	♦ Reviews patient's history and assessment to identify potential allergies, medication interactions, and contraindications
	♦ Identifies patient's culturally based home health remedies and any influence on medication management
	♦ Identifies patient's over-the-counter self-medication use and herbal practices
	♦ Reviews medication orders and understands the medication actions, indications, contraindications, adverse reactions, and emergency management
	♦ Verifies patient identification, medication or solution, dose, route, and time for administration
	♦ Verifies the medication, the doses, and the route of administration with the physician and the scrub person before transferring medication to sterile field
	♦ Verifies patient's written consent before administration of experimental medications
	♦ Verifies verbal orders before administration
	♦ Questions orders that appear to be erroneous, illegible, or incomplete
	♦ Gathers prescribed medications/solutions and necessary supplies and equipment
	♦ Prepares and administers medications/solutions according to facility policy, manufacturers' documented instructions, and federal and state regulations
	♦ Ensures the five rights of medication administration are followed during medication administration:
	  – Right patient, – Right dose – Right time.
	  – Right medication, – Right route, and
	♦ Prepares a written label for all medications placed on the sterile field
	♦ Injects local anesthesia when within of scope of practice (RNFA)
	♦ Recognizes medication reactions, complications, and contraindications
	♦ Determines that specific antidotes and other emergency medication and equipment are available
	♦ Uses resources as needed (eg, product literature, medication bulletins, hospital formulary)
	♦ Communicates with facility's pharmacist as needed
	♦ Offers instruction about medication actions to patient and family as appropriate
	♦ Maintains and follows policies, procedures, guidelines, and/or protocols for safe medication administration
		♦ Direct observation
		♦ Review of patient's medical record
		♦ Demonstration of patient education related to perioperative medication administration
		♦ Verification of accuracy of drug calculations
		♦ Evidence of continuing education related to drug-drug, herb-drug, over-the-counter drug-prescription drug interactions
		♦ Evidence of continuing education modules on moderate sedation/analgesia and/or local anesthesia
		♦ Verification of communication with health care team members
		♦ Education
		Other: _____

Patient Outcome	PNDS Interventions as Measurable Criteria	Recommendations for Validation of Competency
	**Domain 1: SAFETY O2 – O9** *(continued)*	
	*Competency Statement:* The perioperative registered nurse demonstrates the ability to establish an environment of safety for the surgical patient.	

(continued)
O9 The patient receives appropriate medication(s), safely administered during the perioperative period.
	(I7) Administers prescribed antibiotic therapy and immunizing agents as ordered.
	Verifies physician orders for antibiotic therapies and immunizing agents and safely administers.
	♦ Determines if physician orders for antibiotic therapy have been written
	   – Verifies physician orders and determines that orders are appropriate
	   – Determines indications, doses, and intended effects of prescribed medications as well as interactions with other medications that the patient is receiving
	   – Confirms patient compliance with prescribed prophylactic therapies ordered to be self-administered
	   – Assesses patient before administering, delaying, or withholding medication if necessary
	   – Compares physician's order with label on medication container
	   – Confirms correct medication is administered to the right patient at the right dose via the right route at the right time
	   – Notes expiration date
	   – Safely administers antibiotic therapy as prescribed
	   – Recognizes and identifies adverse effects, toxic reactions, and medication allergies
	   – Evaluates the patient's response to medications administered
	♦ Assesses the patient's immunization history for recommended immunizations (eg, vaccines, antisera, immune globulins)
	   – Obtains physician's order for any required immunizations as appropriate
	   – Follows above procedure for safely administering immunizing agents
	   – Safely administers immunization agent as prescribed
	   – Recognizes and identifies adverse effects, toxic reactions, and medication allergies
	♦ Evaluates patient's response to medications administered
		♦ Direct observation
		♦ Review of patient's medical record
		♦ Verification of accuracy of drug calculations
		♦ Evidence of continuing education related to drug-drug, herb-drug, over-the-counter drug-prescription drug interactions
		♦ Verification of communication with health care team members
		Other: _____

	(I51) Evaluates response to medications. Observes for response and adverse reactions to medication administered. ♦ Monitors patient for demonstrated signs of therapeutic effect ♦ Monitors patient for signs of allergic effects ♦ Monitors patient for signs and symptoms of medication toxicity, to include nausea or vomiting ♦ Monitors patient who identifies significant home remedies/over-the-counter medications for potential complications and/or drug interactions ♦ Reports signs or symptoms of adverse reaction to appropriate member of health care team	♦ Direct observation ♦ Review of patient's medical record ♦ Verification of communication with health care team members Other: _____

Patient Outcome	PNDS Interventions as Measurable Criteria	Recommendations for Validation of Competency

Domain 2: PHYSIOLOGIC O10 – O15, O29, O30

Competency Statement: The perioperative registered nurse demonstrates the ability to assess, diagnose, implement, and evaluate treatments and procedures that contribute to the physiological stability of the surgical patient.

Patient Outcome	PNDS Interventions as Measurable Criteria	Recommendations for Validation of Competency
O10 The patient is free from signs and symptoms of infection.	**(I70) Implements aseptic technique.** Initiates the actions necessary related to risks associated with disease-causing microorganisms by creating and maintaining a sterile field, preventing contamination of open wounds, and isolating the operative site from the surrounding nonsterile physical environment. ♦ Establishes and maintains sterile field. ♦ Applies principles of aseptic technique. ♦ Performs skin preparations. ♦ Ensures perioperative environmental sanitation. ♦ Adheres to standard and transmission-based precautions. ♦ Dresses wound at completion of procedure. ♦ Cares for incision sites, invasive-devices wound sites (eg, endotracheal tube, tracheostomy tube, drainage tube, percutaneous catheter, vascular access device), urinary drainage systems, and other drainage systems. ♦ Monitors for wound contamination. ♦ Evaluates implementation of aseptic practices by the health care team.	♦ Direct observation ♦ Review of patient's medical record ♦ Education Other: _____

	(I21) Assesses susceptibility for infection.
	Evaluates the patient's risks for infection related to microbial contamination.
	♦ Identifies the patient's specific risk factors (ie, health problems and situations) for infection.
	  – Identifies pathophysiological risk factors.
	  – Identifies treatment-related risk factors.
	  – Identifies situational (personal, environmental) risk factors.
	  – Identifies patients at high risk for transmitting nosocomial infections (individuals with antibiotic or medication resistant microorganisms, prion diseases, tuberculosis, and/or preoperative nasal colonization of *S. aureus*).
	  – Identifies maturational risk factors.
	  – Identifies recent history of travel within or outside the United States.
	  – Notes American Society of Anesthesiologists (ASA) risk classification.
	♦ Determines if the patient is at high risk for infection (ie, state in which an individual is at risk to be invaded by an opportunistic or pathogenic agent such as virus, fungus, bacteria, protozoa, or other parasite) from endogenous or exogenous sources.
	♦ Identifies the individuals at high risk for nosocomial infections. Considers a person who has one or more contributing factors and one or more predictors to be at high risk.
		♦ Direct observation
		♦ Review of patient's medical record
		♦ Education
		Other: _____

Patient Outcome	PNDS Interventions as Measurable Criteria	Recommendations for Validation of Competency
	**Domain 2: PHYSIOLOGIC O10 – O15, O29, O30** *(continued)*	
	*Competency Statement:* **The perioperative registered nurse demonstrates the ability to assess, diagnose, implement, and evaluate treatments and procedures that contribute to the physiological stability of the surgical patient.**	
(continued) **O10 The patient is free from signs and symptoms of infection.**	**(I22) Classifies the surgical wound.** Designates the appropriate wound classification category for each surgical wound site according to the Centers for Disease Control and Prevention (CDC). <ul><li>Class I/Clean wounds: Uninfected operative wounds in which no inflammation is encountered and the respiratory, alimentary, genital, or uninfected urinary tracts are not entered. Clean wounds are primarily closed, and if necessary, drained with closed drainage. Operative incisional wounds that follow nonpenetrating (blunt) trauma should be included in this category if they meet the criteria.</li><li>Class II/Clean-contaminated wounds: Operative wounds in which the respiratory, alimentary, genital, or urinary tract is entered under controlled conditions and without unusual contamination. Specifically, surgical procedures involving the biliary tract, appendix, vagina, and oropharynx are included in this category, provided no evidence of infection or major beak in technique is encountered.</li><li>Class III/Contaminated wounds: Open, fresh, accidental wounds, surgical procedures with major breaks in sterile technique or gross spillage from the gastrointestinal tract, and incisions in which acute, nonpurulent inflammation is encountered.</li><li>Class IV/Dirty-infected wounds: Old traumatic wounds with retained devitalized tissue and those that involve existing clinical infection or perforated viscera. This definition suggests that organisms causing postoperative infection were present in the operative field before the surgical procedure.</li></ul>	♦ Direct observation ♦ Review of patient's medical record ♦ Education Other: _____
	(I94) Performs skin preparations. Carries out necessary actions to prepare the epidermis for an operative or invasive procedure. <ul><li>Assesses patient's overall health status.</li><li>Assesses patient's skin condition.</li><li>Assesses patient for previous surgery sites (eg, presence of fragile tissue such as scars and/or keloid formation) and exercises caution when preparing the area.</li><li>Assesses operative site before skin preparation.</li><li>Cleans operative site(s) and surrounding areas to remove soil, debris, and transient flora by various methods.</li><li>Determines need for hair removal at the operative site.</li><li>Provides for hair removal if indicated.</li><li>Assembles all equipment and supplies on a sterile field.</li><li>Prepares operative site and surrounding area with antimicrobial agent.</li><li>Implements skin preparation technique suitable for site and condition of skin.</li></ul>	♦ Direct observation ♦ Review of patient's medical record ♦ Verification of communication with health care team members ♦ Documentation of annual equipment review Other: _____

Patient Outcome	PNDS Interventions as Measurable Criteria	Recommendations for Validation of Competency
	**Domain 2: PHYSIOLOGIC O10 – O15, O29, O30** *(continued)*	

Competency Statement: The perioperative registered nurse demonstrates the ability to assess, diagnose, implement, and evaluate treatments and procedures that contribute to the physiological stability of the surgical patient.

Patient Outcome	PNDS Interventions as Measurable Criteria	Recommendations for Validation of Competency

(continued)
O10 The patient is free from signs and symptoms of infection.
	(I88) Monitors for signs and symptoms of infection.
	Observes for manifestations of tissue reaction due to pathogenic microorganism invasion of the body.
	♦ Evaluates patient assessment data noting indications of infection.
	♦ Assesses for signs and symptoms of infection/inflammation.
	♦ Observes for local manifestations of inflammation:
	  – Observes for signs and symptoms of pulmonary infection.
	  – Contacts postoperative patients to determine signs and symptoms of postoperative infection.
	♦ Reports occurrence of surgical wound infection according to approved policy.
		♦ Direct observation
		♦ Review of patient's medical record
		♦ Education
		Other: _____

	(I98) Protects from cross-contamination.
	Applies methodologies that prevent patient exposure to infective agents from endogenous sources (as from one tissue to another within the patient) and from exogenous sources (as acquired from objects, personnel, or other patients).
	♦ Establishes and/or participates in a formalized, multidisciplinary, infection control program.
	♦ Works with facility engineers and managers to provide for ventilation and air filtration systems that meet local, state, and federal regulations and recommendations.
	♦ Promotes personnel health and hygiene.
	  – Excludes personnel with acute infection or skin lesion from the practice setting.
	  – Expects personnel to demonstrate good personal hygiene.
	♦ Helps contain contamination by developing and implementing appropriate traffic patterns based on design of surgical suite.
	
	Equipment/Supplies
	♦ Removes supplies and equipment from external shipping containers before transferring items into surgical suite.
	♦ Separates movement of clean and sterile supplies from contaminated supplies and waste by space, time, and/or traffic patterns.
	♦ Avoids entering elevator with contained or uncontained soiled items when patients, food, or clean/sterile items are present. Uses enclosed soiled linen and trash collection systems in areas separate from corridors, lounges, and other storage areas.
	♦ Moves supplies from restricted area (if present) through ORs to semirestricted corridor. Prevents soiled materials from entering restricted area.
	♦ Maintains unidirectional traffic pattern for items to be reprocessed within surgical suite. Moves items from decontamination area to processing area, and, after processing, to storage areas. Uses clearly identified work areas for each task to minimize cross-contamination.
		♦ Direct observation
		♦ Review of patient's medical record
		♦ Education
		Other: _____

Patient Outcome	PNDS Interventions as Measurable Criteria	Recommendations for Validation of Competency
	Domain 2: PHYSIOLOGIC O10 – O15, O29, O30 *(continued)*	
	Competency Statement: The perioperative registered nurse demonstrates the ability to assess, diagnose, implement, and evaluate treatments and procedures that contribute to the physiological stability of the surgical patient.	
(continued) **O10 The patient is free from signs and symptoms of infection.**	*(continued)* **Personnel** ♦ Wears clean, dry, freshly laundered surgical attire intended for use in the surgical suite. ♦ Wears long-sleeved jacket that is snapped or buttoned closed when not scrubbed. ♦ Covers head and facial hair, including sideburns and neckline, when in semirestricted areas (which include most of the peripheral support areas of the surgical suite that have storage areas for clean and sterile supplies) and restricted areas (where surgical procedures are performed and unwrapped supplies are sterilized) of surgical suite by wearing hat or hood that minimizes microbial dispersal. ♦ Wears single high-efficiency mask when there are open sterile supplies and where scrubbed persons may be located. ♦ Confines or removes all jewelry and watches. ♦ Keeps fingernails short, clean, healthy, and free of artificial or acrylic nails. ♦ Wears shoe covers when gross contamination of the feet can be reasonably expected (eg, orthopedics, neurosurgery, obstetric surgery). ♦ Dons sterile gown and gloves after drying scrubbed hands and arms. ♦ Minimizes cross-contamination by understanding and implementing infection control practices when preparing instruments and supplies for use. – Uses Spaulding classification system to define necessary preparation. – Follows established protocols for high-level disinfection. – Uses category-specific or disease-specific isolation precautions as necessary if infections other than bloodborne infections are diagnosed or suspected.	
	(I85) Minimizes the length of invasive procedure by planning care. Contributes to minimizing operative time by anticipation and advanced preparation; coordinates team members' efforts to set priorities and efficiently accomplish the tasks necessary to achieve a common goal. ♦ Collects and interprets patient data, identifying appropriate nursing diagnoses and desired outcomes. ♦ Plans individualized patient care (a dynamic process that is ongoing and continuous throughout the preoperative, intraoperative, and postoperative phases) based on patient assessment data and an understanding of OR systems, methodologies, and perioperative nursing interventions resulting in desired outcomes. – Applies perioperative nursing principles and knowledge when preparing the OR environment. – Plans and implements intraoperative nursing activities. – Plans and implements postoperative activities.	♦ Direct observation ♦ Review of patient's medical record ♦ Education Other: _____

Patient Outcome	PNDS Interventions as Measurable Criteria	Recommendations for Validation of Competency
	**Domain 2: PHYSIOLOGIC O10 – O15, O29, O30** *(continued)*	
	*Competency Statement:* **The perioperative registered nurse demonstrates the ability to assess, diagnose, implement, and evaluate treatments and procedures that contribute to the physiological stability of the surgical patient.**	
(continued) **O10 The patient is free from signs and symptoms of infection.**	**(I81) Initiates traffic control.** Restricts access to patient care area to authorized individuals only. ♦ Keeps doors to OR or procedure rooms closed except during movement of patients, personnel, supplies, and equipment. ♦ Restricts access to surgical suite to authorized personnel only. ♦ Records names of all individuals who participate in surgical procedure.	♦ Direct observation ♦ Review of patient's medical record ♦ Education Other: _____

	(I10) Administers prescribed prophylactic treatment. Confirms and safely administers orders including dietary regimens, douche, enema, bowel preparation, and/or antimicrobial prophylaxis as ordered.
	♦ Determines if physician orders for prophylactic therapy have been written.
	  – Confirms and implements physician orders.
	  – Confirms patient compliance with prescribed prophylactic therapies to be patient-administered (eg, dietary restrictions, douche, enema, and/or bowel preparation).
	♦ Seeks physician order for parenteral antimicrobial prophylactic therapy as indicated by the CDC guideline for prevention of surgical site infections (1999).
	♦ Ensures timing of antimicrobial administration achieves maximum effectiveness.
	♦ Confirms physician order and discusses any questions with ordering physician.
		♦ Direct observation
		♦ Review of patient's medical record
		♦ Education
		Other: _____

	(I33) Encourages deep breathing and coughing exercises. Encourages use of incentive spirometry (per physician order), diaphragmatic breathing, and coughing. ***Preoperative phase*** ♦ Counsels patient to avoid active and passive cigarette smoking and to avoid smoke-filled rooms. ♦ Counsels patient to avoid exposure to persons with respiratory infections. ♦ Assists patient in practicing incentive spirometry, diaphragmatic breathing, and coughing as appropriate. ♦ Evaluates patient response. ***Postoperative phase*** ♦ Encourages and assists patient in performing incentive spirometry, diaphragmatic breathing, and coughing as appropriate. ♦ Encourages patient's self-use of incentive spirometer approximately 10 to 12 times per hour. ♦ Evaluates effectiveness and patient tolerance of the treatment.	♦ Direct observation ♦ Review of patient's medical record ♦ Education Other: _____

Patient Outcome	PNDS Interventions as Measurable Criteria	Recommendations for Validation of Competency
	**Domain 2: PHYSIOLOGIC O10 – O15, O29, O30 (continued)**	
	*Competency Statement:* **The perioperative registered nurse demonstrates the ability to assess, diagnose, implement, and evaluate treatments and procedures that contribute to the physiological stability of the surgical patient.**	

(continued) **O10 The patient is free from signs and symptoms of infection.**	**(I4) Administers care to wound site.** Examines characteristics of wound sites and provides appropriate wound care.
	♦ Dresses wound at completion of procedure.
	  – Uses sterile gloves when touching wound or dressing materials.
	  – Selects dressing materials based on clinical needs.
	  – Applies sterile dressings.
	  – Secures dressings with tape.
	  – Immobilizes with soft padding, splints, elastic bandages, and/or casting materials as needed.
	  – Applies ostomy bag or other appliance as needed.
	♦ Observes characteristics of any drainage.
	  – Changes dressings over closed wounds and assesses wound if patient has signs or symptoms of infection (eg, fever, unusual wound pain).
	  – Evaluates drainage for signs of infection.
	♦ Checks casting materials for signs of circulatory impairment.
	♦ Examines and compares characteristics of incision regularly.
	♦ Cleans all areas of the wound.
	♦ Aseptically removes skin sutures/staples (per physician order) from the healed wound.
	♦ Covers incisions and/or wounds with appropriate dressing materials.
	♦ Evaluates for signs of infection when dressings are removed.
	♦ Evaluates skin condition when dressings are removed.
		♦ Direct observation
		♦ Review of patient's medical record
		♦ Education
		Other: _____

	(I3) Administers care to invasive device sites. Examines and compares the characteristics of site, drainage, and patency of invasive devices (eg, urinary drainage systems, endotracheal tube, tracheostomy tube, drainage tube, percutaneous catheter, vascular access devices) and provides appropriate wound care.
	♦ Examines and compares the characteristics of invasive device sites regularly.
	  – Changes dressings and evaluates site for signs or symptoms of infection (eg, heat, redness, swelling, odor, drainage, unusual pain).
	  – Applies sterile dressings following site care.
	♦ Maintains patency of invasive devices (eg, tube, catheter).
		♦ Direct observation
		♦ Review of patient's medical record
		♦ Verification of communication with health care team members
		♦ Documentation of annual equipment review
		Other: _____

Patient Outcome	PNDS Interventions as Measurable Criteria	Recommendations for Validation of Competency

Domain 2: PHYSIOLOGIC O10 – O15, O29, O30 *(continued)*

Competency Statement: **The perioperative registered nurse demonstrates the ability to assess, diagnose, implement, and evaluate treatments and procedures that contribute to the physiological stability of the surgical patient.**

Patient Outcome	PNDS Interventions as Measurable Criteria	Recommendations for Validation of Competency
(continued) O10 The patient is free from signs and symptoms of infection.	**(I7) Administers prescribed antibiotic therapy and immunizing agents as ordered.** Verifies physician orders for antibiotic therapies and immunizing agents and safely administers. ♦ Determines if physician orders for antibiotic therapy have been written. – Verifies physician orders and determines that orders are appropriate. – Determines indications, doses, and intended effects of prescribed medications as well as interactions with other medications that the patient is receiving. – Confirms patient compliance with prescribed prophylactic therapies ordered to be self-administered. – Assesses patient before administering, delaying, or withholding medication if necessary. – Compares physician's order with label on medication container. – Confirms correct medication is administered to the right patient at the right dose via the right route at the right time. – Notes expiration date. – Safely administers antibiotic therapy as prescribed. – Recognizes and identifies adverse effects, toxic reactions, and medication allergies. – Evaluates the patient's response to medications administered. ♦ Assesses the patient's immunization history for recommended immunizations (eg, vaccines, antisera, immune globulins). – Obtains physician's order for any required immunizations as appropriate. – Follows above procedure for safely administering immunizing agents. – Safely administers immunization agent as prescribed. – Recognizes and identifies adverse effects, toxic reactions, and medication allergies. – Evaluates patient's response to medications administered.	♦ Direct observation ♦ Review of patient's medical record ♦ Education Other: _____
	(I83) Manages culture specimen collection. Collects, identifies, labels, stores, preserves, and transports specimens for microbiological testing. ♦ Collects specimen using aseptic sampling methods. ♦ Places sample(s) in sterile container with transport medium and/or an inert gas according to type of culture (ie, wound, tissue, blood, urine).	♦ Direct observation ♦ Review of patient's medical record ♦ Education Other: _____

Patient Outcome	PNDS Interventions as Measurable Criteria	Recommendations for Validation of Competency
	**Domain 2: PHYSIOLOGIC O10 – O15, O29, O30** *(continued)*	
	*Competency Statement:* **The perioperative registered nurse demonstrates the ability to assess, diagnose, implement, and evaluate treatments and procedures that contribute to the physiological stability of the surgical patient.**	
(continued) **O10 The patient is free from signs and symptoms of infection.**	**(I128) Maintains continuous surveillance.** Acquires, interprets, and synthesizes patient data so as to detect and prevent potential adverse clinical events. ♦ Continually monitors physiological and psychological indicators to detect discrete changes in overall condition. ♦ Utilizes critical thinking. ♦ Recognizes patients at high risk for complications. ♦ Communicates information about patient's risk status to appropriate member(s) of health care team. ♦ Monitors and controls clinical environment for safety or infection risks and other potential hazards. ♦ Prioritizes nursing actions based on clinical situation and patient's condition. ♦ Monitors patient for changes in status that require immediate nurse attention. ♦ Institutes appropriate care utilizing clinical practice guidelines. ♦ Notes type and amounts of effluent from drainage tube and notifies appropriate member of health care team regarding significant changes. ♦ Troubleshoots surgical equipment and clinical systems.	♦ Direct observation ♦ Review of patient's medical record ♦ Education Other: _____
O11 The patient has wound/tissue perfusion consistent with or improved from baseline levels established preoperatively.	**(I60) Identifies baseline tissue perfusion.** Assesses tissue perfusion and identifies any impairments or risk factors prior to an operative or invasive procedure. ♦ Verifies procedure, recognizes and anticipates fluid loss. ♦ Validates nursing assessment completed preoperatively. ♦ Completes visual inspection and assesses peripheral tissue perfusion. ♦ Follows facility policies, procedures, guidelines, or protocols for skin assessment preoperatively. ♦ Verifies patient's preoperative hydration status, height, weight, skin turgor, and pulses. ♦ Verifies patient's preoperative laboratory results as appropriate (eg, hematocrit [Hct], blood urea nitrogen [BUN], urine specific gravity [SpG]). ♦ Validates variances from norm (eg, edema, ascites, adventitious breath sounds, elevated central venous pressure [CVP]). ♦ Monitors intake and output. ♦ Monitors physiological parameters as indicated: vital signs, CVP, mean arterial pressure (MAP), pulmonary artery pressure (PAP), pulmonary capillary wedge pressure (PCWP), ECG, arterial blood gases (ABG), SaO$_2$, and temperature. ♦ Monitors patient for changes in neurological status (eg, level of consciousness, mentation, speech, reflexes, strength, mobility). ♦ Monitors patient for changes in extremities (eg, pulses, skin color, temperature, turgor, capillary refill, SaO$_2$ as appropriate). ♦ Monitors patient for changes in skin integrity (eg, cuts, abrasions, bruises, edema). ♦ Reports/reviews variance from norm of physiological parameters with appropriate member of health care team.	♦ Direct observation ♦ Review of patient's medical record ♦ Verification of communication with health care team members ♦ Education Other: _____

Patient Outcome	PNDS Interventions as Measurable Criteria	Recommendations for Validation of Competency
	**Domain 2: PHYSIOLOGIC O10 – O15, O29, O30 (continued)**	
	*Competency Statement:* **The perioperative registered nurse demonstrates the ability to assess, diagnose, implement, and evaluate treatments and procedures that contribute to the physiological stability of the surgical patient.**	
(continued) **O11 The patient has wound/tissue perfusion consistent with or improved from baseline levels established preoperatively.**	**(I15) Assesses factors related to risks for ineffective tissue perfusion.** Collects data to evaluate the patient's risk for ineffective tissue perfusion (eg, presence of diabetes, immunosuppression). ♦ Assesses nutritional status for altered nutrition. ♦ Identifies patient's allergies and/or hypersensitivities to medications, tapes, iodine products, soaps, and antimicrobial solutions. ♦ Identifies skin reactions that occur as a result of allergy or sensitivity. ♦ Determines onset and associated symptoms of skin reactions (eg, itching, burning, stinging, numbness, pain, fever, nausea and vomiting, diarrhea, sore throat, cold, stiff neck, exposure to new foods, new soaps or cosmetics, new clothing or bed linens, stressful situations). ♦ Identifies family history of chronic tendencies toward skin disorders. ♦ Identifies previous surgery sites (eg, presence of scars, degrees of keloid formation). ♦ Reviews chart for evidence of: – Diabetes—diminishes circulation to extremities and impairs the body's healing ability. – Cancer—previous irradiation may cause fragile and sensitive skin. – Immunosuppression due to corticosteroids, anti-inflammatory agents, and cytoxic medications. – Vascular disease—diminished circulation. – Hyperthermia. – Impaired physical immmobility. – Urinary/bowel incontinence. – Abnormal lab values (eg, lower hemoglobin). ♦ Individualizes plan of care based on assessment.	♦ Direct observation ♦ Review of patient's medical record ♦ Verification of communication with health care team members ♦ Education Other: _____
	(I46) Evaluates postoperative tissue perfusion. Assesses tissue perfusion throughout postoperative phase of care. ♦ Validates nursing assessment completed preoperatively. ♦ Completes visual inspection and assesses peripheral tissue perfusion. ♦ Follows facility policies, procedures, guidelines, or protocols for skin assessment. ♦ Monitors patient positioning intraoperatively. ♦ Ensures appropriate positioning devices are used. ♦ Monitors patient for changes in neurological status (eg, level of consciousness, mentation, speech, reflexes, strength, mobility). ♦ Monitors patient for changes in extremities (eg, pulses, skin color, temperature, turgor, capillary refill, SaO_2 as appropriate). ♦ Monitors patient for changes in skin integrity (eg, cuts, abrasions, bruises, edema). ♦ Reports variances from norm to appropriate members of health care team.	♦ Direct observation ♦ Review of patient's medical record ♦ Verification of communication with health care team members ♦ Education Other: _____

Patient Outcome	PNDS Interventions as Measurable Criteria	Recommendations for Validation of Competency
	**Domain 2: PHYSIOLOGIC O10 – O15, O29, O30 (continued)**	
	*Competency Statement:* The perioperative registered nurse demonstrates the ability to assess, diagnose, implement, and evaluate treatments and procedures that contribute to the physiological stability of the surgical patient.	
(continued) **O11 The patient has wound/tissue perfusion consistent with or improved from baseline levels established preoperatively.**	**(I130) Evaluates progress of wound healing.** Assesses skin condition, tissue perfusion, and healing process of surgical wound. ♦ Identifies risk factors that impair wound healing. ♦ Assesses wound status (approximation of skin edges, color, warmth, drainage, foul odor) regularly. ♦ Conducts follow-up telephone assessment of wound status in patients discharged within 24 hours of procedure. ♦ Reports signs and symptoms of infection to appropriate member of health care team. ♦ Monitors temperature for elevation. ♦ Provides wound care consistent with wound class.	♦ Direct observation ♦ Review of patient's medical record ♦ Verification of communication with health care team members ♦ Education Other: _____

O12 The patient is at or returning to normothermia at the conclusion of the immediate postoperative period.	**(I131) Assesses risk for inadvertent hypothermia.** Determines patients at risk for loss of body heat and plans appropriate interventions.
	♦ Those at high risk include but are not limited to patients:
	  – With preoperative baseline temperature less than or equal to 36° C.
	  – Receiving general anesthesia (anesthetic agents impair the body's ability to control and conserve heat by inhibiting vasoconstriction and the shivering response).
	  – With open exposed wound for prolonged period of time (eg, trauma, long intraoperative procedure).
	  – Such as infant, neonate, toddler (high body surface/kg and low subcutaneous brown fat for insulation increases rate of heat loss).
	  – Including frail elderly (low basal metabolic rate, limited cardiovascular reserves, thinning of skin, and reduced muscle mass).
	  – With traumatic destruction of skin (burn, industrial accidents).
		♦ Direct observation
		♦ Review of patient's medical record
		♦ Education
		Other: _____

	(I78) Implements thermoregulations measures. Initiates thermoregulation measures and applies devices to cool or warm the patient as indicated. ♦ Selects temperature-monitoring and regulation devices based on identified patient needs. ♦ Determines that devices are readily available, clean, and functioning according to manufacturers' specifications before inserting, attaching, or placing devices on patient. ♦ Inserts or applies temperature-monitoring and regulation devices to patient according to plan of care, facility practice guidelines, and manufacturers' documented instructions. ♦ Operates temperature-monitoring and regulation devices according to manufacturers' documented instructions. ♦ Removes temperature-monitoring and regulation devices from patient when indicated.	♦ Direct observation ♦ Review of patient's medical record ♦ Verification of communication with health care team members ♦ Documentation of annual equipment review Other

Patient Outcome	PNDS Interventions as Measurable Criteria	Recommendations for Validation of Competency
	Domain 2: PHYSIOLOGIC O10 – O15, O29, O30 (continued)	
	Competency Statement: The perioperative registered nurse demonstrates the ability to assess, diagnose, implement, and evaluate treatments and procedures that contribute to the physiological stability of the surgical patient.	
(continued) **O12 The patient is at or returning to normothermia at the conclusion of the immediate postoperative period.**	**(I86) Monitors body temperature.** Inserts, attaches, or applies temperature-monitoring devices. ◆ Measures core body temperature. (Sites that reflect core body temperature include esophagus, nasopharynx, tympanic membrane, bladder, rectum, pulmonary artery.) ◆ Listens for patient verbalization of thermal comfort. ◆ Assesses and documents patient's body temperature at frequent intervals. ◆ Interprets and communicates patient temperature data to appropriate members of health care team for further evaluation and action as appropriate. ◆ Monitors and documents patient's pulse, respirations, blood pressure, and SaO_2. ◆ Assesses patient for signs of shivering. ◆ Monitors patient for intraoperative and immediate postoperative bleeding. ◆ Monitors patient for cardiac dysrhythmia and congestive heart failure. ◆ Reports patient's temperature to PACU nurses for determination of appropriate postoperative treatment methods.	◆ Direct observation ◆ Review of patient's medical record ◆ Verification of communication with health care team members ◆ Documentation of annual equipment review Other:_____
	(I55) Evaluates response to thermoregulation measures. Observes and verifies body temperature and responses to thermoregulation measures, and monitors for adverse effects. ◆ Measures core body temperature (sites that reflect core body temperature include esophagus, nasopharynx, tympanic membrane, bladder, rectum, pulmonary artery). ◆ Listens for patient verbalization of thermal comfort. ◆ Assesses and documents patient's body temperature at frequent intervals. ◆ Interprets and communicates patient temperature data to appropriate members of health care team for further evaluation and action as appropriate. ◆ Monitors and documents patient's pulse, respirations, blood pressure, and SaO_2. ◆ Assesses patient for signs of shivering. ◆ Monitors patient for intraoperative and immediate postoperative bleeding. ◆ Monitors patient for cardiac dysrhythmia and congestive heart failure. ◆ Reports patient's temperature to PACU nurses for determination of appropriate postoperative treatment methods.	◆ Direct observation ◆ Review of patient's medical record ◆ Verification of communication with health care team members ◆ Documentation of annual equipment review Other: _____

Patient Outcome	PNDS Interventions as Measurable Criteria	Recommendations for Validation of Competency
	**Domain 2: PHYSIOLOGIC O10 – O15, O29, O30 *(continued)***	
	*Competency Statement:* The perioperative registered nurse demonstrates the ability to assess, diagnose, implement, and evaluate treatments and procedures that contribute to the physiological stability of the surgical patient.	
O13 The patient's fluid electrolyte and acid base balances are consistent with or improved from baseline levels established preoperatively.	**(I132) Identifies factors associated with an increased risk for hemorrhage or fluid and electrolyte loss.** Identifies individuals at risk for hemorrhage or hypovolemia including those with recent traumatic injury, abnormal bleeding or clotting time, extensive surgical procedure, complicated renal/liver disease, and major organ transplant. ◆ Establishes and verifies nursing assessment. ◆ Identifies and verifies availability of blood/plasma replacement. ◆ Collaborates with blood bank to ensure supply of blood/plasma replacement. ◆ Assures adequate supply of warm intravenous fluids. ◆ Assures adequate supply of suction containers, sponges, and hemostatic agents. ◆ Verifies patient's preoperative hydration status, height, weight, skin turgor, and pulses. ◆ Confers with physician and/or anesthesia care provider if unusual assessment data, or signs and/or symptoms of fluid, electrolyte, and/or acid-base imbalances are noted.	◆ Direct observation ◆ Review of patient's medical record ◆ Verification of communication with health care team members Other: _____
	(I111) Recognizes and reports deviation in diagnostic study results. Identifies critical variances in fluid, electrolyte, and acid-base balances and notifies appropriate members of the health care team. ◆ Obtains patient health data. ◆ Identifies patient's physiological baseline. ◆ Assesses cardiovascular status (eg, pulse, dysrhythmia, edema, ECG, hemodynamic parameters). ◆ Assesses rental status (eg, intake and output, urinalysis, renal function studies). ◆ Assesses nutritional status (eg, NPO status, weight, skin turgor). ◆ Collaborates with other health care providers regarding laboratory or assessment findings related to fluid, electrolyte, and acid-base status. ◆ Plans nursing care based on physiological data. ◆ Communicates physical health status (eg, verbal reports, patient record).	◆ Direct observation ◆ Review of patient's medical record ◆ Verification of communication with health care team members Other: _____
	(I89) Monitors physiological parameters. Monitors physiological parameters including intake and output, arterial blood gases, electrolyte levels, hemodynamic status, and SaO_2. ◆ Assesses and monitors neurologic status (eg, level of consciousness, confusion). ◆ Auscultates breath sounds. ◆ Estimates blood and fluid loss by weighing sponges, measuring suctioned output, and summing fluid amounts from drainage devices (wound drains, chest tubes).	◆ Direct observation ◆ Review of patient's medical record ◆ Verification of communication with health care team members Other: _____

Patient Outcome	PNDS Interventions as Measurable Criteria	Recommendations for Validation of Competency

Domain 2: PHYSIOLOGIC O10 – O15, O29, O30 *(continued)*

Competency Statement: The perioperative registered nurse demonstrates the ability to assess, diagnose, implement, and evaluate treatments and procedures that contribute to the physiological stability of the surgical patient.

Patient Outcome	PNDS Interventions as Measurable Criteria	Recommendations for Validation of Competency
(continued) **O13 The patient's fluid electrolyte and acid base balances are consistent with or improved from baseline levels established preoperatively.**	*(continued)* ♦ Measures urine output. ♦ Monitors vital signs. ♦ Obtains peripheral blood specimen as ordered for monitoring of fluid and electrolyte levels (eg, hematocrit, BUN, protein, sodium, potassium, glucose levels). ♦ Monitors laboratory results relevant to fluid balance (eg, hematocrit, BUN, albumin, serum electrolytes, total protein, serum osmolality, specific gravity levels). ♦ Assists with insertion of invasive hemodynamic monitoring catheters (eg, arterial line, CVP, pulmonary arterial catheter, Swan-Ganz catheter). ♦ Monitors hemodynamic status, including CVP, MAP, PAP, and PCWP levels, if available. ♦ Monitors for signs of hypervolemia/hypovolemia. ♦ Monitors patient's response to prescribed electrolyte/fluid therapy. ♦ Monitors fluid loss (eg, bleeding vomiting, diarrhea, perspiration). ♦ Monitors amount of irrigation fluids administered. ♦ Monitors ABG, as available. ♦ Monitors for loss of acid (eg, vomiting, nasogastric output, diarrhea, diuresis). ♦ Monitors for loss of bicarbonate (eg, fistula drainage, diarrhea). ♦ Monitors respiratory pattern. ♦ Monitors for symptoms of respiratory failure (eg, PaO_2, SaO_2, and elevated $PaCO_2$ levels). ♦ Monitors tissue perfusion (eg, PaO_2, SaO_2, ABG, and hemoglobin levels and cardiac output), if available.	
	(I133) Implements hemostasis techniques. Provides supplies, instrumentation, and appropriate surgical techniques as needed to control hemorrhage. ♦ Provides appropriate supplies (eg, sponges, suction, electrocoagulation unit, instrumentation) to control bleeding. ♦ Applies pressure to bleeding sites as directed.	♦ Direct observation ♦ Education ♦ Verification of communication with health care team members Other: _____
	(I34) Establishes IV access. Establishes and maintains peripheral IV access to administer IV fluids, medications, and blood products per physician order. ♦ Verifies order to establish IV access. ♦ Reviews chart for allergies, laboratory results, and patient history. ♦ Verifies barriers to communication. ♦ Verifies patient's ability to understand information. ♦ Provides information about procedure to be completed and offers emotional support.	♦ Direct observation ♦ Review of patient's medical record ♦ Verification of communication with health care team members ♦ Education Other: _____

Patient Outcome	PNDS Interventions as Measurable Criteria	Recommendations for Validation of Competency
	Domain 2: PHYSIOLOGIC O10 – O15, O29, O30 *(continued)*	
	Competency Statement: **The perioperative registered nurse demonstrates the ability to assess, diagnose, implement, and evaluate treatments and procedures that contribute to the physiological stability of the surgical patient.**	
(continued) **O13 The patient's fluid electrolyte and acid base balances are consistent with or improved from baseline levels established preoperatively.**	*(continued)* ♦ Reviews with patient presence of allergies, clotting disorders, or medications that would affect clotting. ♦ Maintains aseptic technique throughout. ♦ Selects and prepares all items for procedure. ♦ Offers emotional support. ♦ Requests patient hold extremity still. ♦ Avoids placing line in extremity with arteriovenous fistulas or shunts. ♦ Applies warm compresses as appropriate. ♦ Applies tourniquet above insertion site. ♦ Cleanses area with appropriate solution per facility policy or protocol. ♦ Inserts needle per appropriate policy or protocol. ♦ Observes for blood in flash chamber. ♦ Connects needle hub to IV tubing as appropriate. ♦ Applies tape and dressing per facility policy and protocol. ♦ Labels dressing per facility policy and protocol. ♦ Evaluates patient's responses to procedure.	
	(I23) Collaborates in fluid and electrolyte management. Collaborates with other members of the health care team to monitor and implement prescribed treatments (eg, autotransfusion, IV fluids, blood products, medications). ♦ Verifies procedure, recognizes and anticipates fluid loss. ♦ Anticipates replacement requirement for large volume loss procedures. ♦ Verifies patient's preoperative hydration status, height, weight, skin turgor, and pulses. ♦ Verifies patient's preoperative laboratory results as appropriate (eg, Hct, BUN, urine specific gravity). ♦ Validates variances from norm (eg, edema, ascites, adventitious breath sounds, elevated CVP) and reports to appropriate members of health care team. ♦ Monitors vital signs as indicated. ♦ Administers or prepares for administration of IV fluid therapy. ♦ Monitors intake and output. ♦ Considers blood and fluid loss by weighing sponges, measuring suctioned output, and adding fluid amounts from drainage devices (wound drains, chest tubes). ♦ Inserts Foley catheter as ordered. ♦ Monitors physiological parameters: vital signs, CVP, MAP, PAP, PCWP, ECG, ABG, SaO2, and temperature as appropriate. ♦ Reports variances from norm of physiological parameters to appropriate member of health care team. ♦ Retrieves additional fluids and/or supplies as indicated. ♦ Evaluates patient's response to fluid management.	♦ Direct observation ♦ Review of patient's medical record ♦ Verification of communication with health care team members ♦ Education Other: _____

Patient Outcome	PNDS Interventions as Measurable Criteria	Recommendations for Validation of Competency
	**Domain 2: PHYSIOLOGIC O10 – O15, O29, O30** *(continued)*	

Competency Statement: The perioperative registered nurse demonstrates the ability to assess, diagnose, implement, and evaluate treatments and procedures that contribute to the physiological stability of the surgical patient.

Patient Outcome	PNDS Interventions as Measurable Criteria	Recommendations for Validation of Competency
(continued) **O13 The patient's fluid electrolyte and acid base balances are consistent with or improved from baseline levels established preoperatively.**	**(I2) Administers blood product therapy as prescribed.** Arranges for availability and the administration of blood products or blood recovery per physician order. ♦ Validates order as prescribed. ♦ Verifies patient's consent to receive blood product therapy. ♦ Determines blood product has been prepared. ♦ Requests product delivery to area of infusion. ♦ Obtains supplies and prepares administration system for blood product. ♦ Observes standard and transmission-based precautions. ♦ Completes venipuncture with large bore needle. ♦ Follows national standards/guidelines and facility policies, procedures, or protocols for blood administration. ♦ Monitors patient for response to therapy. ♦ Monitors physiological parameters as applicable (eg, vital signs, CVP, MAP, PAP, PCWP, ECG, ABG, SaO_2, and temperature). ♦ Reports variances from norm of physiological parameters to appropriate member of health care team. ♦ Monitors for transfusion reaction, fluid shift to third space, and hypervolemia. ♦ Responds immediately to recognition of transfusion reaction (eg, discontinue infusion, notify physician and blood bank, treat patient's symptoms according to physician's directions and facility policies). ♦ Reports variances from norm to appropriate members of health care team.	♦ Direct observation ♦ Review of patient's medical record ♦ Verification of communication with health care team members ♦ Education Other: _____
	(I9) Administers prescribed medications based on arterial blood gas results. Safely administers prescribed medications related to acid-base balance and monitors for complications resulting from acid-base imbalance. ♦ Validates nursing assessment preoperatively. ♦ Completes a visual inspection, physical examination, and review of laboratory data. ♦ Obtains specimen following facility policies, procedures, and guidelines. ♦ Reviews results with other members of the health care team. ♦ Obtains medications ordered and understands the medication actions, indications, contraindications, adverse reactions, and emergency treatment. ♦ Administers medication as ordered. ♦ Monitors patient for demonstrated signs of therapeutic effect. ♦ Monitors patient for signs of adverse effects. ♦ Monitors applicable physiological parameters (eg, vital signs, SaO_2, ABG, CVP, MAP, PAP, PCWP). ♦ Reports variances from norm to appropriate members of health care team.	♦ Direct observation ♦ Review of patient's medical record ♦ Verification of communication with health care team members ♦ Documentation of annual equipment review Other: _____

Patient Outcome	PNDS Interventions as Measurable Criteria	Recommendations for Validation of Competency
	**Domain 2: PHYSIOLOGIC O10 – O15, O29, O30** *(continued)*	
	*Competency Statement:* The perioperative registered nurse demonstrates the ability to assess, diagnose, implement, and evaluate treatments and procedures that contribute to the physiological stability of the surgical patient.	
(continued) **O13 The patient's fluid electrolyte and acid base balances are consistent with or improved from baseline levels established preoperatively.**	*(continued)* ♦ Retrieves emergency equipment as indicated (eg, intubation equipment, fiber-optic scope). ♦ Evaluates patient's response to medications administered.	
	(I5) Administers electrolyte therapy as prescribed. Administers medications related to electrolyte balance and monitors for complications resulting from abnormal serum electrolyte levels. ♦ Validates order as prescribed. ♦ Verifies patient's preoperative hydration status (eg, weight, height, skin turgor, pulses). ♦ Verifies patient's preoperative laboratory results as applicable (eg, Hct, BUN, urine specific gravity). ♦ Identifies nursing activities necessary for expected outcome (eg, assembles supplies to initiate IV therapy). ♦ Prioritizes nursing actions (eg, correct hypovolemia/ hypervolemia). ♦ Determines availability and coordinates supplies, equipment, and personnel for fluid electrolyte, and blood volume maintenance. ♦ Provides equipment and supplies based on patient's needs. ♦ Anticipates need for equipment and supplies. ♦ Selects equipment and supplies in an organized and timely manner. ♦ Determines all equipment is functioning before use. ♦ Administers electrolyte therapy as prescribed. ♦ Monitors hydration status as appropriate. ♦ Monitors intake and output. ♦ Monitors physiological parameters as appropriate (eg, vital signs, CVP, MAP, PAP, PCWP, ECG, ABG, SaO_2, temperature). ♦ Reports variances from norm of physiological parameters to appropriate members of health care team. ♦ Evaluates patient's response to electrolyte therapy. ♦ Confers with physician and/or anesthesia care provider concerning maintenance and/or corrective therapy (eg, IV fluids, electrolyte replacement, medications to correct acid-base balance). ♦ Determines that emergency equipment and supplies are available at all times (eg, defibrillator/monitor, emergency medication and supply cart).	♦ Direct observation ♦ Review of patient's medical record ♦ Verification of communication with health care team members ♦ Documentation of annual equipment review Other: _____
	(I153) Evaluates response to administered fluids and electrolytes. Observes for signs and symptoms of fluid and electrolyte imbalances. ♦ Monitors intake and output, ABG, electrolyte levels, hemodynamic status, and SaO_2. ♦ Estimates blood and fluid loss.	

Patient Outcome	PNDS Interventions as Measurable Criteria	Recommendations for Validation of Competency
	**Domain 2: PHYSIOLOGIC O10 – O15, O29, O30** *(continued)*	
	*Competency Statement:* The perioperative registered nurse demonstrates the ability to assess, diagnose, implement, and evaluate treatments and procedures that contribute to the physiological stability of the surgical patient.	
(continued) **O13 The patient's fluid electrolyte and acid base balances are consistent with or improved from baseline levels established preoperatively.**	*(continued)* ◆ Monitors for signs and symptoms of fluid volume excess/deficit. ◆ Monitors for signs and symptoms of electrolyte imbalances. ◆ Monitors laboratory results relevant to fluid and electrolyte imbalances. ◆ Monitors patient's response to prescribed fluid/electrolyte therapy. ◆ Reports variances from norm to appropriate members of health care team.	◆ Direct observation ◆ Review of patient's medical record ◆ Verification of communication with health care team members ◆ Education Other:_____
O14 The patient's respiratory status is consistent with or improved from baseline levels established preoperatively.	**(I87) Monitors changes in respiratory status.** Assesses respiratory status and monitors for changes in respiratory status. ◆ Validates nursing assessment completed preoperatively. ◆ Anticipates and assists in maintaining or establishing patent airway. ◆ Monitors rate, rhythm, and depth of respirations. ◆ Monitors chest movement for symmetry and/or any use of accessory muscles. ◆ Monitors for sound of respirations (eg, noisy, wheezy, snoring, crowing). ◆ Auscultates breath sounds for depth and quality and presence of adventitious sounds. ◆ Provides airway maintenance as applicable (eg, suctioning and/or repositioning, chin lift, oral or nasal pharyngeal airway for ineffective airway). ◆ Administers oxygen as needed. ◆ Monitors physiological parameters as applicable (eg, vital signs, ABG, SaO_2). ◆ Monitors for restlessness, agitation, apprehension, or lethargy. ◆ Monitors for airway compromise (ie, laryngospasms unresolved with routine protocols). ◆ Reports variances from norms to appropriate members of health care team. ◆ Has emergency medications and equipment available. ◆ Maintains pharyngeal airway until patient demonstrates return of protective reflexes, then removes assistive airway device to minimize gag reflex. ◆ Extubates patient per facility extubation protocol. ◆ Monitors tidal volume to evaluate patient readiness for extubation. ◆ Positions patient for maximum lung expansion unless contraindicated. ◆ Monitors for pain and anxiety. ◆ Provides pain relief as applicable. ◆ Evaluates patient's responses to respiratory interventions.	◆ Direct observation ◆ Review of patient's medical record ◆ Verification of communication with health care team members ◆ Education Other:_____

Patient Outcome	PNDS Interventions as Measurable Criteria	Recommendations for Validation of Competency
— see below		

Domain 2: PHYSIOLOGIC O10 – O15, O29, O30 *(continued)*

Competency Statement: The perioperative registered nurse demonstrates the ability to assess, diagnose, implement, and evaluate treatments and procedures that contribute to the physiological stability of the surgical patient.

Patient Outcome	PNDS Interventions as Measurable Criteria	Recommendations for Validation of Competency
(continued) O14 The patient's respiratory status is consistent with or improved from baseline levels established preoperatively.	**(I121) Uses monitoring equipment to assess respiratory status.** Assesses respiratory status and SaO$_2$. ♦ Reads and understands manufacturers' documented instructions for all monitoring equipment used by the perioperative nurse. ♦ Recognizes normal and abnormal blood pressure, interprets monitoring device readings, and recognizes abnormal readings. ♦ Validates nursing assessment completed preoperatively. ♦ Completes visual inspection of respiratory functions. ♦ Monitors rate, rhythm, depth, symmetry of chest muscle movement, and use of accessory muscles. ♦ Monitors for audible sounds (eg, noisy, wheezy, snoring, crowing) and auscultates breath sounds. ♦ Applies and operates pulse oximeter according to manufacturers' documented instructions. ♦ Applies, attaches, or inserts a conventional, electronic, or temperature-sensitive patch or tape thermometer according to manufacturer's document instructions. ♦ Attaches ECG leads and operates ECG monitor. ♦ Attaches blood pressure monitoring equipment and operates equipment. ♦ Interprets SaO$_2$. ♦ Interprets temperature readings done with a conventional, electronic, or temperature-sensitive patch or tape thermometer. ♦ Interprets ECG tracings. ♦ Monitors assisted ventilation parameters as appropriate (ie, ventilator settings and alarms). ♦ Maintains pharyngeal airway until patient demonstrates return of protective reflexes, then removes assistive airway device. ♦ Monitors for airway compromise (ie, laryngospasm unresolved with routine protocols). ♦ Positions patient for maximal lung expansion unless contraindicated. ♦ Provides pain relief as applicable. ♦ Has emergency equipment and medications available. ♦ Administers oxygen as needed. ♦ Evaluates patient's response to respiratory-related interventions.	♦ Direct observation ♦ Review of patient's medical record ♦ Verification of communication with health care team members ♦ Documentation of annual equipment review Other: _____

Patient Outcome	PNDS Interventions as Measurable Criteria	Recommendations for Validation of Competency
\multicolumn{3}{c}{**Domain 2: PHYSIOLOGIC O10 – O15, O29, O30** *(continued)*}		

Competency Statement: The perioperative registered nurse demonstrates the ability to assess, diagnose, implement, and evaluate treatments and procedures that contribute to the physiological stability of the surgical patient.

Patient Outcome	PNDS Interventions as Measurable Criteria	Recommendations for Validation of Competency
(continued) O14 The patient's respiratory status is consistent with or improved from baseline levels established preoperatively.	**(I110) Recognizes and reports deviation in arterial blood gas studies.** Identifies critical variances in acid base balance and notifies appropriate members of the health care team. ♦ Validates nursing assessment completed preoperatively. ♦ Reviews preoperative laboratory values. ♦ Monitors physiological parameters as applicable (eg, vital signs, SaO_2, ABG). ♦ Repeats tests whenever indicated. ♦ Reports variances from norms to appropriate members of health care team. ♦ Provides medications or equipment as requested. ♦ Evaluates patient's responses to interventions.	♦ Direct observation ♦ Review of patient's medical record ♦ Verification of communication with health care team members ♦ Education Other: _____
	(I45) Evaluates postoperative respiratory status. Observes and monitors respiratory status throughout postoperative phase of care. ♦ Continually reassesses respiratory status. ♦ Completes visual inspection of respiratory function. ♦ Monitors rate, rhythm, and depth of respirations. ♦ Monitors chest movement for symmetry and/or any use of accessory muscles. ♦ Monitors sounds of respirations (eg, normal, noisy, wheezing, snoring crowing). ♦ Auscultates breath sounds for depth and quality and presence of adventitious sounds. ♦ Monitors airway for patency and secretions. ♦ Provides airway maintenance as indicated. ♦ Monitors physiological parameters as indicated (eg, vital signs, SaO_2, ABG). ♦ Reports variances from norm to the appropriate members of health care team.	
O15 The patient's cardiac status is consistent with or improved from baseline levels established preoperatively.	**(I59) Identifies baseline cardiac status.** Assesses blood pressure, heart rate and rhythm, SaO_2, and other parameters as appropriate. ♦ Validates nursing assessment completed preoperatively. ♦ Completes assessment of tissue perfusion, respiratory function, and cardiac status. ♦ Assesses cognition to include level of consciousness; orientation to person, place and time; and presence of restlessness or agitation. ♦ Assesses respiratory function. ♦ Assesses cardiac function. ♦ Assesses extremities. ♦ Assesses and reviews all pertinent laboratory studies. ♦ Reports variances from norms to appropriate members of health care team.	♦ Direct observation ♦ Review of patient's medical record ♦ Verification of communication with health care team members ♦ Education Other: _____

Patient Outcome	PNDS Interventions as Measurable Criteria	Recommendations for Validation of Competency
	**Domain 2: PHYSIOLOGIC O10 – O15, O29, O30** *(continued)*	
	*Competency Statement:* **The perioperative registered nurse demonstrates the ability to assess, diagnose, implement, and evaluate treatments and procedures that contribute to the physiological stability of the surgical patient.**	
(continued) **O15 The patient's cardiac status is consistent with or improved from baseline levels established preoperatively.**	**(I120) Uses monitoring equipment to assess cardiac status.** Assesses blood pressure, heart rate and rhythm, SaO_2, and other parameters as appropriate. ◆ Reads and understands manufacturers' documented instructions for all monitoring equipment used by the perioperative nurse. ◆ Recognizes normal and abnormal blood pressure, interprets monitoring device readings, and recognizes and reports abnormal readings. ◆ Applies and operates the pulse oximeter according to manufacturer's documented instructions. ◆ Monitors and interprets SaO_2. ◆ Applies, attaches, or inserts a conventional, electronic, or temperature-sensitive patch or tape thermometer according to manufacturer's documented instructions. ◆ Interprets temperature readings obtained with a conventional, electronic, or temperature-sensitive patch or tape thermometer. ◆ Attaches ECG leads and operates ECG monitor. ◆ Interprets ECG tracings. ◆ Attaches blood pressure monitoring equipment and operates equipment. ◆ Validates nursing assessment completed preoperatively. ◆ Completes assessment of peripheral tissue perfusion. ◆ Monitors heart rate, rhythm, and quality. ◆ Monitors respiratory status visually, audibly, and through monitoring indices (eg, SaO_2, ABG). ◆ Monitors physiological parameters as appropriate (eg, vital signs, CVP, MAP, PAP, PCWP, ECG, laboratory studies). ◆ Monitors fluid volume status: initial baseline, estimated blood loss, and fluid replacement therapy. ◆ Monitors mentation and assesses level of consciousness, orientation, presence of restlessness or agitation. ◆ Monitors extremities for warmth, color, dryness, pulse quality, and capillary refill. ◆ Monitors incision site for drainage type and amount. ◆ Recognizes early signs of cardiac complications. ◆ Reports variances from norms to appropriate members of health care team. ◆ Evaluates patient's responses.	◆ Direct observation ◆ Review of patient's medical record ◆ Verification of communication with health care team members ◆ Education Other: _____

Patient Outcome	PNDS Interventions as Measurable Criteria	Recommendations for Validation of Competency
	**Domain 2: PHYSIOLOGIC O10 – O15, O29, O30** *(continued)*	

Competency Statement: **The perioperative registered nurse demonstrates the ability to assess, diagnose, implement, and evaluate treatments and procedures that contribute to the physiological stability of the surgical patient.**

Patient Outcome	PNDS Interventions as Measurable Criteria	Recommendations for Validation of Competency
(continued) **O15 The patient's cardiac status is consistent with or improved from baseline levels established preoperatively.**	**(I58) Identifies and reports the presence of implantable cardiac devices.** Verifies presence of pacemaker and/or automatic implantable cardioverter-defibrillator and notifies the appropriate members of the health care team. ♦ Validates nursing assessment completed preoperatively. ♦ Validates medical history and physical. ♦ Completes baseline cardiac assessment. ♦ Prepares for unplanned cardiac dysfunction due to device (eg, pacemaker magnet, bipolar or battery-operated electrocautery). ♦ Notes any variances from norms (eg, scar tissues). ♦ Requests additional information from patient regarding any variances. ♦ Shares information with appropriate members of health care team.	♦ Direct observation ♦ Review of patient's medical record ♦ Verification of communication with health care team members ♦ Education Other: _____
	(I44) Evaluates postoperative cardiac status. Observes and monitors cardiac status throughout postoperative phase of care. ♦ Monitors mentation and assesses level of consciousness; orientation to person, place, and time; and presence of restlessness or agitation. ♦ Completes visual inspection of tissue perfusion, respiratory function, and cardiac status. ♦ Assesses respiratory function visibly, audibly, and ausculatory. ♦ Assesses cardiac status visibly, ausculatory, and by palpation. ♦ Assesses extremities visually, by palpation, and ausculatory as indicated. ♦ Assesses fluid volume status preoperatively and intraoperatively with estimated blood loss and replacement therapy. ♦ Monitors physiological parameters (eg, vital signs, CVP, SaO_2, MAP, PAP, PCWP, ECG, pertinent laboratory studies). ♦ Reports variances from norms to appropriate members of the health care team.	♦ Direct observation ♦ Review of patient's medical record ♦ Verification of communication with health care team members ♦ Education Other: _____
O30 The patient's neurological status is consistent with or improved from baselines levels established preoperatively.	**(I66) Identifies physiological status.** Assesses current physiological status and reports variances to appropriate members of the health care team. ♦ Establishes/reviews assessment of peripheral tissue perfusion. Assessment includes but is not limited to: – Blood pressure, – Peripheral pulse-equal bilaterally, quality, – Doppler readings, – Cardiac output, and – Presence/absence of deep vein thrombosis.	♦ Direct observation ♦ Review of patient's medical record ♦ Verification of communication with health care team members ♦ Education Other: _____

Patient Outcome	PNDS Interventions as Measurable Criteria	Recommendations for Validation of Competency
	**Domain 2: PHYSIOLOGIC O10 – O15, O29, O30** *(continued)*	
	*Competency Statement:* **The perioperative registered nurse demonstrates the ability to assess, diagnose, implement, and evaluate treatments and procedures that contribute to the physiological stability of the surgical patient.**	

(continued) **O30 The patient's neurological status is consistent with or improved from baselines levels established preoperatively.**	*(continued)*
	♦ Evaluates laboratory values:
	  – Monitors physiological parameters (eg, CBC, PT, PTT).
	  – Monitors drug and alcohol levels.
	♦ Establishes/reviews assessment of respiratory status. Assessment includes but is not limited to:
	  – Rate and depth of respirations,
	  – Use of ventilatory support/oxygen,
	  – Airway patency, and
	  – ABG.
	♦ Assesses temperature.
	♦ Monitors urinary output.
	♦ Reviews pertinent laboratory test results (eg, electrolytes, hormone levels, basal metabolic rate, tissue pathology, culture sensitivities, cerebrospinal fluid analyses, drug/alcohol levels).
	♦ Notes presence of neurological implants (eg, shunts, stimulators, aneurysm clips).	

	(I144) Assesses baseline neurological status.
	Collects data to evaluate patient's current neurological status.
	♦ Assesses patient by scoring the Glasgow coma scale (includes eye response, verbal response, and motor response).
	♦ Assesses while awake preoperatively for:
	  – Presence of nausea and vomiting.
	  – Ability to flex and extend extremities.
	  – Presence of numbness, tingling, or paresthesia in nontargeted areas.
	  – Grip strength and ensures equality bilaterally.
	♦ Validates skin integrity and the presence of any muscle wasting.
	♦ Reviews chart for current neurological status. Review should include:
	  – Latex allergy in patients with spina bifida history, including number of previous surgical procedures.
	  – History of seizure activity-occurrence, variety, frequency, stimulus, medications.
	  – Cranial nerve assessment, including swallowing ability, speech, vision, pupil response.
	  – EEG activity.
	  – Diagnostic test results (eg, x-rays, computed tomography [CT] scans, magnetic resonance imaging [MRI], angiograms).
	♦ Notes presence of tremors, plegia, palsy.
	♦ Reviews history and physical for indications of Creutzfeldt-Jakob disease.
		♦ Direct observation
		♦ Review of patient's medical record
		♦ Verification of communication with health care team members
		♦ Education
		Other: _____

Patient Outcome	PNDS Interventions as Measurable Criteria	Recommendations for Validation of Competency
\multicolumn{3}{c}{**Domain 2: PHYSIOLOGIC O10 – O15, O29, O30** *(continued)*}		

Domain 2: PHYSIOLOGIC O10 – O15, O29, O30 *(continued)*

Competency Statement: The perioperative registered nurse demonstrates the ability to assess, diagnose, implement, and evaluate treatments and procedures that contribute to the physiological stability of the surgical patient.

Patient Outcome	PNDS Interventions as Measurable Criteria	Recommendations for Validation of Competency
(continued) **O30 The patient's neurological status is consistent with or improved from baselines levels established preoperatively.**	*(continued)* ♦ Evaluates current headache/pain/discomfort level using a recognized pain scale (eg, patient with loss of cognition may need the faces scale). ♦ Identifies triggers for patients with seizures or tic douloureux. ♦ Notes presence of decerebrate rigidity in patient posturing. ♦ Notes presence of intracranial pressure monitoring and values prior to surgery. ♦ Notes presence of neurological implants (eg, shunts, stimulators, aneurysm clip). ♦ Assesses psychosocial status.	
	(I145) Implements protective measures during neurosurgical procedures. Protects patient from harm caused by equipment, supplies, or positioning specific to neurological procedures. ♦ Reviews/establishes neurological nursing assessment. ♦ Obtains previous diagnostic tests for comparison during the surgical procedure (eg, x-rays, CT scans, MRI, angiograms). ♦ Prevents potential cross-contamination by prion infection. ♦ Implements latex allergy precautions as necessary (spina bifida cases are high-risk patients). ♦ Implements spine precautions in patients with known or suspected spinal injury. ♦ Implements aneurysm precautions as needed (eg, decrease light stimulus, decrease noise stimulus, maintain medications to lower blood pressure). ♦ Preserves patient dignity by providing privacy for head shave. ♦ Stores hair in labeled container according to facility policy. ♦ Considers safety and surgical visibility when positioning for neurosurgical procedure. ♦ Ensures that drills and perforators used to penetrate the skull are functioning and readily available to relieve intracranial pressure. ♦ Ensures availability of medications to decrease intracranial volume as needed (eg, mannitol, dexamethasone). ♦ Provides suction and warm irrigation continuously to prevent accumulation of fluids/debris in cranium. ♦ Monitors cognition, level of consciousness, orientation to person, place and time, and the presence of restlessness or agitation during awake procedures. ♦ Implements safety precautions when intended hypothermia is required during procedure.	♦ Direct observation ♦ Review of patient's medical record ♦ Verification of communication with health care team members ♦ Documentation of annual equipment review Other: _____

Patient Outcome	PNDS Interventions as Measurable Criteria	Recommendations for Validation of Competency
\multicolumn{3}{Domain 2}		

Domain 2: PHYSIOLOGIC O10 – O15, O29, O30 *(continued)*

Competency Statement: **The perioperative registered nurse demonstrates the ability to assess, diagnose, implement, and evaluate treatments and procedures that contribute to the physiological stability of the surgical patient.**

Patient Outcome	PNDS Interventions as Measurable Criteria	Recommendations for Validation of Competency
(continued) **O30 The patient's neurological status is consistent with or improved from baselines levels established preoperatively.**	*(continued)* ♦ Maintains tissue hydration by covering with wet material or moistening with warm saline. ♦ Provides hemostatic agents to minimize cranial bleeding (eg, local anesthesia for skin edges, skin (Raney) clips, bone wax or equivalent, hemostatic chemical agents). ♦ Observes for signs and symptoms of venous air embolus (eg, end-tidal PCO_2 decline, decreased blood pressure, bradycardia, and convulsions) when patient is placed in the sitting position. ♦ Ensures microdoppler is available and functioning. ♦ Administers care to invasive device sites (eg, ventriculostomy, intracranial pressure monitor [ICP]).	
	(I146) Evaluates postoperative neurological status. Assesses and monitors neurological status throughout postoperative phase of care. ♦ Completes Glasgow coma evaluation post-procedure and compares to preoperative values. ♦ Observes for seizure occurrence, variety, frequency, and duration. ♦ Monitors for changes between preoperative and postoperative cranial nerves function. ♦ Assesses pain/headache/discomfort level using a recognized pain scale. ♦ Evaluates changes in intracranial pressure, levels in skin sensation, and neurological rigidity posturing. ♦ Evaluates physiological parameters (eg, vital signs, ICP, CPP, MAP, SaO_2, ECG, ABG), evoked potentials (BAEP and SSEP), and pertinent laboratory studies. ♦ Reports variances from norms to appropriate members of the health care team. ♦ Inspects location of tong placement and applies ointment and dressing postoperatively.	♦ Direct observation ♦ Review of patient's medical record ♦ Verification of communication with health care team members ♦ Education Other: _____
O29 The patient demonstrates and/or reports adequate pain control throughout the perioperative period.	**(I16) Assesses pain control.** Uses validated pain scale to assess pain control. ♦ Reviews patient assessment for type of pain being treated and medical condition. ♦ Reviews current treatment protocol. ♦ Reviews potential interactions of pain medication(s) with other medications or food. ♦ Requests patient verbalize effectiveness of treatment with recognized assessment tool (eg, numerical scale, faces scale). ♦ Requests verbalization of patient's expectation of acceptable pain score. ♦ Encourages questions related to pain management.	♦ Direct observation ♦ Review of patient's medical record ♦ Verification of communication with health care team members ♦ Education Other: _____

Patient Outcome	PNDS Interventions as Measurable Criteria	Recommendations for Validation of Competency
	**Domain 2: PHYSIOLOGIC O10 – O15, O29, O30** *(continued)*	
	*Competency Statement:* **The perioperative registered nurse demonstrates the ability to assess, diagnose, implement, and evaluate treatments and procedures that contribute to the physiological stability of the surgical patient.**	
(continued) **O29 The patient demonstrates and/or reports adequate pain control throughout the perioperative period.**	*(continued)* ♦ Offers information to patient, family members about pain, pain relief measures, rating scales, and other assessment data to report. ♦ Monitors patient for congruence of verbal and nonverbal cues. ♦ Evaluates patient's responses to pain regimen.	
	(I71) Implements pain guidelines. Provides care consistent with clinical practice guidelines related to pain assessment and management. ♦ Reviews patient assessment for type of pain being treated, medical condition, and health status. ♦ Reviews facility pain guidelines. ♦ Initiates protocols identified in guidelines. ♦ Positions for comfort unless contraindicated. ♦ Determines regimen meets identified need. ♦ Monitors relationship of patient progress to pain control. ♦ Monitors pain guideline effectiveness. ♦ Administers medications as prescribed.	♦ Direct observation ♦ Review of patient's medical record ♦ Verification of communication with health care team members ♦ Education Other: _____
	(I24) Collaborates in initiating patient-controlled analgesia. Identifies and collaborates in identifying patients who will benefit from patient-controlled analgesia. ♦ Reviews assessment for type of pain being treated and patient medical condition. ♦ Reviews with patient goals of pain management therapy. ♦ Reviews treatment protocol for administration. ♦ Encourages titration to effective relief levels. ♦ Monitors administration process. ♦ Provides teaching related to patient-controlled analgesia. ♦ Evaluates patient's response to medication administration.	♦ Direct observation ♦ Review of patient's medical record ♦ Verification of communication with health care team members ♦ Documentation of annual equipment review Other: _____
	(I69) Implements alternative methods of pain control. Uses diversified activities, therapeutic touch, meditation, breathing, and positioning to augment pain control methods. ♦ Reviews patient assessment for type of pain being treated and medical condition. ♦ Reviews current treatment protocol. ♦ Asks patient to verbalize effectiveness of treatment regimen. ♦ Reviews non-medication pain treatments (eg, cold therapy, heat therapy, music distraction, relaxation therapy, physical rehabilitation, visualization, pacing, and transcutaneous electrical nerve stimulation). ♦ Identifies patient's coping style and cultural influences regarding pain management.	♦ Direct observation ♦ Review of patient's medical record ♦ Verification of communication with health care team members ♦ Education Other: _____

Patient Outcome	PNDS Interventions as Measurable Criteria	Recommendations for Validation of Competency
	**Domain 2: PHYSIOLOGIC O10 – O15, O29, O30** *(continued)*	
	*Competency Statement:* The perioperative registered nurse demonstrates the ability to assess, diagnose, implement, and evaluate treatments and procedures that contribute to the physiological stability of the surgical patient.	
(continued) **O29 The patient demonstrates and/or reports adequate pain control throughout the perioperative period.**	*(continued)* ♦ Assesses patient's level of fatigue, cognition, and ability to follow instruction. ♦ Offers information about methods that will assist in pain control. ♦ Includes family/significant other in educational process. ♦ Initiates alternative method following institutional guidelines. ♦ Monitors progress. ♦ Evaluates patient's responses.	
	(I54) Evaluates response to pain management interventions. Assesses patient's responses to pain management interventions including physiological parameters and subjective and objective findings. ♦ Identifies and documents how the patient expresses pain (eg, facial expressions, irritability, restlessness, verbalization). ♦ Observes for clues indicating the patient is in pain (eg, restlessness, increased or decreased blood pressure, pallor, sweating, increased heart rate, nausea, irregular shallow breathing patterns, agitation, crying). ♦ Assesses the nature of the pain and any changes in pain level after pain management interventions. ♦ Uses recognized pain scale to quantify and measure adult patient's pain level in response to pain management interventions. ♦ Uses recognized pain observational scale to quantify and measure change in pediatric/neonate patient's pain level.	♦ Direct observation ♦ Review of patient's medical record ♦ Verification of communication with health care team members ♦ Education Other: _____

Patient Outcome	PNDS Interventions as Measurable Criteria	Recommendations for Validation of Competency

Domain 3A: BEHAVIORAL RESPONSES—KNOWLEDGE O18 – O22, O31

Competency Statement: **The perioperative registered nurse demonstrates knowledge about the psychologic, sociologic, and spiritual responses of patients and their families to the operative or other invasive procedure, including participation of patients in their recovery.**

Patient Outcome	PNDS Interventions as Measurable Criteria	Recommendations for Validation of Competency

O31 The patient demonstrates knowledge of the expected responses to the operative or invasive procedure.	**(I90) Notes sensory impairments.** Determines the patient's ability to see and hear without corrective devices.
	♦ Identifies presence of the following:
	  – Visual impairment,
	  – Auditory impairment, or
	  – Speech impairment
	♦ Modifies plan of care to accommodate sensory impairments
		♦ Direct observation
		♦ Review of patient's medical record
		♦ Verification of communication with health care team members
		♦ Education
		Other: _____

	(I134) Identifies barriers to communication. Assesses factors that could affect ability to communicate, comprehend, and demonstrate understanding of new information.
	♦ Evaluates patient's communication skills.
	♦ Observes and identifies the patient's:
	  – Age and developmental needs;
	  – Understanding of spoken words and ability to hear (presence of hearing aid);
	  – Presence of airway adjuncts (eg, tracheotomy, laryngectomy, endotracheal tube);
	  – Presence of alternative methods of speech (eg, sign language, voice box, keyboard, writing tools);
	  – Nonverbal cues; and
	  – Need for interpreter or provides alternative to direct interpretation (written literature, telephone service) if needed.
	♦ Listens to patient's speech pattern to identify:
	  – Age and developmental needs,
	  – Speech patterns,
	  – Clarity of speech,
	  – Complete thoughts,
	  – Grammar and vocabulary patterns,
	  – Discrepancies between words spoken and tone of voice, and
	  – Patient comprehension from simple to complex.
	♦ Provides the privacy necessary for patient to share confidential information.
	♦ Provides environment that facilitates understanding:
	  – Ensures room is quiet and has adequate lighting with minimal distractions;
	  – Attracts patient's attention before speaking
	  – Looks at patient while speaking;
	  – Speaks clearly and slowly in moderate tone;
	  – Uses facial expressions, touch, and nonverbal cures appropriately to enhance communication; and
	  – Uses visual aids as appropriate to assist with explanations.
	♦ Evaluates patient's responses to teaching.
		♦ Direct observation
		♦ Review of patient's medical record
		♦ Verification of communication with health care team members
		♦ Education
		Other: _____

Patient Outcome	PNDS Interventions as Measurable Criteria	Recommendations for Validation of Competency
\multicolumn{3}{}		

Patient Outcome	PNDS Interventions as Measurable Criteria	Recommendations for Validation of Competency
	Domain 3A: BEHAVIORAL RESPONSES—KNOWLEDGE O18 – O22, O31 (*continued*)	
	Competency Statement: The perioperative registered nurse demonstrates knowledge about the psychologic, sociologic, and spiritual responses of patients and their families to the operative or other invasive procedure, including participation of patients in their recovery.	
(continued) **O31 The patient demonstrates knowledge of the expected responses to the operative or invasive procedure.**	**(I135) Determines knowledge level.** Assesses knowledge and comprehension of new information and ability to apply in self-care activities. ♦ Establish rapport. ♦ Evaluates language and cognitive skills relative to age and developmental stage of growth. ♦ Identifies barriers to communication. ♦ Identifies presence of altered thought processes ♦ Verifies understanding of procedure and perioperative events. ♦ Identifies physiological variables that may interfere with learning, such as central nervous system impairment, confusion, poor cognition, or medicated state. ♦ Assesses behaviors for appropriateness to situation (eg, calm, quiet, attentive, nervous, tense, agitated, apathetic). ♦ Observes for behaviors that demonstrate compliance with an understanding of previous instruction or therapeutic regimens. ♦ Evaluates patient's responses to identify level of knowledge and understanding.	♦ Direct observation ♦ Review of patient's medical record ♦ Verification of communication with health care team members ♦ Education Other: _____
	(I136) Assesses readiness to learn. Evaluates factors that may affect abilities to learn or demonstrate knowledge. ♦ Identifies barriers to communication. ♦ Determines knowledge level. ♦ Identifies deviations from cognitive and psychomotor norms of age group. ♦ Identifies philosophical, cultural, and spiritual beliefs and values. ♦ Assesses coping mechanisms. ♦ Assesses patient's self-perception and self-concept patterns considering self-image, self-worth, and emotional responses. ♦ Identifies barriers to readiness to learn. ♦ Evaluates patient's responses to teaching.	♦ Direct observation ♦ Review of patient's medical record ♦ Evidence of continuing education in cultural competence ♦ Verification of communication with health care team members ♦ Education Other: _____
	(I68) Identifies psychosocial status. Assesses the psychosocial factors that influence that patient's care and develops and implements plan of care to address those needs. ♦ Evaluates psychosocial status relative to age and stage of development. ♦ Verifies psychosocial status. ♦ Identifies barriers to communications. ♦ Determines knowledge level.	♦ Direct observation ♦ Review of patient's medical record ♦ Verification of communication with health care team members ♦ Education Other: _____

Patient Outcome	PNDS Interventions as Measurable Criteria	Recommendations for Validation of Competency
	Domain 3A: BEHAVIORAL RESPONSES—KNOWLEDGE O18 – O22, O31 (*continued*)	
	Competency Statement: **The perioperative registered nurse demonstrates knowledge about the psychologic, sociologic, and spiritual responses of patients and their families to the operative or other invasive procedure, including participation of patients in their recovery.**	
(continued) **O31 The patient demonstrates knowledge of the expected responses to the operative or invasive procedure.**	*(continued)* ♦ Determines patient's ability to understand information offered. ♦ Assesses coping mechanisms. ♦ Identifies patient home profile: household composition, ages, gender, and occupations; and family coping skills, limitations, and roles. ♦ Identifies patient's resources (eg, insurance, home environments, extended family, community). ♦ Identifies patient's religious practices. ♦ Identifies cultural practices and their effect on health behaviors and impending surgical event. ♦ Elicits perceptions of surgery. ♦ Evaluates patient's responses to psychosocial status.	
	(I137) Assesses coping mechanisms. Assesses the influence of coping practices and availability of support from family members. ♦ Reviews patient's coping pattern and its effectiveness. ♦ Identifies barriers to communication. ♦ Determines knowledge level. ♦ Identifies psychosocial status. ♦ Identifies philosophical, cultural, and spiritual beliefs and related practices. ♦ Asks patient to describe current methods of dealing with stress. ♦ Observes for behavior that may indicate ineffective coping (eg, verbalization of anger; depression; ineffective coping; alterations in diet; disruption of sleep pattern; restlessness; absence of eye contact; absence of or reduced participation in plan of care; withdrawal from family or staff; hostility toward family or staff). ♦ Determines when these behaviors became first apparent. ♦ Evaluates patient's potentials for harming/injuring self or others. ♦ Encourages patient to express feelings. ♦ Determines the most effective methods of communication and support. ♦ Evaluates patient's previous and current coping patterns. ♦ Evaluates availability and effectiveness of support system.	♦ Direct observation ♦ Review of patient's medical record ♦ Evidence of continuing education in cultural competence ♦ Verification of communication with health care team members ♦ Education Other: _____

Patient Outcome	PNDS Interventions as Measurable Criteria	Recommendations for Validation of Competency
\[spanning header\]	**Domain 3A: BEHAVIORAL RESPONSES—KNOWLEDGE O18 – O22, O31 (continued)** *Competency Statement:* The perioperative registered nurse demonstrates knowledge about the psychologic, sociologic, and spiritual responses of patients and their families to the operative or other invasive procedure, including participation of patients in their recovery.	
(continued) **O31 The patient demonstrates knowledge of the expected responses to the operative or invasive procedure.**	**(I147) Implements measures to provide psychological support.** Offers assistance, advocates for patient, and provides psychological support during perioperative phases of care. ♦ Assess for signs and symptoms of anxiety/fear (eg, fears and concerns, preoperative insomnia, muscle tenseness, tremors, irritability, change in appetite, restlessness, diaphoresis, tachypmea, tachycardia, elevated blood pressure, facial pallor or flushing, withdrawn behavior). ♦ Orients patient to environment and care routines/practices. ♦ Introduces staff members. ♦ Assures patient that a member of the staff is nearby. ♦ Provides information and answers questions honestly. ♦ Maintains a calm, supportive, confident manner. ♦ Provides an atmosphere of care and concern (privacy, non-judgmental approach, empathy, and respect). ♦ Identifies sociocultural variables such as cultural or religious beliefs, values, and attitudes toward health and health practices. ♦ Observes for increased anxiety demonstrated through behavior (eg, hand tremor, shakiness, restlessness, facial tension, voice quivering, increased perspirations). ♦ Offers alternative methods to minimize anxiety (music, humor). ♦ Reinforces physician's explanations and clarifies any misconceptions. ♦ Explains purpose of preoperative preparations prior to implementations. ♦ Encourages patient participation in decision making and planning for postoperative care.	♦ Direct observation ♦ Review of patient's medical record ♦ Evidence of continuing education in cultural competence ♦ Verification of communication with health care team members ♦ Education Other: _____
	(I47) Evaluates psychosocial response to plan of care. Determines effectiveness of plan and psychosocial responses of patient/family members and modifies plan as indicated. ♦ Identifies barriers to communication. ♦ Determines knowledge level. ♦ Verifies patient's ability to understand information. ♦ Provides necessary time to process information. ♦ Appears relaxed and unhurried in interactions with patient. ♦ Obtains interpreter as appropriate. ♦ Provides culturally sensitive nursing care. ♦ Reviews nursing care plan with patient/family members. ♦ Discusses specific cultural influences (eg, folk medicine/home remedies; religious or spiritual aspects; food preferences or avoidance aspects; socioeconomic aspects; family structure).	♦ Direct observation ♦ Review of patient's medical record ♦ Verification of communication with health care team members ♦ Education Other: _____

Patient Outcome	PNDS Interventions as Measurable Criteria	Recommendations for Validation of Competency
	**Domain 3A: BEHAVIORAL RESPONSES—KNOWLEDGE O18 – O22, O31 (*continued*)** *Competency Statement:* The perioperative registered nurse demonstrates knowledge about the psychologic, sociologic, and spiritual responses of patients and their families to the operative or other invasive procedure, including participation of patients in their recovery.	
(continued) **O31 The patient demonstrates knowledge of the expected responses to the operative or invasive procedure.**	*(continued)* ♦ Provides for continuation of cultural practices and beliefs. ♦ Encourages use of family members as support as appropriate. ♦ Collaborates with patient/family member regarding expectations of care. ♦ Verifies patient's/family member's understanding of plan of care. ♦ Evaluates patient's/family member's response to plan of care.	
	(I32) Elicits perceptions of surgery. Assesses responses to the procedure and ensures access to correct information. ♦ Identifies barriers to communication. ♦ Verifies surgical procedure. ♦ Encourages patient to verbalize understanding of procedure. ♦ Observes behavior for nonverbal cues. ♦ Listens for verbalization of apprehension, uncertainty, fear, distress, or worry. ♦ Encourages patient to verbalize possible outcomes of surgery. ♦ Encourages patient's expression of fear or anxiety related to surgery and the outcomes of surgery. ♦ Evaluates patient's responses.	♦ Direct observation ♦ Review of patient's medical record ♦ Verification of communication with health care team members ♦ Education Other: _____

	(I56) Explains expected sequence of events.
	Describes routines and protocols related to perioperative care.
	♦ Provides preoperative instruction based on age and identified needs.
	♦ Reviews environmental aspects of expected times and location:
	  – Expected time of arrival and location,
	  – Expected time of procedure,
	  – Waiting time and locations,
	  – Directions to facility,
	  – Location of postoperative discussion with physician, and
	  – Anticipated time to see family/family member.
	♦ Reviews preoperative instruction as indicated discussing importance of:
	  – Diet,
	  – Fluids intake (clear liquids allowed or NPO preoperatively, and time frame),
	  – Bowel prep if ordered,
	  – Voiding,
	  – Skin prep,
	  – Clothing, and
	  – Any anticipated transportation/discharge needs and home care.
		♦ Direct observation
		♦ Review of patient's medical record
		♦ Verification of communication with health care team members
		♦ Education
		Other: _____

Patient Outcome	PNDS Interventions as Measurable Criteria	Recommendations for Validation of Competency
	**Domain 3A: BEHAVIORAL RESPONSES—KNOWLEDGE** **O18 – O22, O31 (*continued*)** *Competency Statement:* The perioperative registered nurse demonstrates knowledge about the psychologic, sociologic, and spiritual responses of patients and their families to the operative or other invasive procedure, including participation of patients in their recovery.	
(continued) **O31 The patient demonstrates knowledge of the expected responses to the operative or invasive procedure.**	*(continued)* ♦ Reviews postoperative routines, procedures, and equipment. ♦ Describes potential alterations in comfort levels to be expected postoperatively. ♦ Offers information on how to most effectively minimize postoperative discomfort. ♦ Evaluates patient's responses to teaching.	
	(I114) Screens for substance abuse. Assesses for past or present substance abuse, monitors for and reports defining characteristics of substance abuse or withdrawal, and makes appropriate referrals. ♦ Assess for history of or current substance abuse. ♦ Listens for statements form the patient about how often substance is used and duration and quantity of use. ♦ Determines blood drug/alcohol levels. ♦ Observes behavior for signs and symptoms of substance abuse or withdrawal. ♦ Monitors vital signs. ♦ Offers appropriate referrals. ♦ Notifies appropriate members of health care team regarding history of or present abuse of drugs/alcohol.	♦ Direct observation ♦ Review of patient's medical record ♦ Verification of communication with health care team members ♦ Education Other: _____
	(I113) Screens for physical abuse. Identifies defining characteristics for actual or risk for physical abuse and offers appropriate referrals. ♦ Assesses the patient for impaired skin or tissue integrity such as bruising, cuts, burns, and neuromuscular or skeletal impairment. ♦ Recognizes patient statements indicative of abuse. ♦ Protects the patient from and prevents further abuse. ♦ Provides information related to available resources (eg,, social services, case management). ♦ Reports suspected abuse in accordance with facility policy and state reporting laws.	♦ Direct observation ♦ Review of patient's medical record ♦ Verification of communication with health care team members ♦ Education Other: _____
	(I109) Provides status reports to family members. Reports progress to family members by telephone or in person. ♦ Offers instruction to family members as indicated. ♦ Reviews expected protocols and patient progress through surgical day. ♦ Addresses family members' questions, concerns, and feelings. ♦ Identifies family members' emotional reaction to condition. ♦ Offers messages of assurance to family members. ♦ Provides answers to questions or assists in obtaining answers. ♦ Provides status reports to family members frequently or per facility/physician practice. ♦ Evaluates family members' response to information provided.	♦ Direct observation ♦ Review of patient's medical record ♦ Verification of communication with health care team members ♦ Education Other: _____

Patient Outcome	PNDS Interventions as Measurable Criteria	Recommendations for Validation of Competency
	Domain 3A: BEHAVIORAL RESPONSES—KNOWLEDGE O18 – O22, O31 (continued)	
	Competency Statement: The perioperative registered nurse demonstrates knowledge about the psychologic, sociologic, and spiritual responses of patients and their families to the operative or other invasive procedure, including participation of patients in their recovery.	
(continued) **O31 The patient demonstrates knowledge of the expected responses to the operative or invasive procedure.**	**(I50) Evaluates response to instructions.** Evaluates patient's/family member's understanding of instructions regarding perioperative experience and ongoing care. ♦ Observes patient demonstration of sequential progressive steps of the following appropriate skills: – Deep breathing, – Coughing and wound splinting, – Passive leg exercises, – Progression to ambulation, and – Wound and dressing care. ♦ Assesses the patient's and family members' management skills of: – Medication schedule; – Activity limitations and exercise regimen; – Dietary restrictions or supplements; – Wound care; – Prescribed treatments; – Follow-up appointments, which may include signs and symptoms to report; and – Emergency protocols. ♦ Observes return demonstrations of self-care instruction ♦ Provides patient/family member with written discharge and at-home instructions ♦ Reinforces information provided by other members of health care team ♦ Observes patient's responses to instructions ♦ Requests verbalization of instructions ♦ Clarifies information ♦ Encourages patient/family members to describe in their own words the anticipated physical and psychological effects of surgery, feelings regarding surgery, and expected outcomes ♦ Encourages patient/family members to communicate feelings regarding surgery and expected outcomes ♦ Requests patient/family members communicate understanding of preoperative instructions ♦ Provides time for patient/family members to ask questions ♦ Evaluates patient/family responses to perioperative instruction	♦ Direct observation ♦ Review of patient's medical record ♦ Verification of communication with health care team members ♦ Education Other: _____

Patient Outcome	PNDS Interventions as Measurable Criteria	Recommendations for Validation of Competency
	**Domain 3A: BEHAVIORAL RESPONSES—KNOWLEDGE O18 – O22, O31 (*continued*)**	

Competency Statement: The perioperative registered nurse demonstrates knowledge about the psychologic, sociologic, and spiritual responses of patients and their families to the operative or other invasive procedure, including participation of patients in their recovery.

Patient Outcome	PNDS Interventions as Measurable Criteria	Recommendations for Validation of Competency
O18 The patient demonstrates knowledge of nutritional requirements related to operative or other invasive procedures.	**(I148) Assesses nutritional habits and patterns.** Identifies usual dietary intake, habits, and patterns. ♦ Validates preoperative nutritional assessment including nutritional history and physical examination (eg, 24-hour recall, food record) and laboratory data ♦ Verifies patient's ability to understand information ♦ Provides necessary time to process information ♦ Obtains interpreter if needed ♦ Identifies food allergies ♦ Identifies food preferences, cultural practices, and routine habits ♦ Identifies cultural dietary preferences and practices ♦ Compares usual dietary intake to prescribed postoperative diet ♦ Individualizes postoperative dietary plan ♦ Evaluates nutritional status	♦ Direct observation ♦ Review of patient's medical record ♦ Verification of communication with health care team members ♦ Education Other: _____
	(I18) Assesses psychosocial issues specific to the patient's nutritional status. Identifies any variances in nutritional plan related to psychosocial status. ♦ Identifies barriers to communication ♦ Determines knowledge level ♦ Obtains interpreter if needed ♦ Verifies food preferences and routing practices ♦ Involves patient when planning and providing care ♦ Encourages family member participation in discussions and care processes ♦ Evaluates effects of psychosocial issues on nutritional state	♦ Direct observation ♦ Review of patient's medical record ♦ Verification of communication with health care team members ♦ Education Other: _____
	(I107) Provides instruction regarding dietary needs. Explains dietary needs or restrictions. ♦ Obtains nutritional assessment ♦ Reviews food preferences and routine practices ♦ Obtains interpreter if needed ♦ Provides alternatives to interpreter when appropriate (written material, video, tape recording in primary language) ♦ Verifies any food allergies ♦ Explains purpose of dietary regimen ♦ Provides age-specific, culturally sensitive information about prescribed dietary regimen ♦ Prepares patient for parenteral/enteral feedings when ordered ♦ Instructs patient on appropriate food for the regimen and those prohibited ♦ Reviews applicable food/medication interactions ♦ Answers questions ♦ Provides written instructions ♦ Encourages participation of family members in process	♦ Direct observation ♦ Review of patient's medical record ♦ Verification of communication with health care team members ♦ Education Other: _____

Patient Outcome	PNDS Interventions as Measurable Criteria	Recommendations for Validation of Competency
	**Domain 3A: BEHAVIORAL RESPONSES—KNOWLEDGE O18 – O22, O31 (continued)** *Competency Statement:* The perioperative registered nurse demonstrates knowledge about the psychologic, sociologic, and spiritual responses of patients and their families to the operative or other invasive procedure, including participation of patients in their recovery.	
(continued) **O18 The patient demonstrates knowledge of nutritional requirements related to operative or other invasive procedures.**	**(I52) Evaluates response to nutritional instruction.** Evaluates understanding of nutritional instruction by listening to explanations and observing return demonstrations. ♦ Requests patient/family member verbalize dietary regimen prescribed and review its purpose ♦ Reviews cultural dietary practices ♦ Requests patient/family member verbalize foods allowed and prohibited on prescribed regimen ♦ Requests patient/family member verbalize specific medication/food interactions known from current medical regimen ♦ Encourages and answers questions ♦ Requests patient/family member verbalize understanding of dietary plan	♦ Direct observation ♦ Review of patient's medical record ♦ Verification of communication with health care team members ♦ Education Other: _____
O19 The patient demonstrates knowledge of medication management.	**(I123) Verifies allergies.** Identifies allergies, idiosyncrasies, and sensitivities to medications, latex, chemical agents, foods, and/or adhesives. ♦ Queries patient about allergies or hypersensitivity reaction to adhesives, egg products, or iodine products ♦ Queries patient about medications and foreign proteins that cause anaphylaxis (eg, antibiotics, opiates, vasopressin, protamine, allergen extracts, muscle relaxants, vaccines, local anesthetics, whole blood, cryoprecipitate, immune globulin, and radiocontrast media) ♦ Determines type of food or substance and type of reaction experienced, if any, as reported by the patient ♦ Records and communicates to the anesthesia care provider a patient history of anaphylaxis, asthma, or other respiratory difficulties related to the presence of allergens, toxins, or antigens	♦ Direct observation ♦ Review of patient's medical record ♦ Identification of patient allergies in patient care record and use of facility allergy alert system (eg, arm band) ♦ Verification of communication with health care team members ♦ Education Other: _____
	(I17) Assesses psychosocial issues specific to the patient's medication management. Identifies any variance in medication plan related to psychosocial status. ♦ Identifies barriers to communication ♦ Determines knowledge level ♦ Verifies patient's ability to understand information ♦ Approaches patient in a calm and unhurried manner ♦ Obtains interpreter if needed ♦ Identifies influence of health beliefs and folk practices ♦ Provides culturally sensitive nursing care ♦ Reviews current medication regimens in detail with patient and family members ♦ Reviews factors that may prevent the patient from taking medications as prescribed ♦ Identifies effects of medication use on patient's lifestyle ♦ Evaluates psychosocial issues specific to patient's medication administration	♦ Direct observation ♦ Review of patient's medical record ♦ Verification of communication with health care team members ♦ Education Other: _____

Patient Outcome	PNDS Interventions as Measurable Criteria	Recommendations for Validation of Competency
spanning — see below		

Domain 3A: BEHAVIORAL RESPONSES—KNOWLEDGE
O18 – O22, O31 *(continued)*

Competency Statement: The perioperative registered nurse demonstrates knowledge about the psychologic, sociologic, and spiritual responses of patients and their families to the operative or other invasive procedure, including participation of patients in their recovery.

Patient Outcome	PNDS Interventions as Measurable Criteria	Recommendations for Validation of Competency
(continued) **O19 The patient demonstrates knowledge of medication management.**	**(I104) Provides instruction about prescribed medications.** Provides information about prescribed medications, such as purpose; administration; and desired, side, and adverse effects. ♦ Verifies any allergies and sensitivity reactions. ♦ States names and purpose of medications. ♦ Identifies dose, route, and appropriate times of administration. ♦ Instructs patient/family member of specific procedures necessary before medication administration (eg, checking pulse). ♦ Provides clear, understandable explanations about procedures. ♦ Communicates discharge instructions verbally and in writing. ♦ Communicates instructions that reinforce information provided in the preoperative period. ♦ Assesses patient's/family member's ability to understand information. ♦ Encourages family member participation in the instructional process. ♦ Offers teaching methods relevant to the patient's ability to comprehend information. This could include handouts, audio or video presentations, lecture, discussions, return demonstration, and class/group discussion. ♦ Evaluates the patient's ability to safely and correctly self-administer medications. ♦ Provides detailed instruction about prescribed medications. ♦ Provides written instructions. ♦ Instructs to take a list of all medications to doctor's office appointment. ♦ Evaluates patient's responses to instruction.	♦ Direct observation ♦ Review of patient's medical record ♦ Verification of communication with health care team members ♦ Education Other: _____
	(I48) Evaluates response to instruction about prescribed medications. Evaluates understanding of medication instruction by listening to explanations and observing return demonstrations of activities related to administration and management of medications. ♦ Requests patient/family member verbalize name of medication prescribed and its purpose ♦ Reviews any cultural practices related to medication administration ♦ Requests patient/family member verbalize dose, route, and frequency of medication administration ♦ Requests patient/family member verbalize action to be taken when a dose is missed ♦ Requests patient/family member identify where written instructions will be kept for reference ♦ Requests patient/family member demonstrate specific procedures required prior to medication administration (eg, check pulse) ♦ Encourages and answers questions	♦ Direct observation ♦ Review of patient's medical record ♦ Verification of communication with health care team members ♦ Education Other: _____

Patient Outcome	PNDS Interventions as Measurable Criteria	Recommendations for Validation of Competency
	**Domain 3A: BEHAVIORAL RESPONSES—KNOWLEDGE O18 – O22, O31 (continued)** *Competency Statement:* The perioperative registered nurse demonstrates knowledge about the psychologic, sociologic, and spiritual responses of patients and their families to the operative or other invasive procedure, including participation of patients in their recovery.	
O20 The patient demonstrates knowledge of pain management.	**(I61) Identifies cultural and value components related to pain.** Provides pain control considering cultural factors and manifestations of values (eg, stoicism, alternative therapy, verbalization, meditation). ♦ Reviews records for type of pain being treated, medical condition, demographics, and cultural cues ♦ Establishes rapport ♦ Evaluates language and cognitive skills relative to age and developmental stage ♦ Identifies barriers to communication ♦ Identifies presence of altered thought processes ♦ Determines educational background ♦ Obtains interpreter if needed ♦ Requests patient verbalize pain management protocol and its purpose ♦ Identifies patient's preference of pain therapy and coping methods ♦ Asks patient to describe pain and intensity of pain ♦ Offers assessment tool most appropriate to patient need (ie, numerical scale, color scale, faces scale) ♦ Verifies assessment tool is clearly understood ♦ Provides culturally sensitive nursing care ♦ Identifies mutual goals of care that consider different preferences (eg, alert versus pain free)	♦ Direct observation ♦ Review of patient's medical record ♦ Verification of communication with health care team members ♦ Education Other: _____
	(I108) Provides pain management instruction. Provides information about the purpose; administration; and desired, side, and adverse effects of prescribed medications and nonpharmacological techniques for managing pain. ♦ Reviews action to be taken if a dose is missed ♦ Encourages notification of health care provider when discomfort after pain medication is unrelieved by ordered medications or is worsening ♦ Validates orders for prescribed medication ♦ Verifies patient's ability to understand information ♦ Provides necessary time to process information ♦ Identifies patient's cultural practices ♦ Obtains interpreter if needed ♦ Verifies allergies and any sensitivity reactions ♦ Explains names and purposes of medications ♦ Identifies dose, route, and appropriate times of administration ♦ Instructs patient/family member of specific protocols for medication administration (eg, use of patient-controlled analgesia pump)	♦ Direct observation ♦ Review of patient's medical record ♦ Verification of communication with health care team members ♦ Education Other: _____

Patient Outcome	PNDS Interventions as Measurable Criteria	Recommendations for Validation of Competency
	**Domain 3A: BEHAVIORAL RESPONSES—KNOWLEDGE** **O18 – O22, O31 (*continued*)** *Competency Statement:* The perioperative registered nurse demonstrates knowledge about the psychologic, sociologic, and spiritual responses of patients and their families to the operative or other invasive procedure, including participation of patients in their recovery.	
(continued) **O20 The patient demonstrates knowledge of pain management.**	*(continued)* ♦ Reviews desired, side, and adverse effects ♦ Reviews applicable food/medication interactions ♦ Reviews appropriate storage practices and care of equipment ♦ Provides written instructions ♦ Encourages family member participation in the instruction process ♦ Evaluates patient's understanding of medication administration, purpose, and effects	
	(I53) Evaluates response to pain management instruction. Evaluates understanding of pain management instructions by listening to explanations and observing return demonstrations. ♦ Requests patient/family member verbalize understanding of pain medication and its purpose ♦ Requests feedback on level of pain management achieved using a recognized pain measurement tool (numbers, faces) ♦ Observes patient for nonverbal cues regarding pain (eg, grimacing movement, splinting) ♦ Reviews cultural influences on pain assessment and management ♦ Requests patient/family member verbalize dose, route, and frequency of medication ♦ Requests patient/family member verbalize action to be taken when dose missed ♦ Requests patient/family member identify where written instructions will be kept for reference ♦ Determines patient's understanding to notify health care provider if pain is not controlled or is worsening ♦ Encourages questions and clarifies information	♦ Direct observation ♦ Review of patient's medical record ♦ Verification of communication with health care team members ♦ Education Other: _____
O21 The patient participates in the rehabilitation process.	**(I106) Provides instruction based on age and identified needs.** Provides perioperative instructional activities that promote rehabilitation based on age and developmental and situation-specific needs. ♦ Identifies barriers to communication ♦ Determines knowledge level and psychosocial status ♦ Assesses readiness to learn ♦ Assesses coping mechanisms ♦ Identifies teaching strategies appropriate to age and developmental stage ♦ Encourages family member participation in process ♦ Formulates plan to offer instruction to meet individual need ♦ Provides environment conducive to teaching and learning (ie, room is quiet, with adequate lighting and minimal distraction)	♦ Direct observation ♦ Review of patient's medical record ♦ Verification of communication with health care team members ♦ Education Other: _____

Patient Outcome	PNDS Interventions as Measurable Criteria	Recommendations for Validation of Competency

Domain 3A: BEHAVIORAL RESPONSES—KNOWLEDGE
O18 – O22, O31 (continued)

Competency Statement: The perioperative registered nurse demonstrates knowledge about the psychologic, sociologic, and spiritual responses of patients and their families to the operative or other invasive procedure, including participation of patients in their recovery.

(continued)
 	
O21 The patient participates in the rehabilitation process.
	(continued)
	♦ Uses learning theory and communication skills to facilitate understanding.
	♦ Establishes priorities offering age-appropriate instruction to patient/family focusing on individual need.
	♦ Describes preoperative preparation activities and behaviors expected.
	♦ Describes equipment that may be potentially frightening. Offers child opportunity to hold and explore items (eg, toys, hats, masks, blood pressure cuff, stethoscope)
	♦ Describes how surgical suite environment and surgical experience may affect all senses (eg, noise, coolness, hardness of bed, attire of health care workers, lights, medication taste)
	♦ Describes potential alterations in comfort level to be expected postoperatively (eg, wound pain, soreness, achiness, nausea, bloating, referred pain)
	♦ Offers information regarding how to best minimize discomfort (eg, request pain medication for pain)
	♦ Describes routine activities and equipment
	♦ Identifies resource contact for home care needs (eg, visiting nurse, medical equipment)
	♦ Identifies potential limitations to normal routines and explores solutions to minimize those limitations (eg, may fatigue easily; plan to gradually increase activities)
	♦ Describes postoperative home care instructions to allow for advance preparation (eg, general anesthesia, securing a responsible person to provide transportation from the facility and to provide supportive care for 24 hours postoperatively)
	♦ Uses instruction method that facilitates learning
	♦ Provides adequate time for patient or family member to review information and ask questions.
	♦ Offers demonstrations for the following skills:
	  – Deep breathing,
	  – Coughing and wound splinting
	  – Passive leg exercises,
	  – Progression of diet postoperatively, and
	  – Wound and dressing care.
	♦ Clarifies information
	♦ Selects an alternate teaching method if indicated
	♦ Conducts patient/family learning conferences specific to rehabilitation process
	♦ Provides follow-up rehabilitation instructions as needed	

Patient Outcome	PNDS Interventions as Measurable Criteria	Recommendations for Validation of Competency
	Domain 3A: BEHAVIORAL RESPONSES—KNOWLEDGE O18 – O22, O31 (*continued*)	
	Competency Statement: **The perioperative registered nurse demonstrates knowledge about the psychologic, sociologic, and spiritual responses of patients and their families to the operative or other invasive procedure, including participation of patients in their recovery.**	

(continued) **O21 The patient participates in the rehabilitation process.**	**(I62) Identifies expectations of home care.** Identifies home care needs relative to performing the activities of daily living, managing self-care, and returning to usual activities.
	♦ Assesses the patient's/family members' ability to verbalize feelings about:
	  – Physical changes that occur as a result of surgical intervention and how life will be affected;
	  – Psychological changes that occur as a result of surgical intervention and how life will be affected; and
	  – Concerns about the surgical experience, desired outcomes, or involvement in recovery process
	♦ Identifies nursing diagnoses that describe the patient's needs for postoperative home care
	♦ Identifies expected outcomes for patient for home care following a surgical or invasive procedure
	♦ Assists patient/family member to identify and achieve realistic, measurable goals to attain desired outcomes
	♦ Encourages patient to identify own strengths and weaknesses
	♦ Assists patient/family member develop realistic expectations of themselves in performance of roles
	♦ Assists patient in breaking down complex goals into small, manageable steps and in prioritizing activities leading toward goal achievement
	♦ Assists patient/family member in setting definitive activity targets to achieve goals
	♦ Helps patient with methods to measure progress toward goals
	♦ Explains safety and comfort home care measures appropriate for procedure
	♦ Arranges for home health care and support in the community if indicated
	♦ Provides time for patient to ask questions and discuss concerns
		♦ Direct observation
		♦ Review of patient's medical record
		♦ Verification of communication with health care team members
		♦ Education
		Other: _____

	(I35) Evaluates environment for home care. Identifies needs after discharge by identifying those at risk and the presence of any physical barriers and potential hazards in the home and by collaborating with the patient, family members, and discharge coordinators about home care needs. ♦ Identifies patients who live alone ♦ Identifies patients who may not be able to independently perform activities of daily living ♦ Identifies patients who live in nursing homes or residential facilities ♦ Identifies homeless patients ♦ Identifies patients with special equipment needs ♦ Identifies patients with financial needs	♦ Direct observation ♦ Review of patient's medical record ♦ Verification of communication with health care team members ♦ Education Other: _____

Patient Outcome	PNDS Interventions as Measurable Criteria	Recommendations for Validation of Competency
	Domain 3A: BEHAVIORAL RESPONSES—KNOWLEDGE O18 – O22, O31 (continued)	
	Competency Statement: The perioperative registered nurse demonstrates knowledge about the psychologic, sociologic, and spiritual responses of patients and their families to the operative or other invasive procedure, including participation of patients in their recovery.	
(continued) **O21 The patient participates in the rehabilitation process.**	*(continued)* ♦ Identifies patients with transportation needs ♦ Identifies physical barriers in the home that may interfere with the patient's ability to care for self (eg, stairs, accessibility of bathroom, presence of safety rails in bathroom, potential safety hazards) ♦ Identifies potential safety hazards and risks for injury in the home	
	(I50) Evaluates response to instructions. Evaluates patient's/family member's understanding of instructions regarding perioperative experience and ongoing care. ♦ Observes patient demonstration of sequential progressive steps of the following appropriate skills: – Deep breathing, – Coughing and wound splinting, – Passive leg exercises, – Progression to ambulation, and – Wound and dressing care. ♦ Assesses the patient's and family members' management skills of: – Medication schedule – Activity limitations and exercise regimen; – Dietary restrictions or supplements; – Wound care; – Prescribed treatments; – Follow-up appointments, which may include signs and symptoms to report; and – Emergency protocols ♦ Observes return demonstrations of self-care instruction ♦ Provides patient/family member with written discharge and at-home instructions ♦ Reinforces information provided by other members of health care team ♦ Observes patient's responses to instructions ♦ Requests verbalization of instructions ♦ Clarifies information ♦ Encourages patient/family members to describe in their own words the anticipated physical and psychological effects of surgery, feelings regarding surgery, and expected outcomes ♦ Encourages patient/family members to communicate feelings regarding surgery and expected outcomes ♦ Requests patient/family members communicate understanding of preoperative instructions ♦ Provides time for patient/family members to ask questions ♦ Evaluates patient/family responses to perioperative instruction	♦ Direct observation ♦ Review of patient's medical record ♦ Verification of communication with health care team members ♦ Education Other: _____

Patient Outcome	PNDS Interventions as Measurable Criteria	Recommendations for Validation of Competency
\multicolumn{3}{c}{**Domain 3A: BEHAVIORAL RESPONSES—KNOWLEDGE O18 – O22, O31 (continued)**}		

<table>
<tr><td colspan="3">Domain 3A: BEHAVIORAL RESPONSES—KNOWLEDGE
O18 – O22, O31 (continued)

Competency Statement: The perioperative registered nurse demonstrates knowledge about the psychologic, sociologic, and spiritual responses of patients and their families to the operative or other invasive procedure, including participation of patients in their recovery.</td></tr>
<tr>
<td>O22 The patient demonstrates knowledge of wound management.</td>
<td>(I149) Assesses knowledge regarding wound care and phases of wound healing.
Determines knowledge level about wound care and wound healing process.
♦ Establishes/reviews preoperative assessment and risk for surgical site infection:
  – Wound classification,
  – Age,
  – Cardiovascular status,
  – Nutritional status,
  – Metabolic or systemic disease,
  – History of smoking, and
  – Other immune system disorders
♦ Verifies patient's ability to understand information
♦ Obtains interpreter if needed
♦ Provides necessary time to process information
♦ Identifies patient's cultural practices
♦ Individualizes postoperative wound care plan to accommodate patient's lifestyle</td>
<td>♦ Direct observation
♦ Review of patient's medical record
♦ Verification of communication with health care team members
♦ Education
Other: _____</td>
</tr>
<tr>
<td></td>
<td>(I105) Provides instruction about wound care and phases of wound healing.
Provides necessary information about the phases of wound healing, techniques of wound care, and signs and symptoms to report.
♦ Reviews preoperative nursing assessment data
♦ Reviews procedure for incision site care and dressing application
♦ Discusses phases of wound healing
♦ Discusses protocol for drain care as appropriate
♦ Discusses potential untoward changes in wound signs and symptoms to monitor/report
♦ Demonstrates prescribed procedure for wound care
♦ Encourages family/member participation in instruction process
♦ Provides written instruction</td>
<td>♦ Direct observation
♦ Review of patient's medical record
♦ Verification of communication with health care team members
♦ Education
Other: _____</td>
</tr>
<tr>
<td></td>
<td>(I49) Evaluates response to instruction about wound care and phases of wound healing.
Evaluates understanding of instruction about wound healing and wound care by listening to explanations and observing return demonstrations.
♦ Requests verbalization of procedure for incision site care
♦ Requests verbalization of procedure for dressing application
♦ Requests verbalization of wound progress through healing
♦ Requests verbalization of procedure for drain care as appropriate
♦ Requests verbalization of untoward changes in wound
♦ Encourages questions and offers clarification
♦ Encourages family/member participation in instruction process
♦ Observes return demonstration of incision care and dressing application if indicated.</td>
<td>♦ Direct observation
♦ Review of patient's medical record
♦ Verification of communication with health care team members
♦ Education
Other: _____</td>
</tr>
</table>

Patient Outcome	PNDS Interventions as Measurable Criteria	Recommendations for Validation of Competency
	Domain 3B: BEHAVIORAL RESPONSES—PATIENT AND FAMILY RIGHTS/ETHICS O23 – O28 *Competency Statement:* **The perioperative registered nurse supports patients' rights and ethics by delivering consistent, competent, and ethical care, within legal standards of practice, while maintaining privacy and support of the patient's value system.**	

O23 The patient participates in decision making affecting the perioperative plan of care.	**(I124) Verifies consent for planned procedure.** Determines that informed consent has been granted for planned operative or invasive procedure and any related activities (eg, photographs, investigational studies).
	◆ If consent is present:
	  – Establishes rapport;
	  – Identifies barriers to communication;
	  – Obtains interpreter if needed;
	  – Determines knowledge level;
	  – Identifies psychosocial status;
	  – Elicits perceptions of surgery;
	  – Verifies surgical procedure;
	  – Encourages questions by patient/family members;
	  – Answers patient's/family members' questions;
	  – Refers questions regarding surgical risks, benefits, alternatives, or adverse reactions to physician; and
	  – Ensures documents are filed in appropriate section of medical record.
	◆ If surgery is emergent:
	  – Attempts to establish rapport,
	  – Identifies barriers to communication,
	  – Obtains interpreter if needed,
	  – Determines availability of family members or legal guardian,
	  – Verifies procedure to be completed with physician,
	  – Delegates to another member of health care team notification of appropriate family members, and
	  – Obtains telephone consent from next-of-kin with witnesses listening to and documenting telephone consent
	◆ If consent is not present for alert and oriented patient:
	  – Establishes rapport,
	  – Identifies barriers to communication,
	  – Obtains interpreter if needed,
	  – Determines knowledge level,
	  – Identifies psychosocial status,
	  – Elicits perceptions of surgery,
	  – Verifies surgical procedure,
	  – Contacts surgeon to answer questions regarding surgical risks, benefits, alternatives, or adverse reactions;
	  – Completes consent forms per facility policy and procedure;
	  – Witnesses patient's parent's family member's signature on consent form;
	  – Answers patient's/parent's/family member's questions as appropriate; and
	  – Files documents in appropriate section of medical record.
		◆ Direct observation
		◆ Review of patient's medical record
		◆ Verification of communication with health care team members
		◆ Education
		Other: _____

Patient Outcome	PNDS Interventions as Measurable Criteria	Recommendations for Validation of Competency
	**Domain 3B: BEHAVIORAL RESPONSES—PATIENT AND FAMILY RIGHTS/ETHICS O23 – O28 (*continued*)** *Competency Statement:* The perioperative registered nurse supports patients' rights and ethics by delivering consistent, competent, and ethical care, within legal standards of practice, while maintaining privacy and support of the patient's value system.		

(continued)
O23 The patient participates in decision making affecting the perioperative plan of care.
	(continued)
	♦ If the patient is incompetent:
	  – Attempts to establish rapport
	  – Identifies barriers to communication
	  – Determines knowledge level
	  – Identifies psychosocial status
	  – Attempts to elicit patient's perceptions of surgery
	  – Attempts to verify surgical procedure
	  – Completes consent forms per facility policy and procedure
	  – Witnesses next-of-kin signature on consent form or verifies legal guardianship documents are present and completed
	  – Encourages questions by next-of-kin/legal guardian
	  – Determines that person present is individual identified on consent	

	(I63) Identifies individual values and wishes concerning care. Assesses values, beliefs, and preferences and include in plan of care. ♦ Identifies barriers to communication ♦ Determines knowledge level ♦ Verifies patient's ability to understand information ♦ Provides sufficient time to process the information ♦ Appears relaxed and unhurried in interactions with patient ♦ Identifies influences of beliefs and values ♦ Uses interpreter/family member in a manner that is sensitive to cultural values ♦ Obtains information regarding current philosophical, cultural, and spiritual beliefs and values towards health and health practices. ♦ Recognizes patient's philosophical, cultural, and spiritual beliefs and values and their influences on health and health practices ♦ Encourages family member participation in discussions as appropriate ♦ Encourages family member to remain in attendance preoperatively and postoperatively ♦ Provides culturally sensitive nursing care	♦ Direct observation ♦ Review of patient's medical record ♦ Verification of communication with health care team members ♦ Education Other: _____
	(I79) Includes family members in preoperative teaching. Identifies family member's knowledge and provides education and support. ♦ Establishes rapport with patient/family members ♦ Identifies self and role as perioperative registered nurse ♦ Identifies barriers to communication ♦ Determines knowledge level ♦ Assesses coping mechanisms ♦ Assesses readiness to learn ♦ Encourages verbalization of questions ♦ Encourages verbalization of feelings and expectations ♦ Communicates potential treatment options/choices in perioperative plan (RNFA) ♦ Requests family members verbalize understanding of and return demonstration of preoperative instruction	♦ Direct observation ♦ Review of patient's medical record ♦ Verification of communication with health care team members ♦ Education ♦ Other: _____

Patient Outcome	PNDS Interventions as Measurable Criteria	Recommendations for Validation of Competency
	**Domain 3B: BEHAVIORAL RESPONSES—PATIENT AND FAMILY RIGHTS/ETHICS O23 – O28 (*continued*)**	

Domain 3B: BEHAVIORAL RESPONSES—PATIENT AND FAMILY RIGHTS/ETHICS O23 – O28 (*continued*)

Competency Statement: The perioperative registered nurse supports patients' rights and ethics by delivering consistent, competent, and ethical care, within legal standards of practice, while maintaining privacy and support of the patient's value system.

Patient Outcome	PNDS Interventions as Measurable Criteria	Recommendations for Validation of Competency
(continued) O23 The patient participates in decision making affecting the perioperative plan of care.	**(I80) Includes patient and family members in discharge planning.** Reviews with patient/family members the patient's capabilities, anticipated plan of care, and resources available to facilitate the rehabilitation process. ◆ Identifies availability of family member and encourages their involvement in care ◆ Assesses physical, emotional, and educational resources of family member ◆ Assists family member to understand patient's condition ◆ Provides information to family members in accordance with the patient's preferences ◆ Encourages patient and family members to participate in rehabilitative process ◆ Assesses patient's capabilities, strengths, and limitations ◆ Assesses family members' capabilities, strengths, limitations, perception of situation, and understanding about patient's recovery from surgery ◆ Identifies family member's expectations for patient ◆ Determines patient's level of dependency on family members, considering age and health status ◆ Identifies realistic outcomes ◆ Provides support to patient/family members ◆ Evaluates response to discharge planning	◆ Direct observation ◆ Review of patient's medical record ◆ Verification of communication with health care team members ◆ Education Other: _____
	(I103) Provides information and explains Patient Self-Determination Act. Assesses current knowledge of the Patient Self-Determination Act (eg, the living will, power of attorney for health care, do not resuscitate, informed consent, organ procurement) and provides copy of resources/referral related to the Patient Self-Determination Act. ◆ Verifies presence of advance directive documents in current medical records. If documents are present: – Establishes rapport – Identifies barriers to communication – Obtains interpreter if needed – Determines knowledge level – Identifies psychosocial status – Inquires if patient has considered or desires any changes to current advance directive document – Reassures patient no discrimination in provision of care will occur based on whether patient has provided an advance directive.	◆ Direct observation ◆ Review of patient's medical record ◆ Verification of communication with health care team members ◆ Education Other: _____

Patient Outcome	PNDS Interventions as Measurable Criteria	Recommendations for Validation of Competency

Domain 3B: BEHAVIORAL RESPONSES—PATIENT AND FAMILY RIGHTS/ETHICS O23 – O28 (*continued*)

Competency Statement: **The perioperative registered nurse supports patients' rights and ethics by delivering consistent, competent, and ethical care, within legal standards of practice, while maintaining privacy and support of the patient's value system.**

Patient Outcome	PNDS Interventions as Measurable Criteria	Recommendations for Validation of Competency
(continued) **O23 The patient participates in decision making affecting the perioperative plan of care.**	*(continued)* – Encourages questions regarding the Patient Self-Determination Act – Clarifies information or misinterpretations as requested – Seeks consultation with designated facility resource person for those patients requesting assistance in completion of advance directive documents – Completes proper placement of documentation/forms in patient's records as designated by facility policy and procedure ♦ If documents are not present: – Establishes rapport; – Identifies barriers to communication; – Determines knowledge level; – Identifies psychosocial status; – Verifies patient has received written information regarding Patient Self-Determination Act; – Encourages questions regarding Patient Self-Determination Act; – Clarifies information as requested; – Reassures patient no discrimination in provision of care will occur based on whether patient has provided an advance directive; – Offers assistance in the completion of the documents per facility policy and procedure; – Seeks consultation with designated resource person within facility as requested by patient; – Places documentation/forms in patient's records as designated by facility policy and procedure; and – Evaluates patient's knowledge of the Patient Self-Determination Act.	
O24 The patient's care is consistent with the perioperative plan of care.	**(I30) Develops individualized plan of care.** Considers all assessment information including patient's preferences and unique needs when developing an individualized nursing care plan. ♦ Introduces self and explains role ♦ Establishes/reviews nursing assessment data, preferences individual values, and cultural patterns ♦ Organizes information into concise problem statements/nursing diagnoses ♦ Identifies goals clearly as statements of outcome and congruent with patient's wishes and health status	♦ Direct observation ♦ Review of patient's medical record ♦ Verification of communication with health care team members ♦ Education Other: _____

Patient Outcome	PNDS Interventions as Measurable Criteria	Recommendations for Validation of Competency
	Domain 3B: BEHAVIORAL RESPONSES—PATIENT AND FAMILY RIGHTS/ETHICS O23 – O28 (*continued*) *Competency Statement:* The perioperative registered nurse supports patients' rights and ethics by delivering consistent, competent, and ethical care, within legal standards of practice, while maintaining privacy and support of the patient's value system.	
(continued) **O24 The patient's care is consistent with the periopera-tive plan of care.**	*(continued)* ♦ Provides opportunity for mutual goal setting with patient, family member, and members of health care team as appropriate ♦ Identifies measurable outcome indicators related to goal attainment ♦ Identifies actions to achieve outcomes ♦ Prioritizes nursing actions ♦ Compares individualized plan with standards of care ♦ Reviews plan of care with patient and revises as necessary ♦ Evaluates patient's participation in plan of care ♦ Communicates and coordinates patient's needs ♦ Makes patient care assignments ♦ Identifies and prepares for potential emergency situations ♦ Prepares to implement perioperative plan ♦ Plans for patient's discharge	
	(I92) Obtains consultation from appropriate health care provider to initiate new treatments or change existing treatment. Involves and/or consults other members of the health care team if the patient's condition or planned procedure changes. ♦ Validates nursing assessment completed preoperatively ♦ Continually reassesses physiological parameters as applicable ♦ Reports variances from norm to appropriate members of health care team ♦ Revises treatment regimen at direction of appropriate members of health care team ♦ Monitors emerging treatment modalities potentially appli-cable to perioperative environment ♦ Evaluates new products to determine risk/benefit for patient/facility ♦ Initiates new treatment regimen at the direction of appro-priate members of health care team ♦ Evaluates response to new treatment or change in existing therapy ♦ Documents operative procedure and postoperative orders according to practice guidelines and within institutional policy (RNFA) ♦ Makes postoperative visits to evaluate recovery progress	♦ Direct observation ♦ Review of patient's med-ical record ♦ Verification of communi-cation with health care team members ♦ Education Other: _____

Patient Outcome	PNDS Interventions as Measurable Criteria	Recommendations for Validation of Competency
	**Domain 3B: BEHAVIORAL RESPONSES—PATIENT AND FAMILY RIGHTS/ETHICS O23 – O28 (*continued*)** *Competency Statement:* The perioperative registered nurse supports patients' rights and ethics by delivering consistent, competent, and ethical care, within legal standards of practice, while maintaining privacy and support of the patient's value system.	
(continued) **O24 The patient's care is consistent with the perioperative plan of care.**	**(I119) Uses a clinical pathway.** Actions performed are consistent with predetermined clinical pathway. ♦ Identifies clinical pathway which best correlates with planned procedure and individualized care ♦ Shares clinical pathway with all members of the perioperative team ♦ Implements actions according to prescribed pathway ♦ Evaluates outcomes of actions taken ♦ Recognizes variances from prescribed plan ♦ Modifies actions based on evaluation	♦ Direct observation ♦ Review of patient's medical record ♦ Verification of communication with health care team members ♦ Education Other: _____
	(I27) Ensures continuity of care. Provides for a continuum of care throughout the perioperative phases of care. ♦ Reviews medical records for history and physical and nursing assessment ♦ Identifies barriers to communication ♦ Determines knowledge level ♦ Verifies patient's ability to understand information ♦ Obtains interpreter as appropriate ♦ Validates completed nursing assessment or completes nursing assessment ♦ Identifies potential risk factors ♦ Identifies plan of care to met individual patient needs ♦ Includes patient and family members in establishment of plan of care ♦ Shares plan of care with other members of health care team if appropriate ♦ Implements perioperative plan of nursing care ♦ Monitors patient status throughout the perioperative experience ♦ Reports any variances from norm to appropriate members of health care team ♦ Performs actions or treatments as prescribed ♦ Prioritizes actions based on patient's needs ♦ Evaluates patient's responses to actions and treatments ♦ Evaluates patient's responses to the plan of care ♦ Shares evaluation of plan with appropriate members of the health care team.	♦ Direct observation ♦ Review of patient's medical record ♦ Verification of communication with health care team members ♦ Education Other: _____

Patient Outcome	PNDS Interventions as Measurable Criteria	Recommendations for Validation of Competency
— **Domain 3B: BEHAVIORAL RESPONSES—PATIENT AND FAMILY RIGHTS/ETHICS O23 – O28 (*continued*)**		

Domain 3B: BEHAVIORAL RESPONSES—PATIENT AND FAMILY RIGHTS/ETHICS O23 – O28 (*continued*)

Competency Statement: The perioperative registered nurse supports patients' rights and ethics by delivering consistent, competent, and ethical care, within legal standards of practice, while maintaining privacy and support of the patient's value system.

Patient Outcome	PNDS Interventions as Measurable Criteria	Recommendations for Validation of Competency
O25 The patient's right to privacy is maintained.	**(I81) Initiates traffic control.** Restricts access to patient care area to authorized individuals. ♦ Keeps doors to OR or procedure rooms closed except during movement of patients, personnel, supplies, and equipment ♦ Restricts access to surgical suite to authorized personnel only ♦ Records names of all individuals who participate in surgical procedure	♦ Direct observation ♦ Review of patient's medical record ♦ Education Other: _____
	(I115) Secures patient's records, belongings, and valuables. Protects patient's clinical records and personal property. Releases belongings and valuables to patient or designated individual. ♦ Verifies presence of patient records, belongings, and valuables in secured area ♦ Encourages family member to keep valuables following facility policy, procedure, or protocol ♦ Explains clinical processes to patient/family member ♦ Encourages questions regarding processes ♦ Completes record of disposition of belongings and valuables following facility policy, procedure, or protocol	♦ Direct observation ♦ Review of patient's medical record ♦ Education Other: _____
	(I150) Maintains patient's dignity and privacy. Protects the patient's privacy (eg, keeps OR doors closed, only exposes body as needed for care). Treats the deceased with respect and provides privacy area for family viewing the deceased. ♦ Reviews patient record ♦ Obtains interpreter if needed ♦ Obtains information regarding current philosophical, cultural, and spiritual beliefs and values towards health and health practices ♦ Recognizes patient's philosophical, cultural, and spiritual beliefs and effect on perioperative plan ♦ Responds to patient's questions honestly and in terms the patient can readily understand ♦ Protects patient's privacy by keeping doors closed and only exposing patient's body as needed to provide care ♦ Advocates for respectful conversation during procedure ♦ Provides cover, warmth, and comfort. ♦ Provides and maintains respect for deceased ♦ Provides a protected area for viewing deceased ♦ Evaluates patient's comfort level	♦ Direct observation ♦ Review of patient's medical record ♦ Verification of communication with health care team members ♦ Education Other: _____

Patient Outcome	PNDS Interventions as Measurable Criteria	Recommendations for Validation of Competency
\<td colspan="3" align="center"\>**Domain 3B: BEHAVIORAL RESPONSES—PATIENT AND FAMILY RIGHTS/ETHICS O23 – O28** (*continued*)\<br\>\<br\>*Competency Statement:* The perioperative registered nurse supports patients' rights and ethics by delivering consistent, competent, and ethical care, within legal standards of practice, while maintaining privacy and support of the patient's value system.\</td\>		

(continued)
O25 The patient's right to privacy is maintained.
	(I151) Maintains patient confidentiality.
	Limits access of patient information to appropriate members of health care team.
	♦ Maintains patient's record following facility policy, procedure or protocol
	♦ Obtains consent before engaging in direct patient care activities
	♦ Limits discussion of patient information to:
	  – Appropriate members of the health care team; and
	  – Appropriate areas of facility.
	♦ Restricts access to patient care areas to authorized individuals
	♦ Does not display patient's name with surgical procedure in unrestricted area
	♦ Protects electronic data
	♦ Assures human subjects protection for patients enrolled as research subjects
	♦ Obtains consent before transferring or sharing information to other providers and/or third parties
		♦ Direct observation
		♦ Review of patient's medical record
		♦ Education
		Other: _____

O26 The patient is the recipient of competent and ethical care within the legal standards of practice.	**(I102) Provides care without prejudicial behavior.** Applies standards of nursing practice consistently and without bias (eg, disability, economic background, education, culture, religion, race, age, and gender). ♦ Recognizes personal biases ♦ Identifies barriers to communication ♦ Determines knowledge level ♦ Verifies patient's ability to understand information ♦ Appears relaxed and unhurried in interactions with patient ♦ Provides culturally sensitive nursing care ♦ Obtains interpreter if needed ♦ Offers therapeutic communication techniques such as touch, active listening, and empathy ♦ Maintains the patient's privacy and dignity ♦ Offers comparable care to all patients in all settings ♦ Encourages family member participation in discussions and care processes	♦ Direct observation ♦ Review of patient's medical record ♦ Education Other: _____
	(I100) Provides care respecting worth and dignity regardless of diagnosis, disease process, procedure, or projected outcome. Provides for spiritual comfort, arranges for substitute nursing care when personal values conflict with required care, and respects patient's decision for surgery. ♦ Verifies presence of barriers to communication ♦ Listens to patient and encourages communication ♦ Identifies cultural and spiritual beliefs and values	♦ Direct observation ♦ Review of patient's medical record ♦ Education Other: _____

Patient Outcome	PNDS Interventions as Measurable Criteria	Recommendations for Validation of Competency
	Domain 3B: BEHAVIORAL RESPONSES—PATIENT AND FAMILY RIGHTS/ETHICS O23 – O28 (*continued*) *Competency Statement:* **The perioperative registered nurse supports patients' rights and ethics by delivering consistent, competent, and ethical care, within legal standards of practice, while maintaining privacy and support of the patient's value system.**	
(continued) **O26 The patient is the recipient of competent and ethical care within the legal standards of practice.**	*(continued)* ♦ Provides an environment that facilitates understanding ♦ Obtains interpreter as appropriate ♦ Demonstrates consistency in delivery of care to all patients ♦ Fosters patient/family member participation in development and implementation of care plan ♦ Maintains confidentiality of patient information ♦ Provides privacy through physical protection ♦ Evaluates patient's responses	♦ Direct observation ♦ Review of patient's medical record ♦ Education Other: _____
	(I116) Shares patient information only with those directly involved in care. Protects patient information by completing operative record accurately and shares information in a manner that ensures patient confidentiality. ♦ Maintains patient confidentiality ♦ Discusses patient information only with members of health care team who need the information ♦ Refrains from discussing patients in public areas ♦ Obtains patient consent before initiating direct care activities ♦ Protects patient information ♦ Completes records accurately and objectively ♦ Honors patient's request to withhold information from family member ♦ Releases patient information only to properly identified individuals and in compliance with established policies, mandates, or protocols	♦ Direct observation ♦ Review of patient's medical record ♦ Education Other: _____

	(I1) Acts as a patient advocate by protecting the patient from incompetent, unethical, or illegal practices.
	Respects the "Patient's Bill of Rights," complies with facility policies of competent performance; complies with federal regulations (eg, Occupational Safety and Health Administration), state nurse practice acts, accrediting agencies (eg, Joint Commission); adheres to professional standards of practice (eg, AORN); and confirms clinician's privileges and credentials. Intervenes to protect the patient's safety.
	♦ Demonstrates competency to function in a professional role as a registered professional nurse in the OR as evidenced by the following:
	  – Demonstrates competence to assess patient's physiological health status.
	  – Demonstrates competence to assess the psychosocial health status of the patient/family/significant other.
		♦ Direct observation
		♦ Review of patient's medical record
		♦ Education
		Other: _____

Patient Outcome	PNDS Interventions as Measurable Criteria	Recommendations for Validation of Competency
\multicolumn{3}{c}{**Domain 3B: BEHAVIORAL RESPONSES—PATIENT AND FAMILY RIGHTS/ETHICS O23 – O28 (continued)**}

Domain 3B: BEHAVIORAL RESPONSES—PATIENT AND FAMILY RIGHTS/ETHICS O23 – O28 (continued)

Competency Statement: The perioperative registered nurse supports patients' rights and ethics by delivering consistent, competent, and ethical care, within legal standards of practice, while maintaining privacy and support of the patient's value system.

Patient Outcome	PNDS Interventions as Measurable Criteria	Recommendations for Validation of Competency
(continued) **O26 The patient is the recipient of competent and ethical care within the legal standards of practice.**	*(continued)* – Demonstrates competence to formulate nursing diagnosis based on health status data. – Demonstrates competence to establish patient goals based on nursing diagnosis. – Demonstrates competence to implement nursing actions according to prescribed plan. – Demonstrates competence to participate in patient/family members teaching. – Demonstrates competence to create and maintain multiple sterile fields. – Demonstrates competence to provide equipment and supplies based on patient needs. – Demonstrates extensive knowledge of anatomy and physiology. (RNFA) – Demonstrates competence to perform sponge, sharps, and instrument counts. – Demonstrates competence to administer medications and solutions as prescribed. – Demonstrates competence to physiologically monitor patient during surgery. – Demonstrates competence to act in emergency situations – Demonstrates competence to monitor and control the environment. – Demonstrates competence to respect patient rights. – Demonstrates competence to perform nursing actions that demonstrate accountability. – Demonstrates competence to evaluate patient outcomes. – Demonstrates competence to measure effectiveness of nursing care. – Demonstrates competence to continuously modify plan of care based on new data. ♦ Functions within scope of nursing practice in accordance with state nurse practice act ♦ Delegates duties only to competent appropriate personnel	
O27 The patient receives consistent and comparable levels of care from all caregivers regardless of the situation or setting.	**(I99) Provides care in a nondiscriminatory, nonprejudicial manner regardless of the setting in which care is given.** Adheres to AORN, Joint Commission, and other standards of care. Provides comparable levels of care regardless of the setting in which care is given (eg, inpatient, outpatient, public, private, home, emergency department). ♦ Identifies barriers to communication ♦ Determines knowledge level ♦ Verifies patient's ability to understand information	♦ Direct observation ♦ Review of patient's medical record ♦ Verification of communication with health care team members ♦ Education Other: _____

Patient Outcome	PNDS Interventions as Measurable Criteria	Recommendations for Validation of Competency
	Domain 3B: BEHAVIORAL RESPONSES—PATIENT AND FAMILY RIGHTS/ETHICS O23 – O28 (continued)	
	Competency Statement: The perioperative registered nurse supports patients' rights and ethics by delivering consistent, competent, and ethical care, within legal standards of practice, while maintaining privacy and support of the patient's value system.	
(continued) **O27 The patient receives consistent and comparable levels of care from all caregivers regardless of the situation or setting.**	*(continued)* ♦ Appears relaxed and unhurried in interactions with patient ♦ Obtains interpreter as appropriate ♦ Offers therapeutic communication techniques such as touch, active listening, and empathy ♦ Offers explanation of each action ♦ Maintains the patient's privacy and dignity ♦ Offers comparable care to all patients in all settings ♦ Encourages family member participation in discussions and care processes	
	(I97) Preserves and protects the patient's autonomy, dignity, and human rights. Confirms consent, implements facility advance directive policy, and supports patient's participation in decision making. ♦ Establishes rapport ♦ Identifies barriers to communication ♦ Determines knowledge level ♦ Verifies patient's ability to understand new information ♦ Appears unhurried ♦ Identifies values and beliefs ♦ Provides care in a nonjudgmental manner ♦ Offers therapeutic communication techniques such as touch, active listening, and empathy ♦ Offers explanation of each action ♦ Encourages family member participation in discussions and care processes ♦ Evaluates patient's response to care provided ♦ Provides culturally sensitive nursing care ♦ Obtains interpreter as appropriate ♦ Verifies patient's understanding of American Hospital Association's "Bill of Rights" and do not resuscitate (DNR) orders ♦ Provides information as needed ♦ Includes family members in teaching and decision making according to patient preference ♦ Ensures communication of patient's decisions and preferences to members of health care team ♦ Provides privacy ♦ Maintains confidentiality	♦ Direct observation ♦ Review of patient's medical record ♦ Verification of communication with health care team members ♦ Education Other: _____

Patient Outcome	PNDS Interventions as Measurable Criteria	Recommendations for Validation of Competency
\multicolumn{3}{}		

Patient Outcome	PNDS Interventions as Measurable Criteria	Recommendations for Validation of Competency
Domain 3B: BEHAVIORAL RESPONSES—PATIENT AND FAMILY RIGHTS/ETHICS O23 – O28 (*continued*) *Competency Statement:* **The perioperative registered nurse supports patients' rights and ethics by delivering consistent, competent, and ethical care, within legal standards of practice, while maintaining privacy and support of the patient's value system.**		
(continued) **O27 The patient receives consistent and comparable levels of care from all caregivers regardless of the situation or setting.**	**(I102) Provides care without prejudicial behavior.** Applies standards of nursing practice consistently and without bias (eg, disability, economic background, education, culture, religion, race, age and gender). ♦ Identifies barriers to communication ♦ Determines knowledge level ♦ Verifies patient's ability to understand information ♦ Appears relaxed and unhurried in interactions with patient ♦ Provides culturally sensitive nursing care ♦ Obtains interpreter as appropriate ♦ Offers therapeutic communication techniques such as touch, active listening, and empathy to allay patient's anxiety ♦ Maintains patient's privacy and dignity ♦ Offers comparable care to all patients in all settings ♦ Encourages family member participation in discussions and care processes	♦ Direct observation ♦ Review of patient's medical record ♦ Education Other: _____
O28 The patient's value system, lifestyle, ethnicity and culture are considered, respected and incorporated in the perioperative plan of care as appropriate	**(I57) Identifies and reports philosophical, cultural, and spiritual beliefs and values.** Assesses philosophical, cultural, and spiritual factors valued by the patient. Incorporates pertinent information in the plan of care and reports to other members of health care team as appropriate. ♦ Identifies barriers to communication ♦ Determines knowledge level ♦ Verifies patient's ability to understand information ♦ Provides sufficient time for patient to process the information ♦ Appears relaxed and unhurried in interactions with patient ♦ Provides culturally sensitive nursing care ♦ Validates current beliefs and values ♦ Obtains interpreter as appropriate ♦ Obtains information regarding philosophical, cultural, and spiritual beliefs and values towards health and health practices ♦ Recognizes varying philosophical, cultural, and spiritual practices and beliefs and their effects on health and health practices ♦ Encourages family members' participation in discussions as appropriate ♦ Encourages family members to remain in perioperative area while patient is receiving care ♦ Assesses influence of cultural and spiritual practices that may affect individual behavior and incorporates them in plan of care ♦ Integrates value system/cultural beliefs into plan of care	♦ Direct observation ♦ Review of patient's medical record ♦ Verification of communication with health care team members ♦ Education Other: _____

94

Patient Outcome	PNDS Interventions as Measurable Criteria	Recommendations for Validation of Competency
	Domain 4: HEALTH SYSTEM OUTCOMES	
	Competency Statement: **The perioperative nurse demonstrates knowledge of the health system environment and administrative issues that impact job performance, patient safety, and ethical considerations.**	
	The perioperative nurse should demonstrate knowledge and competence in the following areas: *Professional* ♦ Maintains current licensure ♦ Maintains certifications as required ♦ Completes continuing education as required ♦ Acknowledges career advancement opportunities ♦ Acknowledges scope of practice ♦ Demonstrates critical thinking skills ♦ Participates in research and evidence based practice *Regulatory* ♦ Demonstrates understanding of regulatory issues ♦ Follows employee safety policies and procedures ♦ Identifies employee rights and obligations ♦ Participates in disaster planning ♦ Demonstrates awareness of environmental issues ♦ Follows fire safety policies and procedures *Organizational* ♦ Follows organizational code of conduct ♦ Participates in committees ♦ Demonstrates good communication skills, including conflict resolution ♦ Demonstrates awareness of legal and ethical issues ♦ Understands organizational structure and lines of authority ♦ Participates in performance improvement activities ♦ Describes team roles ♦ Demonstrates knowledge of medical terminology ♦ Understands and follows vendor policies and procedures ♦ Demonstrates fiscal responsibility	♦ Direct observation ♦ Review of patient's medical record ♦ Verification of communication with health care team members ♦ Successful completion of annual safety skills ♦ Education Other: _____

Originally published 1982, revised 1986; revised 1992. Revised and reformatted in 2005.

Perioperative Advanced Practice Nurse Competency Statements

I n 1994, the Nursing Practices Committee completed the first version of the perioperative advanced practice nurse (APN) competency statements.[1] The five statements were derived from the model of expert practice by Patricia E. Benner, RN, PhD, FAAN;[2] the competency of clinical nurse specialists by Mary V. Fenton, RN, DrPH;[3] and the model of advanced nursing practice by Joy D. Calkin, RN, PhD.[4] The committee also used the National Organization of Nurse Practitioner Faculties curriculum guidelines when defining the measurable criteria for the perioperative APN competency statements.[5] A sampling of activities a perioperative APN might perform in the role was presented.

The Validation Study

The Nursing Research Committee conducted a validation study in 1994 using purposive sampling of 62 AORN members who had expanded practice skills (ie, clinical nurse specialists, nurse practitioners/RN first assistants) or knowledge of advanced practice.[1] The competency statements were mailed with instructions to indicate

- whether the statement and measurable criteria were appropriate and clearly stated, and
- the extent to which the activities listed were important to advanced perioperative practice (1=not at all important, 4=very important).

Respondents confirmed their expert status (ie, 91% had earned master's or doctoral degrees; 92% had more than 10 years of perioperative experience). Approximately two-thirds (ie, 68%) of the respondents listed their job title as clinical nurse specialist.

Results. The opinion of the responding experts was that the statements were appropriate and the activities were significant. The most frequent comment was that the activities were too basic for the expected role of the advanced practitioner.

The first revision. The Nursing Practices Committee revised the document based on the validation study results and comments from respondents. A specific effort was made to elevate the level of performance expectation and to clarify statements considered vague or confusing. The Nursing Practices Committee believes the following competencies will need to be revisited as the role of the perioperative APN evolves.

The second revision. In 2005, the Advanced Practice Issues Task Force was charged to review and revise the APN competency statements. They integrated the competency statements from the 1995 "Perioperative advanced practice nurse competency statements"[6] and the Perioperative Nursing Data Set (PNDS).[7] The task force also conducted a literature review and adapted competency statements shared by other advanced practice nurse organizations. The task force used the PNDS framework to organize the competency statements. The competency statements were divided into four domains:

- **Domain 1:** Safety,
- **Domain 2:** Physiologic Outcomes,
- **Domain 3A:** Behavioral Responses,
- **Domain 3B:** Behavioral Responses—Patient and Family Rights/Ethics, and
- **Domain 4:** Health System (Organizational) Outcomes.

Portions of the Hamric model were used to organize the competencies in Domain 4.[8]

Content validity for the 2005 APN competency statements was established through an extensive literature review, input from the Advanced Practice Issues Task Force, and expert reviewers from the APN Specialty Assembly, Nursing Practices Committee, National Committee on Education, and additional APN experts identified by the task force. All Advanced Practice Issues Task Force members hold advanced nursing degrees; the task force consisted of clinical nurse specialists and nurse practitioners. Members of the task force possess extensive and varied perioperative nursing experience, including hospital, ambulatory surgery, academic, and perioperative nursing and health care consultation in the United States and abroad.

The task force collaborated with PNDS experts and research consultants during the development of the competency statements. The subjects identified for the literature review included APN competencies, clinical nurse specialist competencies, nurse practitioner (NP) competencies, documents from the American Nurses Association on APN competencies, and subspecialty organizations (eg, pediatric NP, family NP, geriatric NP, American Association of Critical-Care Nurses, American Association of Clinical Nurse Specialists). The task force reviewed 74 documents and three chapters in APN textbooks and extensively utilized the PNDS manual. The document cites 24 documents as footnotes and 22 other documents as resources. The total number of expert reviewers was 54, which consisted of

♦ identified APNs currently practicing in a variety of settings, including university and community hospitals, ambulatory surgery centers, and several perioperative subspecialties (eg, orthopedics, neurosurgery, cardiovascular surgery);

♦ APN Specialty Assembly members;

♦ Nursing Practices Committee (these members are appointed by the President-elect based on their perioperative clinical expertise);

♦ National Committee on Education (these members are appointed by the President-elect based on their knowledge of perioperative education); and

♦ PNDS experts.

The Advanced Practice Issues Task Force asked the experts to review the competency statements and provide feedback. There were minor changes recommended to add clarity to several items listed in the "Recommendations for Validation of Competency" column. No major content changes were recommended.

The document was designed so the reader can examine one measurable criteria and view the corresponding recommendations for validation without looking at the entire document.

The competency statements are not exhaustive, nor is the perioperative APN required to implement all activities. The statements are intended for use in a variety of settings, and perioperative APNs may adapt the use of these statements to individual practice settings and patient populations. Individuals in each practice setting are encouraged to develop more detailed tools to measure the desired "Recommendations for Validation."

NOTES

1. Nursing Research Committee, *Validation Study* (Denver: AORN, Inc, 1994) unpublished.

2. P Benner, *From Novice to Expert: Excellence and Power in Clinical Nursing Practice* (Menlo Park, Calif: Addison-Wesley Publishing Co, 1984).

3. M V Fenton, "Identifying competencies of clinical nurse specialists," *Journal of Nursing Administration* 15 (December 1985) 31-37.

4. J D Calkin, "A model for advanced nursing practice," *Journal of Nursing Administration* 14 (January 1984) 24-30.

5. National Organization of Nurse Practitioner Faculties, *Advanced Nursing Practice: Nurse Practitioner Curriculum Guidelines* (Washington, DC: National Organization of Nurse Practitioner Faculties, 1990).

6. "Perioperative advanced practice nurse competency statements," in *Standards and Recommended Practices* (Denver: AORN, Inc, 1995), 87-92.

7. S Beyea, *Perioperative Nursing Data Set: The Perioperative Nursing Vocabulary,* second ed (Denver: AORN, Inc, 2002).

8. A B Hamric, "A definition of advanced practice nursing," in *Advanced Practice Nursing: An Integrative Approach,* third ed, A B Hamric, J A Spross, C M Hanson, eds (St Louis: Saunders, 2005) 85-108.

The 2005 competency statements were approved by the AORN Board of Directors in November 2005 and are the work of the Advanced Practice Issues Task Force. Task force members are listed below.

Advanced Practice Issues Task Force 2005–2006
Barbara J. Gruendemann, RN, MS, CNOR, FAAN
Juliana J. Mower, RN, MSN, CNS, CNOR
Jeannemarie Hennessey, RN, MS, CNS, CNOR
Naomi F. Teperow, RN, MS, CNOR, CRNFA, ACNP
Stephanie C. Reitman-Swiss, ARNP, CNOR, JD
Teresa A. Watson, MSN, ARNP, BC

Committee Chair
Jacklyn J. Schuchardt, RN, MSN, CNOR, CNS

Board Liaison
Richard G. Cuming, RN, MSN, CNOR, CPAN

Staff Consultant
Debra T. Moore, ARNP, MSN, CNOR

Perioperative Advanced Practice Nurse Competency

The perioperative advanced practice registered nurse (APN) is a clinical expert in the management of individual and groups of surgical patients. The APN anchors nursing practice to evidence-based science to achieve patient-sensitive outcomes. Multidisciplinary collaboration to effect positive changes in surgical patient care is a hallmark of this specialized role. The APN consults, teaches, mentors, and role-models desirable behaviors and evaluates the results of nursing interventions on patients. The APN meets established criteria and manages resources to attain high quality, cost-effective care. Productive collegial relationships, acute assessment of organizational culture, and exemplary leadership skills are essential for successful APN practice in the organization. The APN possesses a wealth of knowledge concerning applicable standards, guidelines, and regulations and uses this knowledge to analyze, direct, and facilitate the preoperative, intraoperative, and postoperative phases of superior surgical patient care.

To function in this role, the APN must possess a master's degree in nursing concentrated in a recognized area of advanced clinical nursing practice (ie, nurse practitioner [NP], clinical nurse specialist [CNS], certified registered nurse anesthetist [CRNA], or certified nurse-midwife [CNM]) and must have met state regulations that govern APN practice. Certification is highly recommended.

Patient Outcome	PNDS Interventions as Measurable Criteria	Recommendations for Validation of Competency
Domain 1: SAFETY		
Competency Statement: **Protective measures developed, instituted, and monitored by perioperative APNs reduce and prevent injury to individual surgical patients and groups of patients and thus help to assure patient safety.**		
Individuals and groups of patients are free from injuries due to extraneous objects, chemical products, electrical current, positioning, lasers, radiation, transfer/transport, allergic responses, and medication administration.[1]	**Clinical expertise/autonomy of practice** ♦ Assesses signs and symptoms of injury to individuals or groups of patients.[2]	♦ Portfolio of quality improvement/performance improvement (QI/PI) activities ♦ Portfolio of educational projects ♦ Measured observation ♦ Written material (eg, tests, checklists) ♦ Peer review ♦ Committee participation/ leadership (eg, policy and procedure, safety, disaster preparedness, bioterrorism, purchasing, surgical infection prevention [SIP], infection control, PI ♦ Documentation review Other:_____

Patient Outcome	PNDS Interventions as Measurable Criteria	Recommendations for Validation of Competency
	Domain 1: SAFETY *(continued)*	
	Competency Statement: **Protective measures developed, instituted, and monitored by perioperative APNs reduce and prevent injury to individual surgical patients and groups of patients and thus help to assure patient safety.**	
	◆ Evaluates protective measures to prevent injury to individuals and groups at risk.[3]	◆ Portfolio of QI/PI activities ◆ Portfolio of educational projects ◆ Measured observation ◆ Written material (eg, tests, checklists) ◆ Peer review ◆ Committee participation/ leadership (eg, policy and procedure, safety, disaster preparedness, bioterrorism, purchasing, SIP, infection control, PI) Other _____
	◆ Incorporates current evidence-based practice, specialty, and community standards in plan of care.[4]	◆ Portfolio of QI/PI activities ◆ Portfolio of educational projects ◆ Measured observation ◆ Written material (eg, tests, checklists) ◆ Peer review ◆ Committee participation/ leadership (eg, policy and procedure, safety, disaster preparedness, bioterrorism, purchasing, SIP, infection control, PI) Other: _____

Patient Outcome	PNDS Interventions as Measurable Criteria	Recommendations for Validation of Competency
	Domain 1: SAFETY *(continued)*	
	Competency Statement: **Protective measures developed, instituted, and monitored by perioperative APNs reduce and prevent injury to individual surgical patients and groups of patients and thus help to assure patient safety.**	
(continued)	**Clinical expertise/autonomy of practice *(continued)*** ◆ Ensures competent care during treatment of patient injuries.	◆ Portfolio of QI/PI activities ◆ Portfolio of educational projects ◆ Measured observation ◆ Written material (eg, tests, checklists) ◆ Peer review ◆ Committee participation/ leadership (eg, policy and procedure, safety, disaster preparedness, bioterrorism, purchasing, SIP, infection control, PI) Other:_____
	Critical thinking/analysis/clinical judgment/decision making/problem solving ◆ Diagnoses, monitors, and manages signs and symptoms of physical injury.[5]	◆ Critical pathways (eg, develops, implements, evaluates) ◆ Assessment/evaluation tools ◆ Portfolio of QI/PI activities ◆ Benchmarks (eg, compare, implement, evaluate) ◆ Patient satisfaction surveys (eg, develop, synthesize results, suggest changes) ◆ Directs and evaluates patient care ◆ Other: _____
	◆ Synthesizes knowledge of therapeutic regimens and patient response for evaluation of care.	◆ Critical pathways (eg, develops, implements, evaluates) ◆ Assessment/evaluation tools ◆ Portfolio of QI/PI activities ◆ Benchmarks(eg, compare, implement, evaluate) ◆ Patient satisfaction surveys (eg, develop, synthesize results, suggest changes) ◆ Directs and evaluates patient care ◆ Other: _____

Patient Outcome	PNDS Interventions as Measurable Criteria	Recommendations for Validation of Competency
	**Domain 1: SAFETY** *(continued)*	
	*Competency Statement:* **Protective measures developed, instituted, and monitored by perioperative APNs reduce and prevent injury to individual surgical patients and groups of patients and thus help to assure patient safety.**	
(continued)	**Critical thinking/analysis/clinical judgment/decision making/problem solving** *(continued)* ♦ Develops and/or implements systems to ensure safe practices at the point of delivery to the patient.	♦ Critical pathways (eg, develops, implements, evaluates) ♦ Portfolio of QI/PI activities ♦ Benchmarks (eg, compare, implement, evaluate) ♦ Patient satisfaction surveys (eg, develop, synthesize results, suggest changes) ♦ Directs and evaluates patient care Other:_____
	♦ Analyzes human factors and human-technology interfaces involved in adherence to policies, procedures, standards of care, and documentation.	♦ Critical pathways (eg, develops, implements, evaluates) ♦ Portfolio of QI/PI activities ♦ Benchmarks (eg, compare, implement, evaluate) ♦ Patient satisfaction surveys (eg, develop, synthesize results, suggest changes) ♦ Directs and evaluates patient care Other:_____
	Leadership/management ♦ Incorporates strategies of risk analysis and reduction, screening, and disease prevention and detection.	♦ Consultant for multidisciplinary health care team ♦ Committee participation/leadership ♦ Continuing education/inservice programs ♦ Publications/speeches ♦ Evaluations from participants of education programs ♦ Interpretation of regulations/guidelines/surveys Other:_____

Patient Outcome	PNDS Interventions as Measurable Criteria	Recommendations for Validation of Competency
	Domain 1: SAFETY *(continued)*	
	Competency Statement: **Protective measures developed, instituted, and monitored by perioperative APNs reduce and prevent injury to individual surgical patients and groups of patients and thus help to assure patient safety.**	
(continued)	**Leadership/management *(continued)*** ♦ Validates the effects of risk analysis and reduction initiatives.	♦ Consultant for multidisciplinary health care team ♦ Committee participation/ leadership ♦ Continuing education/ inservice programs ♦ Evaluations from participants of education programs ♦ Interpretation of regulations/guidelines/surveys Other:_____
	♦ Actively collaborates with infection control and epidemiology personnel to prevent and reduce the incidence of surgical site infections, health care-associated infections, and other adverse events related to surgical patients.	♦ Consultant for multidisciplinary health care team ♦ Committee participation/ leadership ♦ Continuing education/ inservice programs ♦ Evaluations from participants of education programs ♦ Interpretation of regulations/guidelines/surveys ♦ Other: _____
	♦ Promotes a culture of safety in the organization.	♦ Consultant for multidisciplinary health care team ♦ Committee participation/ leadership ♦ Continuing education/ inservice programs ♦ Mentor/teacher/role model ♦ Evaluations from participants of education programs ♦ Interpretation of regulations/guidelines/surveys ♦ Other: _____
	♦ Participates in legislative and policy-making activities that influence health services/practices.	♦ Consultant for multidisciplinary health care team ♦ Committee participation/ leadership ♦ Interpretation of regulations/guidelines ♦ Continuing education/ inservice programs ♦ Evaluations from participants of education programs ♦ Other: _____

Patient Outcome	PNDS Interventions as Measurable Criteria	Recommendations for Validation of Competency
	**Domain 1: SAFETY** *(continued)*	
	*Competency Statement:* Protective measures developed, instituted, and monitored by perioperative APNs reduce and prevent injury to individual surgical patients and groups of patients and thus help to assure patient safety.	
(continued)	**Leadership/management** *(continued)* ♦ Interprets and/or facilitates staff access to and compliance with current state, local and federal safety regulations and accreditation standards (eg, facility, Joint Commission, Occupational Safety and Health Administration [OSHA], and others).	♦ Interpretation of regulations/guidelines ♦ Committee participation/leadership ♦ Review of literature (eg, evidenced-based practice) ♦ Inservice programs ♦ Consultant for multidisciplinary health care team ♦ Portfolio of QI/PI activities ♦ Written material (eg, tests/checklists) ♦ Measured observation Other:_____
	♦ Identifies risk management strategies and develops performance improvement programs to establish and maintain a safe therapeutic environment.	♦ Interpretation of regulations/guidelines ♦ Committee participation/leadership ♦ Portfolio of QI/PI activities ♦ Educational programs ♦ Evaluation of care ♦ Other: _____
	Education and research ♦ Analyzes ideas for research projects that promote patient safety.	♦ Consultant for multidisciplinary health care team ♦ Preceptor/mentor/teacher/role model ♦ Review of literature (eg, evidenced-based practice) ♦ Inservice programs ♦ Portfolio of education projects ♦ Other: _____
	♦ Synthesizes current and emerging research findings that contribute to positive patient outcomes.	♦ Consultant for multidisciplinary health care team ♦ Preceptor/mentor/teacher/role model ♦ Review of literature (eg, evidenced-based practice) ♦ Inservice programs ♦ Portfolio of education projects ♦ Other: _____

Patient Outcome	PNDS Interventions as Measurable Criteria	Recommendations for Validation of Competency
	**Domain 1: SAFETY** *(continued)*	
	*Competency Statement:* **Protective measures developed, instituted, and monitored by perioperative APNs reduce and prevent injury to individual surgical patients and groups of patients and thus help to assure patient safety.**	
(continued)	**Education and research** *(continued)* ♦ Conducts research studies that culminates in evidence-based practice.	♦ Consultant for multidisciplinary health care team ♦ Preceptor/mentor/teacher/role model ♦ Review of literature (eg, evidenced-based practice) ♦ Inservice programs ♦ Portfolio of education projects Other:_____
	♦ Organizes and/or participates in multidisciplinary educational programs for health care professionals and the community.	♦ Consultant for multidisciplinary health care team ♦ Preceptor/mentor/teacher/role model ♦ Review of literature (eg, evidenced-based practice) ♦ Inservice programs ♦ Portfolio of education projects ♦ Other: _____
	Program development ♦ Designs patient safety protocols that minimizes the risk of injury.[6]	♦ Committee participation/leadership ♦ Preceptor/mentor/teacher/ role model ♦ Consultant for multidisciplinary health care team ♦ Educational programs ♦ Critical pathways (eg, develops, implements, evaluates) ♦ Poster presentations ♦ Assessment/evaluation tools ♦ Portfolio of QI/PI activities ♦ Other: _____
	♦ Evaluates the outcomes of patient safety initiatives and incorporates positive outcomes into patient care.	♦ Committee participation/leadership ♦ Preceptor/mentor/teacher/role model ♦ Consultant for multidisciplinary health care team ♦ Educational programs ♦ Critical pathways (eg, develops, implements, evaluates) ♦ Poster presentations ♦ Assessment/evaluation tools ♦ Portfolio of QI/PI activities ♦ Other: _____

Patient Outcome	PNDS Interventions as Measurable Criteria	Recommendations for Validation of Competency
	Domain 1: SAFETY *(continued)*	
	Competency Statement: **Protective measures developed, instituted, and monitored by perioperative APNs reduce and prevent injury to individual surgical patients and groups of patients and thus help to assure patient safety.**	
(continued)	**Program development** *(continued)* ♦ Raises performance standards and expectations for improvement in safety practices.	♦ Committee participation/ leadership ♦ Preceptor/mentor/ teacher/role model ♦ Consultant for multidisciplinary health care team ♦ Educational programs ♦ Critical pathways (eg, develops, implements, evaluates) ♦ Poster presentations ♦ Assessment/evaluation tools ♦ Portfolio of QI/PI activities Other:_____
	Communication/consultation/collaboration ♦ Serves as resource on safety issues for perioperative staff, surgeons, ancillary departments, other patient care areas, and outreach community projects requiring current clinical expertise.	♦ Assessment/evaluation tools ♦ Consultant for multidisciplinary health care team ♦ Portfolio of QI/PI activities ♦ Critical pathway (eg, develops, implements, evaluates) ♦ Policies and procedures ♦ Case management ♦ Interpretation of regulations/guidelines/surveys ♦ Other: _____
	♦ Analyzes and/or disseminates information regarding local, state, and national health issues that impact safety (eg, outbreaks of disease, disasters, medical errors, mandatory reporting of data by health care institutions).	♦ Assessment/evaluation tools ♦ Consultant for multidisciplinary health care team ♦ Portfolio of QI/PI activities ♦ Critical pathway (eg, develops, implements, evaluates) ♦ Policies and procedures ♦ Case management ♦ Interpretation of regulations/guidelines/surveys ♦ Other: _____

Patient Outcome	PNDS Interventions as Measurable Criteria	Recommendations for Validation of Competency
	**Domain 1: SAFETY (continued)**	
	*Competency Statement:* Protective measures developed, instituted, and monitored by perioperative APNs reduce and prevent injury to individual surgical patients and groups of patients and thus help to assure patient safety.	
(continued)	**Communication/consultation/collaboration (continued)** ♦ Facilitates new product evaluation process.	♦ Assessment/evaluation tools ♦ Consultant for multidisciplinary health care team ♦ Portfolio of QI/PI activities ♦ Critical pathway (eg, develops, implements, evaluates) ♦ Policies and procedures ♦ Case management ♦ Interpretation of regulations/guidelines/surveys Other:_____
	**Domain 2: PHYSIOLOGICAL OUTCOMES**	
	*Competency Statement:* Measured observation and intervention by APNs lead to optimal physiologic patient outcomes.	
The physical, biochemical, and functional responses to the intended therapeutic effects of an operative or other invasive procedure of individuals and groups of patients are consistent with expectations or improved from baseline levels established preoperatively (eg, surgical wound/tissue perfusion; normothermia; fluid-electrolyte and acid-base balances; respiratory, cardiac, and neurological status; pain; infection and inflammation).[7]	**Clinic expertise/autonomy of practice/ critical thinking/analysis/clinical judgment/ decision making/problem solving.** ♦ Assesses, diagnoses, treats, implements, and manages, independently or collaboratively, the comprehensive and individualized physiologic responses utilizing in-depth knowledge of principles of medicine, surgery, nursing process, and science as a foundation of care.	♦ Measured observation ♦ Documentation ♦ Consultant for multidisciplinary health care team ♦ Directing and evaluating patient care ♦ Critical pathways (eg, develops, implements, evaluates) ♦ Continuing education ♦ Review of literature (eg, evidenced-based practice) ♦ Return demonstration of skills ♦ Institutional privileges/ scope of practice ♦ Other: _____

Patient Outcome	PNDS Interventions as Measurable Criteria	Recommendations for Validation of Competency
	**Domain 2: PHYSIOLOGICAL OUTCOMES** *(continued)*	
	*Competency Statement:* Measured observation and intervention by APNs lead to optimal physiologic patient outcomes.	
(continued)	**Clinic expertise/autonomy of practice/ critical thinking/analysis/clinical judgment/ decision making/problem solving** *(continued)* ♦ Assesses, monitors, and recognizes complex physiologic responses (ie, continuous surveillance).[8]	♦ Measured observation ♦ Documentation ♦ Consultant for multidisciplinary health care team ♦ Directing and evaluating patient care ♦ Critical pathways (eg, develops, implements, evaluates) ♦ Continuing education ♦ Review of literature (eg, evidenced-based practice) ♦ Return demonstration of skills ♦ Institutional privileges/ scope of practice ♦ Other: _____
	♦ Integrates specialized knowledge and skills, critical thinking, and analytical skills, as well as clinical judgment and decision-making, to synthesize pathophysiology and related physiologic processes to formulate perioperative diagnostic hypotheses and differential diagnoses.[9]	♦ Measured observation ♦ Documentation ♦ Consultant for multidisciplinary health care team ♦ Directing and evaluating patient care ♦ Critical pathways (eg, develops, implements, evaluates) ♦ Continuing education ♦ Review of literature (eg, evidenced-based practice) ♦ Return demonstration of skills ♦ Institutional privileges/ scope of practice ♦ Other: _____
	♦ Demonstrates complex clinical judgment and reasoning as evidenced by preoperatively performing history and physical examination; selecting, ordering, and interpreting diagnostic tests; assigning ASA classification; and performing procedures to compare and contrast clinical findings to ensure optimal patient outcomes.[10]	♦ Measured observation ♦ Documentation ♦ Consultant for multidisciplinary health care team ♦ Directing and evaluating patient care ♦ Critical pathways (eg, develops, implements, evaluates) ♦ Continuing education ♦ Review of literature (eg, evidenced-based practice) ♦ Return demonstration of skills ♦ Institutional privileges/ scope of practice ♦ Other: _____

Patient Outcome	PNDS Interventions as Measurable Criteria	Recommendations for Validation of Competency
	**Domain 2: PHYSIOLOGICAL OUTCOMES** *(continued)*	
	*Competency Statement:* **Measured observation and intervention by APNs lead to optimal physiologic patient outcomes.**	
(continued)	**Leadership/management/communication consultation/ collaboration** ◆ Collaborates and coordinates with medical, nursing, and other disciplines to plan and implement monitoring of physiologic responses for individuals or specific groups of patients.[11]	◆ Discussion and review ◆ Written material (eg, tests, checklists) ◆ Peer review ◆ Committee participation/ leadership ◆ Institutional privileges/ scope of practice ◆ Patient advocacy ◆ Other Other:_____
	◆ Independently integrates and applies in-depth principles of traditional, complementary, and alternative medicine, to ensure optimal patient outcomes.[12]	◆ Discussion and review ◆ Written material (eg, tests, checklists) ◆ Peer review ◆ Committee participation/leadership ◆ Institutional privileges/scope of practice ◆ Patient advocacy ◆ Other: _____
	◆ Orders, prescribes, or initiates diagnostic, therapeutic and/or pharmacologic interventions.[13]	◆ Discussion and review ◆ Written material (eg, tests, checklists) ◆ Peer review ◆ Committee participation/ leadership ◆ Institutional privileges/ scope of practice ◆ Patient advocacy ◆ Other: _____
	Education and research/program development ◆ Systematically evaluates physiologic responses to interventions and revises differential diagnoses and interventions as needed.[14]	◆ Portfolio of educational projects ◆ Review of literature (eg, evidenced-based practice) ◆ Policies and procedures ◆ Peer review ◆ Review of outcomes ◆ Evidence of appropriate length of stay

Patient Outcome	PNDS Interventions as Measurable Criteria	Recommendations for Validation of Competency
	Domain 3A: BEHAVIORAL RESPONSES	
	Competency Statement: Individualized collaborative treatment plans for surgical patients promote patient responses that are inherent in optimal recovery processes.	
Individuals and groups of patients and families have knowledge about the psychological, socio-logic, and spiritual responses to opera-tive and other inva-sive procedures; this includes participation of patients in their recovery.[15]	**Critical thinking/analysis/clinical judgment/decision making/problem solving** ♦ Appraises behavioral responses utilizing an in-depth knowledge of learning theories, human behavior, change theory, stress and coping mechanisms, crisis management, human family development/ interaction, culturally appro-priate care, diversity, and health issues.	♦ Measured observation ♦ Assessment/evaluation tools ♦ Documentation ♦ Peer review Other:_____
	♦ Elicits an understanding of the interpretations of individu-als, groups of patients, and families regarding health, ill-ness, and the operative or other invasive procedure.[16]	♦ Measured observation ♦ Assessment/evaluation tools ♦ Documentation ♦ Peer review ♦ Other: _____
	♦ Formulates individualized treatment plan and implements measures of psychological support.	♦ Measured observation ♦ Assessment/evaluation tools ♦ Documentation ♦ Peer review ♦ Other: _____
	♦ Provides anticipatory guidance for expected and potential situational changes.	♦ Measured observation ♦ Assessment/evaluation tools ♦ Documentation ♦ Peer review ♦ Other: _____
	♦ Provides an in-depth interpretation of conditions and gives rationale for procedure.	♦ Measured observation ♦ Assessment/evaluation tools ♦ Documentation ♦ Peer review ♦ Other: _____
	♦ Evaluates psychosocial responses to treatment plan.	♦ Measured observation ♦ Assessment/evaluation tools ♦ Documentation ♦ Peer review ♦ Other: _____

Patient Outcome	PNDS Interventions as Measurable Criteria	Recommendations for Validation of Competency
	**Domain 3A: BEHAVIORAL RESPONSES** *(continued)*	
	*Competency Statement:* **Individualized collaborative treatment plans for surgical patients promote patient responses that are inherent in optimal recovery processes.**	

(continued)	**Critical thinking/analysis/clinical judgment/decision making/problem solving** *(continued)*
	♦ Performs a comprehensive and individualized assessment of
	  – psychosocial issues specific to medication management;[17]
	  – sensory impairments, barriers to communication, knowledge level, readiness to learn, psychosocial status, coping mechanisms, perceptions of surgery, history of substance abuse, and history of physical abuse;[18]
	  – presence and adequacy of support system;
	  – pain control and cultural and value components related to pain;[19]
	  – philosophical, cultural, and spiritual beliefs and values, and the individual's values and wishes concerning care;[20]
	  – nutritional habits, patterns, and psychosocial issues specific to the patients' nutritional status;[21]
	  – knowledge regarding wound care and phases of wound healing;[22]
	  – expectations of home care and the environment for home care; and
	  – those at risk or in the presence of physical barriers or potential hazards in the home.
		♦ Measured observation
		♦ Assessment/evaluation tools
		♦ Documentation
		♦ Peer review
		♦ Other: _____

	♦ Collaborates with patients, families, and discharge coordinators.[23]	♦ Measured observation ♦ Assessment/evaluation tools ♦ Documentation ♦ Peer review ♦ Other: _____
	Communication/consultation/collaboration ♦ Develops guidelines.[24]	♦ Critical pathways (eg, develops, implements, evaluates) ♦ Documentation ♦ Peer review ♦ Committee participation/leadership ♦ Case management ♦ Other: _____
	♦ Designs systems to meet the psychosocial needs of individual patients, groups of patients, and families.	♦ Documentation ♦ Peer review ♦ Committee participation/leadership ♦ Consultant for multidisciplinary health care team ♦ Directing and evaluating patient care ♦ Other: _____

Patient Outcome	PNDS Interventions as Measurable Criteria	Recommendations for Validation of Competency
\multicolumn3 **Domain 3A: BEHAVIORAL RESPONSES (continued)**		

Domain 3A: BEHAVIORAL RESPONSES (continued)

Competency Statement: Individualized collaborative treatment plans for surgical patients promote patient responses that are inherent in optimal recovery processes.

Patient Outcome	PNDS Interventions as Measurable Criteria	Recommendations for Validation of Competency
(continued)	**Communication/consultation/collaboration** *(continued)* ♦ Consults with the appropriate health care providers to initiate new treatments or change existing treatment.[25]	♦ Documentation ♦ Peer review ♦ Committee participation/ leadership ♦ Consultant for multidisciplinary health care team ♦ Directing and evaluating patient care Other: _____
	♦ Refers to other health professionals and community agencies.	♦ Referrals (eg, social services, rehabilitation, physical therapy, occupational therapy) Other: _____
	Education ♦ Develops, coordinates, implements, and evaluates educational programs for individual patients, groups of patients, and families based on identified needs.[26]	♦ Portfolio of patient educational materials ♦ Peer review ♦ Assessment/evaluation tools ♦ Patient satisfaction surveys (eg, develop, synthesize results, suggest changes) Other: _____

Domain: 3B: BEHAVIORAL RESPONSES
Patient and Family Rights/Ethics

Competency Statement: Superior individualized plan of care directed by an APN assures ethical, legal, and competent surgical patient care.

Patient Outcome	PNDS Interventions as Measurable Criteria	Recommendations for Validation of Competency
Individuals and groups of patients receive consistent, competent, and ethical care, within legal standards of practice, while maintaining privacy and support for the patient's value system.[27]	**Communication/consultation/collaboration** ♦ Operationalizes and promotes the concepts of caring, support, advocacy, and ethics in interpersonal transactions.	♦ Measured observation ♦ Reports incompetent, unethical, or illegal practices ♦ Peer review ♦ Performance evaluations ♦ Committee participation/ leadership ♦ Continuing education ♦ Review of literature (eg, evidenced-based practice) Other: _____

Patient Outcome	PNDS Interventions as Measurable Criteria	Recommendations for Validation of Competency
	Domain: 3B: BEHAVIORAL RESPONSES **Patient and Family Rights/Ethics** *(continued)* *Competency Statement:* **Superior individualized plan of care directed by an APN assures ethical, legal, and competent surgical patient care.**	
(continued)	**Communication/consultation/collaboration** *(continued)* ♦ Explains and interprets the Patient Self-Determination Act.[28]	♦ Measured observation ♦ Reports incompetent, unethical, or illegal practices ♦ Peer review ♦ Performance evaluations ♦ Committee participation/ leadership ♦ Continuing education ♦ Review of literature (eg, evidenced-based practice) Other: _____
	♦ Informs patients of risks, benefits, and expected outcomes of planned procedures and obtains informed consent.[29]	♦ Measured observation ♦ Reports incompetent, unethical, or illegal practices ♦ Peer review ♦ Performance evaluations ♦ Committee participation/leadership ♦ Continuing education ♦ Review of literature (eg, evidenced-based practice) Other: _____
	♦ Designs protocols for preoperative teaching and discharge planning.[30]	♦ Measured observation ♦ Reports incompetent, unethical, or illegal practices ♦ Peer review ♦ Performance evaluations ♦ Committee participation/ leadership ♦ Continuing education ♦ Review of literature (eg, evidenced-based practice) Other: _____
	♦ Uses an ethical framework to evaluate issues regarding patient care.	♦ Measured observation ♦ Reports incompetent, unethical, or illegal practices ♦ Peer review ♦ Performance evaluations ♦ Committee participation/ leadership ♦ Continuing education ♦ Review of literature (eg, evidenced-based practice) Other: _____

Patient Outcome	PNDS Interventions as Measurable Criteria	Recommendations for Validation of Competency
	**Domain: 3B: BEHAVIORAL RESPONSES** **Patient and Family Rights/Ethics** *(continued)* *Competency Statement:* Superior individualized plan of care directed by an APN assures ethical, legal, and competent surgical patient care.	
(continued)	**Communication/consultation/collaboration** *(continued)* ♦ Advocates care without prejudicial behavior.[31]	♦ Measured observation ♦ Reports incompetent, unethical, or illegal practices ♦ Peer review ♦ Performance evaluations ♦ Committee participation/ leadership ♦ Continuing education ♦ Review of literature (eg, evidenced-based practice) Other:_____
	♦ Shares patient information only with those directly involved in the patient's care (eg, Health Care Portability and Accountability Act).[32]	♦ Measured observation ♦ Reports incompetent, unethical, or illegal practices ♦ Peer review ♦ Performance evaluations ♦ Committee participation/ leadership ♦ Continuing education ♦ Review of literature (eg, evidenced-based practice) Other: _____
	**Domain 4: HEALTH SYSTEM (*Organizational*) OUTCOMES** *Competency Statement:* Comprehensive patient care, performed within the parameters of a particular health system, and its multidisciplinary team, is enhanced by APN expertise.	
The health system, with the assistance of the APN, provides comprehensive care that is targeted to unique patient needs.	**Collaborative responsibility** Within integrated health care system: ♦ Promotes use of nationally accepted clinical practice guidelines and standards.	♦ Consultant for multidisciplinary health care team ♦ Committee participation/ leadership ♦ Documentation ♦ Peer review ♦ Interpretation of regulations/surveys Other: _____
	♦ Fosters a collaborative environment and recognizes the value of each provider's contribution to comprehensive health care.	♦ Consultant for multidisciplinary health care team ♦ Committee participation/ leadership ♦ Documentation ♦ Peer review Other: _____

Patient Outcome	PNDS Interventions as Measurable Criteria	Recommendations for Validation of Competency
	Domain 4: HEALTH SYSTEM (*Organizational*) OUTCOMES (*continued*)	
	Competency Statement: **Comprehensive patient care, performed within the parameters of a particular health system, and its multidisciplinary team, is enhanced by APN expertise.**	
(continued)	**Collaborative responsibility** *(continued)* ♦ Facilitates multidisciplinary groups in designing and/or implementing innovative practices and alternative solutions to patient care issues.	♦ Consultant for multidisciplinary health care team ♦ Committee participation/leadership ♦ Documentation ♦ Peer review Other: _____
	♦ Values other disciplines and multidisciplinary activities (eg, education, consultation, management, developing technological or research opportunities) to enhance patient care.	♦ Consultant for multidisciplinary health care team ♦ Committee participation/leadership ♦ Documentation ♦ Peer review Other: _____
	♦ Cultivates system awareness of advancements in health care through membership in professional organizations and dissemination of expert knowledge.	♦ Consultant for multidisciplinary health care team ♦ Committee participation/leadership ♦ Documentation ♦ Peer review Other: _____
	♦ Promotes nursing practice that is visionary and inventive to improve delivery of care.	♦ Consultant for multidisciplinary health care team ♦ Committee participation/leadership ♦ Documentation ♦ Peer review Other: _____
	Ethical responsibility Within integrated health care system: ♦ Fosters an environment of patient and staff safety.	♦ Patient advocacy ♦ Assessment/evaluation tools ♦ Documentation ♦ Peer review ♦ Portfolio of QI/PI activities Other: _____
	♦ Contributes to the development of services that are consistent, comparable in all settings and performed within the legal and ethical scope of practice.	♦ Committee participation/leadership ♦ Assessment/evaluation tools ♦ Documentation ♦ Peer review Other _____

Patient Outcome	PNDS Interventions as Measurable Criteria	Recommendations for Validation of Competency
	Domain 4: HEALTH SYSTEM (*Organizational*) OUTCOMES (*continued*) *Competency Statement:* **Comprehensive patient care, performed within the parameters of a particular health system, and its multidisciplinary team, is enhanced by APN expertise.**	
(continued)	**Ethical responsibility** *(continued)* ♦ Facilitates care that is nondiscriminatory and nonprejudicial regardless of the setting in which care is given.[33]	♦ Patient advocacy ♦ Measured observation ♦ Assessment/evaluation tools ♦ Documentation ♦ Peer review Other: _____
	♦ Designs care that respects the patient and reflects individuals' uniqueness (eg, social or economic status, personal attributes or lifestyle, culture, ethnicity, level of health are considered).	♦ Assessment/evaluation tools ♦ Documentation ♦ Peer review ♦ Publications/speeches Other: _____
	♦ Encourages professionals to work within cultural context of individual, group, or community from diverse cultural/ethnic background.	♦ Measured observation ♦ Assessment/evaluation tools ♦ Documentation ♦ Peer review Other: _____
	♦ Uses an ethical framework to evaluate individual or system issues regarding care.	♦ Assessment/evaluation tools ♦ Documentation ♦ Peer review Other: _____
	♦ Considers ethical implications of scientific advances, cost and clinical effectiveness, patient and family acceptance/satisfaction.	♦ Committee participation/ leadership ♦ Patient satisfaction surveys (eg, develop, synthesize results, suggest changes) Other: _____
	♦ Coaches professionals to provide care that leads to the highest standards of practice.	♦ Continuing education ♦ Preceptor/mentor/ educator ♦ Measured observation Other: _____
	♦ Participates in health policy activities at the local, state, national, and international levels.	♦ Consultant for multidisciplinary health care team ♦ Committee participation/ leadership Other: _____

Patient Outcome	PNDS Interventions as Measurable Criteria	Recommendations for Validation of Competency
	**Domain 4: HEALTH SYSTEM (*Organizational*) OUTCOMES (*continued*)** *Competency Statement:* **Comprehensive patient care, performed within the parameters of a particular health system, and its multidisciplinary team, is enhanced by APN expertise.**	
(continued)	**Ethical responsibility (*continued*)** ♦ Encourages others to remain current with their profession by attending workshops, reading journals, attending association meetings, participating on committees.	♦ Continuing education ♦ Committee participation/ leadership ♦ Review of literature (eg, evidenced-based practice) ♦ Mentoring/role modeling ♦ Staff involvement in perioperative committees ♦ Staff advisement of upcoming association meetings Other: _____
	Regulatory and credentialing requirements Within integrated health care system: ♦ Supports nursing services within the scope of nursing specialty practice for which the APN is educationally prepared and has maintained through educational preparation (eg, academic course work, workshops or seminars, theory and clinical experience).	♦ Institutional privileges/ scope of practice ♦ Licensure Other: _____

	♦ Promotes an environment that protects the patient from incompetent, unethical, or illegal practices and complies with
	  – Patient's Bill of Rights;
	  – institutional personnel performance policies;
	  – applicable federal, state, and local regulations (eg, HIPAA);
	  – accreditation guidelines; and
	  – professional standards.
		♦ Peer review
		♦ Performance evaluation
		♦ Measured observation
		♦ Directing and evaluating patient care
		♦ Institutional privileges/ scope of practice
		♦ Patient advocacy
		♦ Portfolio of QI/PI activities
		♦ Policies and procedures
		Other: _____

	♦ Fosters professional accountability.	♦ Peer review ♦ Patient advocacy Other: _____
	♦ Evaluates care according to professional standards and state nursing regulations.	♦ Continuing education ♦ Review of literature (eg, evidenced-based practice) ♦ Licensure ♦ Peer review Other: _____
	♦ Interprets and/or facilitates staff access to and compliance with current state, local, and federal regulations/accreditation standards (eg, facility, Joint Commission, OSHA).	♦ Continuing education ♦ Preceptor/mentor/ teacher ♦ Consultant for multidisciplinary health care team ♦ Committee participation/ leadership Other: _____

Patient Outcome	PNDS Interventions as Measurable Criteria	Recommendations for Validation of Competency
	**Domain 4: HEALTH SYSTEM (*Organizational*) OUTCOMES (*continued*)** *Competency Statement:* Comprehensive patient care, performed within the parameters of a particular health system, and its multidisciplinary team, is enhanced by APN expertise.	
(continued)	**Business aspects, reimbursement/payment mechanisms** Within integrated health care system: ♦ Provides consultation services to the organization to achieve quality, cost-effective outcomes for populations of patients across settings.	♦ Review of literature (eg, evidenced-based practice) ♦ Continuing education Other:_____
	♦ Promotes system participation in efforts to diminish cost and unnecessary duplication of testing/diagnostic activities and facilitates timely treatment of patients.	♦ Cost of care ♦ Length of stay Other: _____
	♦ Collects and evaluates data regarding effectiveness of care, cost/benefit relationship, and patient satisfaction.	♦ Patient satisfaction surveys (eg, develop, synthesize results, suggest changes) ♦ Morbidity/mortality ♦ Sentinel events ♦ Readmissions/unplanned returns to surgery Other: _____
	♦ Sustains awareness of organization's method of financing delivery of care.	♦ Committee participation ♦ Knowledge of insurance trends and managed care Other: _____
	♦ Implements cost/benefit evaluation of new technology and participates in product review committees.	♦ Committee participation ♦ Literature review of products ♦ Elicit information from area specialists in use of equipment ♦ Review of staff evaluation forms Other: _____
	♦ Supports nursing practice that considers access, fiscal responsibility, efficacy, and quality.	♦ Staff participation in inservice programs/ continuing education ♦ Measured observation Other: _____
	Policy-making Within integrated health care system: ♦ Participates in local, state, national, or international level of policy-making activities, in concert with professional associations, to ensure equitable patient care and to advocate for the APN role.	♦ Professional membership ♦ Evaluation of state and national agendas as related to health care and perioperative practice ♦ Active political involvement Other: _____

Patient Outcome	PNDS Interventions as Measurable Criteria	Recommendations for Validation of Competency
	**Domain 4: HEALTH SYSTEM (*Organizational*) OUTCOMES (*continued*)** *Competency Statement:* **Comprehensive patient care, performed within the parameters of a particular health system, and its multidisciplinary team, is enhanced by APN expertise.**	
(continued)	**Policy-making (*continued*)** ♦ Promotes the dimensions of APN practice to the public, legislators, policy makers, and other health care professionals.	♦ Professional membership ♦ Evaluation of state and national agendas as related to health care and perioperative practice ♦ Active political involvement Other:_____
	Outcome evaluation and performance improvement Within integrated health care system: ♦ Participates in the generation, application and/or dissemination of research.	♦ Outcomes research Other: _____
	♦ Initiates organizational interest in contributing to or sustaining research to explore current practice.	♦ Committee participation at the system level Other: _____
	♦ Formulates research questions based upon knowledge of current practice environment.	♦ Internal data (eg, clinical database; an example is a patient analysis and tracking system [PATS]) Other: _____
	♦ Evaluates health outcomes of advanced practice to assist in shaping health care and nursing practice.	♦ External data Other: _____
	♦ Monitors current system nursing practice and/or surveys existing research for comparison.	♦ Internal data and external data comparison Other: _____
	♦ Utilizes internal and external data in creation of outcome indicators.	♦ Identification of outcomes and interventions Other: _____
	♦ Advocates and performs clinical investigation of system practice through literature review and critical appraisal.	♦ Summary of research appraisal Other: _____
	♦ Provides leadership when applying research in practice innovations to enhance patient care.	♦ Statement of patient benefits and risks ♦ Utilization of knowledge of research appraisal combined with clinical judgment Other: _____
	♦ Utilizes data from clinical investigations to improve the safety, efficiency, and effectiveness of system-wide patient care.	♦ System feasibility assessment ♦ Cost analysis ♦ Other: _____

Patient Outcome	PNDS Interventions as Measurable Criteria	Recommendations for Validation of Competency
	**Domain 4: HEALTH SYSTEM (*Organizational*) OUTCOMES (*continued*)** *Competency Statement:* **Comprehensive patient care, performed within the parameters of a particular health system, and its multidisciplinary team, is enhanced by APN expertise.**	
(continued)	**Outcome evaluation and performance improvement** *(continued)* ♦ Applies theoretical knowledge, research, and assessment data to design, integrate, and evaluate nursing practice.	♦ Clinical protocol design (eg, design a change to current practice) ♦ Pilot test of practice change Other:_____
	♦ Disseminates outcomes of quality-of-care activities throughout the health care system.	♦ Practice change implementation Other: _____
	♦ Integrates scientific evidence into the health management of patients, families, and communities.	♦ Research dissemination Other: _____
	♦ Synthesizes and utilizes the study results to make or recommend changes, including policy, procedure, and protocol documentation.	♦ Policy and procedure revision ♦ Clinical protocol amendments Other: _____
	♦ Provides continuing education and/or consultation to disseminate research findings to system participants.	♦ Continuing education/inservice programs Other: _____
	♦ Submits findings of clinical research to scholarly journals and at conferences.	♦ Publications ♦ Presentation at professional conferences Other: _____
	♦ Encourages the health system to utilize research and promote evidence-based practice to facilitate quality care.	♦ Presentation of research findings and implementation activities at system level ♦ Presentation of financial analysis Other: _____
	♦ Evaluates the organization for limitations and recommends improvements that influence patient health outcomes.	♦ Data from staff evaluation forms Other: _____
	♦ Obtains data from information systems that illustrate variations in outcome to contribute expertise in organizational decisions that improve practice.	♦ Internal data reevaluation Other: _____

Glossary

ASA classification: American Society of Anesthesiologists physical status classification. An anesthesia risk evaluation using predetermined criteria defined by the American Society of Anesthesiologists. This system ranks patient physical status on a scale of one to six to determine appropriate patient selection for anesthesia.[34]

Benchmarks: A standard or reference by which patient care can be measured, judged, or predicted (eg, turnover time, least expensive cost for a particular surgery that is attained with a minimum level of mortality and morbidity).[35-37]

Nursing case management: A systematic approach of coordinating health services for a specific patient population. The approach is dynamic, streamlined, enhances quality and cost-effective patient outcomes, and offers options and services to meet the patient's needs. It involves patient and family participation and utilizes nursing process and interaction.[38]

Clinical practice guidelines: Systematically developed statements to assist practitioner and patient decisions about appropriate health care for specific clinical circumstances.[39]

Competency statement: Represents expected, measurable, perioperative nursing behaviors. Defines the knowledge, skills, and abilities necessary to fulfill the professional role functions of a perioperative registered nurse.[40]

Consultant: An individual who provides expert or professional advice.[41,42]

Consultation: An exchange of information between two professionals where one individual possesses specialized expertise.[43]

Continuing education: Designed professional experiences that add to the quality of a nurse's contributions to the health care of patients.[44]

Critical pathway: The organization and sequencing of patient care interventions for a specified procedure or population by the health care team along a timeline to better manage resources, ensure quality of care, and minimize delays.[45]

Differential diagnosis: To distinguish a disease or condition from others that present similar symptoms.[46]

Evidence-based practice: A complete process that starts with asking clinical questions, seeking the best practice, and evaluating the "evidence" for applicability and validity to a specific care issue. A clinician applies the best evidence that considers a patient's and family values and needs.[47,48]

Indicator: Well-defined, measurable, objective statement related to the structure, process, or outcomes of care; direct attention to problems or opportunities to improve care.[39]

Inservice program: A learning experience that assists staff to perform assigned functions in their workplace. An inservice program can be job-specific. It can assist a person to learn, maintain, and/or increase competency in his or her specific job responsibilities.[44]

Leadership (clinical): Behaviors the APN acquires as a result of working with health team members. They encourage patients and colleagues to be confident and promote team problem-solving. They serve as clinical role models/mentors or change agents that strive to improve patient care and influence others' perceptions regarding the value of the APN.[49]

Literature review: A summary of research on a selected area of interest that places a research problem in context or can form a basis for initiating a research project.[50]

Mentor: One who provides encouragement and acts as a guide and facilitator while modeling professional nursing behaviors.[51]

Outcomes: Patient outcomes are observable, measurable physiologic and psychosocial responses to perioperative nursing interventions.[52]

Preceptor: An experienced registered nurse practicing in the perioperative setting who provides and directs learning opportunities for learners. The preceptor facilitates the learning process to help the learner meet the goals and objectives of a selected educational program or acquire specific knowledge and/or skills needed to perform job responsibilities.[53]

Quality improvement: Examines processes to improve them. The origin of QI is based in industry and has more of a management and process focus.[39]

Peer review: The examination and evaluation by associates of a practitioner's clinical practice. Individuals are evaluated by recognized, established standards. Physicians review physicians, registered nurses review registered nurses, etc.[39]

Performance improvement: A process to address human performance within an organization at the individual, process, and organizational level. PI focuses more on the people, their motivation, and the tools (eg, work design, technical support, supervision, safety) they use to achieve the goals of the organization.[39]

Risk analysis (also hazard analysis.): The process of collecting and evaluating information on the circumstances leading to a higher risk for adverse outcomes. These circumstances or conditions are not related to the disease process or the condition for which the patient is being treated.[39]

Scope of practice: Refers to a legislative framework, as designed by the individual state practice acts and federal laws and regulations that communicates to others the role, competencies (eg, knowledge, skills, attitudes), and professional accountability of the nurse. It is intended to prevent inappropriate provision of services by those who are unqualified.[54-56]

Sentinel event: The Joint Commission states: "A sentinel event is any unexpected occurrence involving death or serious physical or psychological injury, or the risk thereof. Serious injuries specifically include a loss of limb or function. The phrase 'or the risk thereof' includes any process variation for which a recurrence would carry a significant chance of a serious adverse outcome."[57] Such events are called *sentinel* because they signal the need for immediate investigation and response. These unexpected occurrences are subject to individual case review under the sentinel event policy of the Joint Commission.[39,58]

NOTES

Notes 1-33 refer to the Outcomes (O) and Indicators (I) from S Beyea, ed, *Perioperative Nursing Data Set: The Perioperative Nursing Vocabulary,* second ed (Denver: AORN Inc, 2002).

1. O2 to O9
2. I123, I36 to I43
3. I138 to I139, I146, I72 to I77
4. I30
5. I36 to I48, I51
6. I72 to I78
7. O10 to O15, O29, O30
8. I2 to I5, I7, I9, I10, I15, I16, I21, I22, I30, I33, I34, I54, I55, I58, I70, I78, I86 to I89, I98, I110, I111, I120, I121, I128, I131, I145
9. I15, I59, I60, I66, I132, I144
10. I4, I21, I66, I88, I89, I132, I144
11. I23, I24, I85, I110, I111, I120, I129, I133
12. I69, I148
13. I2, I4, I5, I7 to I9, I68, I71, I78, I89, I92, I110, I111, I140, I141
14. I44, I45, I46, I51, I54, I55, I92, I130, I146, I153
15. O18 to O22, O31
16. I32, I135, I136, I137
17. I17
18. I31, I90, I113, I114, I134, I135, I136, I168, I137
19. I16, I61
20. I57, I63
21. I18, I148
22. I149
23. I35, I62
24. I71, I119
25. I92
26. I48 to I50, I52, I53, I56, I79, I80, I104, I105, I106, I107, I108, I134, I135, I136
27. O23 to O28
28. I103
29. I124
30. I63, I79, I80
31. I1, I97, I99, I100, I102
32. I116, I150, I151
33. I99
34. "Recommended practices for managing the patient receiving moderate sedation/analgesia," in *Standards, Recommended Practices, and Guidelines* (Denver: AORN, Inc, 2005) 286.
35. E B Rudy et al, "Benchmarking patient outcomes," *Journal of Nursing Scholarship* 33 no 2 (2001) 185-189.
36. Merriam-Webster Online Dictionary, *http://www.m-w.com/cgi-bin/dictionary?book=Dictionary&va=benchmark* (accessed 16 Oct 2005)
37. "Sentinel event glossary of terms," Joint Commission on the Accreditation of Healthcare Organizations, *http://www.jcaho.org/accredited+organizations/sentinel+event/glossary.htm* (accessed 16 Oct 2005).
38. V A Mahn-DiNicola, D J Zazworsky, "The advanced practice nurse case manager," in *Advanced Practice Nursing: An Integrative Approach,* ed A B Hamric, J A Spross, C M Hanson (St Louis, Mo: Elsevier Saunders, 2005) 621.
39. "Quality and performance improvement standards for perioperative nursing," in *Standards, Recommended Practices, and Guidelines* (Denver: AORN, Inc, 2005) 257-266.
40. "AORN document definitions," in *Standards, Recommended Practices, and Guidelines* (Denver: AORN, Inc, 2005) 20.
41. Dictionary.com, *http://dictionary.reference.com/search?q=consultant* (accessed 16 Oct 05).
42. *The American Heritage Dictionary of the English Language,* fourth ed (New York: Houghton Mifflin Company, 2000.)
43. A Barron, P A White, "Consultation," in *Advanced Practice Nursing: An Integrative Approach,* ed A B Hamric, J A Spross, C M Hanson (St Louis: Saunders, 2005) 225-255.

44. L Brazen, "Nursing staff development," in *Patient Care During Operative and Invasive Procedures,* ed M L Phippen, M P Wells (Philadelphia: W B Saunders, 2000) 737-753.

45. "AORN clinical path template," in *Standards, Recommended Practices, and Guidelines* (Denver: AORN, Inc, 2005) 75-83.

46. Medline Plus Medical Dictionary, *http://www2 .merriam-webster.com/cgi-bin/mwmednlm?book=Medical &va=differential%20diagnosis* (accessed 16 Oct 05).

47. M A Rosswurm, J H Larrabee, "A model for change to evidence-based practice," *Journal of Nursing Scholarship* 31 no 4 (1999) 317-322.

48. Oncology Nursing Society Evidence-Based Practice Resource Center, *http://onsopcontent.ons.org/toolkits/ ebp/definition/definition.htm,* accessed (accessed 16 Oct 2005).

49. C M Hanson, J A Spross, "Clinical and professional leadership," in *Advanced Practice Nursing: An Integrative Approach,* ed A B Hamric, J A Spross, C M Hanson (St Louis: Saunders, 2005) 301-339.

50. D F Polit, B P Hungler, eds, sixth ed, *Nursing Research: Principles and Methods* (Philadelphia: Lippincott, 1995).

51. "AORN resolution on responsibility for mentoring," in *Standards, Recommended Practices, and Guidelines* (Denver: AORN, Inc, 2005) 231.

52. "Perioperative patient outcomes," in *Standards, Recommended Practices, and Guidelines* (Denver: AORN, Inc, 2005) 267.

53. *Preceptor Guide for Perioperative Nursing* (Denver: Association of Operating Room Nurses, 1993).

54. "Health professions regulatory issues," at *http:// nursingworld.org/gova/hod97/regulate.htm#scopes* (accessed 16 Oct 2005).

55. About.com, "Scope of practice," *http://nursing.about .com/od/glossary/g/Scope.htm* (accessed 16 Oct 2005).

56. A B Hamric, "A definition of advanced practice nursing," in *Advanced Practice Nursing: An Integrative Approach,* ed A B Hamric, J A Spross, C M Hanson (St Louis, Mo: Saunders, 2005) 85-108.

57. "Facts about the sentinel event policy," Joint Commission on Accreditation of Healthcare Organizations, *http://www.jcaho.org/accredited+organizations/sentinel +event/sefacts.htm* (accessed 16 Oct 2005).

58. "Sentinel event policy and procedures—Updated: June 2005," Joint Commission on Accreditation of Healthcare Organizations, at *http://www.jcaho.org /accredited+organizations/sentinel+event/se_pp.htm* (accessed 16 Oct 05).

RESOURCES

Domain 1

American Nurses Association. *Scope and Standards of Practice* (Washington, DC: American Nurses Association, 2004).

Davies, B; Hughes, A M. "Clarification of advanced nursing practice: Characteristics and competencies," *Clinical Nurse Specialist* 16 (May 2002) 147-152.

Degrasse, C; Nicklin, W. "Advanced nursing practice: Old hat, new design," *Canadian Journal of Nursing Leadership* 14 (November/December 2001) 7-12.

Klardie, K; et al. "Integrating the principles of evidence-based practice into clinical practice," *Journal of the American Academy of Nurse Practitioners* 16 (March 2004) 98-105.

Domain 2

American Academy of Nurse Practitioners. *Position Statement: Nurse Practitioners as an Advanced Practice Nurse Role* (Austin, Tex: American Academy of Nurse Practitioners, 2002).

American Academy of Nurse Practitioners. *Scope of Practice for Nurse Practitioners* (Austin, Tex: American Academy of Nurse Practitioners, 2002).

American Academy of Nurse Practitioners. *Standards of Practice* (Austin, Tex: American Academy of Nurse Practitioners, 2002).

American Nurses Association. *Scope and Standards of Practice* (Washington, DC: American Nurses Association, 2004).

Beyea, S C, ed. *Perioperative Nursing Data Set: The Perioperative Nursing Vocabulary,* second ed (Denver: AORN, Inc, 2002).

Burman, M. "Complementary and alternative medicine: Core competencies for family nurse practitioners," *Journal of Nursing Education* 42 (January 2003) 28-34.

"Definition of perioperative advanced practice nurse," in *Standards, Recommended Practices, and Guidelines* (Denver: AORN, Inc, 2005) 225.

"What is a nurse practitioner?" American College of Nurse Practitioners, *http://www.npcentral.net/consumer/ about.nps.shtml* (accessed 16 Oct 2005).

Domain 3A

American Academy of Nurse Practitioners. *Standards of Practice* (Austin, Tex: American Academy of Nurse Practitioners, 2002).

Beyea, S C, ed. *Perioperative Nursing Data Set: The Perioperative Nursing Vocabulary,* second ed (Denver: AORN, Inc, 2002).

National Organization of Nurse Practitioner Faculties. *Domains and Core Competencies of Nurse Practitioner Practice* (Washington, DC: National Organization of Nurse Practitioner Faculties, 2000).

"Perioperative advanced practice nurse competencies," in *Standards, Recommended Practices, and Guidelines* (Denver: AORN, Inc, 2005) 35-40.

Domain 3B

Beyea, S C, ed. *Perioperative Nursing Data Set: The Perioperative Nursing Vocabulary,* second ed (Denver: AORN, Inc, 2002).

Perioperative advanced practice nurse competencies," in *Standards Recommended Practices, and Guidelines* (Denver: AORN, Inc, 2005) 35-40.

Domain 4

American Academy of Nurse Practitioners. *Standards of Practice.* (Austin, Tex: American Academy of Nurse Practitioners, 2002).

American Nurses Association. *Scope and Standards of Advanced Practice Registered Nursing* (Washington, DC: American Nurses Association, 2004).

Beyea, S C, ed. *Perioperative Nursing Data Set: The Perioperative Nursing Vocabulary,* second ed (Denver: AORN, Inc, 2002).

Hamric, A B. "A definition of advanced practice nursing," in *Advanced Practice Nursing: An Integrative Approach,* ed A B Hamric, J A Spross, C M Hanson (St Louis: Saunders, 2005) 62, 85-108.

"Model rules and regulations for CNS title protection and scope of practice," National Association of Clinical Nurse Specialists, *http://www.nacns.org/model_language.pdf* (accessed 16 Oct 2005).

National Association of Pediatric Nurse Practitioners. *Scope and Standards of Practice: Pediatric Nurse Practitioner* (Cherry Hill, NJ: National Association of Pediatric Nurse Practitioners, 2004).

National Organization of Nurse Practitioner Faculties. *Domains and Core Competencies of Nurse Practitioner Practice* (Washington, DC: National Organization of Nurse Practitioner Faculties, 2000).

The Women's Health Nurse Practitioner: Guidelines for Practice and Education, fifth ed (Washington, DC: Association of Women's Health, Obstetrics and Neonatal Nurses and National Association of Nurse Practitioners in Women's Health, 2002).

Originally published January 1994, *AORN Journal.* Revised and reformatted in 2005.

Perioperative Care Coordinator Nurse Competency Statements

I n 2005 the Nursing Practices Committee was charged by the AORN Board of Directors to review and revise the existing perioperative care coordinator competency statements to incorporate the Perioperative Nursing Data Set (PNDS).[1] The *perioperative care coordinator* is defined as a perioperative nurse who is responsible and accountable for coordinating and supervising the nursing care provided to patients having a surgical or other invasive procedure. In this expanded role, the perioperative care coordinator is responsible for providing guidance, clinical expertise, mentoring and functional direction to the perioperative team and orchestrates the availability of resources required for safe patient care. The perioperative care coordinator should have mastered the skills outlined in the "Competency statements in perioperative nursing." AORN strongly believes that the best foundation for the perioperative care coordinator role is perioperative nursing. The measurable criteria listed are not exhaustive, nor is the perioperative care coordinator required to perform all activities listed to demonstrate a particular competency.

The Nursing Practices Committee (NPC) members were appointed by the President-elect based on their perioperative clinical and leadership expertise. Members of the NPC possess extensive and varied national and international perioperative clinical and leadership experience including hospital and ambulatory surgery. All NPC members have specialty certification, educational levels include diploma to PhD level, and perioperative experience spanning from 13 years to 36 years.

Building on previous work on the perioperative care coordinator competencies the NPC performed a literature search and obtained input from the NPC members and peer/expert reviewers. The literature search was performed using the subject headings patient care coordinator, perioperative clinical, leadership and professional competencies, and OR case management. The NPC used the PNDS framework to organize the competency statements. The competency statements were divided into four domains:

- **Domain 1:** Safety;
- **Domain 2:** Physiologic Outcomes;
- **Domain 3A:** Behavioral Responses;
- **Domain 3B:** Behavioral Responses—Patient and Family Rights and Ethics; and
- **Domain 4:** Health System (Organizational) Outcomes.[1]

The NPC collaborated with the Advanced Practice Issues Task Force and the National Committee on Education, charged with revising the APN and perioperative nurse competency statements respectively, to coordinate the competency statements. The statements were evaluated for congruency and progression from the core competencies of the perioperative registered nurse. In addition the NPC collaborated with perioperative nurse data set experts and research consultants during the development of the competency statements. The revised perioperative care coordinator competencies were sent to 53 expert reviewers selected for their experience and knowledge. They were asked to review the competency statements and submit comments. The reviewers consisted of the following:

- Perioperative Nursing Data Set experts,
- Advanced Practice Issues Task Force members,
- National Committee on Education members,
- Perioperative RN specialists in the Center for Nursing Practice, and
- Representatives from the following Specialty Assemblies:
  - Nurse Educator/Clinical Nurse Specialist,
  - Leadership, and
  - Nurses in Business, Industry, and Consulting.

The expert comments were reviewed and incorporated into the perioperative care coordinator competency statements. The NPC submitted the completed revised competencies to the AORN Board of Directors in November 2005. The AORN Board reviewed and approved, with minor revisions, the "Perioperative care coordinator nurse competency statements" using the PNDS as a foundation.

NOTES

1. S Beyea, ed, *Perioperative Nursing Data Set: The Perioperative Nursing Vocabulary,* second ed (Denver: AORN Inc, 2002).

Nursing Practices Committee 2005–2006
George D. Allen, RN, PhD, CNOR, CIC
Martine Bouchard, RN, MSc, CPN
Viola E. Farrell, RN, MBA, CNOR
Debby J. Shobe, RN, BSN, CNOR
Raema A. Howell, RN, BSN, CNOR

Committee Chair
Catherine M. Moses, RN, CNOR, CPHQ

Board Liaison
Nathalie F. Walker, RN, BS, MBA

Staff Consultant
Carol Petersen, RN, BSN, MAOM, CNOR

Perioperative Care Coordinator Competency Statements

The perioperative care coordinator (PCC) is a perioperative registered nurse who is responsible and accountable for coordinating and supervising the nursing care provided to patients having a surgical or other invasive procedure. The perioperative care coordinator should have mastered the skills outlined in the "Competency statements in perioperative nursing." In this leadership role, the perioperative nurse is responsible for providing guidance, clinical expertise, mentoring, and functional direction to members of the health care team while optimizing available resources to achieve optimal patient outcomes. This role may include, but is not limited to, surgical case management, perioperative patient care coordination, staff education, and organization of quality/performance improvement activities. In no way should patient safety be compromised in the interest of efficiency.

Patient Outcome	PNDS Interventions as Measurable Criteria	Recommendations for Validation of Competency
	Domain 1: SAFETY	
Competency Statement: **The perioperative care coordinator demonstrates competency to coordinate, facilitate, and manage safe care for perioperative patients.**		
Individuals and groups of patients are free from injuries due to extraneous objects, chemical products, electrical current, positioning, lasers, radiation, transfer/transport, allergic responses, and medication administration.[1]	**Clinical Resource Expert** Acts as clinical resource for perioperative nursing staff and incorporates the following activities: ♦ Utilizes critical thinking skills ♦ Incorporates evidence-based knowledge into decisions for the provision of safe patient care ♦ Participates in the planning and provision of safety-related education with age-specific considerations.	♦ Direct observation ♦ Communication records (eg, staff communication log, staff meetings, daily briefings) ♦ Inservice/education session participant evaluations or attendance sheets ♦ Documentation of required staff competencies Other: _____
	Clinical Coordinator Manages the care provided to multiple patients in one or more services or specialties to ensure that staff properly: ♦ Confirm patient's identity and verify operative site, surgical procedure(s), and NPO status.[2] ♦ Assess the patient's baseline skin condition, body mobility, sensory impairments, allergies, idiosyncrasies, and sensitivities that require additional precautions.[3] ♦ Identify patients' physical alterations that require additional precautions for procedure-specific positioning.[4] ♦ Implement protective measures and appropriately apply safety devices to protect patients during all phases of care.[5] ♦ Evaluate patients for signs and symptoms of physical injuries.[6] ♦ Collaborate with staff and other disciplines to incorporate elements of evidence-based practice and prevailing standards of safety into the individual plan of care.[7] ♦ Administer medications according to safe medication practices as prescribed and monitor patient responses.[8]	♦ Peer review ♦ Direct observation ♦ Written or verbal reports (eg, incident reports, compliance issues) ♦ Quality improvement (QI)/performance improvement (PI) reports ♦ Peer review ♦ Documentation review Other: _____
	Acts in a timely fashion in response to adverse events to assist staff in evaluating the error, near miss, or patient injury.	♦ Direct observation ♦ Peer review ♦ Written or verbal reports (eg, incident reports, QI/PI reports) Other: _____
	Collaborates with other members of the health care team to implement actions to mitigate further injury.	♦ Direct observation ♦ Peer review Other: _____

Patient Outcome	PNDS Interventions as Measurable Criteria	Recommendations for Validation of Competency
	Domain 2: PHYSIOLOGIC	
	Competency Statement: **The perioperative care coordinator demonstrates competency to direct and evaluate the nursing staff's ability to assess their patients' physical, biochemical, and functional responses.**	
The physical, biochemical, and functional responses to the intended therapeutic effects of an operative or other invasive procedure of individuals and groups of patients are consistent with expectations or improved from baseline levels established preoperatively (eg, surgical wound/tissue perfusion; normothermia; fluid-electrolyte and acid-base balances; respiratory, cardiac, and neurological status; pain; infection and inflammation).[9]	**Clinical Resource Expert** Acts as clinical resource for perioperative nursing staff and incorporates the following activities: ♦ Ensures that the appropriate equipment and supplies are available. ♦ Responds promptly to team requests for immediate or emergent assistance.	♦ Direct observation ♦ Communication records (eg, staff communication log, staff meeting minutes, daily report) ♦ Peer review ♦ Incident/variance reports Other:_____
	Participates in the planning and provision of perioperative team education related to age-specific physiologic responses.	♦ Direct observation ♦ Communication records (eg, staff communication log, staff meeting minutes, daily report) ♦ Inservice/education session participant evaluations or attendance sheets ♦ Documentation of required staff competencies ♦ Peer review Other: _____
	Collaborates with staff and other disciplines to incorporate evidence-based practice and prevailing standards into the individual plan of care.[10]	♦ Direct observation ♦ Peer review ♦ QI/PI reports Other: _____

	Clinical Coordinator
	Manages the care provided to multiple patients in one or more services or specialties to ensure that staff properly:
	♦ Assess pain control and respiratory, cardiac, and neurological status to
	  – establish baseline,
	  – continuously monitor, and
	  – report changes throughout the continuum of care.[11]
	♦ Review diagnostic studies and report deviations from normal to appropriate member of the health care team.[12]
	♦ Participate in the management of blood, fluid, and electrolytes.[13]
	♦ Implement pain guidelines, assessing response to pain control and interventions.[14]
	♦ Assess patient susceptibility to infection and plan, implement, and monitor aseptic technique to prevent surgical infection.[15]
	♦ Assess risk for hypothermia and plan, implement, and monitor thermoregulation measures and the patient's temperature.[16]
	♦ Use critical thinking to take action when there is a change in patient status.
	♦ Provide and/or assist in providing status report to family/ support person.
		♦ Direct observation
		♦ Peer review
		♦ Written or verbal reports (eg, incident reports, compliance issues)
		♦ QI/PI reports
		Other: _____

Patient Outcome	PNDS Interventions as Measurable Criteria	Recommendations for Validation of Competency
	**Domain 3A: BEHAVIORAL RESPONSES**	
	*Competency Statement:* **The perioperative care coordinator demonstrates competency to direct and evaluate the nursing staff's ability to assess the psychological, sociologic, and spiritual responses of their patients and families.**	
Patients and their families demonstrate knowledge of the expected responses to a surgical or other invasive procedure.[17]	**Clinical Resource Expert** Acts as clinical resource for perioperative nursing staff, patients, and families to ♦ provide staff support for the provision of patient/ family education, and ♦ provide educational resources for perioperative registered nurses.	♦ Direct observation ♦ Communication records (eg, staff communication log, staff meeting minutes, daily report) ♦ Peer review Other: _____
Patients and their families demonstrate knowledge of the nutrition, medication management, pain management, rehabilitation, and wound healing required for postoperative recovery.[18]	Participates in planning and providing education related to age-specific behavioral responses.	♦ Inservice/education session participant evaluations or attendance sheets ♦ Documentation of required staff competencies ♦ Peer review ♦ Communication records (eg, staff communication log, staff meeting minutes, daily report) ♦ QI/PI reports ♦ Occurrence/variance reports Other: _____
	Clinical Coordinator Collaborates with staff and other disciplines to improve processes related to patient/family teaching and the psychological, sociologic, and spiritual responses of their patients and families using QI/PI tools.	♦ Direct observation ♦ Peer review ♦ Documentation review (eg, chart review, forms review) Other: _____
	Manages the care provided to multiple patients in one or more services or specialties to ensure that staff properly: ♦ Involve patient and family in planning care, education, communication, and provision of support. ♦ Use appropriate assessment skills to determine the patient's/family's ability to comprehend information provided and to incorporate that information into activities. ♦ Instruct patient/family about – medication management, – pain management, and – wound care. ♦ Evaluate patient/family responses to instruction return demonstrations as appropriate.[19]	♦ Direct observation ♦ Peer review ♦ Written or verbal reports (eg, incident reports, compliance issues) ♦ QI/PI reports ♦ Documentation review (eg, chart review) Other: _____

Patient Outcome	PNDS Interventions as Measurable Criteria	Recommendations for Validation of Competency
	Domain 3B: BEHAVIORAL RESPONSES— PATIENT AND FAMILY RIGHTS/ETHICS *Competency Statement:* The perioperative care coordinator demonstrates competency to direct and evaluate the nursing staff's ability to provide consistent, competent, and ethical care.	
Patients receive consistent, competent, and ethical care within standards of professional nursing practice and in compliance with regulations and accreditation standards.[20]	**Clinical Resource Expert** Acts as clinical resource for perioperative health care team, patients, and families.	♦ Direct observation ♦ Communication records (eg, staff communication log, staff meeting minutes, daily report) ♦ Peer review Other: _____
	Facilitates staff compliance with organizational policies, accreditation standards, governmental regulations, and professional standards of care.	♦ QI/PI reports ♦ Direct observation ♦ Occurrence/variance reports Other: _____
	Acts as a role model to preserve and protect patient autonomy, dignity, and human rights, providing care in a nondiscriminatory and nonprejudicial manner.[21]	♦ Direct observation ♦ Peer review Other: _____
	Clinical Coordinator Manages the care provided to multiple patients in one or more services or specialties to ensure that staff properly: ♦ Include patient/family in – consent verification, – preoperative teaching, – discharge planning, and – the perioperative plan of care. ♦ Maintain the patient's dignity, privacy and confidentiality by – initiating traffic control to restrict access to authorized individuals, and – securing records, belongings, and valuables. ♦ Provide care in a nondiscriminatory, nonprejudicial manner regardless of setting. ♦ Preserve and protect patient autonomy, dignity, and human rights. ♦ Provide care without prejudicial behavior. ♦ Identify the patients' beliefs and values and incorporate pertinent information into the plan of care. ♦ Provide perioperative care in a nondiscriminatory manner.[22]	♦ Direct observation ♦ Peer review ♦ Written or verbal reports (eg, incident reports, compliance issues) ♦ QI/PI reports ♦ Chart review Other: _____
	Considers the patient's cultural values, beliefs, preferences, language barriers, and staff competencies when making assignments.[23]	♦ Documentation (eg, staff assignment sheet, case schedule) ♦ Direct observation ♦ Peer review Other: _____

Patient Outcome	PNDS Interventions as Measurable Criteria	Recommendations for Validation of Competency
	Domain 4: HEALTH SYSTEM	
	Competency Statement: The perioperative care coordinator demonstrates competency to direct and evaluate the nursing staff's ability to provide perioperative patient care. The perioperative care coordinator competencies include clinical, operational, and fiscal management skills.	
The health system provides comprehensive care that is targeted to unique patient needs. The perioperative care coordinator utilizes standards of care and evidence-based practices to achieve safe quality patient outcomes while adhering to organizational policies and protocols, regulations, and accreditation guidelines.	**Leadership** Demonstrates collaborative/consultative/negotiation skills by performing the following activities: ♦ Collects and analyzes data required to facilitate collaboration and negotiation with stakeholders. ♦ Reviews the case schedule in advance and initiates interventions and consultation as needed. ♦ Queries physicians and perioperative staff to identify needs. ♦ Demonstrates effectiveness in negotiations and compromise as needed to ensure positive outcome. ♦ Actively collaborates with other health care professionals and departments to improve patient care and prevent negative patient outcomes (eg, infection control department, advanced practice nurse).	♦ Direct observation ♦ Peer review ♦ Verbal and written documentation (eg, incident reports, patient complaints) ♦ Communication records (eg, staff communication log, staff meeting minutes, daily report) ♦ QI/PI reports ♦ Evidence of committee participation/leadership Other: _____
	Demonstrates effective communication with members of the perioperative team and other stakeholders within and outside the organization. ♦ Uses effective written and verbal communication in an organized, logical, and concise manner to convey information to superiors, staff, physicians, patients, and families. ♦ Adapts communication techniques appropriate to the situation. ♦ Incorporates good listening skills. ♦ Evaluates effectiveness of communication. ♦ Identifies barriers to communication. ♦ Guides others to develop effective communication.	♦ Direct observation ♦ Peer review ♦ Verbal and written documentation (eg, incident reports, patient complaints) ♦ Communication records (eg, staff communication log, staff meeting minutes, daily report) ♦ QI/PI reports Other: _____
	Coordinates, facilitates, and manages change by performing the following activities. ♦ Assesses the need, readiness, and environment for change. ♦ Demonstrates knowledge of the change process. ♦ Participates in the development of the project plan. ♦ Assists with the implementation of the change.	♦ Direct observation ♦ Project plan reports ♦ Peer review Other: _____
	Utilizes effective conflict resolution techniques by performing the following activities: ♦ Mediates interdepartmental and intradepartmental conflict ♦ Follows the appropriate chain of command. ♦ Evaluates outcome of conflict resolution.	♦ Direct observation ♦ Peer review ♦ Formal and informal verbal and written reports ♦ Evidence of team accord Other: _____

AORN Bariatric Surgery Guideline

I. Overview

A. Introduction

Assumptions

This document is intended to serve as a guide for perioperative nurses and others currently involved in the care of morbidly obese patients and to assist those working to establish bariatric surgical services in the facilities where they practice. The guideline is designed to assist perioperative practitioners in creating and maintaining an optimal health care environment for bariatric patients. The guideline defines the unique physical and psychosocial needs of the patient population that is morbidly obese and presents guidance for establishing a bariatric surgery program.

The "AORN bariatric surgery guideline" is based on current available research and expert opinion. It is assumed that ongoing research will result in new knowledge, procedures, and medical and nursing interventions for the treatment of morbid obesity. This guideline may require modification based on specific patient and facility needs.

Bariatric surgery is the surgical treatment of morbid obesity. It is a recognized subspecialty in the field of general surgery and is a rapidly growing subspecialty in the United States and throughout the world. The goal of bariatric surgery is to achieve sustained weight loss and reversal of patients' comorbidities. The recent increase in both the popularity of and demand for bariatric surgery can be attributed primarily to two factors: there are no nonsurgical approaches that are effective long term for treating morbid obesity, and the overall success of weight loss surgery has resulted in greater acceptance of surgery as a treatment option.

Definitions

For the purposes of this document, the following definitions apply.

Anastomosis—The surgical connection of two hollow structures (eg, stomach to intestine, intestine to intestine, intestine to colon, bile duct to intestine). The structures can be connected end to end, end to side, or side to end. The connection can be accomplished by use of sutures, surgical staples, or a combination of both.

Band—A constricting device that limits the movement of food from the stomach. The device may be placed around the entire stomach, a portion of the stomach, or a portion of the intestine and may consist of tissue, mesh, silastic tubing, or other material approved for this use.

Bariatric surgery—Any surgical procedure performed for the purpose of producing weight loss.

Biliopancreatic limb—The segment of small bowel connecting the bile duct to the distal end of the Roux limb. This segment follows the Roux limb and is the bile-carrying limb.

Body mass index (BMI)—A mathematical calculation used to determine whether a patient is overweight. It is calculated by dividing a person's body weight in kilograms by his or her height in meters squared (kg/m^2).

Common channel—The segment of small bowel where the biliopancreatic limb and the Roux limb become one and continue to the cecum. Complex proteins, fats, and carbohydrates are digested in the common channel.

Comorbidity—One or more coexisting diseases or conditions in addition to the condition that is the subject of study.

Malabsorption—Incomplete digestion or absorption of food intake.

Morbid obesity—Having a BMI greater than 40 with or without comorbidities.

Pouch—A surgically created portion of the stomach that serves as a reservoir for food immediately after food exits the esophagus.

Restrictive—Decreasing or limiting the amount of food intake.

Roux limb—The segment of small bowel where food exits the stomach and enters the bowel. The Roux limb starts where food enters and ends where the biliopancreatic limb joins it to form the common channel.

Staple line—A row of staples placed in the bowel or stomach by a surgical stapling device. Staples can be used to create an anastomosis, create a partition, or secure the end of the bowel when a side anastomosis is performed.

B. Population Affected

Prevalence

In the twenty-first century, obesity may be the number one US public health problem.[1] The prevalence of obesity is global and ranks high in the United State, as well as in other developed nations.[2] Nearly

Table 1

WEIGHT CATEGORY BASED ON BODY MASS INDEX (BMI)	
BMI (kg/m²)	*Category*
< 18.5	Underweight
18.5 – 24.99	Normal
25 – 26.99	Overweight
27 – 30	Mild obesity
> 30	Moderate obesity
> 35	Severe obesity
> 40	Morbid obesity
> 50	Super obesity

two-thirds of US adults are overweight, including those who are obese.[3,4] Overweight is defined as having excess body weight compared to preset standards. This excess weight can be composed of muscle, bone, fat, or body water. Obesity refers specifically to having an abnormal proportion of body fat. Although it is possible to be overweight without being obese (eg, heavily muscled athletes, body builders), many people who are overweight also are obese. Of all US adults (ie, people 20 years of age or older), 129.6 million (64.5%) are overweight. This includes 64.5 million women (61.9%) and 65.1 million men (67.2%).[3,4] There also has been a continual increase in the number of children and adolescents who are overweight. Approximately 15.3% of children (ie, ages six to 11) and 15.5% of adolescents (ie, ages 12 to 17) were overweight in 2000, a significant increase from approximately 5% in the 1960s and 1970s.[3,4] Of all US adults, 61.3 million (30.5%) are obese. This includes 34.7 million (33.4%) women and 26.6 million (27.1%) men.[2]

Socioeconomic factors

Health care costs associated with being overweight and obese have escalated. Estimated annual medical spending due to overweight and obesity may have been as high as $78.5 billion in 1998, which is $92.6 billion in 2002 dollars.[5] According to one study, this represents 9.1% of US health care expenditures.[5,6]

Costs are divided into direct health care costs and indirect costs. Direct health care costs refer to diagnostic and treatment services (eg, physician costs, medications, hospital and nursing home care) and preventive services. Indirect costs include the cost of wages lost by people unable to work because of illness or disability, as well as the cost of future lost earnings because of premature

death. Americans spend $33 billion annually on weight-loss products and services, including low-calorie foods, artificially sweetened products, and memberships to commercial weight-loss centers.[6]

C. Pathophysiology

Obesity is a life-threatening, genetically related, costly, life-long, progressive, multifactoral disease of excess fat storage. Body mass index is a mathematical calculation used to determine whether a person is overweight. It is calculated by dividing a person's body weight in kilograms by his or her height in meters squared. A person is considered obese if he or she weighs 20% or more above a predetermined ideal weight, or has a BMI greater than or equal to 30 (Table 1).[7]

Morbid obesity, which also is called clinically severe obesity, correlates with a BMI of greater than 40 or with being 100 lbs overweight. Morbid obesity is associated with numerous health problems, which are referred to as comorbidities and is directly related to mortality rates. A 12-year study of 750,000 individuals found that mortality rates for men and women who weighed 50% more than the average weight for their height increased approximately twofold.[8]

Common comorbidities

The most common comorbidities associated with morbid obesity are type II diabetes, hypertension, atherosclerosis, hyperlipidemia, stroke, gallbladder disease, arthritis of weight bearing joints, sleep apnea, alveolar hypoventilation, urinary stress incontinence, gastroesophageal reflux disease, infertility, certain cancers (ie, colorectal, kidney, breast, uterine), and sudden death.[9] To date, long-term medical therapies and regimens have not been effective in treating morbid obesity.

D. History

Bariatric surgery evolved in the 1950s following observation that individuals who had short-bowel syndrome lost weight as a result of inadequate nutrient absorption. Bariatric surgery was introduced by A. J. Kremen, MD, and his associates, who performed and published reports of a jejunoileal bypass procedure.[10] In the procedure, the upper small intestine was anastomosed to the lower small intestine in an attempt to bypass much of the absorptive circuit. At about the same time, a Swedish physician performed a similar procedure, but he excised the redundant portion of the small intestine.

In the 1960s, researchers published reports of 10 jejunalcolic shunt procedures in which the upper small intestine was anastomosed to the colon, with the intent of bypassing even more of the nutrient absorbing gastrointestinal tract.[10] Unfortunately, these patients experienced uncontrollable diarrhea, dehydration, and electrolyte imbalance. Ultimately, the shunts were converted to jejunoileostomies in which the upper portion of the jejunum was anastomosed to the lower portion of the ileum. Nevertheless, patients with jejunoileal bypass continued to experience diarrhea caused by fatty acid irritation of the colon from interference with bile digestion of the ingested fats. This diarrhea resulted in fluid and electrolyte imbalance, which was a major complaint among patients and physicians. Additional complications included mineral and electrolyte imbalances, vitamin depletion, anemia, cholelithiasis, and renal and liver disease. Other procedures were developed, including gastric bypass, because of these complications. The jejunoileal bypass no longer is a recommended bariatric surgical procedure.[10]

In 1966, gastric bypass was developed and introduced by Edward E. Mason, MD, of the University of Iowa. Dr Mason developed the procedure based on the observation that women who had undergone partial gastrectomy for peptic ulcer disease tended to remain underweight after the surgery and that it was difficult to achieve weight gain in this patient population. He applied the principles of partial gastrectomy to women who were obese and found that they lost weight. Using surgical staples, he created a partition across the upper stomach and anastomosed this pouch to the small intestine. Complications of the early gastric bypass procedures led to the further development and refinement of gastroplasty in the late 1960s and early 1970s.

In the mid-1970s, in an effort to simplify gastric restriction, Dr Mason divided the stomach transversely toward the greater curvature where he left a small channel; however, this outlet subsequently enlarged.[11] This led to experimentation with horizontal gastroplasties. Unfortunately, the upper gastric pouch and the outlet tended to enlarge, leading to weight regain.[11] In response, Dr Mason partitioned the stomach vertically (ie, vertical gastroplasty) because the thicker muscle along the lesser curva-

ture was thought to be more resistant to dilatation. In addition, the outlet was banded by a mesh strip or a silastic ring to prevent enlargement.[11]

In the late 1970s, biliopancreatic diversion was developed in Genoa, Italy. The weight loss that occurs after this procedure initially is related to the restriction of food intake from the decreased size of the available gastric pouch, which later enlarges. The weight loss, however, is maintained by a tolerable degree of malabsorption of starches and fats in the common limb. The biliopancreatic diversion provides the greatest loss of excess weight (ie, up to 80% excess weight loss) of any of the bariatric procedures, but it requires surgical expertise and close, long-term follow-up because nutritional deficiencies may develop. In the biliopancreatic diversion, both the Roux limb and the biliopancreatic limb are long with a shortened common channel.

A modification of the biliopancreatic diversion in wide use is the duodenal switch procedure. This is performed by resecting the greater curvature of the stomach, leaving the entire lesser curvature and pylorus in continuity.[10] The biliopancreatic limb is separated from the proximal, food-carrying duodenum and re-anastomosed to the distal portion of the Roux limb to form the common channel. The Roux limb is connected just below the pylorus by means of an end-to-side anastomosis.

In the 1970s and 1980s, gastric banding was developed as another method of limiting food intake.[10] The band is placed near the upper end of the stomach just below the junction of the stomach and the esophagus. Early attempts were unsuccessful because readily available materials, such as arterial grafts, were used for banding. Later, bands were developed specifically for this purpose along with techniques to measure stoma size. Later in the 1980s, the adjustable gastric band—a hollow band with an inflatable balloon as its lining—was developed by Lubomyr I. Kuzmak, MD. The balloon is connected to a small reservoir that is placed under the skin in the upper abdomen. Adjustment of the gastric restriction occurs from injection or withdrawal of saline from the reservoir.[12]

During the past decade, minimally invasive laparoscopic surgery became the technique of choice. These procedures are less invasive, and patients often can return home on the day of surgery. Patients also can return to work and activities of daily living more quickly. Bariatric surgery is a

Table 2

HISTORY OF BARIATRIC SURGERY	
Decade	**Procedure**
1950s	Jejunoileal bypass
1960s	Jejunocolic bypass
	Gastric bypass
1970s	Gastroplasty
	Biliopancreatic diversion
1980s	Gastric banding
	Adjustable gastric banding
1990s	Laparoscopic procedures

serious undertaking, however, and it should be recommended only for patients who meet carefully defined criteria. Table 2 provides a summary of bariatric surgery history.

E. Patient Selection Criteria

The option of surgical treatment should be offered to patients who are morbidly obese, well-informed, and motivated and who have acceptable surgical risks. Patients should be able to participate in treatment and long-term follow-up. Patients with manifest psychopathology that would jeopardize informed consent and cooperation with long-term follow-up may not be candidates for bariatric surgery. A decision to select surgical treatment should be determined on an individual basis according to an in-depth assessment of the risks and benefits for each individual. Increased abdominal fat or central obesity (ie, apple shape as opposed to pear shape) is a significant risk factor associated with major complications from obesity. Functional impairments associated with obesity also are important factors for deciding on treatment via surgery. According to the National Institutes Consensus Development Conference statement on the surgical treatment of obesity,

> Patients judged by experienced clinicians to have a low probability of success with non-surgical measures, as demonstrated, for example, by failure in established weight control programs or reluctance by the patient to enter such a program, may be considered for surgical treatment.[13]

Bariatric surgery standards for candidate qualifications are set by the National Institutes of Health (NIH) and the American Society of Bariatric Surgeons (ASBS). To qualify for surgery and possible compensation by the insurer, patients must

- be determined to make lifestyle and eating habit changes,
- be severely obese (ie, BMI greater than 35) with one or more comorbidities,
- have made numerous attempts at medical weight loss, and/or
- be morbidly obese with a BMI greater than 40 with or without comorbidities.

As noted, treatment must be tailored to the individual concerned. The BMI is only one of many criteria for investigating and selecting a surgical option and weight management goal. The following are other factors to consider.

- Medical comorbidities (eg, diabetes, hypertension, sleep apnea, hypercholesterolemia, infertility, urinary stress incontinence, dysmenorrhea).
- Functional factors—is the patient able to perform activities of daily living, dine out, or travel?
- Psychological comorbidities—an evaluation by a licensed psychologist is advised because patients with manifest psychopathology can jeopardize informed consent and cooperation with long-term follow-up.
- Social factors—many morbidly obese patients face harassment and prejudice due to their size. They may have a limited number of friends, and society as a whole regards obesity in the same context as alcoholism and drug addiction. Will the patient have or need a system of support postoperatively?
- Economic factors—people who are obese find it harder to enroll in school or universities or obtain employment. Will the patient's quality of life improve with the selected bariatric procedure?
- Endocrine status—does the patient have an endocrine condition that contributes to or causes the obesity?
- Substance dependency—is the patient alcohol or drug dependent?
- Eating habits—is the patient a grazer (ie, eats small quantities of food continuously), a sweeter (ie, ingests calories mainly from sweets), or a bloater (ie, eats a huge meal at one sitting)? These different eating behaviors should be approached with different surgical options for successful weight loss and weight management outcomes. Often, patients fit more than one category, making selection of the correct procedure more difficult.

F. Surgical Choices in the New Century

There are three categories of bariatric procedures. These include malabsorptive, restrictive, and combined restrictive and malabsorptive procedures.

Malabsorptive procedures

Malabsorptive procedures are associated with incomplete digestion or absorption of food. Jejunoileal bypass is the classic example of a malabsorptive weight loss procedure. Some modern procedures use a lesser degree of malabsorption combined with gastric restriction to induce and maintain weight loss. Any patient undergoing a procedure involving malabsorption must be considered at risk to develop at least some of the malabsorptive complications created by jejunoileal bypass. The multiple complications associated with jejunoileal bypass, although considerably less severe than those associated with jejunocolic anastomosis, were sufficiently distressing both to patients and physicians to result in its being deemed an undesirable procedure.[10]

Biliopancreatic diversion. Biliopancreatic diversion is a malabsorptive procedure used today. In the biliopancreatic diversion, both the Roux limb and the biliopancreatic limb of the small bowel are quite long with a shortened common channel where digestion of proteins, fats, and carbohydrates takes place (Figure 1).

Advantages of the biliopancreatic diversion include

- greater weight loss than with other procedures;
- greater long-term success from lifelong malabsorption of food;[14]
- a larger stomach pouch that allows a return to fairly normal eating habits, thus improving quality of diet; and
- an increased chance of improving certain comorbidities, such as diabetes and hypertension.[14]

Disadvantages of biliopancreatic diversion include

- longer surgery time (ie, averaging three to four hours);
- greater risks for both surgical and general complications compared to other procedures;
- greater risks for nutritional and functional deficiencies due to high malabsorption of food—these deficiencies include fat soluble vitamins (eg, A, D, E, K);

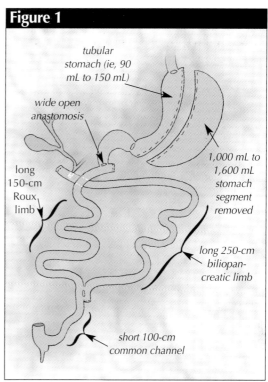

Figure 1

tubular stomach (ie, 90 mL to 150 mL)

wide open anastomosis

long 150-cm Roux limb

1,000 mL to 1,600 mL stomach segment removed

long 250-cm biliopancreatic limb

short 100-cm common channel

Biliopancreatic diversion with duodenal switch and vertical gastroplasty/sleeve gastrectomy.

- risk of liver abnormalities;
- risk of insufficient calcium absorption, resulting in bone disease;
- risk of lactose intolerance;
- risk of severe iron anemia; and
- possible offensive, foul-smelling soft bowel movements and flatus.[14]

Restrictive procedures

Restrictive procedures reduce the size of the stomach to decrease or limit the intake of food so small amounts of food give a feeling of fullness. Examples of restrictive procedures are proximal gastric bypass, vertical banded gastroplasty, and adjustable gastric banding procedures.

Proximal gastric bypass. Proximal gastric bypass primarily is a restrictive procedure, although it does have a minimal absorptive component. Proximal gastric bypass involves creating a small pouch at the top of the stomach. The remainder of the stomach remains intact. The Roux limb of the intestine is attached to the created pouch with a small anastomosis intended to slow emptying of the pouch into the intestine. The Roux limb is relatively

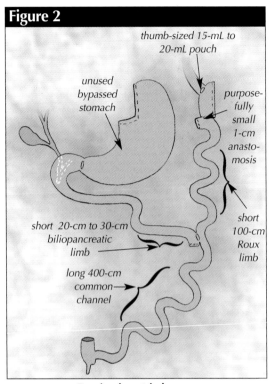

Figure 2

thumb-sized 15-mL to 20-mL pouch

unused bypassed stomach

purposefully small 1-cm anastomosis

short 20-cm to 30-cm biliopancreatic limb

short 100-cm Roux limb

long 400-cm common channel

Proximal gastric bypass.

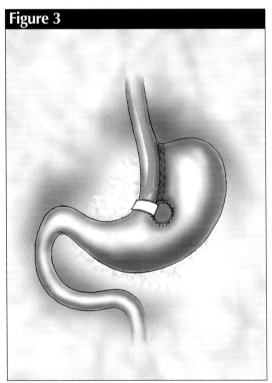

Figure 3

Vertical banded gastroplasty creates a tubular stomach that is restrictive.

short before being joined by the short biliopancreatic limb to create a long common channel. The long common channel allows for absorption of nutrients (Figure 2).

The proximal bypass works for patients who are sweeters and bloaters, but grazers can successfully overcome the restriction by continuously eating small amounts of food. Patients can achieve 60% to 65% loss of excess body weight, but approximately 25% of patients experience a 20% to 30% weight gain after three years.[7] Advantages of the proximal gastric bypass include

- minimized dumping syndrome, which can be partially controlled by avoiding sugars, and
- absence or minimal occurrence of acid reflux.

Disadvantages of proximal gastric bypass include

- the possibility of an anastomotic stricture and
- the possibility of anastomotic ulceration.[7]

Vertical banded gastroplasty. In vertical banded gastroplasty surgery, the stomach is partitioned vertically along the lesser curvature of the stomach. Unless a duodenal switch is performed to lessen absorption, the pylorus and small intestine remain intact. The procedure (without duodenal switch) is purely restrictive, and weight loss is achieved because of the restricted intake of food. Both polypropylene mesh bands and silastic rings have been used to prevent stretching of the newly created stomach outlet. The bands are placed at the stomal outlet to prevent or limit stomal stretching and subsequent weight gain. The band or ring circumference is somewhat larger than the stoma when it is created, so the limiting effect only occurs after the pouch has stretched to some degree (Figure 3).[10]

Vertical banded gastroplasty achieves gastric partitioning, has been widely performed, and generally is associated with satisfactory weight loss. The procedure works well for bloaters, but it often is unsuccessful for sweeters and grazers. Advantages of vertical banded gastroplasty include that

- it has lower perioperative complication rates than other restrictive procedures,
- it technically is easier to perform, and
- it has a low mortality rate.

Disadvantages of vertical banded gastroplasty include

- rare staple line leaks, which can be dangerous if not diagnosed immediately;

♦ vertical line disruption due to vomiting caused by overeating;
♦ risk of infection;
♦ possible incisional hernia; and
♦ risk of band erosion, usually caused by ulcer formation near the restrictive device.[7]

Adjustable gastric band. Adjustable gastric banding is a restrictive procedure in which the surgeon places an inflatable silicone band completely around the upper portion of the stomach. This band usually is placed endoscopically. The band constricts the stomach, thus producing a small pouch with a narrow opening into the lower stomach. The small pouch size decreases food intake and creates a feeling of fullness. With the adjustable band, there are no anatomical removals or rearrangements. The inflatable band is connected to a small reservoir that is placed under the skin in the upper abdomen. Adjustment of the gastric restriction occurs from injection or withdrawal of saline from the reservoir.[7,10] The adjustable gastric band works best for bloaters. Sweeters and grazers simply must avoid sweets and snacks to achieve success with the adjustable band (Figure 4).

Advantages of adjustable banding include
♦ use of a minimally invasive approach;
♦ shorter average length of stay (ie, usually 24 hours);
♦ faster recovery period (ie, usually less than two weeks);
♦ no staple line to break down;
♦ that the band can be adjusted;
♦ that the procedure is reversible with normal stomach restoration; and
♦ that the band is easily deflated if necessary.
Disadvantages of adjustable banding include
♦ risk of foreign body reaction,
♦ that the band position can slip with subsequent tissue erosion,
♦ the possibility of access port leakage and infection, and
♦ that some insurance companies will not cover this procedure.

Combined restrictive and malabsorptive procedures
Both restrictive and malabsorptive procedures can result in complications. Combining the two, however, can have less drastic adverse effects on the body's gastrointestinal (GI) function.

Roux-en-Y gastric bypass. Roux-en-Y gastric bypass combines gastric restriction with a small

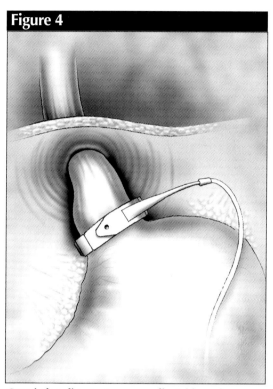

Figure 4

Gastric banding systems are adjustable and reversible and can be placed laparoscopically.

amount of malabsorption. In this procedure, the stomach is divided into two compartments with the upper part consisting of a small pouch capable of holding 1 oz to 2 oz. The lower compartment, approximately 90% of the original stomach, no longer stores food, but it continues to secrete digestive juices that flow into the duodenum. The jejunum is transected from the duodenum, and the upper jejunum then is connected to the pouch to allow food to pass from the pouch. The lower end of the jejunum is anastomosed to the biliopancreatic limb from which gastric and other digestive juices are delivered to the common channel where absorption takes place. Depending on the length of the Roux limb and the point of anastomosis forming the common channel, more or less absorption will occur. The decrease in absorption occurs because the food is not exposed to the digestive juices until the point of anastomosis.

If the anastomosis point creates a long common channel, the procedure is considered a proximal gastric bypass, and absorption will be greater (Figure 5). If the anastomosis creates a short common channel,

Figure 5

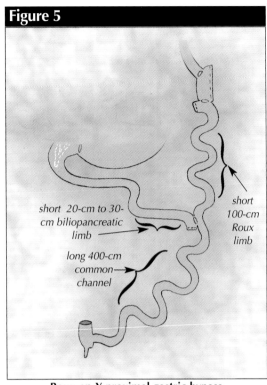

short 20-cm to 30-cm biliopancreatic limb

short 100-cm Roux limb

long 400-cm common channel

Roux-en-Y proximal gastric bypass.

Figure 6

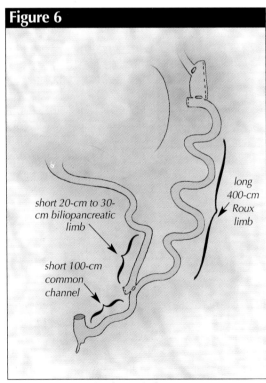

short 20-cm to 30-cm biliopancreatic limb

long 400-cm Roux limb

short 100-cm common channel

Distal gastric bypass.

the procedure is considered a distal gastric bypass, and less absorption will take place (Figure 6).

Advantages of the Roux-en-Y gastric bypass include

♦ both food restriction and malabsorption;

♦ optimal long-term weight loss results compared to restrictive only procedures; and

♦ documented improvement in comorbidities, especially type II diabetes.

Disadvantages of the Roux-en-Y gastric bypass include

♦ painful dumping syndrome that occurs with sugar consumption;

♦ longer average length of stay than with a restrictive only procedure;

♦ risk for nutritional complications, such as vitamin (eg, A, B12, D, E) and mineral (eg, calcium, iron, folic acid) deficiencies;

♦ risk for stomal stenosis requiring dilation;

♦ risk for Y-limb obstruction requiring surgical intervention;

♦ risk for anastomosis leakage;

♦ risk for marginal ulceration at the stomach to intestine anastomosis site; and

♦ risk for ventral incisional hernia.

Minimally invasive approach

In the 1990s, use of laparoscopic or minimally invasive surgery gained prominence in bariatric surgery. The development of specialized instruments, which obviate the need for the traditional abdominal incision, has advanced laparoscopic surgery. To perform laparoscopic bariatric procedures, surgeons must be competent and experienced in both open bariatric procedures and in laparoscopic procedures. Every bariatric procedure can be performed laparoscopically.

Laparoscopic surgery involves placing trocars through the skin. These trocars allow for passage of long, fiber-optic telescopes and narrow instruments, such as graspers, scissors, babcocks, and staplers, to perform the surgical procedure. Fiber-optic cameras and videotaping equipment also are used. Most laparoscopic bariatric surgery begins by inflating the patient's abdomen with carbon dioxide to allow the surgeon more visibility and space within the abdomen for greater ease of trocar placement. Advantages of a laparoscopic approach include

♦ enhanced visualization of anatomy;

♦ decreased surgical complications (eg, incisional hernia, infection);

♦ less postoperative pain; and

♦ shorter average length of stay.

Disadvantages of a laparoscopic approach include

♦ increased surgical time compared to an open approach,

♦ increased exposure to anesthetic agents and gases,

♦ added surgical costs because of additional supplies and equipment,

♦ risk of organ perforation, and

♦ possible necessity for conversion to an open approach.

G. Results

Weight loss usually reaches a maximum between 18 and 24 months postoperatively. Mean percent excess weight loss at five years ranges from 48% to 74% after gastric bypass and from 50% to 60% after vertical banded gastroplasty.[8] A study of more than 600 patients who underwent gastric bypass that had a 96% follow-up rate found that mean percent excess weight loss exceeded 50% at 14 years.[15] A 10-year follow-up series from the University of Virginia reported weight loss of 60% of excess weight at five years and more than 50% between years six and 10.[16] Other authors have reported five- and six-year follow-up of their patients with similar weight loss results.[15,17-22]

Weight reduction surgery has been reported to improve several comorbid conditions, including glucose intolerance and diabetes mellitus,[15] sleep apnea, obesity associated hypoventilation,[23,24] hypertension,[25] and serum lipid abnormalities.[23,24] One study demonstrated that type II diabetics treated medically had a mortality rate three times that of a comparable group that underwent gastric bypass surgery.[26] Improved heart function, decreased ventricular wall thickness, and decreased ventricular chamber size have been observed with sustained weight loss. Some patients experience improved mobility and stamina after surgical treatment for morbid obesity. Many patients report a better mood, greater self-esteem, improved interpersonal effectiveness, and enhanced quality of life.[27] They are less self-conscious[28] and are able to explore social and vocational activities formerly unavailable to them. Patients also are less inclined to be disparaging about their body image. If marital satisfaction existed before surgery, that satisfaction is likely to increase after surgery. If the couple experienced marital discord before surgery, the patient's improved self-image may lead to divorce postoperatively.[28]

II. Nursing Process Application

A. Perioperative Nursing Vocabulary

The perioperative nursing vocabulary is a clinically relevant and empirically validated standardized nursing language. It relates to the delivery of care in perioperative settings. This standardized language consists of a collection of data elements (ie, the Perioperative Nursing Data Set [PNDS]), and includes perioperative nursing diagnoses, interventions, and outcomes.[29] In 1999, the PNDS was recognized by the American Nurses Association's Committee on Nursing Practice Information Infrastructure as a data set useful in the practice of nursing. The perioperative patient focused model provides the conceptual framework for the PNDS and the model for perioperative nursing practice. The patient and his or her family members are at the core of the model. The model depicts perioperative nursing in four domains and illustrates the relationship between the patient, his or her family members, and care provided by the perioperative professional nurse. The patient-centered domains are

♦ D1—safety,

♦ D2—physiological responses to surgery,

♦ D3—patient and family member behavioral responses to surgery, and

♦ D4—health system in which perioperative care is provided.

Each data element in the PNDS is represented by a unique identifier. The domains are represented by the letter "D" followed by numbers one to four to indicate the particular domain being addressed. Nursing diagnoses are represented by the letter "X" and a number unique to the diagnosis; interventions are represented by the letter "I" and a unique number; and outcomes are represented by the letter "O" and a unique number. These designations are used in this document as appropriate.

B. Assessment

Perioperative nurses assess, document, and communicate patient status to all members of the health care team. Data collection involves the patient and his or her significant others. Patient assessment begins when the patient initially consults the bariatric physician or surgeon. The anesthesia care provider then should review the patient's medical history and develop a plan of care. Bariatric surgery patients should be assessed for the following risk factors:

- ◆ psychopathology—
  - may jeopardize informed consent, and
  - may jeopardize cooperation with long-term follow-up;
- ◆ body type—increased abdominal fat (ie, "central tendency");
- ◆ potential airway problems—
  - bariatric patients may need an awake intubation,
  - an airway cart should be available, and
  - bariatric patients desaturate quickly;
- ◆ circulation problems;
- ◆ skin integrity/breakdown; and
- ◆ medical comorbidities, including
  - diabetes,
  - hypertension,
  - sleep apnea,
  - hypercholesterolemia, and
  - stress incontinence.

C. Nursing Diagnoses

The perioperative nurse analyzes the assessment data to determine nursing diagnoses. Following is a partial list of nursing diagnoses that may be associated with patients undergoing bariatric surgery.

- ◆ X 30 (D3)—knowledge deficit;
- ◆ X 1 (D2)—activity intolerance;
- ◆ X 34 (D1)—physical mobility, impaired;
- ◆ X 4 (D3)—anxiety;
- ◆ X 37 (D2)—imbalanced nutrition (ie, more than body requirements);
- ◆ X 28 (D1)—infection, risk for;
- ◆ X 7 (D2)—breathing pattern, ineffective—related to morbid obesity and/or comorbidities;
- ◆ X 20 (D2)—fluid volume, risk for imbalance—related to altered nutritional state;
- ◆ X 26 (D2)—hypothermia; and
- ◆ X 33 (D3)—therapeutic regime management, ineffective—related to necessary lifestyle changes.

D. Outcome Identification

To develop a plan of care for the patient, the perioperative nurse identifies desired patient outcomes collaboratively with the patient. Following is a partial list of nursing outcomes that may be associated with patients having bariatric surgery.

- ◆ O 31 (D3)—The patient demonstrates knowledge of the expected responses to the operative or other invasive procedure.
- ◆ O 5 (D1)—The patient is free from signs and symptoms of injury related to positioning.
- ◆ O 10 (D2)—The patient is free from signs and symptoms of infection.
- ◆ O 13 (D2)—The patient's fluid, electrolyte, and acid-base balances are consistent with or improved from the baseline levels established preoperatively.
- ◆ O 18 (D3)—The patient demonstrates knowledge of nutritional requirements related to the operative or other invasive procedure.
- ◆ O 20 (D3)—The patient demonstrates knowledge of medication management.

E. Planning

The perioperative nurse develops a plan of care for the patient undergoing bariatric surgery that prescribes nursing interventions to attain expected outcomes. Interventions and activities are selected according to individual patient needs and the type of procedure to be performed. Following is a partial list of interventions that may be associated with patients having bariatric surgery.

- ◆ I 30—Develops an individualized plan of care.
- ◆ I 32—Elicits perceptions of surgery.
- ◆ I 56—Explains expected sequence of events.
- ◆ I 124—Verifies consent for planned procedure.
- ◆ I 64—Identifies physical alterations that require additional precautions for procedure-specific positioning.
- ◆ I 96—Positions the patient.
- ◆ I 38—Evaluates for signs and symptoms of injury as a result of positioning.
- ◆ I 46—Evaluates postoperative tissue perfusion.
- ◆ I 88—Monitors for signs and symptoms of infection.
- ◆ I 18—Administers prescribed prophylactic treatments.
- ◆ I 107—Provides instruction regarding dietary needs.
- ◆ I 108—Provides pain management instruction.
- ◆ I 150—Maintains patient's dignity and privacy.

F. Implementation

Interventions can be and usually are composed of many different activities. Implementation refers to the actual performance of the activities comprising the interventions in the individualized plan of care. The following are provided as examples of activities performed when caring for bariatric surgery patients. This is a multidisciplinary team approach (eg, includes members from medical, nursing, laboratory, radiology, nutrition, pharmacy staffs).

Preoperative

During the preadmission process, the nurse ensures that all laboratory work, x-rays, and other tests are performed before the day of admission for surgery. The anesthesia care provider reviews the patient's history and develops an anesthesia care plan. Other preoperative activities include the following.

♦ Perform a preoperative assessment, noting any circulatory or skin integrity problems and the patient's body type. Body type will affect positioning.

♦ Assess for comorbidities (eg, diabetes, hypertension, urinary incontinency) and initiate activities to address individual comorbidities.

♦ Weigh the patient on admission.
– Scales should be large enough to obtain an accurate weight.
– Do not use freight scales. This is demoralizing to the patient.

♦ Use only floor-mounted toilets for these patients. Wall-mounted units can break away when subjected to the patient's weight unless they are reinforced with grab bars.

♦ Supply larger patient gowns to ensure comfort and protect modesty.

♦ Perform continuous positive airway pressure procedures according to physician orders.

♦ Provide a gastric stretcher or gurney for bariatric patients. Other stretchers or gurneys have weight limits and may not be of sufficient dimension to accommodate the patient.

♦ Ensure that doorways are large enough, especially restroom doorways.

Intraoperative

The following activities should be performed in the OR.

♦ Place side attachments on the OR bed, if needed, for patients with extra-wide girth.

♦ Secure the patient to the OR bed.

♦ Protect skin integrity and circulation.

♦ Use two straps—one across the patient's thighs and the second across the lower legs.

♦ Provide emotional support to the patient.

♦ Assist the anesthesia care provider as necessary.

♦ Insert a Foley catheter, and attach it to a urimeter.

♦ Place an electrosurgical grounding pad on the patient's thigh or other appropriate location.

♦ Apply lower limb sequential compression devices or arterial venous compression boots.
– Apply to the lower legs only.
– Avoid devices that will roll and interfere with circulation.

♦ Position the patient.
– Place a padded footboard on the foot of the bed to prevent the patient from slipping when the bed is placed in the reverse Trendelenburg position. Ensure that the patient's feet and ankles are in an anatomically neutral position and secure them to the footboard.
– Place the patient's arms on extended arm boards. Wedges may be used if needed. Some procedures may require the patient's arms to be tucked securely at his or her sides to facilitate the surgeon's positioning (eg, when measuring the small bowel during the duodenal switch procedure).
– Pay special attention to the breasts of both male and female patients. Secure the patient in a manner to avoid injury.
– Pad all pressure points.
– Place padding between the patient and any positioning device attached to the OR bed.
– Place the patient in reverse Trendelenburg's position to facilitate access to the stomach area according to physician preference.

♦ Assess extremities for circulatory compromise.

♦ Place upper and lower temperature-regulating blankets on the patient to maintain his or her body temperature.[30]

Postoperative

The following activities should be performed postoperatively.

♦ Assess skin integrity, particularly at pressure points.

♦ Assess extremities for circulatory compromise.

♦ Move the patient to an appropriately sized bed for transport.

♦ Continue to perform continuous positive airway pressure procedures according to the physician's orders.

♦ Continue use of sequential compression devices, if ordered.

♦ Check dressings as appropriate for the procedure performed.

G. Evaluation of Outcomes

The perioperative nurse evaluates the patient's progress toward attainment of outcomes. This evaluation should be systematic, ongoing, and documented using the recognized, standardized perioperative nursing vocabulary. Outcome indicators will vary according to the specific desired outcome and may include

♦ physiological indicators (eg, nausea, vomiting, anastomosis leak, stricture, skin condition, deep vein thrombosis);

♦ cognitive indicators (eg, repeats instructions correctly, asks appropriate questions);

♦ affective indicators (eg, verbalizes individual needs and whether they are met, verbalizes and demonstrates willingness to comply with the treatment regimen);

♦ supportive resources (eg, family members participate in care planning and delivery); and

♦ patient satisfaction.

Evaluation of patient progress is based on observations of the patient's responses to nursing interventions and the effectiveness of interventions in moving the patient toward the desired outcome. Desired patient outcomes, nursing interventions, and potentially applicable nursing diagnoses are articulated in the standardized perioperative nursing vocabulary, which provides the basis for documentation of perioperative nursing practice. Ongoing assessment should be used to revise diagnoses, outcomes, and the plan of care as needed. Revisions in diagnoses, outcomes, and the plan of care should be documented. The patient, his or her significant others, and other health care providers should be involved in the evaluation process when appropriate.

III. Developing a Program

A. Financial Implications

When a facility begins a bariatric program, it is a significant financial commitment. It is important that the facility and its physicians understand the impact and begin discussion with payers to determine whether the procedures are covered and, if

so, what number of patients each insurer will cover at what reimbursement rates. If insurance companies do not cover the procedure, a self-pay schedule for these procedures needs to be determined based on total cost per procedure. This information will be used when developing the business plan.

With the increase in the number of bariatric procedures performed, the market has been flooded with new products. It is important for health care providers and administrators to be educated about what is available and to benchmark the facility's program with other programs to be competitive in the marketplace. Many companies help promote programs and surgeons and can help ensure the program is as cost-effective as possible.

Staffing is another significant financial consideration. Additional staffing will be needed to support a bariatric program. Patients who undergo bariatric surgery require more assistance. The surgeon may require additional personnel in the OR. After the patient is on the nursing unit, he or she will need assistance ambulating and with other activities of daily living for a period of time. Staff member availability is a serious consideration.

B. Rationale for a Bariatric Surgery Program

Careful consideration should be given to the driving forces for implementing a bariatric surgery program. Often a decision is made in an effort to differentiate the facility in the marketplace. An absence of such a program in the geographic area represents an opportunity for the facility to distinguish itself in the community. Surgeons with bariatric surgery expertise may be present on the staff of the facility, or it may be necessary to recruit these surgeons from elsewhere. Another driving force for program implementation is the potential return on investment. If bariatric surgeons already are present on staff, implementing a bariatric surgery program can represent new or expanded revenue. Even if the facility must recruit these surgeons, revenue potential exists. In addition, it is likely that a portion of patients having bariatric surgery will be self-pay clients, representing previously untapped revenue. Finally, patient demand may be the primary driving force for developing and implementing a program, provided it can be shown that such a program would be fiscally sound.

C. Elements of a Financially Successful Program

A successful bariatric surgery program will be multidisciplinary and comprehensive, offering all the necessary services within the program. There must be commitment to the program from the top of the organization down, beginning with the governing body and facility administrators. An accounting system capable of providing information about revenues and actual costs of the program will be essential. Knowledge about payers and reimbursement also will be necessary. As noted, it may be necessary to negotiate with third-party payers to determine exactly what services will be covered and to what extent they will be covered. Based on this knowledge, careful control of case mix will be important to maintain fiscal viability of the program. An appropriate mix of insured, partially insured, and self-pay clients can contribute to a successful program. Program marketing strategies also can play a role in the financial success of a program. This is especially important when there are multiple programs in an area. It will be important for the program to distinguish itself from others.

D. The Business Plan

A business plan should be developed for any new program, a change in an existing program, or for physician recruitment. The planning process will vary according to protocols in the individual facility or system. A bariatric surgery program should be thoroughly planned before procedures are performed. Many departments will be involved in some way in the care of patients having bariatric surgery, so the planning team may be quite large. At a minimum the team should include a

♦ facility administrator,
♦ chief financial officer,
♦ director of business development or marketing,
♦ director or vice president of clinical program management,
♦ director or chief of surgery and the sponsoring chief of service,
♦ director of perioperative services,
♦ director or vice president of patient care services, including nursing, and
♦ director of purchasing/contracting.

After completing the business plan and deciding to go forward with the program, others will join in making the plan operational and in actual plan implementation.

The business plan will vary according to the protocols and needs of the individual facility or system. The mission, vision, and strategic plan of the facility should be reviewed to determine that the proposed program fits within those parameters. If it does not, the program may not be appropriate for the facility, or the mission, vision, and strategic plan may require modification for congruency with the proposed program. The business plan should contain a description of the proposed program, including both clinical and educational components. An assessment of the internal environment and external environments will be an important part of the business plan. The internal assessment will consist of identifying strengths, weaknesses, opportunities, and threats (ie, SWOT analysis) of the system as it exists. The external assessment will consider things such as identified need, target market, competition, market share or potential market share, and regulatory or legislative issues.

Finally, the business plan will have a financial component in which projected costs and revenues will be identified. Costs will include the cost of program development and marketing; personnel, including physician recruitment if necessary; and technology and equipment. Space also must be considered, along with that needed for other systems that may be put into place or upgraded. The following list can be used to consider components to be included in the business plan:

♦ service description with clinical and educational components;
♦ program objectives;
♦ program incentives;
♦ service continuum;
♦ technology or equipment required for the program;
♦ timeline (ie, length of time to increase to full incremental volume);
♦ competition;
♦ target market and market share, including
  – inpatient surgeries,
  – diagnosis-related groups, and
  – outpatient visits;
♦ pricing and contracting;
♦ financial investment (eg, capital and operational costs), including
  – physician full-time equivalents (FTEs);
  – nonphysician FTEs;
  – equipment and supplies;
  – marketing;

- information systems;
- length and volume of OR procedures; and
- effects on the postanesthesia care unit (PACU), intensive care unit, and medical/surgical unit;
- ◆ regulatory issues; and
- ◆ barriers and obstacles.

When the business plan has been formulated, top administrative personnel should evaluate the plan and determine whether to proceed. When a decision is made to proceed, the plan should be reviewed with all stakeholders and those who will implement the plan. The plan should be familiar to these participants because their input was sought during creation of the business plan. It is important to include operations personnel during the planning process. The plan can be refined and some detail provided at this point in the process, but substantial changes should not be made without the approval of top administrators.

The plan should be funded from both the operational and capital budgets. After final approval and funding have been secured, staff members can be educated and the program launched. Periodic review and performance measurement will be essential to keep the program on track and viable. Program adjustments can be made based on performance reviews.

E. Operational Planning

After a commitment is made to move forward with a bariatric program, it is helpful to create a multidisciplinary operational planning team. Members of this team should include, but not be limited to,

- ◆ OR and PACU managers to coordinate program implementation;
- ◆ nurse educators to provide staff member education;
- ◆ anesthesia care provider(s) to collaborate on the development of the perioperative care pathway and coordinate education and equipment needs for the anesthesia department;
- ◆ surgeon(s) to collaborate on the development of the perioperative plan of care;
- ◆ a nutritionist to provide preoperative and postoperative teaching and support patients' nutritional needs;
- ◆ a respiratory therapist to promote best possible ventilation;
- ◆ a physical therapist to provide services, as needed;

- ◆ a medical/surgical nursing representative to plan for postoperative patient care;
- ◆ a pharmacist to ensure pharmaceutical needs are met;
- ◆ radiology and endoscopy representatives to provide for their role in the program, if required;
- ◆ a clinical psychologist for patient evaluation; and
- ◆ a materials manager to negotiate contracts and ensure adequate inventory.

The goal of the team is to plan program operation and create timelines and a plan for implementation. The size of the operational planning team and the magnitude of the project makes it useful to develop a team charter as a working document. This charter will provide clarity and a framework for the operational team. The charter should be written and should describe the mission of the team and how the mission will be accomplished. The charter directs the operational planning process, establishes key milestones for the process, and identifies desired outcomes. Elements of the team charter will vary depending on circumstances in the facility. Table 3 contains an example of elements to be included in a team charter.

F. Impact on the Workplace

To achieve a successful bariatric program, there must be a demonstrated commitment to provide adequate facilities and equipment. There also must be a multifaceted approach throughout the institution.

Physical plant considerations

All support areas of the hospital should have adequate equipment and furnishings to accommodate bariatric patients. The waiting area should contain

- ◆ appropriate furniture,
- ◆ love seats or chairs with extra width and side reinforcements,
- ◆ accessible bathrooms with floor-mounted or reinforced wall-mounted toilets at elevated levels with reinforced grab bars, and
- ◆ extra large wheelchairs.

The preoperative area should contain

- ◆ wide stretchers with fully functional hydraulics,
- ◆ extra large gowns with shoulder snaps,
- ◆ large and extra large blood pressure cuffs, and
- ◆ a wheelchair-accessible large scale.

The OR should contain

- an OR bed for bariatric procedures with the capacity to hold up to 1,000 lbs with 600 lbs tilt capacity—attachments to extend the sides of the bed should be included;
- a footboard with holders to attach to the bariatric OR bed;
- a hydraulic lift or appropriate moving device to ensure easy positioning of the patient and easier transfer back to the bed after surgery—this device should be ergonomically safe for staff members and protect them from back injuries;
- sequential compression devices (ie, knee high) or arterial-venous compression boots with appropriate motor units;
- a blanket on the bottom portion of the OR bed to wrap lower extremities to ensure thigh adduction while maintaining physiologic external rotation of the feet;
- foam padding for arms, heels, and feet;
- cotton cast padding to wrap the patient's arms on the arm board because the hook and loop fastener strap normally used alone may not be sufficient;
- a draw-sheet long enough to tuck the patient's arms at his or her sides;
- Hurst or Maloney dilators per the physician's preference (ie, sizes 30 to 60) to ensure adequate size of anastomosis;
- an endoscopy cart with an upper GI endoscope; and
- upper and lower body temperature-regulating blankets to ensure adequate body temperature.

Special instrumentation should include

- esophageal dilators,
- long instruments for open procedures, and
- long instruments for laparoscopic procedures.

Patients must be transported to the PACU in a bed appropriate to the patient's size and weight. The majority of patients will have a nasogastric (NG) tube in place. Within 12 to 24 hours, most patients will be taken to radiology to test the anastomosis for leaks. Some physicians prefer a leak test using methylene blue in sodium chloride via the NG tube.

Integrated services/multidisciplinary participation

A number of departments should be involved in the patient's care. The patient may need psychological, nutritional, and follow-up support.

Table 3

ELEMENTS TO INCLUDE IN A TEAM CHARTER

- Team name (eg, bariatric task force)
- Subject (eg, executing the bariatric business plan), which clarifies the purpose of the team
- Plan/version number—tracks versions as they are developed and accepted by the team
- Team sponsor—the senior leader who supports this effort and will be expected to break down barriers for the team
- Team leader—an individual who will guide the team to a successful outcome and will communicate with senior leadership
- Team facilitator—an optional support person who may be needed to promote effective group dynamics and provide structure and guidance
- Team members and areas of expertise—who will be on the team and why
- Team member time commitments—the team's meeting schedule and allowances for team members' planning
- Problem/opportunity statement—why this effort was initiated and what will be affected by the outcome
- Strategic alignment—how the development of this program aligns with organizational and departmental goals
- Scope—boundaries of the project
- Objectives—specific and measurable objectives
- Available resources—who and what is available to support the team
- Considerations (ie, assumptions, constraints, obstacles, risks)—identifies positive and negative factors and clarifies expectations
- Customers—patient population and customer needs
- Key stakeholders—who will be affected by the team and its work
- Key milestones/dates—specific expectations and deliverables
- Communication/action plan—who, how, and when
- Performance improvement—focus and a way to measure progress

Psychology. Of great concern is the lack of respect that people who are morbidly obese experience. A survey of individuals who were severely obese found that nearly 80% reported being treated disrespectfully by medical professionals.[31] There are widespread negative attitudes that adults who are morbidly obese are weak-willed, ugly, awkward, self-indulgent, and immoral. This intense prejudice cuts across age, gender, religion, race, and socioeconomic status. Numerous studies have documented the stigma people who are obese experience in most areas of social functioning. This can promote psychological distress and increase the risk of developing a psychological disorder. Patients who are morbidly obese are at risk for affective, anxiety, and substance abuse disorders. People who are obese often consider their condition to be a greater handicap than deafness, dyslexia, or blindness.[32,33]

Nutritional implications. Nutrients needed by all patients include water, protein, carbohydrates, fat, and vitamins. Dieticians play a pivotal role preoperatively and postoperatively in bariatric surgery. Preoperatively, the dietitian determines whether patients meet the NIH Consensus Panel's weight criteria calculations.[34] A full nutritional assessment is performed followed by a discussion of postoperative diet. Preoperative diet education classes have proven to be very successful. Postoperatively, the dietitian's role includes monitoring weight loss progress (ie, number of pounds lost; percentage of excess weight loss; percentage of weight loss; adequacy of dietary intake; exercise) and psychological and social support of the multiple changes that can occur in the patient's life.

Follow-up support groups. According to an NIH statement from September 1998, "An integrated program must be in place to provide guidance on diet, physical activity, and behavioral therapy, as well as to provide social support before and after surgery."[34] Patients are encouraged to consider joining a support group. These programs may be offered by the surgeon's office, the hospital, or a third party. Many patients find that a support group helps them deal with the challenges that may occur as a result of life and health changes. In one study, patients who regularly attended group meetings tended to lose more weight, and increased frequency of attendance was associated with greater weight loss.[35] It is critical that a support group leader have a full understanding of and be in compliance with the guidelines set forth by the surgeon. Everything that a support group leader says or does is perceived to be the surgeon's point of view. Great caution should be taken to ensure that support group leaders know and understand what kind of influence they have and are willing to assume the responsibility.

Employee education and competency

Staff members from all disciplines providing perioperative care to bariatric patients should participate in a comprehensive education program. The education plan for different disciplines will vary. For example, the education plan for nursing and specified disciplines should include, but not be limited to,

- an overview of the disease of morbid obesity and its associated comorbidities;
- the procedures performed and the associated complications during each phase of the perioperative period;
- obesity sensitivity training that focuses on the rights of each patient to be treated with dignity and the need to prevent obesity discrimination;
- obesity and bariatric surgery-related nutrition; and
- training and familiarity with all patient education materials, including
  - preoperative preparation materials,
  - nutrition materials,
  - postoperative care, and
  - long-term follow-up care postoperatively.

Nursing staff members who provide patient education should have a clear understanding of the preoperative evaluation process, including the preoperative testing regimen (eg, psychiatric screening, sleep studies, laboratory tests, upper GI series). Perioperative staff members should communicate to other caregivers along the continuum the patient's weight and BMI to individualize patient care needs (ie, gown size, bed selection, OR bed selection, patient transportation needs, other size-related aspects of care).

Intraoperative patient safety concerns, including positioning patients who are morbidly obese, should be reviewed, and competency should be validated. Intraoperative methods for measuring the integrity of the gastrojejunostomy should be the subject of an inservice program, and competency should be validated. Staff members should be knowledgeable about the quality indicators that will be used to monitor bariatric surgery, and results of this monitoring should be made available to staff members as part of a performance improvement process.

Staff members who provide care to bariatric patients would benefit from attending at least one of the classes patients are required to attend, as well as a support group meeting. It is suggested that these classes provide contact hours for hospital staff members who attend.

Physician education and competency

Bariatric surgeons, like those in other subspecialty areas, must be formally educated in bariatric surgery, acquire clinical experience, and demonstrate expertise in performing bariatric surgery before being granted privileges. The ASBS has published guidelines for granting privileges to surgeons who perform bariatric surgery.[36] The ASBS is a recognized educational professional medical society; it is not a credentialing body. Each facility should develop criteria and define acceptable credentials required for general surgeons to be eligible for privileges.

G. Inpatient Outcome Indicators

Each facility should identify and monitor outcome indicators to be reviewed by the hospital-wide process improvement committee. Such criteria should include, but not be limited to,

- average BMI of patients having bariatric surgery;
- postoperative admission to surgical intensive care;
- ambulation on the day of surgery;
- complications (eg, postoperative fever, nausea, vomiting, diarrhea, surgical site infection, deep vein thrombosis, pulmonary embolism, pneumonia);
- need to return to surgery (eg, anastomotic leak, small bowel obstruction, inguinal hernia, stricture);
- average length of stay; and
- readmission within 30 days.

IV. Conclusion

This guideline was developed to promote safe care for morbidly obese patients undergoing bariatric surgery. This surgery is complex and requires a special understanding of the needs of this patient population to ensure optimal outcomes. This document addresses prevalence, history, pathophysiology, program fundamentals, patient considerations, nursing process applications, and impact on the workplace. It is AORN's intent that practitioners will use this document in their facilities to develop policies, procedures, and protocols specific to bariatric surgery and care of patients who are morbidly obese. This guideline may require alteration based on specific patient and facility needs.

NOTES

1. "Overweight and obesity threaten US health gains," HHS News, *http://www.surgeongeneral.gov/news/pressreleases/pr_obesity.PDF* (accessed 9 Feb 2004).

2. "Statistics related to overweight and obesity," National Institute of Diabetes and Digestive and Kidney Diseases, Weight Control Information Network, *http://www.niddk.nih.gov/health/nutrit/pubs/statobes.htm* (accessed 9 Feb 2004)

3. C L Ogden et al, "Prevalence and trends in overweight among US children and adolescents, 1999-2000," *JAMA* 288 (Oct 9, 2002) 1728-1732.

4. R P Troiano, K M Flegal, "Overweight children and adolescents: Description, epidemiology, and demographics," *Pediatrics* 101 (March 1998) 497-504.

5. E A Finkelstein, I C Fiebelkorn, G Wang, "National medical spending attributable to overweight and obesity: How much, and who's paying?" *Health Affairs* Web exclusive, *http://content.healthaffairs.org/cgi/reprint/hlthaff.w3.219v1.pdf* (accessed 9 Feb 2004).

6. A M Wolf, G A Colditz, "Current estimates of the economic cost of obesity in the United States," *Obesity Research* 6 (March 1998) 97-106.

7. P Graling, H Elariny, "Perioperative care of the patient with morbid obesity," *AORN Journal* 77 (April 2003) 803.

8. "Rationale for the surgical treatment of morbid obesity," American Society for Bariatric Surgery, *http://www.asbs.org/html/rationale/rationale.html* (accessed 9 Feb 2004).

9. F Pi-Sunyer, "Comorbidities of overweight and obesity: Current evidence and research issue," *Medical Science Sports and Exercise* 31 suppl (November 1999) 602-608.

10. A MacGregory, "The story of surgery for obesity," American Society for Bariatric Surgery, *http://www.asbs.org/html/story/chapter 1.html* (accessed 9 Feb 2004)

11. M Deitel, S A Shikora, "The development of the surgical treatment of morbid obesity," *Journal of the American College of Nutrition* 21 (October 2002) 365-371.

12. L I Kuzmak et al, "Surgery for morbid obesity using an inflatable gastric band," *AORN Journal* 51 (May 1990) 1307-1324.

13. "Gastrointestinal surgery for severe obesity. Proceedings of a National Institutes of Health Consensus Development Conference. March 25-27, 1991, Bethesda, MD," *American Journal of Clinical Nutrition* 55 suppl (February 1992) 487S-619S.

14. B G Woodward, "Bariatric surgery options," *Critical Care Nursing Quarterly* 26 (April-June 2003) 89-100.

15. W J Pories et al, "Who would have thought it? An operation proves to be the most effective therapy for adult-onset diabetes mellitus," *Annals of Surgery* 222 (September 1995) 339-352.

16. H J Sugerman et al, "Gastric bypass for treating severe obesity," *American Journal of Clinical Nutrition* 55 suppl (February 1992) 560S-566S.

17. W C Willett et al, "Weight, weight change, and coronary heart disease in women. Risk within the 'normal' weight range," *JAMA* 273 (Feb 8, 1995) 461-465.

18. J H Linner, R L Drew, "Why the operation we prefer is the Roux-Y gastric bypass," *Obesity Surgery* 1 (September 1991) 305-306.

19. E E Mason, "Gastric surgery for morbid obesity," *Surgery Clinics of North America* 72 (April 1992) 501-513.

20. C E Yale, "Gastric surgery for morbid obesity. Complications and long-term weight control," *Archives of Surgery* 124 (August 1989) 941-946.

21. L D MacLean, B M Rhode, R A Forse, "Late results of vertical banded gastroplasty for morbid and super obesity," *Surgery* 107 (January 1990) 20-27.

22. J C Hall et al, "Gastric surgery for morbid obesity. The Adelaide Study," *Annals of Surgery* 211 (April 1990) 419-427.

23. R E Brolin, "Results of obesity surgery," *Gastroenterology Clinics of North America* 16 (June 1987) 317-338.

24. J J Gleysteen, "Results of surgery: Long-term effects on hyperlipidemia," *American Journal of Clinical Nutrition* 55 suppl (February 1992) 591S-593S.

25. P N Benotti et al, "Heart disease and hypertension in severe obesity: The benefits of weight reduction," *American Journal of Clinical Nutrition* 55 suppl (February 1992) 586S-590S.

26. K G MacDonald, Jr, et al, "The gastric bypass operation reduces the progression and mortality of non-insulin-dependent diabetes mellitus," *Journal of Gastrointestinal Surgery* 1 (May 1997) 213-220.

27. J G Kral, L V Sjostrom, M B Sullivan, "Assessment of quality of life before and after surgery for severe obesity," *American Journal of Clinical Nutrition* 55 suppl (February 1992) 611S-614S.

28. C S Rand, A Macgregor, G Hankins, "Gastric bypass surgery for obesity: Weight loss, psychosocial outcome, and morbidity one and three years later," *Southern Medical Journal* 79 (December 1986) 1511-1514.

29. S Beyea, ed, *Perioperative Nursing Data Set* (Denver: AORN, Inc, 2002).

30. *Health Implications of Obesity* (Rockville, Md: US Department of Health and Human Services, Public Health Service, National Institutes of Health, Office of Medical Applications of Research, 1985).

31. G L Maddox, V Leiderman, "Overweight as a social disability with medical implications," *Journal of Medical Education* 44 (March 1969) 214-220.

32. C S Rand, A M Macgregor, "Morbidly obese patients' perceptions of social discrimination before and after surgery for obesity," *Southern Medical Journal* 83 (December 1990) 1390-1395.

33. C S Rand, A M Macgregor, "Successful weight loss following obesity surgery and the perceived liability of morbid obesity," *International Journal of Obesity* 15 (September 1991) 577-579.

34. National Institutes of Health, "Health Implications of Obesity," *NIH Consensus Statement Online*, http://consensus,nih.gov/cons/049/049_statement.htm (accessed 9 Feb 2004).

35. S E Hildebrandt, "Effects of participation in bariatric support group after Roux-en-Y gastric bypass," *Obesity Surgery* 8 (October 1998) 535-542.

36. "Guidelines for granting privileges in bariatric surgery," American Society for Bariatric Surgery, http://www.asbs.org/html/story/chapter 4.html (accessed 7 Feb 2004)

RESOURCES

Bennett, P H, et al. "Epidemiologic studies of diabetes in the Pima Indians," *Recent Progress in Hormone Research* 32 (1976) 333-376.

Benotti, P N, et al. "Gastric restrictive operations for morbid obesity," *American Journal of Surgery* 157 (January 1989) 150-155.

Bierman, E L; Bagdade, J D; Porte, D, Jr. "Obesity and diabetes: The odd couple," *American Journal of Clinical Nutrition* 21 (December 1968) 1434-1437.

Bouchard, C. *The Genetics of Obesity* (Boca Raton, Fla: CRC Press, 1994) 245.

Breaux, C W. "Obesity surgery in children," *Obesity Surgery* 5 (August 1995) 279-284.

Build and Blood Pressure Study (Chicago: Society of Actuaries, 1959).

Calle, E E, et al. "Body mass index and mortality in a prospective cohort of US adults," *The New England Journal of Medicine* 341 (Oct 7, 1999) 1097-1105.

Charuzi, I, et al. "Bariatric surgery in morbidly obese sleep-apnea patients: Short- and long-term follow-up," *American Journal of Clinical Nutrition* 55 suppl (February 1992) 594S-596S.

Colditz, G A, et al. "Weight as a risk factor for clinical diabetes in women," *American Journal of Epidemiology* 132 (September 1990) 501-513.

Dixon, J B; Chapman, L; O'Brien, P. "Marked improvement in asthma after Lap-Band surgery for morbid obesity," *Obesity Surgery* 9 (August 1999) 385-389.

Drenick, E J, et al. "Excessive mortality and causes of death in morbidly obese men," *JAMA* 243 (Feb 1, 1980) 443-445.

Francke, S, et al. "Genetic studies of the leptin receptor gene in morbidly obese French Caucasian families," *Human Genetics* 100 (October 1997) 491-496.

Freidman, J M; Halaas, J L. "Leptin and the regulation of body weight in mammals," *Nature* 395 (Oct 22, 1998) 763-770.

Garfinkel, L. "Overweight and cancer," *Annals of Internal Medicine* 103 (December 1985) 1034-1036.

Hartz, A J, et al. "Relationship of obesity to diabetes: Influences of obesity level and body fat distribution," *Prevention Medicine* 12 (March 1983) 351-357.

"Health implications of obesity. National Institutes of Health Consensus Development Conference statement," *Annals of Internal Medicine* 103 (December 1985) 1073-1077.

Higa, K D; Boone, K B; Ho, T. "Complications of the laparoscopic Roux-en-Y gastric bypass: 1,040 patients—what have we learned?" *Obesity Surgery* 10 (December 2000) 509-513.

Hubert, H B, et al. "Obesity as an independent risk factor for cardiovascular disease: A 26-year follow-up of participants in the Framingham Heart Study," *Circulation* 67 (May 1983) 968-977.

Kalkhoff, R K, et al. "Relationship of body fat distribution to blood pressure, carbohydrate tolerance, and plasma lipids in healthy obese women," *The Journal of Laboratory and Clinical Medicine* 102 (October 1983) 621-627.

Kanders, B S, et al. "Weight loss outcome and health benefits associated with the Optifast program in the treatment of obesity," *International Journal of Obesity* 13 no 2 suppl (1989) 131-134.

Kuczmarski, R J. "Prevalence of overweight and weight gain in the United States," *American Journal of Clinical Nutrition* 55 suppl (February 1992) 495S-502S.

Kuczmarski, R J, et al. "Varying body mass index cutoff points to describe overweight prevalence among US adults: NHANES III (1988 to 1994)," *Obesity Research* 5 (November 1997) 542-548.

Lew, E A; Garfinkel, L. "Variations in mortality by weight among 750,000 men and women," *Journal of Chronic Diseases* 32 no 8 (1979) 563-576.

Linner, J H; Drew, R L. "Reoperative surgery—Indications, efficacy, and long-term follow-up," *American Journal of Clinical Nutrition* 55 suppl (February 1992) 606S-610S.

Macgregor, A M; Greenberg, R A. "Effect of surgically induced weight loss on asthma in the morbidly obese," *Obesity Surgery* 3 (February 1993) 15-21.

Macgregor, A M; Rand, C S. "Gastric surgery in morbid obesity. Outcome in patients aged 55 years and older," *Archives of Surgery* 128 (October 1993) 1153-1157.

Macgregor, A M; Rand, C S. "Revision of staple line failure following Roux-en-Y gastric bypass for obesity: A follow-up of weight loss," *Obesity Surgery* 1 (June 1991) 151-154.

Mason, E E; Renquist, K; Jiang, D. "Predictors of two obesity complications: Diabetes and hypertension," *Obesity Surgery* 2 (August 1992) 231-237.

Murr, M M; Siadati, M R; Sarr, M G. "Results of bariatric surgery for morbid obesity in patients older than 50 years," *Obesity Surgery* 5 (November 1995) 399-402.

Powers, P S, "Conservative treatments for morbid obesity," in *Surgery for the Morbidly Obese Patient*, ed M Deitel (Philadelphia: Lea & Febiger, 1989) 27-37.

Rand, C S; Macgregor, A M. "Adolescents having obesity surgery: A 6-year follow-up," *Southern Medical Journal* 87 (December 1994) 1208-1213.

Rand, C S; Macgregor, A M. "Medical care and pregnancy outcome after gastric bypass surgery for obesity," (letter) *Southern Medical Journal* 82 (October 1989) 1319-1320.

Rand, C S; Macgregor, A M; Hankins, G C. "Eating behavior after gastric bypass surgery for obesity," *Southern Medical Journal* 80 (August 1987) 961-964.

Safer, D J. "Diet, behavior modification, and exercise. A review of obesity treatments from a long-term perspective," *Southern Medical Journal* 84 (December 1991) 1470-1474.

Sjostrom, C D, et al. "Reduction in incidence of diabetes, hypertension and lipid disturbances after intentional weight loss induced by bariatric surgery: The SOS Intervention Study," *Obesity Research* 7 (September 1999) 477-484.

Sjostrom, L, et al. "Swedish obese subjects (SOS). Recruitment for an intervention study and a selected description of the obese state," *International Journal of Obesity and Related Metabolic Disorders* 16 (June 1992) 465-479.

Stevens, J, et al. "The effect of age on the association between body-mass index and mortality," *The New England Journal of Medicine* 338 (Jan 1, 1998) 1-7.

Strauss, R S; Bradley, L J; Brolin, R E. "Gastric bypass surgery in adolescents with morbid obesity," *The Journal of Pediatrics* 138 (April 2001) 499-504.

Stunkard, A J. "An overview of current treatments for obesity," in *Treatment of the Seriously Obese Patient*, ed T A Wadden, T B Van Itallie (New York: Guilford Press, 1992) 34.

Sugerman, H J, et al. "Long-term effects of gastric surgery for treating respiratory insufficiency of obesity," *American Journal of Clinical Nutrition* 55 suppl (February 1992) 597S-601S.

Vallis, M T; Ross, M A. "The role of psychological factors in bariatric surgery for morbid obesity: Identification of psychological predictors of success," *Obesity Surgery* 4 (November 1993) 346-359.

Van Itallie, T B. "Health implications of overweight and obesity in the United States," *Annals of Internal Medicine* 103 (December 1985) 983-988.

"Very low calorie diets. National Task Force on the Prevention and Treatment of Obesity, National Institutes of Health," *JAMA* 270 (Aug 25, 1993) 967-974.

Weintraub, M, et al. "Long-term weight control study. IV (weeks 156-190). The second double-blind phase," *Clinical Pharmacology and Therapeutics* 51 (May 1992) 608-614.

Westlund, K; Nickolaysen, R. "Ten-year mortality and morbidity related to serum cholesterol. A follow-up of 3,751 men aged 40-49," *Scandinavian Journal of Clinical and Laboratory Investigation Supplementum* 127 (1972) 1-24.

Wittgrove, A C; Clark, G W. "Laparoscopic gastric bypass, Roux-en-Y—500 patients: Technique and results, with 3-60 month follow-up," *Obesity Surgery* 10 (June 2000) 233-239.

Wittgrove, A C, et al. "Pregnancy following gastric bypass for morbid obesity," *Obesity Surgery* 8 (August 1998) 461-466.

York, D A. "Peripheral and central mechanisms regulating food intake and macronutrient selection," *Obesity Surgery* 9 (October 1999) 471-479.

Originally published May 2004, *AORN Journal.*

AORN Clinical Path Template

Introduction

The clinical path is the organization and sequencing of patient care interventions for a specified procedure or population by the health care team along a timeline to better manage resources, ensure quality of care, and minimize delays (Spath, 1995). A clinical path is not a mandatory treatment plan, a standard of care, a substitute for clinical judgment, or a substitute for physician orders. The intraoperative clinical path should serve as an integrated documentation tool to stabilize the intraoperative process of patient care (Patterson, 1997) and effectively manage clinical and financial outcomes (Windle, 1994). The purpose of this template is to assist perioperative nurses in understanding and developing clinical paths with an emphasis on the intraoperative portion of patient care.

Before Building a Clinical Path

Before using this template, the clinical path design team should complete the following tasks:

1. Gather and review relevant clinical literature on pathway development (Spath, 1996).
2. Organize the multidisciplinary clinical path design team.
3. Identify the goals and objectives you wish to achieve as a result of implementing this path (Spath, 1996). Be as specific as possible. For example, is the objective to decrease turnover time, to standardize orthopedic prosthesis, or to lower costs on high-volume diagnosis related groups (DRGs)? Keep these goals in mind when using the template.
4. Select a path format. The matrix format is used in this document because it provides the best conceptualization of care intervention sequencing. However, the algorithm format may be used when the objective is to assist caregivers with the complexity of clinical decision making (Spath, 1996). If clinical paths already exist in your facility, assess their adaptability to the intraoperative setting.

Building the Clinical Path

1. Name the focus of the clinical path you wish to develop. What is the focus of this path (Spath, 1996)? Consider the following points:
   A. Will this path target a specific procedure such as modified radical mastectomy, total hip replacement, or coronary artery bypass graft?
   B. Will this path target general types of procedures such as all types of bowel resections or vascular procedures?
   C. Will this path target a group of patients? For example, is this a generic path for all day surgery patients, ambulatory surgery patients, or patients admitted for a 23-hour stay?
   D. What kinds of patients or procedures are beyond the scope of this path?
2. Define the desired timeline. The timeline refers to "clinically relevant increments of time" (Spath, 1996). AORN describes perioperative nursing practice as performing "nursing activities in the preoperative, intraoperative, and postoperative phases of the patient's surgical experience" (AORN, 1992). Depending on how the path will be used in your facility, the timeline can be in hours, minutes, phases, or levels of care within the preoperative, intraoperative, and postoperative phases (Spath, 1996). Consider the following points:
   A. Determine precisely how much of the patient's surgical experience the path will encompass. Where do you want this path to start and stop?
   B. In what practice setting will the path be used?
      (1) Ambulatory or day surgery facilities may wish to develop paths that include admission into the facility in the preoperative phase, the intraoperative phase, and discharge in the postoperative phase.
      (2) Acute care facilities may wish to develop paths for the immediate preoperative phase (ie, while the patient is in the preoperative holding or preanesthesia area), the intraoperative phase, and the immediate postoperative phase (ie, while the patient is in the postanesthesia care unit).
   C. Can existing clinical paths in your facility be modified to include the perioperative period?
   D. Does a new clinical path have the potential to be "plugged in" to a clinical path already being used in the surgical nursing unit or intensive care unit for preoperative and postoperative patient care? If so, how does this affect the timeline selected?

E. Is the purpose of the timeline in your facility to encourage the team to achieve "best practices," to reflect current practice, or both?

3. List the most commonly encountered or anticipated patient care problems for the target condition or population on which this path is focused. Actual or potential medical and nursing diagnoses are appropriate patient care problems, as are problems identified by other members of the health care team. Consider the following points:
   A. Who will be using the path (Spath, 1996)? In facilities where the path is strictly a nursing tool, nursing diagnoses may be used exclusively. However, in facilities where the path is developed, implemented, and used by a multidisciplinary team, patient care problems should be defined by the multidisciplinary team members caring for the patient. The success of the clinical path depends on the input of and acceptance by the multidisciplinary team.
   B. Nurses and physicians may see the same or similar patient care problems for any given procedure or population but describe them differently. The surgeon may write an order, "Needs preop teaching," while the perioperative nurse would refer to the patient's "knowledge deficit." Flexibility with terminology may be to your advantage.
   C. Some medical and nursing problems overlap. For example, "hypothermia" or "hyperthermia" can be a medical or nursing diagnosis, as can "fluid volume excess, decreased cardiac output."
   D. Patient care problems can be standardized by target procedure or population, left blank to be customized by the perioperative nurse, or a combination of both.
   E. Patient care problems can be subcategorized by their location in the timeline (ie, preoperative, intraoperative, postoperative).

4. Identify patient care interventions by the multidisciplinary team. Interventions can be considered critical elements of care that if not completed can adversely affect outcomes (Spath, 1996). Consider the following points:
   A. Interventions can be considered critical elements of care, tasks (eg, gathering equipment and supplies), diagnostic tests (eg, electrocardiogram), nursing activities (eg, perioperative nursing assessment, safety, positioning), medical activities (eg, history and physical), laboratory tests (eg, SMA 6), radiologic tests (eg, arteriograms), medications (eg, preoperative sedation), fluids, patient teaching, and discharge planning.
   B. Some nurses believe there should be an intervention for each patient problem listed (see Sample 1); others disagree (see Sample 2).
   C. Some matrix paths have a separate row for specific interventions to emphasize certain aspects of care, to logically organize interventions, or to facilitate documentation. For example, under the broad heading of "interventions," there may be separate rows for diagnostic/laboratory tests, nursing activities/treatments, medications, and patient teaching/discharge planning.
   D. Interventions can be subcategorized by their location in the timeline (ie, preoperative, intraoperative, postoperative).
   E. AORN's "Competency statements in perioperative nursing" and "Standards of perioperative clinical practice" may assist in delineating perioperative nursing interventions (AORN, 1997).
   F. Using standardized language and/or common data elements may be useful.

5. Specify expected outcomes in measurable terms. Outcomes should be correlated to patient care performance measures (Spath, 1996). Consider the following points:
   A. Outcomes can be clinical, functional, financial, and/or related to patient satisfaction.
   B. Outcomes can be immediate, occurring either after or during an intervention. Did the intervention achieve the desired goal?
   C. Outcomes can be those achieved by discharge or at the completion of this episode of care.
   D. Outcomes can be subcategorized by their location in the timeline (ie, preoperative, intraoperative, postoperative).

E. AORN's "Patient outcomes: Standards of perioperative care" may be used to assist in delineating appropriate clinical outcomes (AORN, 1997). Standards of other professional groups also should be considered.

6. Define variances and how to track them. Variances can be viewed as performance measures. Performance measures can be documented during the episode of care and undergo concurrent review and intervention or be reviewed retrospectively.

   A. Depending on the facility in which the clinical path is used, the variance record may be part of the patient's permanent record or a separate document removed from the patient record for quality improvement activities.

   B. Variances can be subcategorized by their location in the timeline (ie, preoperative, intraoperative, postoperative).

   C. Variances also can be subcategorized by patient and family, clinician, or system.

   D. Patient variances can be used to document changes in the patient's condition that prevent adherence to the path. Clinician variances can be used to evaluate caregivers' performance and establish best practices. System variances can identify breakdowns in the system (eg, unavailability of the history and physical on the chart) that cause patients to vary from the desired timeline.

   E. Can variance tracking assist the quality improvement department by modifying or replacing quality assurance audits?

   F. For ease of documentation, variances can be coded with a key posted in each OR or can be developed into a checklist format. Variance tracking can be enhanced with a computer documentation system.

Now That the Clinical Path Has Been Built

1. Design accessory tools to complement the implementation of the path (Spath, 1996). Preprinted orders, family/patient paths for education purposes, and integrated documentation tools are examples of such tools.

2. Anticipate the difficulties. Common difficulties with clinical paths include the following (Musfeldt, 1995):

   ♦ Inadequate physician involvement from the beginning of clinical path design.

   ♦ Ineffective sharing of quality and financial data with physicians.

   ♦ Unavailability of the clinical path document for the physician to examine.

   ♦ Meetings that last too long, or having too many meetings about one clinical path.

   ♦ Inadequate variance tracking.

   ♦ Ineffective communication with individual caregivers, including physicians, regarding their own most frequent variances from the path.

   ♦ Ineffective communication with individual caregivers regarding their personal improvements in financial or clinical outcomes.

REFERENCES

Association of Operating Room Nurses, Inc. (1992). A model for perioperative nursing practice. In *AORN Standards and Recommended Practices for Perioperative Nursing.* Denver: Author, I:1-1 to I:1-3.

Association of Operating Room Nurses, Inc. (1997). *AORN Standards, Recommended Practices, and Guidelines.* Denver: Author.

Musfeldt, C. (February 1995). A clinical look at critical pathways. *Healthcare Informatics* 12 (2) 44–48.

Patterson, P. (February 1997). Pathways: What role do they play in the OR? *OR Manager* 13 (2) 1, 14–15.

Spath, P L. (1996). Critical path development process. Unpublished manuscript.

Spath, P L. (March/April 1995). Critical paths: Maximizing patient care coordination. *Today's OR Nurse* 17 (2) 13–20.

Windle, P E. (September 1994). Critical pathways: An integrated documentation tool. *Nursing Management* 25 (9) 80F–80P.

RESOURCES

Bueno, M M, and Hwang, R F. (November 1993). Understanding variances in hospital stay. *Nursing Management* 24 (11) 51–57.

Choosing high-volume, high-cost DRGs for pathways not always the best bet. (October 1995). *Hospital Peer Review* 20 (10) 137–140.

Critical paths conflict with MDs' traditional ethics. (October 1995). *Hospital Peer Review* 20 (10) 140–141.

Garbin, B A. (November/December 1995). Introduction to clinical pathways. *Journal of Healthcare Quality* 17 (6) 6–9.

Hogan, P. (January 1995). Pulling it all together: Critical paths, outcomes, variance analysis, and accountability. *Inside Case Management* 1 (10) 3–4.

Make your paths more cost efficient. (April 1996). *Hospital Case Management* 4 (4) 53–54.

Moss, M T. (January 1994). Practical implementation of outcomes oriented case management. *Seminars in Perioperative Nursing* 3 (1) 40–45.

Moss, M T. (November/December 1993). Outcomes management in perioperative services. *Nursing Economics* 11 (6) 364–369.

Nolin, C E, and Clougherty, L A. (September 1994). Will critical paths keep you out of trouble? *Inside Case Management* 1 (6) 4–5.

Patterson, P. (July 1994). Critical pathways: ORs streamline patient care, control resource utilization. *OR Manager* 10 (7) 1, 6–7.

Patterson, P. (July 1994). Critical pathways: Perioperative case managers redesign processes. *OR Manager* 10 (7) 8–10.

Patterson, P. (July 1994). Critical pathways: Care paths cut length of stay, reduce charges. *OR Manager* 10 (7) 12.

Patterson, P. (August 1994). Critical pathways: Hospital shortens cataract stays, boosts satisfaction. *OR Manager* 10 (8) 19.

Rothrock, J C. (1996). *Perioperative Nursing Care Planning* (2nd ed). St. Louis: Mosby.

Royer, K. (January 1994). A case management experience with cholecystectomies. *Seminars in Perioperative Nursing* 3 (1) 3–12.

Perioperative paths buck the trend, produce results for hospital CMs. (June 1994). *Hospital Case Management* 2 (6) 89–94.

Spath, P L. (November/December 1995). Path-based patient care should build quality into the process. *Journal of Healthcare Quality* 17 (6) 26–29.

Which perioperative variances should you track? (June 1994). *Hospital Case Management* 2 (6) 95.

Williams, D B. (January 1995). Case management without walls: Breaking down traditional barriers among organizations. *Inside Case Management* 1 (10) 1–3.

The ideas and concepts presented in this template were developed by the Clinical Paths Work Group, which was appointed by the Professional Practice Issues Project Team and chaired by Vicki J. Fox, RN, MSN, CNOR, CNS, CRNFA, in 1996–1997.

AORN Clinical Path Template

1. **Focus of Clinical Path:** _____

2. **Timeline:** _____

3. **Patient Care Problems**		Preoperative:	Intraoperative:	Postoperative:
A. B. C. D. E. F.	4. I N T E R V E N T I O N S			
5. O U T C O M E D S		Immediate:	Discharge:	
6. V A R I A N C E S		For concurrent intervention:	For retrospective analysis:	

AORN Clinical Path Sample 1

1. Focus of Clinical Path: Laparoscopic cholecystectomy

2. Timeline: Preoperative: 120 minutes   Intraoperative: 60–90 minutes   Postoperative: 2–23 hours

3. Patient Care Problems		Preoperative:	Intraoperative:	Postoperative:
A. Knowledge deficit	**4. INTERVENTIONS**	◆ Reinforce patient/family teaching; use materials/booklet PRN ◆ Review clinical pathway ◆ Discuss informed consent ◆ Reinforce Patient Bill of Rights	◆ Reinforce knowledge; explain new events in OR ◆ Answer questions ◆ Provide emotional support	◆ Reinforce and provide details of postop care ◆ Answer questions ◆ Provide emotional support ◆ Reinforce discharge teaching: diet, activity, medications, wound care, and follow-up
B. High risk for injury		◆ Confirm patient ID ◆ Confirm NPO status ◆ Nursing assessment for risk factors ◆ Allergies documented ◆ Check equipment and supplies in OR	◆ Assist with induction ◆ Supine position ◆ Prepare incision site ◆ Monitor CO_2 insufflation/expulsion ◆ Antibiotic irrigation ◆ Heparin irrigation ◆ Insert NG ◆ Urinary catheter PRN ◆ Place electrodispersive pad	◆ PACU discharge criteria met ◆ DC, NG, and urinary catheter ◆ Safe transfer of patient to PACU ◆ Postop assessment
C. High risk for altered physiologic function		◆ H&P, preop lab, ECG, x-rays complete (as needed) and documented ◆ Nursing assessment documented	◆ Physiologic monitoring ◆ Warm IV/irrigation fluids ◆ DVT prophylaxes	◆ Physiologic monitoring ◆ OOB to chair with assistance ◆ Progress ambulation ◆ Ice chips/liquids; advance as tolerated ◆ VS q 15 min x 2 hrs, then q 4 hrs ◆ Turn, cough, deep breathing

AORN Clinical Path Sample 1, continued

3. Patient Care Problems	Preoperative:	Intraoperative:	Postoperative:
D. Pain	◆ Pain assessment and intervention as needed (biliary colic) ◆ Patient/family teaching regarding postop pain (shoulder and incisions) and control options	◆ Provide comfort/privacy measures ◆ Local anesthetic agent at incision sites	◆ Provide comfort/privacy measures ◆ Pain assessment and intervention ◆ Reinforce preop teaching regarding types of pain and home pain management options
5. OUTCOMES	Immediate: A. The patient verbalizes understanding of procedures and sequence of events. B. The patient is free of electrical, chemical, or mechanical injury. C. The patient is free of significant alterations in physiologic functioning. D. The patient has adequate pain control.	Discharge: A. Patient/family understands postop care of incisions, activity level, and time and location of clinic follow-up. B. The patient remains free of injury. C. Vital signs within normal limits; free of nausea; able to perform ADL with little assistance. D. Adequate pain control; understands use of home pain medicines; understands activity limits.	
6. VARIANCES	For concurrent intervention: A. Knowledge deficit: Consent signed/correct; patient/family perception of adequacy of preop/postop teaching. B. Injury: Skin integrity; neuromotor integrity; oral/pharyngeal/dental integrity; visceral integrity. C. Presence of assessment data on chart at time of surgery (eg, H&P, preop lab, ECG, x-rays, nursing assessment); significant changes in physiologic function; DVT; significant VS changes associated with pneumoperitoneum; significant VS changes associated with reverse Trendelenburg. D. Adequacy of pain control; adequacy of teaching regarding use of home pain meds.	For retrospective analysis: A. Knowledge deficit: Patient/family perception of adequacy of preop/postop teaching within 3–6 weeks after surgery. B. Injury: Neuromotor integrity within first postop week. C. DVT within 24–48 hours postoperative. D. Adequacy of pain control 24–72 hours postop; adequacy of teaching regarding use of home pain meds within 3–6 weeks of surgery.	

AORN Clinical Path Sample 2

1. Focus of Clinical Path: Carotid endarterectomy

2. Timeline: Preoperative: 60–90 minutes   Intraoperative: 90–120 minutes   Postoperative: 60–90 minutes

3. Patient Care Problems		Preoperative:	Intraoperative:	Postoperative:

A. Carotid stenosis
List existing neuro deficit _____
	4.
	I
	N
	T
	E
	R
	V
	E
	N
	T
	I
	O
	N
	S
		◆ Identify patient
		
		◆ Reinforce patient/family teaching
		
		◆ Confirm operative site
		
		◆ Secure results of Dx tests: arteriogram, labs, ECG
		
		◆ Document baseline neuro assessment
		
		◆ Assess skin integrity
			◆ Utilize safety measures
			◆ Safe transport/transfer
			◆ Head/neck/arm positioning with appropriate aids
			◆ Electrosurgical dispersive pad
			◆ Containment of surgical prep solutions
			
			◆ Assist anesthesia provider
			  – With induction
			  – With hemodynamic monitoring
			
			◆ Prepare skin at surgical incision site
			
			◆ Appropriate use of intraoperative medication/fluids/devices
			  – Heparin
			  – Surgicel
			  – Xylocaine
			  – IV fluids
			  – Shunts
			
			◆ Create/maintain sterile field
			
			◆ Perform counts
			
			◆ Communicate with family
				◆ VS q 15 min
				
				◆ Neuro check q 30 min
				
				◆ Assess wound drainage q 30 min
				
				◆ Observe for signs of tracheal edema q 30 min
				
				◆ Assess skin integrity

B. High risk for altered cerebral perfusion				
C. High risk for fluid volume excess				
D. High risk for injury				

AORN Clinical Path Sample 2, continued

5. OUTCOMES	Immediate: ◆ Free from physical, chemical, or electrical injury ◆ Normothermic ◆ Maintain preoperative level of neuro function ◆ Free of hematoma at incision site	Discharge from PACU: ◆ Maintain VS within acceptable baseline limits ◆ Free of hematoma at incision site ◆ Freedom from or slight tracheal edema
6. VARIANCES	For concurrent intervention: ◆ Preoperative and postoperative neuro function ◆ Impaired skin integrity ◆ Return to OR for hemostasis	For retrospective analysis: ◆ New postoperative onset of neuro deficit ◆ Impaired skin integrity ◆ Return to OR for hemostasis

AORN Explications for Perioperative Nursing

Editor's note: *The following is reprinted with permission from American Nurses Association,* Code of Ethics for Nurses with Interpretive Statements, © *2001 American Nurses Publishing, American Nurses Foundation/ American Nurses Association, Washington, DC.*

ANA Code of Ethics for Nurses With Interpretive Statements

Preface

Ethics is an integral part of the foundation of nursing. Nursing has a distinguished history of concern for the welfare of the sick, injured, and vulnerable and for social justice. This concern is embodied in the provision of nursing care to individuals and the community. Nursing encompasses the prevention of illness, the alleviation of suffering, and the protection, promotion, and restoration of health in the care of individuals, families, groups, and communities. Nurses act to change those aspects of social structures that detract from health and well-being. Individuals who become nurses are expected not only to adhere to the ideals and moral norms of the profession but also to embrace them as a part of what it means to be a nurse. The ethical tradition of nursing is self-reflective, enduring, and distinctive. A code of ethics makes explicit the primary goals, values, and obligations of the profession.

The *Code of Ethics for Nurses* serves the following purposes:
- ♦ It is a succinct statement of the ethical obligations and duties of every individual who enters the nursing profession.
- ♦ It is the profession's nonnegotiable ethical standard.
- ♦ It is an expression of nursing's own understanding of its commitment to society.

There are numerous approaches for addressing ethics; these include adopting or subscribing to ethical theories, including humanist, feminist, and social ethics, adhering to ethical principles, and cultivating virtues. The *Code of Ethics for Nurses* reflects all of these approaches. The words "ethical" and "moral" are used throughout the *Code of Ethics.* "Ethical" is used to refer to reasons for decisions about how one ought to act, using the above mentioned approaches. In general, the word "moral" overlaps with "ethical" but is more aligned with personal belief and cultural values. Statements that describe activities and attributes of nurses in this *Code of Ethics* are to be understood

AORN Explications

Preamble

The American Nurses Association (ANA) *Code of Ethics for Nurses with Interpretive Statements* expresses the moral commitment to uphold the goals, values, and distinct ethical obligations of all nurses. As nursing is practiced in a changing social context, the *Code of Ethics for Nurses* becomes a dynamic document. AORN's Ethics Task Force detailed the specific perioperative nursing explications that correspond to the nine provisions from the ANA *Code of Ethics for Nurses with Interpretive Statements* (ANA, 2001). The primary goals and values of a profession are made explicit in a code of ethics.

Together, the ANA code, reprinted here with permission from ANA, and the explications for perioperative nursing provide the framework within which perioperative nurses can make ethical decisions. The code establishes the profession's nonnegotiable ethical standard. This document demonstrates accountability and responsibility to the public, to other members of the health care team, and to the profession. This document helps perioperative nurses relate the ANA *Code of Ethics* to their own areas of practice and provides examples of behaviors that reflect the ethical obligations of perioperative nurses.

Introduction

Ethical decisions for the perioperative nurse are often difficult but necessary during the care of the surgical patient. Additionally, perioperative nurses need to be able to recognize ethical dilemmas and take action. Perioperative nurses are responsible for nursing decisions that are not only clinically and technically sound but also morally appropriate and suitable for the specific problems of the particular patient being treated. The technical or medical aspects of the decision answer the question, "What can be done for this patient?" The moral component involves the patient's wishes and answers the question, "What should be done for this patient?"

The strength of the ethical perspective is its resolute nature. It promotes an action guide for nurses to follow in the realm of patient care. Ethics, as a branch of philosophy, incorporates multiple approaches to take when dealing with or applying actions to real life situations. Thus, each

as normative or prescriptive statements expressing expectations of ethical behavior.

The *Code of Ethics for Nurses* uses the term *patient* to refer to recipients of nursing care. The derivation of this word refers to "one who suffers," reflecting a universal aspect of human existence. Nonetheless, it is recognized that nurses also provide services to those seeking health as well as those responding to illness, to students and to staff, in health care facilities as well as in communities. Similarly, the term *practice* refers to the actions of the nurse in whatever role the nurse fulfills, including direct patient care provider, educator, administrator, researcher, policy developer, or other. Thus, the values and obligations expressed in this *Code of Ethics* apply to nurses in all roles and settings.

The *Code of Ethics for Nurses* is a dynamic document. As nursing and its social context change, changes to the *Code of Ethics* are also necessary. The *Code of Ethics* consists of two components: the provisions and the accompanying interpretive statements. There are nine provisions. The first three describe the most fundamental values and commitments of the nurse, the next three address boundaries of duty and loyalty, and the last three address aspects of duties beyond individual patient encounters. For each provision, there are interpretive statements that provide greater specificity for practice and are responsive to the contemporary context of nursing. Consequently, the interpretive statements are subject to more frequent revision than are the provisions. Additional ethical guidance and detail can be found in ANA or constituent member association position statements that address clinical, research, administrative, educational, or public policy issues.

The *Code of Ethics for Nurses with Interpretive Statements* provides a framework for nurses to use in ethical analysis and decision-making. The *Code of Ethics* establishes the ethical standard for the profession. It is not negotiable in any setting, nor is it subject to revision or amendment except by formal process of the House of Delegates of the ANA. The *Code of Ethics for Nurses* is a reflection of the proud ethical heritage of nursing, a guide for nurses now and in the future.

1 : The nurse, in all professional relationships, practices with compassion and respect for the inherent dignity, worth, and uniqueness of every individual, unrestricted by considerations of social or economic status, personal attributes, or the nature of health problems.

perioperative nurse may experience a situation differently, as well as addressing the situation and identifying the ethical conflict issues, his or her feelings, behaviors, actions, analysis, and resolution of the situation differently.

Health care delivery provided via a team format, such as the surgical team, does not necessarily create ethical conflicts, but it may highlight the conflicts if the values of the team members emphasize different priorities. Additionally, new roles of health care team members may carry expectations about how members should interact with each other and how standards of care should be met.

The perioperative nurse, by virtue of the nurse-patient relationship, has an obligation to provide safe, professional, and ethical patient care. It is important that nurses know how to manage ethical decisions appropriately so that patients' beliefs can be honored without compromising the nurse's own moral conscience. Ethical practice is thus a critical aspect of nursing care, and the development of ethical competency is paramount for present and future nursing practice.

1.1 Respect for human dignity

A fundamental principle that underlies all nursing practice is respect for the inherent worth, dignity, and human rights of every individual. Nurses take into account the needs and values of all persons in all professional relationships.

Perioperative Explications

The perioperative nurse is morally obligated to respect the dignity and worth of each individual patient. Perioperative nursing care is provided to each patient undergoing a surgical or other invasive procedure in a manner that preserves and protects patient autonomy, dignity, and human rights.[1] Each nurse has an obligation to be knowledgeable about the moral and legal rights of all patients and to protect and support those rights. As health care does not occur in a vacuum, the perioperative nurse must take into account both the individual rights and the interdependence of individuals in decision-making.

Perioperative examples

- Respects patient's decision for surgery.
- Respects patient's wishes (eg, advance directives, end-of-life choices).
- Implements institutional advance directive policy in the practice setting.
- Restrains patient only when patient poses a direct or potential danger to self or others.

1.2 Relationships to patients

The need for health care is universal, transcending all individual differences. The nurse establishes relationships and delivers nursing services with respect for human needs and values, and without prejudice. An individual's lifestyle, value system, and religious beliefs should be considered in planning health care with and for each patient. Such consideration does not suggest that the nurse necessarily agrees with or condones certain individual choices, but that the nurse respects the patient as a person.

Perioperative Explications

It is the responsibility of the perioperative nurse to provide care for each patient without prejudicial behavior. The care should be planned with consideration for the patient's values, religious beliefs, lifestyle choices, and age. The perioperative nurse respects the worth and dignity of the patient regardless of the diagnosis, disease process, procedure, or projected outcome. When the perioperative nurse is ethically opposed to interventions or procedures in a particular case, the nurse is justified in refusing to participate if the refusal is made known in advance and in time for other appropriate arrangements to be made for the patient's nursing care. When the patient's life is in jeopardy, the perioperative nurse is obliged to provide for the patient's safety, to avoid abandonment, and to withdraw only when assured that alternative sources of nursing care are available to the patient.

Perioperative examples

- Applies standards of nursing practice consistently to all patients with sensitivity to disability and economic, educational, cultural, religious, racial, age, and sexual differences.[2]
- Provides nursing care respecting the worth and dignity regardless of diagnosis, disease process, procedure, or projected outcome.[3]

♦ Respects the Patient's Bill of Rights.
♦ Refrains from derogatory comments about patients, families and significant others, colleagues, and other associates.
♦ Seeks guidance for resolving personal belief conflicts with the patient (eg, from supervisor, ethics committee, colleagues with appropriate authority).
♦ Uses principles of ethical analysis and moral reasoning to resolve ethical questions.[4]
♦ Provides spiritual comfort, arranges for appropriate substitute nursing care if personal beliefs conflict with required care, and respects the patient's decision for surgery.

1.3   The nature of health problems

The nurse respects the worth, dignity, and rights of all human beings irrespective of the nature of the health problem. The worth of the person is not affected by disease, disability, functional status, or proximity to death. This respect extends to all who require the services of the nurse for the promotion of health, the prevention of illness, the restoration of health, the alleviation of suffering, and the provision of supportive care to those who are dying.

The measures nurses take to care for the patient enable the patient to live with as much physical, emotional, social, and spiritual well-being as possible. Nursing care aims to maximize the values that the patient has treasured in life and extends supportive care to the family and significant others. Nursing care is directed toward meeting the comprehensive needs of patients and their families across the continuum of care. This is particularly vital in the care of patients and their families at the end of life to prevent and relieve the cascade of symptoms and suffering that are commonly associated with dying.

Nurses are leaders and vigilant advocates for the delivery of dignified and humane care. Nurses actively participate in assessing and assuring the responsible and appropriate use of interventions in order to minimize unwarranted or unwanted treatment and patient suffering. The acceptability and importance of carefully considered decisions regarding resuscitation status, withholding and withdrawing life-sustaining therapies, forgoing medically provided nutrition and hydration, aggressive pain and symptom management, and advance directives are increasingly evident. The nurse should provide interventions to relieve pain and other symptoms in the

Perioperative Explications

Perioperative nurses provide nursing care directed to meet the comprehensive needs of all patients, regardless of diagnosis, taking into consideration aspects of culture, language, perception of pain, significant others, values, and beliefs.[5] Nurses, as individuals, bring to their practice assumptions from their own culture, as well as about the cultures of others. In order to provide care that is culturally relevant to a diverse patient population, it is vital that nurses recognize the importance of each patient's values, beliefs, and health practices. In many instances, nurses provide care across cultures; thus, it becomes an ethical imperative for nurses to develop the skill of culturally competent caring.

To most effectively care for patients of other cultures, the nurse must be a conscientious observer, a perceptive listener, and thorough assessor. Acquiring information about the patient's culture and gaining further personal insight provides the nurse with an increased understanding of culture and values from both perspectives (the patient's and the nurse's) as they relate to providing culturally competent care.

Perioperative examples
♦ Provides nursing care respecting the patient's worth and dignity regardless of diagnosis, disease process, procedure, or projected outcome.[6]
♦ Overcomes communication barriers to allow patients and their significant others to express preferences for care, providing interpreters when necessary.[7]

dying patient even when those interventions entail risks of hastening death. However, nurses may not act with the sole intent of ending a patient's life even though such action may be motivated by compassion, respect for patient autonomy, and quality of life considerations. Nurses have invaluable experience, knowledge, and insight into care at the end of life and should be actively involved in related research, education, practice, and policy development.

1.4 The right to self-determination

Respect for human dignity requires the recognition of specific patient rights, particularly, the right of self-determination. Self-determination, also known as autonomy, is the philosophical basis for informed consent in health care. Patients have the moral and legal right to determine what will be done with their own person; to be given accurate, complete, and understandable information in a manner that facilitates an informed judgment; to be assisted with weighing the benefits, burdens, and available options in their treatment, including the choice of no treatment; to accept, refuse, or terminate treatment without deceit, undue influence, duress, coercion, or penalty; and to be given necessary support throughout the decision-making and treatment process. Such support would include the opportunity to make decisions with family and significant others and the provision of advice and support from knowledgeable nurses and other health professionals. Patients should be involved in planning their own health care to the extent they are able and choose to participate.

Each nurse has an obligation to be knowledgeable about the moral and legal rights of all patients to self-determination. The nurse preserves, protects, and supports those interests by assessing the patient's comprehension of both the information presented and the implications of decisions. In situations in which the patient lacks the capacity to make a decision, a designated surrogate decision-maker should be consulted. The role of the surrogate is to make decisions as the patient would, based upon the patient's previously expressed wishes and known values. In the absence of a designated surrogate decision-maker, decisions should be made in the best interests of the patient, considering the patient's personal values to the extent that they are known. The nurse supports patient self-determination by participating in discussions with surrogates, providing guidance and referral to other resources as necessary, and

Perioperative Explications

Patients have the right to self-determination (ie, the ability to decide for oneself what course of action will be taken in various circumstances). The perioperative nurse provides care to each patient undergoing surgical intervention in a manner that preserves and protects patient autonomy, dignity, and human rights. The patient's autonomy in the decision-making process is acknowledged and supported by the perioperative nurse, who provides accurate, appropriate, and reasonable information to assist the patient in making an informed choice.[8] The perioperative nurse elicits the patient's response regarding perception of the surgical procedure and the implications of decisions. The perioperative nurse ensures that the patient has access to additional and accurate information.[9]

When individual rights must be temporarily overridden to preserve the life of the patient or of another person, the suspension of those rights must be considered a deviation to be tolerated as briefly as possible.

Perioperative examples

- Provides information and explains the Patient Self-Determination Act (eg, informed consent, living will, power of attorney for health care, do-not-resuscitate order, organ procurement).[10]
- Confirms that informed consent has been granted for planned procedure;[11] when possible, obtains surrogate's permission for emergency surgery.
- Explains procedures before initiating action.
- Restrains patient only when patient poses a direct danger to self or others.
- Respects advance directives and end-of-life choices.
- Implements institutional advance directive policy in practice setting.
- Participates in perioperative teaching; answers patient's questions accurately and honestly.

identifying and addressing problems in the decision-making process. Support of autonomy in the broadest sense also includes recognition that people of some cultures place less weight on individualism and choose to defer to family or community values in decision-making. Respect not just for the specific decision but also for the patient's method of decision-making is consistent with the principle of autonomy.

Individuals are interdependent members of the community. The nurse recognizes that there are situations in which the right to individual self-determination may be outweighed or limited by the rights, health, and welfare of others, particularly in relation to public health considerations. Nonetheless, limitation of individual rights must always be considered a serious deviation from the standard of care, justified only when there are no less restrictive means available to preserve the rights of others and the demands of justice.

1.5 Relationships with colleagues and others

The principle of respect for persons extends to all individuals with whom the nurse interacts. The nurse maintains compassionate and caring relationships with colleagues and others with a commitment to the fair treatment of individuals, to integrity-preserving compromise, and to resolving conflict. Nurses function in many roles, including direct care provider, administrator, educator, researcher, and consultant. In each of these roles, the nurse treats colleagues, employees, assistants, and students with respect and compassion. This standard of conduct precludes any and all prejudicial actions, any form of harassment or threatening behavior, or disregard for the effect of one's actions on others. The nurse values the distinctive contribution of individuals or groups, and collaborates to meet the shared goal of providing quality health services.

♦ Allows choices within RN scope of practice (eg, child's preference for transport to the operating room, wagon versus cart).
♦ Formulates ethical decisions with assistance of available resources (eg, ethics committee, ethicists).

Perioperative Explications

Perioperative nurses must recognize the individuality not only of their patients, but also of their colleagues and others. As health care is not provided in a vacuum, nurses must be able to interact with a variety of other professionals and ancillary providers in the perioperative environment. In working with colleagues, perioperative nurses display the same nondiscriminatory and nonjudgmental behavior as they do with their patients. Treating others with professionalism and respect will enhance the performance of the health care team.

Perioperative nurses are compelled to treat colleagues and all people in a just and fair manner regardless of disability, economic status, level of education, culture, religion, race, age, and sexuality. Just as nurses have the right not to be abused or harassed in the workplace, so must they treat others in their workplace with respect and compassion. The nurse recognizes the contributions of each member of the health care team and works to collaborate to achieve quality patient care.

Perioperative examples
♦ Integrates cultural differences of coworkers.
♦ Recognizes and respects the value of all team members, including students and ancillary and support staff members.
♦ Provides education and information to coworkers, including ancillary and support staff.

♦ Promotes comparable levels of care in all practice settings in which invasive procedures are performed.

♦ Uses medical devices in a safe manner and complies with the Safe Medical Devices Act and other laws and regulations.

2 : The nurse's primary commitment is to the patient, whether an individual, family, group or community.

2.1 Primacy of the patient's interests

The nurse's primary commitment is to the recipient of nursing and health care services—the patient—whether the recipient is an individual, a family, a group, or a community. Nursing holds a fundamental commitment to the uniqueness of the individual patient; therefore, any plan of care must reflect that uniqueness. The nurse strives to provide patients with opportunities to participate in planning care, assures that patients find the plans acceptable, and supports the implementation of the plan. Addressing patient interests requires recognition of the patient's place in the family or other networks of relationship. When the patient's wishes are in conflict with others, the nurse seeks to help resolve the conflict. Where conflict persists, the nurse's commitment remains to the identified patient.

Perioperative Explications

The perioperative nurse supports both the interdependence and the individual rights of the patient when making decisions. The perioperative nurse collaborates in a manner that preserves and protects the patient's autonomy, dignity, and human rights. When individual rights must be temporarily overridden to preserve the life of the patient or of another person (eg, in the case of violent patients or patients with communicable diseases), the suspension of those rights must be considered a deviation to be tolerated as briefly as possible.

Perioperative examples

♦ Collaborates with patient regarding health care whenever possible.

♦ Collects patient health data.

♦ Analyzes assessment data and utilizes the *Perioperative Nursing Data Set* (PNDS) to formulate a nursing diagnosis and plan nursing care.

♦ Identifies expected outcomes unique to the patient.[12]

♦ Considers assessment information, including patient preferences and unique needs, when developing an individualized plan of care to attain designated patient outcomes.[13]

♦ Includes family/significant others in planning care.[14]

♦ Provides for spiritual comfort to the patient and significant others (eg, contacts religious counselor).

♦ Acts as patient advocate.

♦ Provides interpreters when necessary.

♦ Respects patient's decision to choose or refuse care or interventions.

2.2 Conflict of interest for nurses

Nurses are frequently put in situations of conflict arising from competing loyalties in the workplace, including situations of conflicting expectations from patients, families, physicians, colleagues, and in

Perioperative Explications

Conflicts may arise from financial considerations in the perioperative setting that may contribute to conflicting loyalties between the perioperative nurse and the patient. While the perioperative

many cases, health care organizations and health plans. Nurses must examine the conflicts arising between their own personal and professional values, the values and interests of others who are also responsible for patient care and health care decisions, as well as those of patients. Nurses strive to resolve such conflicts in ways that ensure patient safety, guard the patient's best interests, and preserve the professional integrity of the nurse.

Situations created by changes in health care financing and delivery systems, such as incentive systems to decrease spending, pose new possibilities of conflict between economic self-interest and professional integrity. The use of bonuses, sanctions, and incentives tied to financial targets are examples of features of health care systems that may present such conflict. Conflicts of interest may arise in any domain of nursing activity, including clinical practice, administration, education, or research. Advanced practice nurses who bill directly for services and nursing executives with budgetary responsibilities must be especially cognizant of the potential for conflicts of interest. Nurses should disclose to all relevant parties (eg, patients, employers, colleagues) any perceived or actual conflict of interest and in some situations should withdraw from further participation. Nurses in all roles must seek to ensure that employment arrangements are just and fair and do not create an unreasonable conflict between patient care and direct personal gain.

2.3 Collaboration

Collaboration is not just cooperation, but it is the concerted effort of individuals and groups to attain a shared goal. In health care, that goal is to address the health needs of the patient and the public. The complexity of health care delivery systems requires a multidisciplinary approach to the delivery of services that has the strong support and active participation of all the health professions. Within this context, nursing's unique contribution, scope of practice, and relationship with other health professions needs to be clearly articulated, represented, and preserved. By its very nature, collaboration requires mutual trust, recognition, and respect among the health care team, shared decision-making about patient care, and open dialogue among all parties who have an interest in and a concern for health outcomes. Nurses should work to assure that the relevant parties

nurse needs to be fiscally responsible, the perioperative nurse's primary responsibility is to ensure that the patient's safety is maintained.

The perioperative nurse does not give or imply endorsement to advertising, promotion, or sale of commercial products or services in a manner that may be interpreted as reflecting the opinion or judgment of the profession as a whole.

Perioperative examples

- Identifies and resolves conflicts of interest effectively.
- Abstains from influencing purchasing decisions involving companies in which nurses have ownership to make financial gains (eg, stocks, other equity interest).
- The perioperative nurse does not solicit or accept gifts, gratuities, or other items of value that reasonably could be interpreted by others as influencing impartiality.

Perioperative Explications

The perioperative nurse respects the interdependence of all health care providers in achieving positive outcomes for patients undergoing a surgical or other invasive procedure. As a fundamental member of the surgical team, the perioperative nurse actively participates with other health care professionals when planning and providing patient care. The perioperative nurse, nurse managers, educators, and researchers need to participate in direct and indirect multidisciplinary planning and decision-making regarding patient care protocols and activities.

Perioperative examples

- Collaborates with the surgeon and anesthesia care provider to plan care specific to the procedure and the patient's needs.

are involved and have a voice in decision-making about patient care issues. Nurses should see that the questions that need to be addressed are asked and that the information needed for informed decision-making is available and provided. Nurses should actively promote the collaborative multidisciplinary planning required to ensure the availability and accessibility of quality health services to all persons who have needs for health care.

Intraprofessional collaboration within nursing is fundamental to effectively addressing the health needs of patients and the public. Nurses engaged in nonclinical roles, such as administration or research, while not providing direct care, nonetheless are collaborating in the provision of care through their influence and direction of those who do. Effective nursing care is accomplished through the interdependence of nurses in differing roles—those who teach the needed skills, set standards, manage the environment of care, or expand the boundaries of knowledge used by the profession. In this sense, nurses in all roles share a responsibility for the outcomes of nursing care.

2.4   Professional boundaries

When acting within one's role as a professional, the nurse recognizes and maintains boundaries that establish appropriate limits to relationships. While the nature of nursing work has an inherently personal component, nurse-patient relationships and nurse-colleague relationships have, as their foundation, the purpose of preventing illness, alleviating suffering, and protecting, promoting, and restoring the health of patients. In this way, nurse-patient and nurse-colleague relationships differ from those that are purely personal and unstructured, such as friendship. The intimate nature of nursing care, the involvement of nurses in important and sometimes highly stressful life events, and the mutual dependence of colleagues working in close concert all present the potential for blurring of limits to professional relationships. Maintaining authenticity and expressing oneself as an individual, while remaining within the bounds established by the purpose of the relationship, can be especially difficult in prolonged or long-term relationships. In all encounters, nurses are responsible for retaining their professional boundaries. When those professional boundaries are jeopardized, the nurse should seek assistance from peers or supervisors or take appropriate steps to remove her/himself from the situation.

- ◆ Collaborates and consults with nursing colleagues in the perioperative setting and practicing in other specialty areas (eg, RN first assistant [RNFA], critical care, psychiatry, pain management, pediatrics, postanesthesia care, home health).
- ◆ Demonstrates collaborative practice among subspecialties within and outside the perioperative arena.
- ◆ Collaborates with ancillary and support staff to enhance communication and work patterns that are mutually beneficial for staff and for efficient patient care.
- ◆ Collaborates with the public, industry, and health care workers regarding environmental and cost-containment issues
- ◆ Formulates ethical decisions with assistance of available resources (eg, ethics committee, counselors, and ethicists).

Perioperative Explications

Perioperative nurses promote and maintain professional relationships with patients, peers, coworkers, and all members of the surgical team. Perioperative nurses are aware of the intimate nature of nursing care, the highly stressful nature of the surgical environment, and the collegial nature of the surgical team. The perioperative nurse respects professional boundaries in the nurse-patient relationship and does not convey undue influence on patient decisions. Perioperative nurses play a critical role in providing information to patients so that decisions affecting that patient will be appropriate and effective.

The nurse should seek the assistance of peers or supervisors, without hesitation, when professional boundaries are unclear or in jeopardy. Perioperative nurses deliver patient care in a nondiscriminatory and nonjudgmental manner according to published, legal, agency, professional, and regulatory standards.[15]

Perioperative examples

- ◆ Plans for appropriate substitute nursing care if personal beliefs conflict with required care.
- ◆ Avoids unprofessional behavior toward patients, coworkers, and other health care professionals.

- ◆ Demonstrates respect toward colleagues and students.
- ◆ Recognizes the professional nature of the nurse-patient relationship and its inherent boundaries.

3: The nurse promotes, advocates for, and strives to protect the health, safety, and rights of the patient.

3.1 Privacy

The nurse safeguards the patient's right to privacy. The need for health care does not justify unwanted intrusion into the patient's life. The nurse advocates for an environment that provides for sufficient physical privacy, including auditory privacy for discussions of a personal nature and policies and practices that protect the confidentiality of information.

Perioperative Explications

The perioperative nurse has an obligation to protect patients from undue exposure or unwarranted invasions of privacy. Maintaining the patient's privacy is essential to preserving the trust developed in the nurse-patient relationship. Actions demeaning the dignity of the individual could destroy this relationship and jeopardize the patient's welfare. Maintaining the patient's privacy is reflected by securing mechanisms to protect the patient's physical privacy, all forms of identifiable personal information (ie, verbal, written, electronic), personal belongings, and valuables.

Perioperative examples

- ◆ Avoids needless exposure of patient's body.
- ◆ Keeps doors to OR or procedure rooms closed except during movement of patients, personnel, supplies, or equipment.[16]
- ◆ Restricts access to patient care areas to designated, authorized personnel only.
- ◆ Provides cover, warmth, and comfort during transfer from unit to surgical suite as well as during transfer to postoperative unit.
- ◆ Provides and maintains respect for deceased.
- ◆ Provides protected area for viewing deceased by family/significant others.[17]
- ◆ Provides auditory privacy for patient and staff conversations.

3.2 Confidentiality

Associated with the right to privacy, the nurse has a duty to maintain confidentiality of all patient information. The patient's well-being could be jeopardized and the fundamental trust between patient and nurse destroyed by unnecessary access to data or by the inappropriate disclosure of identifiable patient information. The rights, well-being, and safety of the individual patient should be the primary factors in arriving at any professional judgment concerning the disposition of confidential information received from or about the patient, whether oral, written or electronic. The standard of nursing practice and the

Perioperative Explications

In concert with privacy is the professional responsibility to maintain the confidentiality of the patient's personal information. The perioperative nurse has a duty to safeguard the confidentiality of all patient information. Measures must be taken to protect the confidentiality of patient information, including oral, written, and electronic forms. Information pertinent to the patient's treatment and welfare is shared only with members of the health care team directly concerned with the patient's care. While relevant patient information must be shared in an expeditious manner with other members of the

nurse's responsibility to provide quality care require that relevant data be shared with those members of the health care team who have a need to know. Only information pertinent to a patient's treatment and welfare is disclosed, and only to those directly involved with the patient's care. Duties of confidentiality, however, are not absolute and may need to be modified in order to protect the patient, other innocent parties, and in circumstances of mandatory disclosure for public health reasons.

Information used for purposes of peer review, third-party payments, and other quality improvement or risk management mechanisms may be disclosed only under defined policies, mandates, or protocols. These written guidelines must assure that the rights, well-being, and safety of the patient are protected. In general, only that information directly relevant to a task or specific responsibility should be disclosed. When using electronic communications, special effort should be made to maintain data security.

health care team in order to provide safe patient care, the patient must have trust and confidence in the nurse that information related to his or her care will be protected. Safeguarding private information about patients is a core belief of nursing; however, new technologies such as electronic records have added a challenge to protecting patient information.

Perioperative examples
- Maintains confidentiality of patient information within scope of practice.
- Closes patient record and logs off whenever leaving the computer unattended to protect patient information.
- Follows facility policies regarding electronic information documentation and storage.
- Is aware of and complies with local, state, and federal privacy and security regulations.
- Limits access to patient's record and information (eg, surgery schedule) to appropriate members of the health care team.
- Shares and discusses patient information only with appropriate health care providers and those directly involved in care.
- Protects all forms of confidential patient information (ie, verbal, written, electronic).
- Secures patient's records, belongings, and valuables.
- Maintains patient's record following agency policy, procedure, or protocol.
- Completes record of disposition of belongings and valuables following agency policy, procedure, or protocol.
- Completes operative records accurately and in an objective and nonjudgmental manner.
- Releases patient information only to individuals properly identified and in compliance with established policies, mandates, or protocols.
- Uses information for quality improvement purposes in a manner that protects patient confidentiality.[18]
- Follows regulations regarding disposal of printed records (eg, perioperative schedules, laboratory reports, face sheets).

3.3 Protection of participants in research
Stemming from the right to self-determination, each individual has the right to choose whether or not to participate in research. It is imperative that the patient or legally authorized surrogate receive

Perioperative Explications
The nurse acts to protect the rights of patients involved in clinical research.[19] These rights include the right of adequately informed consent, the right of freedom from risk of injury, the right of privacy, and the right to

sufficient information that is material to an informed decision, to comprehend that information, and to know how to discontinue participation in research without penalty. Necessary information to achieve an adequately informed consent includes the nature of participation, potential harms and benefits, and available alternatives to taking part in the research. Additionally, the patient should be informed of how the data will be protected. The patient has the right to refuse to participate in research or to withdraw at any time without fear of adverse consequences or reprisal.

Research should be conducted and directed only by qualified persons. Prior to implementation, all research should be approved by a qualified review board to ensure patient protection and the ethical integrity of the research. Nurses should be cognizant of the special concerns raised by research involving vulnerable groups, including children, prisoners, students, the elderly, and the poor. The nurse who participates in research in any capacity should be fully informed about both the subject's and the nurse's rights and obligations in the particular research study and in research in general. Nurses have the duty to question and, if necessary, to report and to refuse to participate in research they deem morally objectionable.

3.4   Standards and review mechanisms

Nursing is responsible and accountable for assuring that only those individuals who have demonstrated the knowledge, skill, practice experiences, commitment, and integrity essential to professional practice are allowed to enter into and continue to practice within the profession. Nurse educators have a responsibility to ensure that basic competencies are achieved and to promote a commitment

the preservation of dignity. The perioperative nurse respects the patient's right to decline or discontinue participation in research. The perioperative nurse should be knowledgeable about the rights of the nurse as well as the patient regarding research studies.

Perioperative nurses have an obligation to (a) ensure that research is conducted by qualified people, (b) obtain information about the intent and nature of the research, and (c) confirm that the study is approved by appropriate review bodies. The researcher should disclose the rights and obligations of the patient and the perioperative nurse. Furthermore, the researcher has an obligation to provide information about the nature of the study to the staff members providing care to the participants. Perioperative nurses should be able to question, report, or refuse to participate in research to which they are morally opposed.

Perioperative examples

- ◆ Confirms informed consent of patient, by physician or responsible researcher, prior to initiation of study and before use of patient information for research.
- ◆ Safeguards patient's rights as a research subject.
- ◆ Submits research proposals to the institutional review board.
- ◆ Follows recommended guidelines and protocols when using investigational devices or when engaging in new procedures.
- ◆ Follows federal guidelines for treatment of human and animal subjects.
- ◆ Provides for patient confidentiality during data collection.
- ◆ Seeks guidance from supervisor to resolve issues regarding any research project that conflict with the nurse's personal beliefs.
- ◆ Plans for appropriate substitute nursing care if personal beliefs conflict with the research project.

Perioperative Explications

The perioperative nurse's primary obligation is to promote the health, welfare, and safety of the patient. The perioperative nurse is responsible for implementing and maintaining standards of perioperative nursing practice. The nurse follows policies, practice guidelines, and laws to safeguard the health and safety of the patient. The nurse participates in the establishment and evaluation of mechanisms to

to professional practice prior to entry of an individual into practice. Nurse administrators are responsible for assuring that the knowledge and skills of each nurse in the workplace are assessed prior to the assignment of responsibilities requiring preparation beyond basic academic programs.

The nurse has a responsibility to implement and maintain standards of professional nursing practice. The nurse should participate in planning, establishing, implementing, and evaluating review mechanisms designed to safeguard patients and nurses, such as peer review processes or committees, credentialing processes, quality improvement initiatives, and ethics committees. Nurse administrators must ensure that nurses have access to and inclusion on institutional ethics committees. Nurses must bring forward difficult issues related to patient care and/or institutional constraints upon ethical practice for discussion and review. The nurse acts to promote inclusion of appropriate others in all deliberations related to patient care.

Nurses should also be active participants in the development of policies and review mechanisms designed to promote patient safety, reduce the likelihood of errors, and address both environmental system factors and human factors that present increased risk to patients. In addition, when errors do occur, nurses are expected to follow institutional guidelines in reporting errors committed or observed to the appropriate supervisory personnel and for assuring responsible disclosure of errors to patients. Under no circumstances should the nurse participate in, or condone through silence, either an attempt to hide an error or a punitive response that serves only to fix blame rather than correct the conditions that led to the error.

3.5 Acting on questionable practice

The nurse's primary commitment is to the health, well-being, and safety of the patient across the life span and in all settings in which health care needs are addressed. As an advocate for the patient, the nurse must be alert to and take appropriate action regarding any instances of incompetent, unethical,

review practice. Competency validation is an essential component to providing safe and effective patient care. Perioperative nurses need to be aware of their own educational and clinical capabilities and seek the assistance of colleagues without hesitation when patient care needs require additional skills. The perioperative nurse uses personal, institutional, professional, and regulatory resources to assist with the resolution of incompetent, unethical, and illegal practices in the work setting.

Perioperative examples

♦ Uses institutional ethics committee, practice committee, and peer review.

♦ Supports and participates in institutional ethics committee and institutional review boards.

♦ Participates in educational programs that enhance patient care (eg, morbidity/mortality conferences, ethics grand rounds, patient care conferences).

♦ Participates in quality and performance improvement processes.

♦ Participates in development and revision of professional standards of practice.

♦ Adheres to professional standards of practice, such as AORN's "Standards of perioperative clinical practice" and "Standards of perioperative professional performance."[20]

♦ Participates in multidisciplinary review of patient outcomes.

♦ Complies with institutional policies and procedures regarding competent performance of nursing activities.

♦ Complies with federal and state regulations such as Occupational Safety and Health Administration regulations, the Americans with Disabilities Act, and state boards of nursing regulations.

♦ Complies with accrediting agencies such as the Joint Commission and state regulatory agencies.

♦ Confirms clinicians' practice privileges and credentials (eg, RN first assistants, physicians, physician's assistants).

Perioperative Explications

Care providers in the perioperative environment provide health services within the scope of legitimate and ethical practice and safeguard the health and safety of their patients. The perioperative nurse is responsible for meeting legal, institutional, professional, and regulatory standards. It is the ethical

illegal, or impaired practice by any member of the health care team or the health care system or any action on the part of others that places the rights or best interests of the patient in jeopardy. To function effectively in this role, nurses must be knowledgeable about the *Code of Ethics*, standards of practice of the profession, relevant federal, state and local laws and regulations, and the employing organization's policies and procedures.

When the nurse is aware of inappropriate or questionable practice in the provision or denial of health care, concern should be expressed to the person carrying out the questionable practice. Attention should be called to the possible detrimental affect upon the patient's well-being or best interests as well as the integrity of nursing practice. When factors in the health care delivery system or health care organization threaten the welfare of the patient, similar action should be directed to the responsible administrator. If indicated, the problem should be reported to an appropriate higher authority within the institution or agency, or to an appropriate external authority.

There should be established processes for reporting and handling incompetent, unethical, illegal, or impaired practice within the employment setting so that such reporting can go through official channels, thereby reducing the risk of reprisal against the reporting nurse. All nurses have a responsibility to assist those who identify potentially questionable practice. State nurses associations should be prepared to provide assistance and support in the development and evaluation of such processes and reporting procedures. When incompetent, unethical, illegal, or impaired practice is not corrected within the employment setting and continues to jeopardize patient well-being and safety, the problem should be reported to other appropriate authorities such as practice committees of the pertinent professional organizations, the legally constituted bodies concerned with licensing of specific categories of health workers and professional practitioners, or the regulatory agencies concerned with evaluating standards or practice. Some situations may warrant the concern and involvement of all such groups. Accurate reporting and factual documentation, and not merely opinion, undergird all such responsible actions. When a nurse chooses to engage in the act of responsible reporting about situations that are perceived as unethical, incompetent, illegal, or

obligation of the perioperative nurse to identify and appropriately report questionable practices by any member of the health care team. There should be an established process for reporting and handling incompetent, unethical, or illegal practice within the employment setting so that such reporting can go through official channels without causing fear of reprisal. The perioperative nurse should be knowledgeable about the process and be prepared to use it if necessary. Written documentation of the observed practices or behaviors must be available to the appropriate authorities.

When incompetent, unethical, or illegal practice on the part of anyone concerned with the patient's care is not corrected within the employment setting and continues to jeopardized the patient's welfare and safety, the problem should be reported to other appropriate authorities, such as practice committees of the pertinent professional organizations or the legally constituted bodies concerned with licensing of specific categories of health workers or professional practitioners. Accurate reporting and documentation undergird all action.

Perioperative examples

♦ Acts as a patient advocate by protecting the patient from incompetent, unethical, or illegal practices.

♦ Questions care that appears inappropriate or substandard.

♦ Expresses concern to person carrying out the questionable practice.

♦ Reports incompetent, unethical, or illegal practice to responsible administrative person.

♦ Consults with colleagues and supervisors to resolve concerns.

♦ Documents observations and occurrences in an objective manner according to institutional policy.

♦ Complies with institutional policies in resolving problems.

♦ Reports verbal, psychological, and physical harassment or abuse.

♦ Intervenes appropriately to protect patient safety.

impaired, the professional organization has a responsibility to provide the nurse with support and assistance and to protect the practice of those nurses who choose to voice their concerns. Reporting unethical, illegal, incompetent, or impaired practices, even when done appropriately, may present substantial risks to the nurse; nevertheless, such risks do not eliminate the obligation to address serious threats to patient safety.

3.6 Addressing impaired practice

Nurses must be vigilant to protect the patient, the public, and the profession from potential harm when a colleague's practice, in any setting, appears to be impaired. The nurse extends compassion and caring to colleagues who are in recovery from illness or when illness interferes with job performance. In a situation where a nurse suspects another's practice may be impaired, the nurse's duty is to take action designed both to protect patients and to assure that the impaired individual receives assistance in regaining optimal function. Such action should usually begin with consulting supervisory personnel and may also include confronting the individual in a supportive manner and with the assistance of others or helping the individual to access appropriate resources. Nurses are encouraged to follow guidelines outlined by the profession and policies of the employing organization to assist colleagues whose job performance may be adversely affected by mental or physical illness or by personal circumstances. Nurses in all roles should advocate for colleagues whose job performance may be impaired to ensure that they receive appropriate assistance, treatment, and access to fair institutional and legal processes. This includes supporting the return to practice of the individual who has sought assistance and is ready to resume professional duties.

If impaired practice poses a threat or danger to self or others, regardless of whether the individual has sought help, the nurse must take action to report the individual to persons authorized to address the problem. Nurses who advocate for others whose job performance creates a risk for harm should be protected from negative consequences. Advocacy may be a difficult process, and the nurse is advised to follow workplace policies. If workplace policies do not exist or are inappropriate—that is, they deny the nurse in question access to due legal process or demand resignation—the reporting nurse may

Perioperative Explications

The perioperative nurse has an ethical responsibility to protect the patient, the public, and the profession from potential harm that could result from a colleague's impairment. It is both caring and compassionate to take action to protect the patient and ensure that the impaired person receives appropriate assistance. Nurse should follow guidelines outlined by the profession and the policies and procedures of the employing agency.

Perioperative examples

- ◆ Uses institutional procedural mechanisms to report substance abuse or impairment of colleagues.
- ◆ Consults with supervisory personnel.
- ◆ Confronts the individual in a supportive, caring manner.
- ◆ Use agency resources for helping individual to access treatment and care.
- ◆ Acts as patient advocate and takes action to ensure patient safety (eg, makes arrangements to remove unsafe practitioner and replace with appropriate practitioner to continue patient care).

obtain guidance from the professional association, state peer assistance programs, employee assistance program, or a similar resource.

4: The nurse is responsible and accountable for individual nursing practice and determines the appropriate delegation of tasks consistent with the nurse's obligation to provide optimum patient care.

4.1 Acceptance of accountability and responsibility

Individual registered nurses bear primary responsibility for the nursing care that their patients receive and are individually accountable for their own practice. Nursing practice includes direct care activities, acts of delegation, and other responsibilities such as teaching, research, and administration. In each instance, the nurse retains accountability and responsibility for the quality of practice and for conformity with standards of care.

Nurses are faced with decisions in the context of the increased complexity and changing patterns in the delivery of health care. As the scope of nursing practice changes, the nurse must exercise judgment in accepting responsibilities, seeking consultation, and assigning activities to others who carry out nursing care. For example, some advanced practice nurses have the authority to issue prescription and treatment orders to be carried out by other nurses. These acts are not acts of delegation. Both the advanced practice nurse issuing the order and the nurse accepting the order are responsible for the judgments made and accountable for the actions taken.

4.2 Accountability for nursing judgment and action

Accountability means to be answerable to oneself and others for one's own actions. In order to be accountable, nurses act under a code of ethical conduct that is grounded in the moral principles of fidelity and respect for the dignity, worth, and self-determination of patients. Nurses are accountable for judgments made and actions taken in the course of nursing practice, irrespective of health care organizations' policies or providers' directives.

Perioperative Explications

The individual professional licensee protects the public by ensuring the basic competencies of the professional nurse. Moreover, society grants the nursing profession the right to regulate its own practice. Perioperative nurses bear primary responsibility for perioperative nursing care and are individually accountable for their own practice. The nurse is responsible for nursing decisions made regarding care and is accountable for individual actions. Perioperative nursing practice may include direct patient care, delegation, teaching, research, or administration. Nurses are responsible for judgments they make regarding care and accountable for actions taken.

Perioperative examples

♦ Maintains nursing licensure and certification.
♦ Accepts responsibility and accountability for perioperative nursing practice, staffing schedules, and on-call assignments.
♦ Assumes responsibility for continued education.

Perioperative Explications

Accountability refers to being answerable to one's self, patients, peers, the profession, and society for judgments made and actions taken as a perioperative nurse. Neither physicians' orders nor the employing agency's policies relieve the perioperative nurse of accountability for those actions and judgments. Professional accountability to society is reflected in the ANA *Code of Ethics for Nurses*, standards of practice, educational requirements for practice, certification, and a performance evaluation.

Perioperative examples

♦ Provides safe and competent patient care.
♦ Accounts for sponges, needles, instruments, and other potential foreign bodies.

♦ Practices according to the ANA *Code of Ethics for Nurses;* AORN's *Standards, Recommended Practices, and Guidelines;* and hospital and departmental policies and procedures.
♦ Practices within scope of practice.
♦ Evaluates own performance and solicits peer review.
♦ Alerts surgeon and colleagues to potential risks to patients (eg, positioning, electrical hazards, blood loss, inadvertent laceration of blood vessel).
♦ Questions orders that appear incorrect or inappropriate.

4.3 Responsibility for nursing judgment and action

Responsibility refers to the specific accountability or liability associated with the performance of duties of a particular role. Nurses accept or reject specific role demands based upon their education, knowledge, competence, and extent of experience. Nurses in administration, education, and research also have obligations to the recipients of nursing care. Although nurses in administration, education, and research have relationships with patients that are less direct, in assuming the responsibilities of a particular role, they share responsibility for the care provided by those whom they supervise and instruct. The nurse must not engage in practices prohibited by law or delegate activities to others that are prohibited by the practice acts of other health care providers.

Individual nurses are responsible for assessing their own competence. When the needs of the patient are beyond the qualifications and competencies of the nurse, consultation and collaboration must be sought from qualified nurses, other health professionals, or other appropriate sources. Educational resources should be sought by nurses and provided by institutions to maintain and advance the competence of nurses. Nurse educators act in collaboration with their students to assess the learning needs of the student, the effectiveness of the teaching program, the identification and utilization of appropriate resources, and the support needed for the learning process.

Perioperative Explications

Responsibility refers to carrying out the duties associated with perioperative nursing. Perioperative nurse obligations are reflected in AORN's *Standards, Recommended Practices, and Guidelines.* The acceptance of responsibility for care is determined by an individual's educational preparation, professional competence, and work experience. Nurses in administration, education, and research also are responsible for care through the people they supervise.

Each perioperative nurse is responsible for maintaining competence of professional knowledge and technical skills. It is the nurse's responsibility to assess when care required is beyond an individual's knowledge and to report it to the appropriate support person.

Perioperative examples

♦ Consults other health care providers for assistance when necessary.
♦ Identifies and develops a plan of corrective action related to deficits and limitations in knowledge.
♦ Assumes responsibility for continuous education through personal study; attendance at institutional inservice programs, staff orientation workshops, seminars, AORN chapter and other professional meetings; and reading the *AORN Journal* and other perioperative professional journals.
♦ Remains current on new procedures affecting practice.
♦ Uses the AORN competency statements in perioperative practice.
♦ Provides unit-based orientation.
♦ Provides competency-based orientation.

- Practices adult learning theory.
- Demonstrates competency in use of new technologies.
- Engages in continued professional learning.

4.4 Delegation of nursing activities

Since the nurse is accountable for the quality of nursing care given to patients, nurses are accountable for the assignment of nursing responsibilities to other nurses and the delegation of nursing care activities to other health care workers. While delegation and assignment are used here in a generic moral sense, it is understood that individual states may have a particular legal definition of these terms.

The nurse must make reasonable efforts to assess individual competence when assigning selected components of nursing care to other health care workers. This assessment involves evaluating the knowledge, skills, and experience of the individual to whom the care is assigned, the complexity of the assigned tasks, and the health status of the patient. The nurse is also responsible for monitoring the activities of these individuals and evaluating the quality of the care provided. Nurses may not delegate responsibilities such as assessment and evaluation; they may delegate tasks. The nurse must not knowingly assign or delegate to any member of the nursing team a task for which that person is not prepared or qualified. Employer policies or directives do not relieve the nurse of responsibility for making judgments about the delegation and assignment of nursing care tasks.

Nurses functioning in management or administrative roles have a particular responsibility to provide an environment that supports and facilitates appropriate assignment and delegation. This includes providing appropriate orientation to staff, assisting less experienced nurses in developing necessary skills and competencies, and establishing policies and procedures that protect both the patient and nurse from the inappropriate assignment or delegation of nursing responsibilities, activities, or tasks.

Nurses functioning in educator or preceptor roles may have less direct relationship with patients. However, through assignment of nursing care activities to learners they share responsibility and accountability for the care provided. It is imperative that the knowledge and skills of the learner be sufficient to provide the assigned nursing care and that appropriate supervision be provided to protect both the patient and the learner.

Perioperative Explications

Perioperative nurses are accountable for patient outcomes resulting from nursing care rendered to patients during the perioperative experience. Perioperative nurses are accountable for the assignment of nursing responsibilities to other nurses and for the delegation of nursing care activities to other health care workers. The nurse retains accountability for patient outcomes resulting from delegated nursing tasks. Only the perioperative registered nurse plans and directs the nursing care of every patient undergoing operative and other invasive procedures. The core activities of perioperative nursing are assessment, diagnosis, outcome identification, planning, implementation, and evaluation. The perioperative nurse may delegate certain nursing care tasks, but the nursing activities that cannot be delegated are assessment diagnosis, outcome identification, planning, and evaluation.[21]

The nurse must be aware of specific state legal definitions and guidelines regarding delegation and assignment. The perioperative nurse follows facility policies or directives in delegating functions, but these do not relieve the nurse of accountability for making judgments about the competency of personnel and the appropriateness of delegated activities. Before delegation of patient care tasks, the perioperative nurse uses professional clinical judgment to decide to whom and under what circumstances to delegate appropriate patient care activities.[22] Prior to delegation, consideration also should be given to the patient's condition, the complexity of the procedure, the predictability of the outcome, the level of preparation and competence of the person accepting the delegation, and the amount of supervision needed.[23]

The perioperative work environment supports orientation to less experienced staff. It also provides policies to prevent nurses from accepting inappropriate assignments. This is to protect both the patient and the nurse.

Perioperative examples

- Knows state regulations and definitions regarding delegation and assignment.
- Knows organizational guidelines regarding assignment and delegation.

♦ Delegates nursing functions to nurses.
♦ Allows assistive personnel to assist with delegated nursing tasks only when competency has been established and when allowed by state scope of practice.
♦ Bases delegation and assignments on individual competency, patient acuity, complexity of the procedure, predictability of outcomes, amount of supervision required, staffing pattern, and staff availability.[24]
♦ Follows institutional policies for modifying patient care assignments that the nurse or other health care provider does not feel competent in performing.
♦ Participates in perioperative competency-based orientation.
♦ Perioperative nurses define and supervise the training of unlicensed assistive personnel to perform the delegated nursing care tasks.

5 **: The nurse owes the same duties to self as to others, including the responsibility to preserve integrity and safety, to maintain competence, and to continue personal and professional growth.**

5.1 Moral self-respect

Moral respect accords moral worth and dignity to all human beings irrespective of their personal attributes or life situation. Such respect extends to oneself as well; the same duties that we owe to others we owe to ourselves. Self-regarding duties refer to a realm of duties that primarily concern oneself and include professional growth and maintenance of competence, preservation of wholeness of character, and personal integrity.

Perioperative Explications

Perioperative nurses deliver care in a manner that is respectful not only to patients but also to themselves and their colleagues. Nurses identify areas for personal and professional development and assist others in their development. Nurses participate actively in community education about surgery, invasive procedures, and perioperative nursing, and they correct misinformation and misunderstanding about perioperative patient care.

Perioperative examples

♦ Promotes a positive image of nursing in the media and the community.
♦ Promotes professional autonomy and self-regulation of practice.
♦ Uses nursing titles according to demonstrated professional achievement (eg, CNOR, CRNFA).
♦ Corrects inaccurate portrayals of and misinformation about the profession.
♦ Promotes an environment that does not tolerate harassment and abuse.
♦ Provides an environment that optimizes the occupational health and safety of all employees.
♦ Promotes empowerment and team building.
♦ Supports the nurse's role as a patient advocate.

5.2 Professional growth and maintenance of competence

Though it has consequences for others, maintenance of competence and ongoing professional growth involves the control of one's own conduct in a way that is primarily self-regarding. Competence affects one's self-respect, self-esteem, professional status, and the meaningfulness of work. In all nursing roles, evaluation of one's own performance, coupled with peer review, is a means by which nursing practice can be held to the highest standards. Each nurse is responsible for participating in the development of criteria for evaluation of practice for using those criteria in peer and self-assessment.

Continual professional growth, particularly in knowledge and skill, requires a commitment to lifelong learning. Such learning includes, but is not limited to, continuing education, networking with professional colleagues, self-study, professional reading, certification, and seeking advanced degrees. Nurses are required to have knowledge relevant to the current scope and standards of nursing practice, changing issues, concerns, controversies, and ethics. Where the care required is outside the competencies of the individual nurse, consultation should be sought or the patient should be referred to others for appropriate care.

5.3 Wholeness of character

Nurses have both personal and professional identities that are neither entirely separate, nor entirely merged, but are integrated. In the process of becoming a professional, the nurse embraces the values of the profession, integrating them with personal values. Duties to self involve an authentic

Perioperative Explications

The perioperative nurse is accountable to society and the profession for appropriate, effective, and efficient nursing practice. Mechanisms are established to demonstrate professional accountability and responsibility for maintaining clinical competence. Knowledge and skill related to technological advances and surgical interventions should be incorporated into the perioperative nurse's practice. The perioperative nurse maintains responsibility for his or her own continuing education.

Perioperative examples

- ♦ Incorporates AORN's competency statements in perioperative nursing education.
- ♦ Remains current on new procedures related to perioperative clinical practice.
- ♦ Participates in certification processes (eg, CNOR, CRNFA, advanced cardiac life support).
- ♦ Acquires new knowledge from continuous education through personal study; attendance at institutional inservice programs, staff orientation workshops, seminars, AORN Congress, AORN chapter and other professional meetings; and reading the *AORN Journal, Surgical Services Management,* and other perioperative and professional literature.
- ♦ Supports competency-based orientation and annual review process.
- ♦ Demonstrates competency in use of new technologies.
- ♦ Participates in self-evaluation and peer evaluation of clinical competence, decision-making skills, and professional judgment.
- ♦ Seeks consultation as necessary to provide patient care.
- ♦ Confirms clinical privileges of all caregivers.
- ♦ Promotes individual accountability for maintaining competence.
- ♦ Promotes patient safety and other forms of patient advocacy initiatives recommended by professional organizations, legislation, and regulations.

Perioperative Explications

The perioperative nurse must be genuine, open, and honest in interactions with patients and other health care providers. Nurses are aware of their powerful influence and offer their opinions based on scientific principles, evidence-based practices, and clinical experiences.

expression of one's own moral point of view in practice. Sound ethical decision-making requires the respectful and open exchange of views between and among all individuals with relevant interests. In a community of moral discourse, no one person's view should automatically take precedence over that of another. Thus, the nurse has a responsibility to express moral perspectives, even when they differ from those of others, and even when they might not prevail.

This wholeness of character encompasses relationships with patients. In situations where the patient requests a personal opinion from the nurse, the nurse is generally free to express an informed personal opinion as long as this preserves the voluntariness of the patient and maintains appropriate professional and moral boundaries. It is essential to be aware of the potential for undue influence attached to the nurse's professional role. Assisting patients to clarify their own values in reaching informed decisions may be helpful in avoiding unintended persuasion. In situations where nurses' responsibilities include care for those whose personal attributes, condition, lifestyle, or situation is stigmatized by the community and are personally unacceptable, the nurse still renders respectful and skilled care.

5.4 Preservation of integrity

Integrity is an aspect of wholeness of character and is primarily a self-concern of the individual nurse. An economically constrained health care environment presents the nurse with particularly troubling threats to integrity. Threats to integrity may include a request to deceive a patient, to withhold information, or to falsify records, as well as verbal abuse from patients or coworkers. Threats to integrity also may include an expectation that the nurse will act in a way that is inconsistent with the values or ethics of the profession, or more specifically a request that is in direct violation of the *Code of Ethics.* Nurses have a duty to remain consistent with both their personal and professional values and to accept compromise only to the degree that it remains an integrity-preserving compromise. An integrity-preserving compromise does not jeopardize the dignity or well-being of the nurse or others. Integrity-preserving compromise can be difficult to achieve, but is more likely to be accomplished in situations where there is an open forum for moral discourse and an atmosphere of mutual respect and regard.

Perioperative examples

♦ Assists patients in formulating decisions affecting care as appropriate.
♦ Facilitates patient participation in perioperative plan of care.
♦ Integrates personal philosophy of nursing into practice setting.
♦ Helps peers to be assertive and emotionally healthy.
♦ Respects views of others, but clarifies misinformation.
♦ Applies standards of nursing practice consistently to all patients regardless of disability, economic status, culture, religion, race, age, lifestyle choices, or sexuality.
♦ Plans for appropriate substitute care provider if personal beliefs conflict with required care.

Perioperative Explications

The perioperative registered nurse does not compromise professional or personal integrity. Additionally, the perioperative nurse knows that the use of the title *Registered Nurse (RN),* as granted by state licensure, carries with it the responsibility to act in the public interest. The title *RN* and all other symbols of academic degrees or other earned or honorary professional symbols of recognition may be used in all ways that are legal and appropriate

The pressure to reduce costs, especially in surgical services, reflects the current emphasis on financial well-being. Perioperative nurses can be financially prudent and at the same time discharge their clinical, educational, and administrative duties in a manner that is consistent with ethical principles.

When the perioperative nurse is ethically and morally opposed to interventions or procedures in a particular case, the nurse is justified in refusing to participate if the refusal is made known in advance and in time for other appropriate arrangements to be made for the patient's nursing care. When the patient's life is in jeopardy, the perioperative nurse is

Where nurses are placed in situations of compromise that exceed acceptable moral limits or involve violations of the moral standards of the profession, whether in direct patient care or in any other forms of nursing practice, they may express their conscientious objection to participation. Where a particular treatment, intervention, activity, or practice is morally objectionable to the nurse, whether intrinsically so or because it is inappropriate for the specific patient, or where it may jeopardize both patients and nursing practice, the nurse is justified in refusing to participate on moral grounds. Such grounds exclude personal preference, prejudice, convenience, or arbitrariness. Conscientious objection may not insulate the nurse against formal or informal penalty. The nurse who decides not to take part on the grounds of conscientious objection must communicate this decision in appropriate ways. Whenever possible, such a refusal should be made known in advance and in time for alternate arrangements to be made for patient care. The nurse is obliged to provide for the patient's safety, to avoid patient abandonment, and to withdraw only when assured that alternative sources of nursing care are available to the patient.

Where patterns of institutional behavior or professional practice compromise the integrity of all its nurses, nurses should express their concern or conscientious objection collectively to the appropriate body or committee. In addition, they should express their concern, resist, and seek to bring about a change in those persistent activities or expectations in the practice setting that are morally objectionable to nurses and jeopardize either patient or nurse well-being.

6: The nurse participates in establishing, maintaining, and improving health care environments and conditions of employment conducive to the provision of quality health care and consistent with the values of the profession through individual and collective action.

6.1 Influence of the environment on moral virtues and values

Virtues are habits of character that predispose persons to meet their moral obligations; that is, to do what is right. Excellences are habits of character that predispose a person to do a particular job or task well. Virtues such as wisdom, honesty, and courage are habits or attributes of the morally good person. Excellences such as compassion, patience,

obliged to provide for the patient's safety, to avoid abandonment, and to withdraw only when assured that alternative sources of nursing care are available to the patient.

Perioperative examples
- Facilitates a working environment conducive to learning, teaching, and education.
- Makes purchasing decisions equitably and justly to provide cost-effective, quality care.
- Uses and maintains supplies and equipment according to manufacturers' instructions.
- Resterilizes and reprocesses instruments and supplies in a manner consistent with standards and regulations.
- Accepts responsibility and accountability for perioperative nursing practices.
- Is aware of limitations and accepts assignments only when competent to function safely.
- Uses nursing titles (eg, CNOR, CRNFA) according to demonstrated professional achievement.
- Participates in risk management efforts and quality process improvement.
- Plans for appropriate substitute care provider if personal beliefs conflict with required care.

Perioperative Explications
The perioperative nurse is responsible for developing a caring environment that promotes the well-being of patients. This is accomplished by doing what is right and doing it well. The nurse provides a compassionate and therapeutic environment by promoting comfort and preventing unnecessary suffering. The working environment necessary to accomplish these goals supports the growth of virtues and excellences.

and skill are habits of character of the morally good nurse. For the nurse, virtues and excellences are those habits that affirm and promote the values of human dignity, well-being, respect, health, independence, and other values central to nursing. Both virtues and excellences, as aspects of moral character, can be either nurtured by the environment in which the nurse practices or they can be diminished or thwarted. All nurses have a responsibility to create, maintain, and contribute to environments that support the growth of virtues and excellences and enable nurses to fulfill their ethical obligations.

6.2 Influence of the environment on ethical obligations

All nurses, regardless of role, have a responsibility to create, maintain, and contribute to environments of practice that support nurses in fulfilling their ethical obligations. Environments of practice include observable features, such as working conditions, and written policies and procedures setting out expectations for nurses, as well as less tangible characteristics such as informal peer norms. Organizational structures, role descriptions, health and safety initiatives, grievance mechanisms, ethics committees, compensation systems, and disciplinary procedures all contribute to environments that can either present barriers or foster ethical practice and professional fulfillment. Environments in which employees are provided fair hearing of grievances, are supported in practicing according to standards of care, and are justly treated allow for the realization of the values of the profession and are consistent with sound nursing practice.

6.3 Responsibility for the health care environment

The nurse is responsible for contributing to a moral environment that encourages respectful interactions with colleagues, support of peers, and identification of issues that need to be addressed. Nurse administrators have a particular responsibility to assure that employees are treated fairly and that nurses are involved in decisions related to their practice and working conditions. Acquiescing and accepting unsafe or inappropriate practices, even if the individual does not participate in the specific practice, is equivalent to condoning unsafe practice. Nurses should not remain employed in facilities that routinely violate patient rights or require nurses to severely and repeatedly compromise standards of practice or personal morality.

Perioperative examples
♦ Interacts with patients in a compassionate manner.
♦ Demonstrates empathy, sensitivity, and patience in difficult or stressful situations.
♦ Uses therapeutic communication.
♦ Assists families with challenging issues.
♦ Develops relationships with patients that support mutual involvement in planning care.
♦ Helps to answer patients' questions related to their care.
♦ Listens attentively and, when appropriate, refers patient to other resources.

Perioperative Explications
Perioperative nurses create, maintain, and contribute to a work environment that supports individuals in their nursing practice. This environment is safe and has policies, procedures, guidelines, and standards for practice. The nurse is knowledgeable about the various processes and committees to support and promote a professional working environment.

Perioperative examples
♦ Follows process for addressing unsafe practice.
♦ Follows process for addressing ethical issues.
♦ Participates in developing policies, procedures, and standards.
♦ Maintains knowledge of policies and procedures.
♦ Promotes a positive work environment.
♦ Facilitates a working atmosphere conducive to education.

Perioperative Explications
The perioperative nurse treats colleagues and peers respectfully and fairly. The nurse, in all roles, participates in decisions that will affect practice and working conditions. The perioperative nurse identifies and supports conditions of employment that promote practice in accordance with AORN standards and recommended practices. This environment also meets accrediting and other regulatory standards. As a moral agent, if the work environment does not routinely support high quality patient care and safe practice, the nurse should seek employment elsewhere.

Perioperative nurses may need to address concerns about the work environment through appropriate channels. Perioperative nurses may need

As with concerns about patient care, nurses should address concerns about the health care environment through appropriate channels. Organizational changes are difficult to accomplish and may require persistent efforts over time. Toward this end, nurses may participate in collective action such as collective bargaining or workplace advocacy, preferably through a professional association such as the state nurses association, in order to address the terms and conditions of employment. Agreements reached through such action must be consistent with the profession's standards of practice, the state law regulating practice, and the *Code of Ethics for Nurses*. Conditions of employment must contribute to the moral environment, the provision of quality patient care, and the professional satisfaction for nurses.

The professional association also serves as an advocate for the nurse by seeking to secure just compensation and humane working conditions for nurses. To accomplish this, the professional association may engage in collective bargaining on behalf of nurses. While seeking to assure just economic and general welfare for nurses, collective bargaining nonetheless seeks to keep the interests of both nurses and patients in balance.

7: The nurse participates in the advancement of the profession through contributions to practice, education, administration, and knowledge development.

7.1 Advancing the profession through active involvement in nursing and in health care policy

Nurses should advance their profession by contributing in some way to the leadership, activities, and the viability of their professional organizations. Nurses can also advance the profession by serving in leadership or mentorship roles or on committees within their places of employment. Nurses who are self-employed can advance the profession by serving as role models for professional integrity. Nurses can also advance the profession through participation in civic activities related to health care or through local, state, national, or international initiatives. Nurse educators have a specific responsibility to enhance students' commitment to professional and civic values. Nurse administrators have a responsibility to foster an employment environment that facilitates nurses' ethical integrity and professionalism, and

to participate in collective activities (eg, collective bargaining, workplace advocacy) to address concerns about patient care, work environment, or just compensation. These activities should be consistent with AORN standards and recommended practices, accrediting standards, state nurse practice acts, and the ANA *Code of Ethics for Nurses*. In this process, the interests of both nurses and patients must be kept in balance.

Perioperative examples
♦ Knows chain of command.
♦ Promotes environment that does not tolerate harassment and abuse.
♦ Facilitates work environment conducive to learning.
♦ Collaborates with all health care team members.
♦ Questions unfair employee practices.
♦ Identifies and reports unsafe patient practices.
♦ Participates in strategic planning and development of departmental and institutional goals.
♦ Promotes empowerment.
♦ Belongs to state nursing organization.
♦ Maintains membership in AORN.

Perioperative Explications
The perioperative nurse has a personal responsibility to contribute to the advancement of the profession by participating in professional organizations. There are various activities within employment agencies and local, state, and national organizations by which one can contribute to the profession. Perioperative educators and managers are additionally responsible for providing an environment conducive to advancing the profession. Nurses can contribute to the advancement of the profession and health care policy by participating in civic activities.

Perioperative examples
♦ Maintains membership in AORN.
♦ Serves as a committee member at place of employment.
♦ Actively participates in AORN local and national initiatives.

nurse researchers are responsible for active contribution to the body of knowledge supporting and advancing nursing practice.

7.2 Advancing the profession by developing, maintaining, and implementing professional standards in clinical, administrative, and educational practice

Standards and guidelines reflect the practice of nursing grounded in ethical commitments and a body of knowledge. Professional standards and guidelines for nurses must be developed by nurses and reflect nursing's responsibility to society. It is the responsibility of nurses to identify their own scope of practice as permitted by professional practice standards and guidelines, by state and federal laws, by relevant societal values, and by the *Code of Ethics.*

The nurse as administrator or manager must establish, maintain, and promote conditions of employment that enable nurses within that organization or community setting to practice in accord with accepted standards of nursing practice and provide a nursing and health care work environment that meets the standards and guidelines of nursing practice. Professional autonomy and self regulation in the control of conditions of practice are necessary for implementing nursing standards and guidelines and assuring quality care for those whom nursing serves.

The nurse educator is responsible for promoting and maintaining optimum standards of both nursing education and of nursing practice in any settings where planned learning activities occur. Nurse educators must also ensure that only those students who possess the knowledge, skills, and competencies that are essential to nursing graduate from their nursing programs.

♦ Volunteers at schools of nursing (eg, teaching, mentoring).
♦ Actively seeks opportunity to be involved in activities related to patient care at place of employment (eg, patient care, product selection, safety initiatives, strategic planning, risk management, infection control, and ethics committees).
♦ Supports perioperative preceptor programs.
♦ Serves as leader or mentor on committees.
♦ Maintains awareness of changing health care policy at the local, state, and national levels.
♦ Participates in defining and revising scope of practice acts.
♦ Consults and collaborates with individuals who shape health care policy.

Perioperative Explications

Perioperative nurses are responsible for monitoring standards of practice pertinent to their role(s) and for fostering optimal standards of practice at the local, regional, state, and national levels of the health care system: "The perioperative nurse systematically evaluates the quality and appropriateness of nursing practice."[25] Perioperative educators and managers are equally responsible to provide an environment conducive to implementing and improving standards and recommended practices.

Perioperative examples
♦ Uses standards in nursing practice.
♦ Contributes to the work of AORN committees and projects to develop standards.
♦ Reviews and critiques practice standards (eg, responds to proposed AORN recommended practices).
♦ Participates in development and revision of standards of practice.
♦ Participates in quality and process improvement processes.
♦ Participates in multidisciplinary review of patient outcomes.
♦ Follows investigational device protocol and regulations.

7.3 Advancing the profession through knowledge development, dissemination, and application to practice

The nursing profession should engage in scholarly inquiry to identify, evaluate, refine, and expand the body of knowledge that forms the foundation of its discipline and practice. In addition, nursing knowledge is derived from the sciences and from the humanities. Ongoing scholarly activities are essential to fulfilling a profession's obligations to society. All nurses working alone or in collaboration with others can participate in the advancement of the profession through the development, evaluation, dissemination, and application of knowledge in practice. However, an organizational climate and infrastructure conducive to scholarly inquiry must be valued and implemented for this to occur.

8: The nurse collaborates with other health professionals and the public in promoting community, national, and international efforts to meet health needs.

8.1 Health needs and concerns

The nursing profession is committed to promoting the health, welfare, and safety of all people. The nurse has a responsibility to be aware not only of specific health needs of individual patients but also of broader health concerns such as world hunger, environmental pollution, lack of access to health care, violation of human rights, and inequitable distribution of nursing and health care resources. The availability and accessibility of high quality health services to all people require both interdisciplinary planning and collaborative partnerships among health professionals and others at the community, national, and international levels.

8.2 Responsibilities to the public

Nurses, individually and collectively, have a responsibility to be knowledgeable about the health status of the community and existing threats to health and safety. Through support of and participation in

Perioperative Explications

The perioperative nurse has an obligation to the patient and to society to engage in activities that promote scholarly inquiry to identify, verify, and expand the body of perioperative nursing knowledge. Perioperative nursing roles include investigation to further knowledge, participation in research, and application of theoretical and empirical knowledge. Perioperative nurses can support the research process as content experts, data collectors, research subjects, or researchers.

Perioperative examples

- Uses research findings to support and improve clinical practice.
- Fosters an environment of intellectual curiosity.
- Identifies problems amenable to the research process (eg, questions outmoded practices).
- Disseminates research findings to colleagues.

Perioperative Explications

Availability of health care involves not only addressing specific health needs, but also factors that affect well-being. These factors include world hunger, environmental pollution, lack of access to care, violation of human rights, and rationing of health care. The perioperative nurse recognizes the interdependence and collaboration of all health care workers to provide quality health care to everyone.

Perioperative examples

- Collaborates with members of other professional organizations at international, national, and state levels (eg, joint education offerings, joint patient safety legislative efforts).
- Communicates with elected officials about health care needs.
- Educates elected officials about health care needs.
- Donates to health care-related charities.
- Participates in international nursing societies.

Perioperative Explications

The perioperative nurse is knowledgeable about the health status of the community and factors that threaten well-being and safety. The nurse participates in educating the public about the various community organizations and groups, the nurse assists in efforts to educate the public, facilitates informed choice, identifies conditions and circumstances that contribute to illness, injury, and disease, fosters healthy lifestyles, and participates in institutional and legislative efforts to promote health and meet national health objectives. In addition, the nurse supports initiatives to address barriers to health, such as poverty, homelessness, unsafe living conditions, abuse and violence, and lack of access to health services.

The nurse also recognizes that health care is provided to culturally diverse populations in this country and in all parts of the world. In providing care, the nurse should avoid imposition of the nurse's own cultural values upon others. The nurse should affirm human dignity and show respect for the values and practices associated with different cultures and use approaches to care that reflect awareness and sensitivity.

9: The profession of nursing, as represented by associations and their members, is responsible for articulating nursing values, for maintaining the integrity of the profession and its practice, and for shaping social policy.

9.1 Assertion of values
It is the responsibility of a professional association to communicate and affirm the values of the profession to its members. It is essential that the professional organization encourages discourse that supports critical self-reflection and evaluation within the profession. The organization also communicates to the public the values that nursing considers central to social change that will enhance health.

factors influencing health care. The perioperative nurse recognizes cultural differences of various populations and does not allow his or her own beliefs and values to influence the care provided to patients of different beliefs and values. Nursing needs to adequately represent cultural diversity to promote the welfare and safety of all patients.

Perioperative examples
- Volunteers to teach wellness classes.
- Educates members of community about perioperative nursing.
- Collaborates with consumer, service, and support organizations related to health care.
- Fosters collaboration with and education of the public on local, state, and national health care issues.
- Prepares for disasters and threat to community.
- Provides explanations and answers to questions in the patient's primary language.
- Incorporates patient requests regarding religious preferences into practice as much as possible.
- Integrates cultural differences into patient care.
- Incorporates requests for alternative therapies into care, as appropriate.

Perioperative Explications
AORN's mission is to support perioperative registered nurses in achieving optimal outcomes for patients undergoing operative and other invasive procedures. To further its goals, AORN is committed to excellence in support of its mission and values education, representation, and standards that are research based, current, timely, comprehensive, applicable, and achievable.[26]

Perioperative examples
- Participates in educational programs to promote life-long learning.
- Reads professional journals and newsletters.
- Incorporates AORN's *Standards, Recommended Practices, and Guidelines* into practice.
- Uses the *Perioperative Nursing Data Set* (PNDS) to link perioperative nursing care to positive patient outcomes.

♦ Applies "Patient Safety First" principles to perioperative patient care.

♦ Provides consultative and other services to support perioperative nursing and patient care.

♦ Engages in legislative activities to support perioperative nursing and patient care.

♦ Promotes interaction with regulatory agencies (eg, FDA, CMS) to advance safe, quality patient care.

♦ Maintains membership in AORN.

♦ Participates in AORN chapters, state councils, specialty assemblies, and other organizational units to support AORN and perioperative nursing.

9.2 The profession carries out its collective responsibility through professional associations

The nursing profession continues to develop ways to clarify nursing's accountability to society. The contract between the profession and society is made explicit through such mechanisms as (a) the *Code of Ethics for Nurses,* (b) the standards of nursing practice, (c) the ongoing development of nursing knowledge derived from nursing theory, scholarship, and research in order to guide nursing actions, (d) educational requirements for practice, (e) certification, and (f) mechanisms for evaluating the effectiveness of professional nursing actions.

Perioperative Explications

AORN's purpose is to unite perioperative registered nurses for the purpose of maintaining an association dedicated to the constant endeavor of promoting the highest professional standards of perioperative nursing practice for optimum patient care. AORN cooperates with other professional associations, health care facilities, universities, industries, technical societies, research organizations, and governmental agencies in matters affecting the goals and purposes of AORN.[27]

Perioperative examples

♦ Practices perioperative nursing incorporating AORN's *Standards, Recommended Practices, and Guidelines.*

♦ Participates in nursing research.

♦ Becomes knowledgeable about the ANA *Code of Ethics for Nurses* and the "AORN explications for perioperative nurses."

♦ Collaborates with other organizations (eg, American College of Surgeons, American Association of Nurse Anesthetists, American Society of Anesthesiologists) to foster optimal perioperative patient care.

♦ Collaborates with other nursing organizations (eg, Nursing Organizations Alliance, American Nurses Association) to enhance the nursing profession.

♦ Identifies partnering opportunities with educational, health care, governmental, payer, business, and professional organizations to promote mutually beneficial patient care initiatives.

9.3 Intraprofessional integrity

A professional association is responsible for expressing the values and ethics of the profession and also for encouraging the professional organization and its members to function in accord with those values and ethics. Thus, one of its fundamental responsibilities is to promote awareness of and adherence to the *Code of Ethics* and to critique the activities and ends of the professional association itself. Values and ethics influence the power structures of the association in guiding, correcting, and directing its activities. Legitimate concerns for the self-interest of the association and the profession are balanced by a commitment to the social goods that are sought. Through critical self-reflection and self-evaluation, associations must foster change within themselves, seeking to move the professional community toward its stated ideals.

9.4 Social reform

Nurses can work individually as citizens or collectively through political action to bring about social change. It is the responsibility of a professional nursing association to speak for nurses collectively in shaping and reshaping health care within our nation, specifically in areas of health care policy and legislation that affect accessibility, quality, and the cost of health care. Here, the professional association maintains vigilance and takes action to influence legislators, reimbursement agencies, nursing organizations, and other health professions. In these activities, health is understood as being broader than delivery and reimbursement systems, but extending to health-related sociocultural issues such as violation of human rights, homelessness, hunger, violence, and the stigma of illness.

Perioperative Explications

The ANA *Code of Ethics for Nurses,* together with the "AORN explications for perioperative nursing," expresses the values and ethics of perioperative nursing. Use of the title *RN* carries with it the individual's responsibility to act in public's best interest. The title *RN* and all other academic degrees or other earned or honorary professional symbols of recognition may be used in all ways that are legal and reflect professional achievement.

Perioperative examples

♦ Promotes a positive image of nursing in the media and the community.
♦ Promotes professional autonomy and self-regulation of practice.
♦ Uses nursing titles (eg, CNOR, CRNFA) according to professional achievement.
♦ Identifies and resolves conflicts of interest effectively.
♦ Corrects inaccurate portrayals of and misinformation about the profession.
♦ Incorporates the ANA *Code of Ethics for Nurses* into daily practice.

Perioperative Explications

To promote the welfare and safety of all people, nurses need adequate representation to support effective health care delivery. Individual patients and society as whole benefit from nursing participation in decisions made about health care.

Perioperative examples

♦ Participates in lobbying efforts affecting health care.
♦ Supports political candidates that advance health care issues.
♦ Participates in electoral process at the local, state, and national levels.
♦ Participates in institutional decision-making.
♦ Participates in the electoral process.
♦ Volunteers in community health services.
♦ Supports political candidates, governmental programs, and legislation agenda for improving patient care.
♦ Educates members of the community about perioperative nursing (eg, through health fairs, Perioperative Nurse Week activities, educational programs).

- Collaborates with consumer, service, and support organizations (eg, Lions Club, Reach to Recovery, AARP).
- Collaborates with the public, industry, and health care workers regarding environmental and cost containment issues.
- Fosters collaboration with and education of the public regarding local, state, and national issues (eg, the environment, health care costs).

Conclusion

Perioperative nurses must be familiar with the ethical issues inherent to their practice. To develop familiarity with the issues, one can discuss them with peers and ethics committee members or consult other knowledgeable resources. Nurses may find it beneficial to have a file on ethics available in the department for review. Inservice programs focusing on ethical issues can be implemented for the department by utilizing members of the hospital's nursing ethics and/or medical ethics committees. Other departments and contacts, such as social services, also can be a resource, especially in the area of advance directives. Nurses can use values clarification to identify and understand their moral beliefs and attitudes.

Ethics provides guidelines of action for behavior with others. Such guidelines are both important and necessary when dealing with issues in the context of health care. To effectively deal with ethical situations in practice, nurses must be cognizant of limitations to scope of practice and never jeopardize patient care. Nurses need to realize they have a personal accountability to the care of the patient. As guidelines for practice, nurses can utilize many resources such as the ANA *Code of Ethics for Nurses* and knowledge of patient and individual rights, policies and procedures, standards of care, and community norms. Ultimately, the nurse must provide ethical care for all patients. Utilizing guidelines and recommended practices is a means to an end—safe, competent, and ethical patient care.

NOTES

1. S Beyea, ed, *Perioperative Nursing Data Set,* second ed (Denver: AORN, Inc, 2002) 182.

2. *Ibid.*

3. *Ibid.*

4. S Beyea, L Nicoll, "Using ethical analysis when there is no research," *AORN Journal* 69 (June 1999) 1261-1263.

5. S Beyea, ed, *Perioperative Nursing Data Set* (Denver: AORN, Inc, 2000) 150.

6. Beyea, *Perioperative Nursing Data Set,* second ed, 182.

7. *Ibid,* 184.

8. "ANA code for nurses with interpretive statements—Explications for perioperative nursing," in *Standards, Recommended Practices, and Guidelines* (Denver: AORN, Inc, 2002) 54.

9. Beyea, *Perioperative Nursing Data Set,* second ed, 178.

10. *Ibid,* 182.

11. *Ibid,* 183.

12. *Ibid,* 175-176.

13. *Ibid,* 178, 180.

14. *Ibid,* 179, 181.

15. Beyea, *Perioperative Nursing Data Set,* 125.

16. "Recommended practices for traffic patterns," in *Standards, Recommended Practices, and Guidelines* (Denver: AORN, Inc, 2002) 350.

17. Beyea, *Perioperative Nursing Data Set,* second ed, 184.

18. Beyea, *Perioperative Nursing Data Set,* second ed, 183.

19. A Orb, L Eisenhauer, D Wynaden, "Ethics in qualitative research," *Journal of Nursing Scholarship* 33 (2001) 93-96.

20. *Standards, Recommended Practices, and Guidelines* (Denver: AORN, Inc, 2002) 157-162.

21. "AORN official statement on unlicensed assistive personnel," in *Standards, Recommended Practices, and Guidelines* (Denver: AORN, Inc, 2002) 141.

22. *Ibid.*

23. *Ibid.*

24. *Ibid.*

25. "Standards of perioperative professional performance," in *Standards, Recommended Practices, and Guidelines* (Denver: AORN, Inc, 2002) 160.

26. "AORN vision, mission, philosophy, and values," in *Standards, Recommended Practices, and Guidelines* (Denver: AORN, Inc, 2002) 5.

27. "AORN national bylaws," in *Standards, Recommended Practices, and Guidelines* (Denver: AORN, Inc, 2002) 7.

Originally published in the 1994 edition of the AORN *Standards and Recommended Practices.*

Revised; approved by the AORN Board of Directors in November 2002.

AORN Latex Guideline

I. Overview

A. Introduction

Preamble

Natural rubber latex allergy is a significant medical concern because it affects health care workers, as well as the general population. It crosses racial and ethnic boundaries, and it can affect males or females anytime during their lives.

There is no cure at this time, only prevention. Three types of reactions are associated with latex products. In order of frequency of occurrence they are an irritant reaction, a delayed hypersensitivity reaction (ie, type IV), and an immediate hypersensitivity reaction (ie, type I) (Table 1). Any individual who experiences any type of latex-associated reaction should be evaluated by a qualified health care practitioner.

Assumptions

Natural rubber latex allergy can be a serious and potentially life-threatening condition. Health care workers and others who experience repeated exposure to latex allergens can develop a latex sensitivity or allergy. Several hundred cases of severe allergic reactions and anaphylaxis and 17 deaths have been reported to the US Food and Drug Administration (FDA).[1,2]

Sensitivity can be described as development of an immunologic memory to the specific latex proteins; however, the affected individual may be asymptomatic. Allergy is the demonstrated outward expression of the sensitivity (eg, hives, rhinitis, conjunctivitis, anaphylaxis). Sensitivity to natural rubber latex is more common than the actual allergy; however, any individual sensitized to natural rubber latex is at risk of a life-threatening reaction and should be treated in the same way as an allergic individual.

Powdered latex gloves are the most common item contributing to the latex load in health care facilities. Recent estimates have shown a 20-fold increase in medical glove use (in billions of pairs) since the introduction of universal precautions in 1987.[3] During the manufacturing process, powder usually is applied to the glove as cornstarch slurry when the glove still is on the mold or former. When the powder slurry is applied to the glove, the extractable, water-soluble proteins leach from the surface of the glove onto the cornstarch particle. When dry, the glove powder then acts as a vector that carries latex proteins from the glove into the environment.

Health care facilities and providers have an ethical responsibility to prevent latex sensitization in patients and employees by creating an environment in which it is safe to be treated and to work. Many facilities in the United States consciously have moved toward a latex-safe environment by switching from powdered latex gloves (eg, examination, surgical) and other latex products to powder-free products with reduced latex protein content. High-protein, powdered latex gloves and other products that create aerosolization can contaminate a facility's environment with latex allergens.

In 1998, Sussman et al reported a 1% annual incidence of sensitization among powdered latex-glove users, whereas users of powder-free, low-protein, latex glove reported a 0% sensitization rate.[4] In 1999, Levy et al studied a group of dental students in both France and England, reporting that students who wore protein-rich (ie, high protein), powdered latex gloves had a 15% and a 5% sensitization rate, respectively, while students who wore powder-free, protein-poor (ie, low protein) gloves had a 0% sensitization rate.[5]

It is unsafe to treat latex-allergic individuals in an environment laden with latex allergens. Individuals who have been clinically diagnosed as either sensitive or allergic to natural rubber latex should be treated or work in an environment that is latex-safe, with additional measures taken for the immediate vicinity (ie, room) in which the individual receives or provides care. If the entire care facility is maintained as a latex-safe environment, few additional precautions will be needed for latex-allergic individuals. If the facility is not maintained as latex-safe, comprehensive latex precautions will be required each time a latex-allergic individual presents for care or services.

This revised "AORN latex guideline" is based on research and expert opinion available at the time of its revision. Ongoing and future research likely will enhance and expand current knowledge about this topic.

Review of this document has been solicited from content experts at the American Association of Nurse Anesthetists (AANA), the American College of Surgeons (ACS), the American Society of Anesthesiologists (ASA), the American Academy of Allergy, Asthma, and Immunology (AAAAI), the American College of Allergy, Asthma, and Immunology (ACAAI), the American Nurses Association (ANA),

Table 1

TYPES OF LATEX AND OTHER GLOVE-ASSOCIATED REACTIONS

Mechanism	Terms Used	Cause	Signs and Symptoms
Irritation	Irritant contact dermatitis (nonallergic irritation)	Hand washing, insufficient rinsing, scrubs, antiseptics, glove occlusion, glove powder.	Dry, crusty hard bumps, sores, and horizontal cracks on skin may manifest as itchy dermatitis on the back of the hands under the gloves.
Type IV hypersensitivity; cell-mediated	Delayed type hypersensitivity; allergic contact dermatitis; chemical allergy	Exposure to chemicals used in latex manufacturing, mostly thiurams.	Red, raised, palpable area with bumps, sores, and horizontal cracks may extend up the forearm. Occurs after a sensitization period. Appears several hours after glove contact and may persist many days.
Type I hypersensitivity; immunoglobulin-mediated	Immediate type hypersensitivity; latex allergy; protein allergy	Exposure to proteins in latex on glove surface and/or bound to powder and suspended in the air, settled on objects, or transferred by touch.	Wheal and flare response or itchy redness on the skin under the glove. Occurs within minutes, fades away rapidly after removing the glove. In chronic form, may mimic irritant and allergic contact dermatitis. Symptoms can include facial swelling, rhinitis, eye symptoms, generalized urticaria, respiratory distress, and asthma. In rare cases, anaphylactic shock may occur.

Reprinted with permission from *Latex Allergy: Protect Yourself, Protect Your Patients* © 1996 American Nurses Association. For the complete text of this brochure, call (800) 274-4ANA and ask for WP-7, or visit the ANA Web site at http://www.nursingworld.org.

the Association of Practitioners of Infection Control, Inc (APIC), the Spina Bifida Association, and the National Institute of Occupational Safety and Health (NIOSH) division of the Centers for Disease Control and Prevention, as well as the AORN Board of Directors and other recognized experts. This guideline may not apply to every individual and may require modification based on specific needs of a given patient, health care provider, or situation.

Definitions

For purposes of this document the following definitions apply.

♦ *Allergen:* A substance that in some individuals can cause an allergic or hypersensitivity reaction but is not normally considered harmful.[6]

♦ *Allergenic:* A substance that can elicit a hypersensitivity reaction in certain individuals.[7]

♦ *Allergy:* An immune reaction to an environmental agent that results in a symptomatic reaction.[6,7]

♦ *Antigen:* Any molecule or substance, more often a protein, that has the ability to bind to an antibody.[6,7] "The name arises from their ability to generate antibodies."[6]

♦ *Irritant contact dermatitis:* A nonallergic, cutaneous response to an irritant. Normally this reaction is primarily localized to the site of exposure. This is not a latex allergy.

♦ *Allergic contact dermatitis (type IV: T-cell mediated/delayed hypersensitivity):* A delayed, T-cell mediated hypersensitivity response attributed to chemicals (ie, antigens) used in the latex and some synthetic manufacturing processes and absorbed through the skin.[6] This reaction generally is localized to the contact area.

♦ *Latex:* Also known as natural rubber latex, this milky cytosol is acquired by tapping the commercial rubber tree, *Hevea brasiliensis.*

♦ *Latex allergy (type immunoglobulin E [IgE]-mediated/immediate hypersensitivity response):* A localized or systemic allergic response to one or more specific proteins (ie, antigens)[6] found in latex to which the individual has been sensitized and has developed antibodies.

♦ *Latex-free environment:* An environment in which all latex-containing products, not simply gloves, have been removed. This state is considered unattainable due to the ubiquitous nature of latex products.

♦ *Latex-safe environment:* An environment in which every reasonable effort has been made to remove high-allergen and airborne latex sources from coming into direct contact with affected individuals. The airborne latex protein load should be less than 0.6 ng per cubic meter.[8]

♦ *Latex precautions:* Interventions to prevent reactions in people (eg, patients, health care workers) allergic to latex proteins.

♦ *Reactions associated with latex:* Irritant contact dermatitis, allergic type IV cell-mediated contact dermatitis, and type I IgE-mediated latex allergy. Only the type I IgE-mediated response constitutes a true latex allergy.

♦ *Sensitization:* The development of immunological memory in response to exposure to an antigen.

♦ *Sensitivity:* A clinical manifestation of symptoms or response that develops after sensitization.

Prevalence

Numerous studies indicate prevalence rates for IgE-mediated latex allergy from 0.8% to 6.5% of the general population.[1,9-13] Latex allergy is believed to be responsible for 70% of anaphylactic reactions occurring in anesthetized children with myelodysplasia (eg, spina bifida).[12] Further, there is a large population of latex-sensitive individuals. Varying sensitization rates have been reported for both patients with myelodysplasia and health care workers.[14-17] According to Sussman, the prevalence rate of latex sensitization among patients with spina bifida is between 35% and 70%. The sensitization rate for health care

workers with significant exposure to latex is reported to be 10% to 17%.[18] Although latex-sensitive individuals do not always present with clinical symptoms, these individuals should be assessed for latex allergy. For those who are latex-sensitive but have yet to manifest frank symptoms, there is no predictor of whether or when they will react; therefore, all individuals presenting with natural rubber latex sensitivity should be treated as if they are allergic.

In 1992, Lagier et al reported a 10.7% latex allergy rate in French perioperative nurses.[19] A study of Canadian perioperative nurses by Mace et al, in 1997, reported a 6.9% latex allergy prevalence.[20] Studies of perioperative personnel demonstrate sensitivity rates between 2.5% and 15.8%. In 1992, Arellano et al reported a 9.9% latex sensitization rate in a study of 101 anesthesiologists, radiologists, and surgeons.[21] In 1996, Grzybowski reported an 8.9% rate for hospital RNs in general, but showed perioperative nurses to be less affected than nurses in other areas. One possible explanation for this disparity was that nurses in the OR who were latex sensitive or allergic may have transferred to other nursing units.[22] In 1997, Konrad et al reported a 15.8% positive skin prick test rate for anesthesiologists.[23] In 1998, Brown et al identified 12.5% of anesthesiologists at a tertiary care hospital as sensitized (ie, IgE antibody positive by skin test or serology) with only 2.5% expressing symptoms.[24]

B. Pathophysiology

The major component of natural rubber latex is the hydrocarbon, cis-1, 4 polyisoprene. Chemicals such as sulfur, ammonia, mercaptobenzothiazole, thiuram, and antioxidants may be added during the manufacturing process. Latex protein content and residual chemical levels differ among producers due to variations in manufacturing processes.

Several natural rubber latex proteins responsible for allergenic reactions have been identified (Table 2), and sensitivity appears to differ among risk groups.[25-28] Proteins in natural rubber latex may cause a range of mild to severe or even life-threatening type I allergic reactions. Dipped products made from liquid natural rubber latex (eg, gloves, balloons, condoms) contain a greater amount of soluble proteins than dry gum rubber or heat molded latex products and, therefore, can release more allergen.[2,9,29]

Several types of synthetic materials also may be referred to as latex (eg, butyl, petroleum-based materials) but these do not contain the proteins

Table 2

KNOWN LATEX ALLERGENS				
Name	*Description*	*MW (kD)*	*Plant family*	*Cross-food*
Hev b 1	Rubber elongation factor	14.6		Papain
Hev b 2	Beta one=third gluconase	34-36	PR2	
Hev b 3	Prenyltransferase	24-27		
Hev b 4	Microhelix	110/50		
Hev b 5	Acidic protein	16-24		Kiwi
Hev b 6.02	Hevein protein	4.7	PR3	Kiwi, avocado, banana
Hev b 7	Patatin homologue	43-46		Potato
Hev b 8	Hevea profilin	14-14.2	Profilin	Pollens, celery
Hev b 9	Hevea enolase	51		Molds
Hev b 10	Mn superoxide dismutase	22-26		Molds
Hev b 11	Class I chitinase	33	PR3	Banana, avocado
Hev b 12	Lipid transfer protein	9.4	PR-14	Peach, stone fruit
Hev b 13	Esterase	42		

Suggested by Robert Hamilton, PhD, Latex Committee, Chairman, American Academy of Asthma, Allergy, and Immunology.

that cause allergic reactions. There have been case reports, however, of individuals having a type I natural rubber latex-allergic reaction because synthetic materials may have been mixed with or contaminated with natural rubber latex.[29] Water extractable, residual chemicals found in both latex and synthetic gloves usually are implicated in the development of allergic contact dermatitis in individuals who are presensitized.[30-33]

C. Reactions Associated With Latex and Synthetic Products

Reactions associated with latex and synthetic products include irritant contact dermatitis, allergic contact dermatitis (type IV), and immediate IgE hypersensitivity reactions (type I).[34,35] Only the type I hypersensitivity reaction constitutes a latex allergy. Some individuals may present with a single complaint or a combination of all three reactions listed above. Irritant and allergic contact dermatitis are the most common clinical reactions associated with latex and other additives.[34,35]

Irritant contact dermatitis is the result of damage to the skin, but it is not an allergic reaction. Soaps and cleansers, multiple hand washings, inadequate hand drying, or mechanical irritation (ie, sweating, rubbing inside powdered gloves) may cause skin irritation. It also can be caused by chemicals added during glove manufacture. An acute localized response is evidenced by redness, swelling, burning, and itching. Chronic exposure to the irritant can lead to dry, thickened, and cracked skin. Health care workers experiencing irritant contact dermatitis or skin breakdown should be referred to an occupational health practitioner, allergist, dermatologist, or immunologist for further diagnostic testing. This type of dermatitis is reduced by removing the irritant source after it is identified. Thoroughly washing and drying hands, using only powder-free gloves, changing gloves more frequently, or changing glove types can reduce skin irritation.[11,36,37]

Other palliative measures include using only water- or silicone-based moisturizing creams, lotions, or topical barrier agents. Avoid using oil- or petroleum-based skin agents with latex products. These agents may cause breakdown of the latex product. Some skin care agents may help reduce glove-related problems and have been clinically formulated not to interfere with the glove's barrier integrity. Always check with the manufacturer of the skin care agent to verify that the chosen agent is latex compatible before putting the product into use.[38]

Allergic contact dermatitis (ie, delayed hypersensitivity) is a type IV immune reaction. It is a T-cell mediated allergic reaction and usually is localized to the area of contact. Chemical additives used in the manufacturing processes (eg, accelerators) and not the latex itself causes previously sensitized T-cell lymphocytes to stimulate proliferation of other lymphocytes and mononuclear cells, resulting in tissue inflammation and dermatitis.

Table 3

ANAPHYLACTIC REACTION ASSESSMENT CRITERIA

Decreased cardiac output
Assess physical status and document changes. Report:
♦ Vital signs, including, temperature, pulse rate, blood pressure, cardiac rhythm, respiratory rate.
♦ Lung sounds (eg, rales, wheezing, stridor).
♦ Jugular vein distention, pulmonary pressures.
♦ Skin color, rashes, temperature, moisture.
♦ Changes in level of consciousness or mentation.
♦ Changes in patient's level of anxiety.
Defining characteristics: Hypotension, tachycardia, decreased central venous pressure, decreased pulmonary pressures, decreased cardiac output, oliguria.

Ineffective breathing pattern
♦ Monitor respiratory status and observe for changes.
♦ Monitor arterial blood gases and note changes.
♦ Check breath sounds and report changes.
♦ Monitor chest x-ray reports.
Defining characteristics: Dyspnea, wheezing, tachypnea, cyanosis, stridor, tightness of chest.

Impaired skin integrity
♦ Observe for signs of local or generalized flushing.
♦ Watch for development of rashes; note character.
♦ Assess for swelling/edema.
Defining characteristics: Urticaria, pruritus, edema, angioedema, eczema hypersensitivity, dermatitis erythema, swelling, inflammation, vesiculation, blister formation.

Fluid volume deficit
♦ Assess fluid balance (I & O) every hour.
♦ Assess for edema.
Defining characteristics: Decreased urine output, concentrated urine, decreased venous filling, hypotension, thirst, tachycardia.

Altered renal perfusion
♦ Monitor serum and urine electrolytes and osmolarity and document.
♦ Monitor urine output every hour; document changes.
♦ Monitor laboratory data for elevation in BUN (blood urea nitrogen) and creatinine levels, acid-base imbalances, particularly sodium (Na+) and potassium (K+).
Defining characteristics: Decreased urine output, decreased venous filing, hemoconcentration.

Altered level of consciousness
♦ Obtain neurological checks; report and record any changes.
♦ Observe for seizure activity; report and record changes.
♦ Monitor vital signs.
Defining characteristics: Fainting, changes in alertness, changes in orientation.

Gastrointestinal
Defining characteristics: Abdominal cramping, diarrhea, nausea, and vomiting.

Potential anxiety/fear
♦ Recognize patient's level of anxiety and note signs and symptoms.
♦ Assess patient's coping mechanisms.

Knowledge deficit
♦ Assess patient's knowledge of his or her condition and allergens.

The onset of type IV reactions is slow, usually occurring during 18 to 24 hours and peaking at 48 hours after exposure. Reactions may present as pruritis, erythema, swelling, crusty thickened skin, pimples, blisters, and other skin lesions. Symptoms usually resolve within three to four days after exposure.[39,40] Each exposure may lead to increased sensitization and a more severe reaction. Diagnosis is made by a health care provider experienced in chemical allergy testing—patch tests commonly are used. Treatment involves education; thoroughly drying hands; using water- or silicone-based moisturizing creams, lotions, or topical barrier agents; avoiding oil- or petroleum-based products unless they are latex compatible; and avoiding the identified causative agent.[38,41,42] Continued use of latex prod-

ucts when there are breaks in the wearer's skin is believed to contribute to latex protein sensitization. This is due to absorption of solubilized latex proteins associated with the product.[43,44]

Latex allergy (ie, immediate hypersensitivity) is a systemic type I IgE-mediated response to plant proteins in natural rubber latex. In sensitized individuals, an anti-latex IgE antibody stimulates mast cell proliferation and basophil histamine release, leading to local swelling, redness, edema, itching, and systemic reactions, including anaphylaxis.[39,44] Type I reactions are immediate, with the onset of symptoms usually occurring in minutes.[39] Symptoms include rhinitis, conjunctivitis, urticaria, laryngeal edema, bronchospasm, asthma, angioedema, anaphylaxis, and death.[39,45-48] These responses can

Table 4

SAMPLE LATEX ALLERGY QUESTIONNAIRE	Yes	No
1. Have you ever had allergies, asthma, hay fever, eczema, or problems with rashes?	❏	❏
2. Have you ever had respiratory distress, rapid heart rate, or swelling?	❏	❏
3. Have you ever had swelling, itching, hives, or other symptoms after contact with a balloon?	❏	❏
4. Have you ever had swelling, itching, hives, or other symptoms after a dental examination or procedure?	❏	❏
5. Have you ever had swelling, itching, hives, or other symptoms following a vaginal or rectal examination or after contact with a diaphragm or condom?	❏	❏
6. Have you ever had swelling, itching, or hives during or within one hour after wearing rubber gloves?	❏	❏
7. Have you ever had a rash on your hands that lasted longer than one week?	❏	❏
8. Have you ever had swelling, itching, hives, runny nose, eye irritation, wheezing, or asthma after contact with any latex or rubber product?	❏	❏
9. Have you ever had swelling, itching, or hives after being examined by someone wearing rubber or latex gloves?	❏	❏
10. Has a physician ever told you that you had rubber or latex allergy?	❏	❏
11. Are you allergic to bananas, papaya, avocados, kiwifruits, other stone fruits, tomatoes, raw potatoes, or chestnuts?	❏	❏
12. Have you ever had an unexplained anaphylactic episode? If so, please describe.	❏	❏

occur when materials containing latex come into contact with the skin, mucous membranes, or internal tissues. Aerosolization of very small amounts of natural rubber latex proteins may cause some individuals to react after inhaling traces of powder from latex gloves or balloons.[49,50] The severity of repeat reactions is unpredictable; therefore, individuals who have suffered any type I reaction are considered to be at high risk for anaphylaxis.

Latex allergy is diagnosed by a history of type I reactions to latex products, such as gloves, balloons, or condoms, and a skin prick test—no FDA-approved reagent is yet approved in the United States—or serum test to identify IgE antibodies to latex. Individuals may experience irritant, type IV, and type I reactions simultaneously. If a patient or health care worker experiences any form of reaction to a medical device that may contain latex (eg, medical gloves), the individual should be carefully evaluated by a health care provider experienced in latex allergy diagnosis and management. Table 3 provides anaphylactic reaction assessment criteria with which health care workers should be familiar.

D. Population Affected/Risk Factors

Children with myelodysplasia or a history of multiple surgeries beginning in infancy and any individual with a past history of type I reaction or positive test results to natural rubber latex are at high risk for developing anaphylaxis. People at risk for developing latex sensitization include individuals occupationally exposed to latex (eg, health care workers, food service workers); atopic individuals with a history of asthma, eczema, and rhinitis; people who react to medications; and individuals with multiple environmental allergies. People with a history of type I allergic reactions to certain foods (eg, banana, avocado, chestnut, kiwi) also are at

Table 5

LATEX ALLERGY RISK GROUPS

Persons at high risk for systemic reactions

♦ Children with a history of frequent surgeries or use of instrumentation, particularly if begun in early infancy, as with congenital malformations like myelodysplasia (eg, spina bifida) or genitourinary problems.

♦ Verifiable history of latex allergic reactions, particularly if intraoperative or asthmatic.

♦ Positive test results to serum latex antibody test (eg, radioallergosorbent/enzyme-linked immunosorbent assay) or skin prick test.

♦ History of any immunoglobulin E-mediated symptoms, (eg, urticaria, rhino-conjunctivitis, asthma, bronchospasm) when in contact with natural rubber latex products.

Persons at risk for developing latex allergy

♦ Occupational exposure to latex products, particularly to powdered products such as gloves, or to aerosolized latex proteins.

♦ History of latex-fruit syndrome or progressive reactions to foods known to cross-react with NRL—including bananas, kiwifruits, avocados, stone fruits, raw potato, tomato, papaya, or chestnuts—or a history of a latex glove-associated contact dermatitis.

Persons who should be evaluated for latex allergy

♦ History of any unexplained anaphylaxis—particularly if occurring in a medical or dental setting.

♦ History of hives or itching after incidental latex exposure, such as dental or gynecological examinations, or on contact with balloons, condoms, or natural rubber latex gloves.

♦ History of multiple surgical procedures.

Risks suggested by Dr. B. Lauren Charous, Milwaukee Medical Clinic

increased risk for latex sensitization. This is because of a cross reactivity that exists between natural rubber latex proteins and certain food allergens.[10,22,24,51] Table 4 provides a sample questionnaire suitable for assessing patients and others for their risk of latex allergy or sensitization.

The ACAAI recommends that individuals with known latex allergy and those at high risk for allergy be treated in a latex-safe environment. Individuals designated as at risk for developing latex sensitization should be assessed carefully, and health care facility protocol should be followed in determining the need for testing for immediate hypersensitivity to natural rubber latex (Table 5).[10,12,52,53]

E. Exposure

Systemic exposure to latex can occur through the following routes: mucous membrane, ingestion, inhalation, or intravascular or cutaneous contact. The majority of severe latex reactions result from latex proteins coming in contact with internal tissues during invasive procedures or after contact with mucous membranes of the mouth, vagina, urethra, or rectum.[45,46] Triggering items include latex gloves, latex glove powder, orthodontic elastic, dental dams, nasogastric tubes, balloons, pacifiers, urinary catheters, enema kits, barium enema catheters, condoms, and balloon catheters. Case reports describe intraoperative anaphylaxis after the peritoneum or other internal tissues are contacted by surgical gloves.[39,45-48]

Inhalation of latex proteins can lead to bronchospasm or laryngeal edema. Aerosolized glove powder is the most common source of latex protein inhalation.[49,50] Latex proteins bind to the glove starch powder during the manufacturing process and are expelled into the air when gloves are opened, donned, or removed.[50] Latex proteins, particularly when bound to starch glove powder and then aerosolized, can and have caused serious health problems for both patients and employees.[3] Use of powdered latex gloves in the same room as a sensitized individual can produce an allergic reaction. Use of powder-free gloves results in only small or negligible amounts of latex in the air.[8,50,54-56]

Cutaneous exposure to latex products can trigger serious systemic reactions in highly sensitized individuals. Examples of products that have triggered reactions include gloves, condoms, anesthesia masks, tourniquets, electrocardiogram electrodes, adhesive tape, elastic bandages, condom catheters, rubber shoes, elastic in clothing, balloons, and racquet handles.

F. Prevention

The goals of prevention are twofold: to prevent reactions in individuals who are latex-sensitized and to prevent initial sensitization of nonsensitized persons. The only effective preventive strategy at this time is latex avoidance. Working in an environment that is free of powdered, high-allergen latex gloves and products will help minimize sensitization of health care workers.[4,5] The NIOSH, AAAAI, ACAAI, and others recommend and encourage the use of low-allergen, powder-free latex gloves as an important factor in developing a latex-safe environment.[8,37,38,41,50,53,55-65] For patients or staff members with a known allergy to natural rubber latex proteins, additional precautions are necessary. The presence of even small amounts of residual aerosolized latex in the air or on surfaces can trigger a life-threatening reaction. Latex-allergic individuals should be treated or work in an environment using strict latex avoidance. Although it is impossible to remove all latex from the environment (eg, wheels on carts), all latex that may potentially contact the individual should be removed.

When establishing a latex-safe environment, pertinent clinical data should be obtained on every latex or latex-containing product used in the facility, with an emphasis placed on the protein and powder content of each product, if powdered gloves or other powdered items are used. Latex products selected for use should be low-allergen and powder-free. The protein content should be less than 50 µg/dm² using the American Society for Testing and Materials (ASTM) D5712 total protein test[66] and less than 10 µg per dm² by the ASTM D6499 antigen test.[67]

AORN's "Recommended practices for product selection in perioperative practice settings" provides guidance to assist practitioners with product evaluation and selection.[68] A master list or directory of products containing latex and appropriate latex-free substitutes for those products should be maintained by the health care facility and be readily accessible to all health care providers. Since September 30, 1998, the FDA has required that all FDA-cleared medical devices containing natural rubber latex carry a warning statement.[69-71] This statement reads "Caution: This product contains natural rubber latex which may cause allergic reactions." This label warning will facilitate alternative product selection for latex-allergic individuals. This ruling does not include pharmaceuticals or products that are not regulated by the FDA.

A latex-free cart may be helpful for consolidating latex-free items in a single place for ease of location and use. Specialty patient care areas, such as the OR, emergency, and labor and delivery departments, should develop a list of items to meet their special care needs. Emergency carts (ie, code carts) also should contain latex-free items (eg, syringes, latex-free gloves, resuscitation equipment). Manufacturer documentation should be obtained to ensure the latex-free status of contents for all carts (eg, code, latex, other specialty carts). It is important that each cart be latex-free as emergency situations can occur without respect for any individual patient considerations. A sample of items to be included in a latex-free cart can be found in Table 6.

Pretreating latex-allergic individuals with certain medication regimens (eg diphenhydramine, ranitidine, corticosteroids) may prevent initial allergy symptoms, but it also may give care providers with a false sense of security.[9,34,39,53] This practice remains controversial. Pretreated latex-allergic individuals may present with anaphylaxis as the first sign observed by the health care team.[72]

The use of medication vials with rubber stoppers also is controversial when caring for latex-sensitive or allergic patients. Protein can be leached from the vial stopper. Even when the single-puncture or the pop-the-top-off method is used, individuals already sensitized to natural rubber latex can react.[73] One study reported that the amount of latex found in a medication vial after 40 punctures was below the level of detection using standardized methods.[74] Another study suggested that medication vials should be changed to synthetic vial tops or be clearly labeled as is required for other medical devices.[75] Coring of the stopper also is a concern. Coring may occur from repetitive puncturing of a multi-use vial stopper. This raises a concern about latex-containing particulate matter potentially contaminating the medication. In two studies, the use of sharp needles reportedly caused coring fragments in 73% of solutions in test vials using multi-dose insulin stoppers.[75,76] Whenever possible, medications should be used from a latex-free vial. When this is not possible, arrangements with the pharmacy should be made in advance so medications can be drawn into a latex-free delivery device under aseptic conditions (eg, inside the pharmacy's hood). If neither of these solutions is possible, the stopper should be removed and the medication withdrawn using a latex-free syringe. AORN does not recommend this practice unless all other options have been exhausted.

Reprocessing instruments previously processed in steam and potentially exposed to latex contamination via sterilization tape, container gaskets, or gloves worn in processing is considered unnecessary by most experts because proteins are denatured by heat and steam.[53,77,78] Health care facilities are cautioned not to heat sterilize a known latex product in an attempt to render it safe for use on a latex-allergic individual.

Sterilization of medical products by means other than heat has not been well studied in relation to latex allergy. Each facility should contact the manufacturer of the sterilizing agent or technology to verify its safe use for individuals with a latex allergy.

G. Managing Latex-Allergic Individuals

Patients

Preparing a health care facility to care for latex-allergic patients is a complex process that can be costly and labor intensive. A multidisciplinary task force to address latex issues should be formed and may include representatives from the following areas:

- administration,
- risk management,
- quality management,
- safety management,
- surgical services,
- sterile processing,
- distribution,
- anesthesia services,
- materiel management,
- pharmacy,
- laboratory,
- infection control,
- family medicine,
- department of surgery,
- department of allergy and immunology, and
- various nursing departments (eg, intensive care unit, emergency, medical-surgical, home care, education, occupational health).

Table 6

SUGGESTED CONTENTS FOR A LATEX-SAFE CART
Note: All items must be latex-free.

Safety needles (25 g through 15 g)
Syringes (multiple sizes)
3-way stopcocks
IV tubing
Blood tubing
Tourniquets
Assorted tape (.5", 1", 1.5")
Underpads and small chux
100% silicone or polyvinyl chloride (PVC) urinary catheters
Silicone or PVC external catheters—pediatric and adult
Urinary drainage system
Feeding tubes (5 Fr to 10 Fr)
Feeding pump bag and tubing
Bulb syringe (60 cc)
Blood pressure cuffs and connecting tubing
Stethoscope
Examination gloves
Sterile gloves
Oxygen delivery supplies (eg, cannula, masks)
Anesthesia breathing bag

The role of the task force is to develop a protocol for creating a latex-safe environment for patients who are latex-allergic. Removing devices and supplies with high latex protein content and discontinuing use of powdered latex products should be an integral part of the protocol. The possible increase in purchase costs for nonlatex items must be weighed against the costs of potential anaphylactic episodes or patient death. The protocol also should include a mechanism for patient education about latex allergy and its management.

Patient safety cannot be compromised. If a facility is maintained as latex-safe, additional preparation for latex-allergic patients may not be necessary. If a facility makes the conscious decision not to continuously maintain a latex-safe environment, special preparation and precautions will be required every time a latex-allergic individual presents for care.[64,79-82]

Employees

Latex-allergic individuals should be counseled about the risk of working in environments with high latex use. They should use only nonlatex gloves and avoid all products containing latex. The ACAAI suggests that these individuals wear an allergic identification bracelet or tag, always carry an epinephrine auto-injector device, and avoid environments where powdered latex gloves are used or balloons are allowed.[52]

For both facility and employee protection, employees new to a facility should be assessed to determine the risk or presence of latex-related problems. This can be done through the employee health service or a similar mechanism during the pre-employment history and physical examination. A simple questionnaire can be used as part of the initial assessment. People at high risk for latex sensitivity should have further evaluation for latex allergy. Individuals considered at high risk

- have existing allergies, particularly to fruits (eg, latex-fruit syndrome)[83];
- have hand dermatitis or eczema; and
- use gloves regularly.

Low-risk employees with a negative clinical history of latex reactions do not need allergy testing, but they should be evaluated if symptoms suggestive of latex sensitivity develop during their employment. For people with contact dermatitis, the causative agent should be identified and avoided if possible. If the dermatitis appears on the hands, the use of glove liners under latex or nonlatex gloves that do not contain the triggering agent has been found to be helpful.[41,52]

All employees should be educated about latex sensitivity and allergy and be able to recognize the symptoms of a latex reaction. Employees should be encouraged to report development of any symptoms to the facility's employee health service or other designated mechanism.

II. Nursing Process Application

A. Perioperative Nursing Vocabulary

The perioperative nursing vocabulary is a clinically relevant and empirically validated standardized nursing language. It relates to the delivery of care in the perioperative setting. This standardized language consists of a collection of data elements (ie, the Perioperative Nursing Data Set [PNDS]) and includes perioperative nursing diagnoses, interventions, and outcomes. In 1999, the PNDS was recognized by the ANA committee on nursing practice

information infrastructure as a data set useful in the practice of nursing. The perioperative patient-focused model provides the conceptual framework for the PNDS and the model for perioperative nursing practice.[84] The patient and his or her family members are at the core of the model. The model depicts perioperative nursing in four domains and illustrates the relationship between the patient, family members, and care provided by the perioperative professional nurse. The patient-centered domains are

- D1—safety,
- D2—physiological responses to surgery,
- D3—patient's and family members' behavioral responses to surgery, and
- D4—health system in which perioperative care is provided.

Each data element in the PNDS is represented by a unique identifier. The domains are represented by the letter "D" followed by numbers one to four to indicate the particular domain being addressed. Nursing diagnoses are represented by the letter "X" and a number unique to the diagnosis; interventions are represented by the letter "I" and a unique number; and outcomes are represented by the letter "O" and a unique number. These designations are used in this document as appropriate.

B. Assessment

Perioperative nurses assess, document, and communicate patient status to all members of the health care team. Data collection involves the patient and his or her significant others. Assess for the following risk factors:

- history of multiple surgeries beginning at an early age (eg, spina bifida, urinary malformations);
- food allergies (eg, latex-fruit syndrome);[83]
- exposure to latex; and
- history of allergic reaction to latex.

Assess for inadvertent latex exposure and impending anaphylaxis. Table 7 provides a summary of symptoms of latex exposure and possible anaphylaxis for both conscious and anesthetized patients.

C. Nursing Diagnosis

The perioperative nurse analyzes the assessment data when determining nursing diagnoses. Following is a partial list of nursing diagnoses that may be associated with latex-allergic individuals ("X" = nursing diagnosis, "D" = domain).

- ◆ X 32 (D2)—latex allergy response (risk for);
- ◆ X 30 (D3)—knowledge deficient related to latex hypersensitivity (risk for/actual);
- ◆ X 50 (D1)—skin integrity, impaired, related to manifestations of allergic reaction (risk for/actual);
- ◆ X 7 (D2)—breathing pattern, ineffective, related to facial angioedema, bronchospasm, and laryngeal edema (risk for/actual);
- ◆ X 8 (D2)—cardiac output, decreased, related to severe latex-allergic reaction (risk for/actual);
- ◆ X 61 (D2)—tissue perfusion, ineffective, renal, related to hypotension and decreased cardiac output (risk for/actual);
- ◆ X 18 (D2)—fluid volume, risk for deficient
- ◆ X 11 (D2)—acute confusion related to physiologic condition and decreased circulation;
- ◆ X 64 (D3)—verbal communication, impaired, related to hypotension and decreased cardiac output (risk for/actual);
- ◆ X 47 (D1)—sensory perception, disturbed, related to hypotension and decreased cardiac output (risk for/actual); and
- ◆ X 4 (D1)—anxiety, related to change in physiological status in response to latex.

D. Outcome Identification

The following is a partial list of nursing outcomes that may be associated with the latex-allergic individual ("O" = outcome, "D" = domain).

- ◆ O 2 (D1)—The patient is free from signs and symptoms of injury caused by extraneous objects.
- ◆ O 3 (D2)—The patient is free from signs and symptoms of chemical injury.
- ◆ O 11 (D2)—The patient has wound/tissue perfusion consistent with or improved from baseline levels established preoperatively.
- ◆ O 13 (D2)—The patient's fluid, electrolyte, and acid-base balances are consistent with or improved from baseline levels established preoperatively.
- ◆ O 14 (D2)—The patient's respiratory status is consistent with or improved from baseline levels established preoperatively.
- ◆ O 15 (D2)—The patient's cardiac status is consistent with or improved from baseline levels established preoperatively.
- ◆ O 23 (D3)—The patient participates in decision making affecting the perioperative plan of care.

Table 7

SYMPTOMS OF LATEX EXPOSURE AND POSSIBLE ANAPHYLAXIS	
Conscious Patient	**Anesthetized Patient**
Itchy eyes	Facial edema
Generalized pruritis	Urticaria
Shortness of breath	Rash
Sneezing	Skin flushing
Wheezing	Bronchospasm
Nausea	Laryngeal edema
Edema	Edema
Vomiting	Hypotension
Abdominal cramping	Tachycardia
Diarrhea	Cardiac arrest
Faintness	
Feeling of impending doom	

E. Planning

The perioperative nurse develops a plan of care for the latex-allergic patient that prescribes interventions to attain expected outcomes. Interventions and activities are selected according to the procedure to be performed as well as to address the latex allergy. The following is a partial list of interventions that may be associated with the latex-allergic individual ("I" = interventions).

- ◆ I 30—Develops individualized plan of care.
- ◆ I 139—Implements latex-allergy precautions as needed.
- ◆ I 27—Ensures continuity of care.

The natural rubber latex-allergic individual should be identified by the admitting practitioner, and this information should be made available to the entire health care team, thus providing a continuous safe level of care. The latex-allergic individual should be treated in a latex-safe environment with emphasis placed on the removal of all latex-containing devices and products within the immediate care environment. Figure 1 provides a simple flow chart to assist with planning for a latex-safe procedure.

F. Implementation

Implementation refers to actually performing the activities comprising the interventions identified in the individualized plan of care. This includes taking latex-allergy precautions as appropriate. If the patient is to be cared for in a facility-wide, latex-

Figure 1

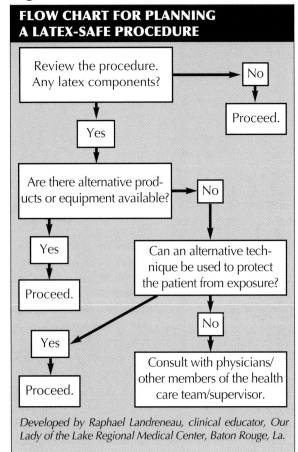

FLOW CHART FOR PLANNING A LATEX-SAFE PROCEDURE

Review the procedure. Any latex components? → No → Proceed.

Yes ↓

Are there alternative products or equipment available? → No

Yes ↓

Proceed.

Can an alternative technique be used to protect the patient from exposure?

Yes → Proceed.

No ↓

Consult with physicians/ other members of the health care team/supervisor.

Developed by Raphael Landreneau, clinical educator, Our Lady of the Lake Regional Medical Center, Baton Rouge, La.

safe environment, no additional latex precautions should be needed. If latex or latex-containing products remain in the patient's immediate care environment, those products should be removed.

Nursing interventions are composed of many and varied activities. To care for the latex-allergic individual, some or all the following activities will be appropriate, particularly if the patient is not in a facility-wide latex-safe environment.

Preoperative activities

The following activities should take place before the surgical procedure.

- ◆ Notify OR of potential or known latex-allergic patient 24 to 48 hours (or as soon as possible) before scheduled procedure.
- ◆ Identify the patient's risk factors for latex allergy and communicate same to health care team.
- ◆ Schedule procedure as first case of the day if the facility is not latex-safe.

- ◆ Notify all other care providers of patient's allergy status.
- ◆ Educate patient about latex-safe plan and ensure involvement of all providers.
- ◆ Involve patient, family members, and significant others in planning patient's care.
- ◆ Plan for a latex-safe environment of care.
- ◆ Secure latex-free products for all latex-containing items on surgeon's preference card and those used by anesthesia care provider.
- ◆ Notify surgeon if no alternative product is available.
- ◆ Notify anesthesia care provider if latex-containing product is to be used, and develop plan for emergency care if needed.
- ◆ Remove all latex items from OR unless no nonlatex alternative exists.
  - Remove boxes of latex gloves and replace with nonlatex gloves (eg, sterile, nonsterile).
  - Double-check all supplies and equipment for latex and remove any latex-containing items.

Intraoperative activities

The following activities should be performed during the surgical procedure.

- ◆ Continue implementing the perioperative latex-safe plan of care.
- ◆ Mark the OR room doors with "Latex precautions" signs.
- ◆ Mark the patient's admitting bed and transport vehicles.
- ◆ Provide latex-sensitive patients with a "latex allergy" identification band and ensure that the bed and chart also are clearly labeled.
- ◆ Remind all health care team members of the necessity for following latex avoidance procedures.
- ◆ Restrict traffic flow in the room before and during the procedure.
- ◆ Use latex-free IV tubing or replace injection ports with three-way stopcocks. Tape over any remaining ports to prevent inadvertent use.
- ◆ Use medication in ampules or latex-free vials when available.
- ◆ Use latex-free syringes.
- ◆ Use latex-free blood pressure cuffs and connecting tubing. If they are not available, wrap the patient's arm to prevent blood pressure cuff tubing or tourniquet cuff tubing from coming into contact with the patient's skin.

◆ Do not use latex tourniquets (eg, Penrose drains) to start IV lines or as drains in a wound.

◆ Use a 100% silicone (ie, not silicone coated) or polyvinyl chloride catheter if a urinary catheter is ordered for a procedure.

◆ Verify that additional items requested after the case is in progress are latex-free before delivering them to the sterile field.

◆ Be prepared for the possibility that the procedure may require more than the scheduled equipment (eg, laparoscopy to open).

◆ Monitor for anaphylactic reactions to latex throughout the procedure as reactions may occur immediately after induction (eg, IV exposure) or up to 40 minutes later.

◆ Have IV fluids and medications for treatment of allergic reaction available immediately.

◆ Inform postanesthesia care unit (PACU) staff members in advance of the patient's arrival time.

Postoperative activities

The following activities should be performed after the surgical procedure.

◆ Continue the perioperative latex-safe plan of care.

◆ Ensure that latex-free supplies are available to follow the patient to all future locations within the health care facility.

◆ Provide a latex-free resuscitation bag, oxygen mask, and supplies.

◆ Transport the patient to a latex-safe area.

◆ Provide education for patient and his or her family members or significant others.

If the latex-allergic patient is not cared for in a facility-wide, latex-safe environment, he or she is at risk for reaction upon arrival in the PACU. When the patient re-enters the mainstream care environment, he or she is at risk because of the aerosolized powder-containing latex proteins being transferred through the air or shed from scrub attire of individuals working with or near powdered latex products. In a nonlatex-safe facility, it may be necessary to use a positive pressure isolation room if a latex-safe environment of care has not been previously established in preparation for the patient.

G. Evaluation of Outcomes

The perioperative nurse evaluates the patient's progress toward attainment of outcomes. The perioperative nurse's evaluation should be systematic and ongoing. The patient's progress toward attainment of outcomes should be documented using the recognized, standardized perioperative nursing vocabulary.[84] Outcome indicators will vary according to the specific desired outcome and may include

◆ physiological indicators (eg, neurological status, cardiovascular status);

◆ cognitive indicators (eg, repeats instructions correctly, asks appropriate questions);

◆ affective indicators (eg, verbalizes and demonstrates willingness to comply with treatment regimen); and

◆ supportive resources (eg family members participate in care planning and delivery).

Patient satisfaction

Evaluation of patient progress is based on observations of the patient's responses to nursing interventions and the effectiveness of interventions in moving the patient toward the desired outcome. Desired patient outcomes, nursing interventions, and potentially applicable nursing diagnoses are articulated in the standardized perioperative nursing vocabulary which provides the basis for documentation of perioperative nursing practice. Ongoing assessment should be used to revise diagnoses, outcomes, and the plan of care as needed. Revisions in diagnoses, outcomes, and the plan of care should be documented. The patient, his or her significant others, and other health care providers should be involved in the evaluation process when appropriate.

III. Conclusion

This guideline has been designed to promote a safe health care environment for latex-sensitive and latex-allergic patients and health care workers. The document addresses prevalence, history, pathophysiology, risk factors, prevention, and nursing process applications. This guideline can be used as a resource by facilities developing latex-safe policies, procedures, and protocols. The guideline may not apply to every individual and may require alteration based on specific needs.

NOTES

1. P C A Kam, M S M Lee, J F Thompson, "Latex allergy: An emerging clinical and occupational health problem," *Anaesthesia* 52 (June 1997) 570-575.

2. S Reddy, "Latex allergy," *American Family Physician* 57 (Jan 1, 1998) 93-100.

3. M Swanson, D W Olson, "Latex allergen affinity for starch powders applied to natural rubber gloves and released as an aerosol: From dust to don," *Canadian Journal of Allergy and Clinical Immunology* 5 no 8 (2000) 328-336.

4. G L Sussman et al, "Incidence of latex sensitization among latex glove users," *Journal of Allergy and Clinical Immunology* 101 (February 1998) 171-178.

5. D A Levy et al, "Powder-free protein-poor natural rubber latex gloves and latex sensitization," (Research Letters) *JAMA* 281 (March 17, 1999); also available at http://jama.amaassn.org/issues/v281n11/ffull/jlt0317-5.html (accessed 5 July 2003).

6. C A Janeway et al, "The induction, measurement, and manipulation of the immune response," *Immuno Biology: The Immune System in Health and Disease,* fourth ed (New York: Elsevier Science Ltd/Garland Publishing, 1999) 33-75.

7. *Mosby's Medical and Nursing Dictionary* (St Louis: The C V Mosby Co, 1983)

8. X Bauer, Z Chen, H Allmers, "Can a threshold limit value for natural rubber latex airborne allergens be defined?" *Journal of Clinical Allergy and Immunology* 101 (January 1998) 24-27.

9. *Latex Allergy Protocol* (Park Ridge, Ill: American Association of Nurse Anesthetists, 1993) 1-2.

10. G L Sussman, D H Beezhold, "Latex allergy: A clinical perspective," *Surgical Services Management* 3 (February 1997) 25-28.

11. V J Tomazic, "Adverse reactions to natural rubber latex," *FDA User Facility Report* 19 (Spring 1997) 2.

12. F Porri et al, "Prevalence of latex sensitization in subjects attending health screening: Implications for a perioperative screening," *Clinical and Experimental Allergy* 27 (April 1997) 413-417.

13. R Bernardini et al, "Prevalence and risk factors of latex sensitization in an unselected pediatric population," *Journal of Allergy and Clinical Immunology* 101 (May 1998) 621-625.

14. American College of Allergy and Immunology, "Latex allergy: An emerging healthcare problem," *Annals of Allergy, Asthma, and Immunology* 75 (July 1995) 19-21.

15. P Patterson, "Latex allergy: Managers' actions can aid latex-sensitive employees," *OR Manager* 13 (February 1997) 1-10

16. M Veach, "Latex gloves hand health workers a growing worry," *Latex Allergy News* 4 (December 1997) 1-4.

17. T Kibby, M Akl, "Prevalence of latex sensitization in a hospital employee population," *Annals of Allergy, Asthma, and Immunology* 78 (January 1997) 41-44.

18. G L Sussman, "Latex allergy: An overview," *Canadian Journal of Allergy and Clinical Immunology* 5 (May 2000) 317-322.

19. F Lagier et al "Prevalence of latex allergy in operating room nurses," *Journal of Allergy and Clinical Immunology* 90 (September, 1992) 319-322.

20. S R Mace et al "Latex allergy in operating room nurses," *Annals of Allergy, Asthma, and Immunology* 80 (March 1998) 252-256.

21. R Arellano, J Bradley, G Sussman, "Prevalence of latex sensitization among hospital physicians occupationally exposed to latex gloves," *Anesthesiology* 77 (November 1992) 905-908.

22. M Grzybowski et al "The prevalence of anti-latex IgE antibodies among registered nurses," *Journal of Allergy and Clinical Immunology* 98 (September 1996) 535-544.

23. C Konrad et al, "The prevalence of latex sensitivity among anesthesiology staff," *Anesthesia and Analgesia* 84 (March 1997) 629-633.

24. R H Brown, J A Schauble, R G Hamilton, "Prevalence of latex allergy among anesthesiologists: Identification of sensitized but asymptomatic individuals," *Anesthesiology* 89 (August 1998) 292-299.

25. H Alenius et al, "IgE reactivity to 14-kD and 27-kD natural rubber proteins in latex-allergic children with spina bifida and other congenital anomalies," *International Archives of Allergy & Immunology* 102 no 1 (1993) 61-66.

26. J E Slater, S K Chhabra "Latex antigens," *Journal of Allergy and Clinical Immunology* 89 (March 1992) 673-678.

27. B L Charous, "The puzzle of latex allergy: Some answers, still more questions," *Annals of Allergy* 73 (October 1994) 277-281.

28. H Y Yeang et al, "The 14.6 kd rubber elongation factor (Hev b 1) and 24 kd (Hev b 3) rubber particle proteins are recognized by IgE from patients with spina bifida and latex allergy," *Journal of Allergy and Clinical Immunology* 98 (September 1996) 629-639.

29. J W Yunginger, "Natural rubber latex," *Immunology and Allergy Clinics of North America* 15 (August 1995) 583-595.

30. E M Warshaw, "Continuing medical education: Latex allergy," *Journal of the American Academy of Dermatology* 39 (July 1998) 1-24

31. R M Adams, "Reflecting on developments in occupational dermatitis," *Clinics in Dermatology* 15 (July-August 1997) 473-477

32. S M Wilkinson, M H Beck, "Allergic contact dermatitis from latex rubber," *British Journal of Dermatology* 134 (May 1996) 910-914.

33. M Wyss et al, "Allergic contact dermatitis from natural latex without contact urticaria," *Contact Dermatitis* 28 (March 1993) 154-156.

34. K P Bensky, "Latex allergy: Who, what, when, where, why, and how," *CRNA: The Clinical Forum for Nurse Anesthetists* 6 (November 1995) 177-182.

35. N M Strzyzewski, "Latex allergy: Everyone is at risk," *Plastic Surgical Nursing* 15 (Winter 1995) 204-206.

36. H Zhai, H I Maibach, "Moisturizers in preventing irritant contact dermatitis: An overview," *Contact Dermatitis* 38 (May 1998) 241-244.

37. "Latex allergy: Protect yourself, protect your patients," *Work Place Information Series Brochure,* American Nurses Association, http://www.nursingworld.org/dlwa/osh/wp7.htm (accessed 17 Oct 2003).

38. National Institute for Occupational Safety and Health, *NIOSH Alert: Preventing Allergic Reactions to Natural Rubber Latex in the Workplace.* DHHS Publ 97-135 (Cincinnati: National Institute for Occupational Safety and Health, August 1997).

39. D L Hancock, "Latex allergy: Prevention and treatment," *Anesthesiology Review* 21 (September/October 1994) 153-163.

40. A Heese et al, "Allergic and irritant reactions to rubber gloves in medical health services," *Journal of the American Academy of Dermatology* 25 (November 1991) 831-841.

41. ECRI, "Latex sensitivity: Clinical and legal issues," in *Operating Room Risk Management* (Plymouth Meeting, Pa: ECRI, September 1997) 1-9.

42. W Wigger-Alberti, P Elsner, "Preventive measures in contact dermatitis," *Clinics in Dermatology* 15 (July-August 1997) 661-665.

43. M Evangelisto, "Latex allergy: The downside of standard precautions," *Today's Surgical Nurse* (September/October 1997) 28-33.

44. V M Steelman, "Latex allergy precautions: A research-based protocol," *Nursing Clinics of North America* 30 (September 1995) 475-493.

45. G Sussman, S Tarlo, J Dolovich, "The spectrum of IgE-mediated responses to latex," *JAMA* 265 (June 5, 1991) 2844-2847.

46. J G K Axelsson, S G O Johansson, K Wrangsjo, "IgE-mediated anaphylactoid reactions to rubber," *Allergy* 42 (January 1987) 46-50.

47. T Carrillo et al, "Contact urticaria and rhinitis from latex surgical gloves," *Contact Dermatitis* 15 (August 1986) 69-72.

48. A C Gerber et al, "Severe intraoperative anaphylaxis to surgical gloves: Latex Allergy, an unfamiliar condition," *Anesthesiology* 7 (November 1989) 800-802.

49. K J Kelly, G Sussman, J N Fink, "Stop the sensitization," *Journal of Allergy and Clinical Immunology* 98 (November 1996) 857-858.

50. D K Heilman et al, "A prospective, controlled study showing that rubber gloves are the major contributor to latex aeroallergen levels in the operating room," *Journal of Allergy and Clinical Immunology* 98 (August 1996) 325-330.

51. M Ahlroth et al, "Cross-reacting allergens in natural rubber latex and avocado," *Journal of Allergy and Clinical Immunology* 96 (August 1995) 167-173.

52. G Sussman, M Gold, *Guidelines for the Management of Latex Allergies and Safe Latex Use in Health Care Facilities* (Arlington Heights, Ill: American College of Allergy, Asthma, and Immunology, March 1996) 1-25.

53. K T Kim et al, "Implementation recommendations for making health care facilities latex safe," *AORN Journal* 67 (March 1998) 615-632.

54. O Vandenplas et al, "Prevalence of occupational asthma due to latex among hospital personnel," *American Journal of Respiratory Critical Care Medicine* 151 (January 1995) 54-60.

55. O Vandenplas et al, "Latex gloves with a lower protein content reduce bronchial reactions in subjects with occupational asthma caused by latex," *American Journal of Respiratory and Critical Care Medicine* 151 (March 1995) 887-889.

56. B L Charous, P J Scheunemann, M C Swanson, "Dispersion of latex aeroallergen," (Abstract) *Journal of Allergy and Clinical Immunology* suppl (January 1998) S160-S161.

57. American College of Allergy, Asthma and Immunology, American Academy of Allergy, Asthma and Immunology, "AAAAI and ACAAI joint statement concerning the use of powdered and non-powdered natural rubber latex gloves," *Annals of Allergy, Asthma, and Immunology* 79 (December 1997) 487.

58. *Interim Recommendations to Health Professionals and Organizations Regarding Latex Allergy Precautions* (Arlington Heights, Ill: American College of Allergy and Immunology, March 1992) 1-4.

59. D H Beezhold, G L Sussman, "Determining the allergenic potential of latex gloves," *Surgical Services Management* 3 (February 1997) 35-41.

60. C L Romig, "The powdered latex glove war," (Health Policy Issues) *AORN Journal* 66 (July 1997) 152-153.

61. D M Korniewicz, K J Kelly, "Barrier protection and latex allergy associated with surgical gloves," *AORN Journal* 61 (June 1995) 1037-1044.

62. E F O'Boyle, B Brochard, "Latex allergy: Be prepared," *Surgical Services Management* 4 (March 1998) 34-37.

63. M A Young, "Strategies for a latex-safe environment," *Surgical Services Management* 4 (March 1998) 19-24.

64. V M Steelman, "Is it really necessary to go powder-free?" *Infection Control Today* 2 no 4 29-30.

65. R S Holzman, J D Katzk, "Occupational latex allergy: The end of innocence," *Anesthesiology* 89 (August 1998) 287-289.

66. *Standard Test Method for the Analysis of Aqueous Extractable Protein in Natural Rubber and Its Products Using the Modified Lowry Method,* D 5712 (West Conshohocken, Pa: American Society for Testing and Materials, 1999) 1-7.

67. *Standard Test Method for the Immunological Measurement of Antigenic Protein in Natural Rubber and Its Products,* D 6499 (West Conshohocken, Pa: American Society for Testing and Materials, 2003) 1-6.

68. "Recommended practices for product selection in perioperative practice settings," in *Standards, Recommended Practices, and Guidelines* (Denver: AORN, Inc, 2004) 347-350.

69. "Natural rubber-containing medical devices: User labeling, Final rule," *Federal Register* 62 (Sept 30, 1997) 51021-51030.

70. "Guidance on the content and format of pre-market notification [510(k)] submissions for testing for skin sensitization to chemicals in latex products, draft document" (Rockville, Md: US Department of Health and Human Services Center for Devices and Radiological Health, Feb 13, 1998) 1-14.

71. "Latex allergy position statements, guidelines, and resources," (Trends) *Surgical Services Management* 4 (March 1998) 56.

72. *Natural Rubber Latex Allergy: Considerations for Anesthesiologists* (Park Ridge, Ill: American Society of Anesthesiologists, 1999).

73. S A Vassallo et al, "Allergic reaction to latex from stopper of a medication vial," *Anesthesia & Analgesia* 80 (May 1995) 1057-1058.

74. J W Yunginger et al, "Latex allergen contents of medical and consumer rubber products," *Journal of Allergy Clinical Immunology* 91 (1993) 241.

75. M N Primeau, N F Adkinson, Jr, R G Hamilton, "Natural rubber pharmaceutical vial closures release latex allergens that produce skin reactions," *Journal of Allergy and Clinical Immunology* 107 (June 2001) 958-962.

76. T Asakura, "Occurrence of coring in insulin vials and possibility of rubber piece contamination by self injection," *Journal of the Pharmaceutical Society of Japan* 121 (June 2001) 459-463.

77. S A Sherman, "Precautions reduce risk of latex reactions," *OR Manager* 9 (August 1993) 17-20.

78. B D Zehr, S Gromelski, D Beezhold, "Reduction of antigenic protein levels in latex gloves after gamma irradiation," *Biomedical Instrumentation and Technology* 28 (November/December 1994) 481-483.

79. G Weinert, "Health care latex allergy costs," *Surgical Services Management* 4 (March 1998) 27-30.

80. K Catalano, "Risk management and latex allergies," *Surgical Services Management* 3 (February 1997) 42-46.

81. C Johns, "A call to action: Latex allergy in the workplace," *Surgical Services Management* 4 (March 1998) 41-44.

82. "Natural rubber latex sensitivity: An AAOHN position statement," American Association of Occupational Health Nurses, Inc, http://www.aaohn.org/natrubr.htm#latex (accessed 16 May 1998) 1-3.

83. S Wagner, H Breiteneder, "The latex-fruit syndrome," *Biochemical Society Transactions* 30 (November 2002) 935-940.

84. S Beyea, ed, *Perioperative Nursing Data Set*, second ed (Denver: AORN, Inc, 2002).

RESOURCES

Kim, K, et al. "Implementation recommendations for making health care facilities latex safe," *AORN Journal* 67 (March 1998) 615-632.

Latex Allergy Links, http://latexallergylinks.tripod.com/ (accessed 19 Oct 2003).

"Natural rubber latex allergy: Considerations for anesthesiologists," American Society of Anesthesiologists, http://www.asahq.org/publicationsAndServices/latexallergy.html (accessed 19 Oct 2003).

Phillips, V; Goodrich, M; Sullivan, T. "Health care worker disability due to latex allergy and asthma: A cost analysis," *American Journal of Public Health* 89 (July 1999) 1024-1028.

Steelman, V. "Latex allergy precautions: A research-based protocol," *Nursing Clinics of North America* 30 (September 1995) 475-493.

Sussman, G. "Latex allergy: An overview," *Canadian Journal of Allergy and Clinical Immunology* 5 no 8 (2000) 317-322.

Originally approved by the AORN Board of Directors in November 1998.

Revised; approved by the AORN Board of Directors in November 2003.

Revised November 2003; published March 2004, *AORN Journal.*

AORN Malignant Hyperthermia Guideline

I. Introduction

Assumptions

1. The "AORN malignant hyperthermia guideline" is a translation and not a new guideline. *Rationale: The Malignant Hyperthermia Association of the United States (MHAUS) has a nationally recognized protocol that is viewed as the national guideline or standard of care for the malignant hyperthermia (MH) patient. This protocol has been developed by a panel of known experts and based on scientific research.*

2. The "AORN malignant hyperthermia guideline" is specific to perioperative care for patients confirmed to have or thought to be susceptible to MH.

3. Content experts (ie, MHAUS, American Society of PeriAnesthesia Nurses, American Society of Anesthesiologists, American Association of Colleges of Nursing, American Association of Nurse Anesthetists) will be requested to review the final guideline document for comments.

4. The "AORN malignant hyperthermia guideline" is based on current available research. It is assumed that ongoing research will expand current knowledge to include other causative agents and treatment modalities.

5. This guideline may not apply to every patient and may require alteration based on specific patient needs.

Definition

Malignant hyperthermia is a potentially lethal syndrome caused by a hypermetabolic state that can be precipitated by the administration of volatile inhalation anesthetic agents and depolarizing muscle relaxants, such as succinylcholine.[1] The triggering agent causes an increase in intracellular calcium ion concentration. This elevated calcium level produces a chain of reactions. Emphasis is placed on the rapid recognition of signs and symptoms related to hypermetabolism. These include, but are not limited to, tachycardia, dysrhythmias, tachypnea, hypercarbia, respiratory acidosis, metabolic acidosis, masseter muscle rigidity, generalized muscle rigidity, elevated body temperature, myoglobinuria, rhabdomyolysis, cyanosis, skin mottling, hyperkalemia, diaphoresis, rapid temperature elevation, hemodynamic instability, and coagulopathy. Potential triggering agents include, but are not limited to, volatile inhalation agents and succinylcholine.

History

The history of MH as a known and described disorder is relatively short. In 1960, Denborough reported the case of a young man with a compound leg fracture who feared general anesthesia because relatives had died while undergoing ether anesthesia. He was given a new inhalation anesthetic agent, halothane. Intraoperatively, he experienced fever, tachycardia, cyanosis, and hypotension, but survived.[2]

Since that time, much progress has been made in the diagnosis and treatment of MH. In 1962, an autosomal dominant mode of inheritance was suggested, leading to the thesis that increased skeletal muscle metabolism, not abnormal central temperature regulation, accounted for the hyperthermia seen in MH. *In vitro* muscle biopsy testing done by Kalow and Ellis in 1970 showed that freshly cut muscle demonstrated contracture responses to caffeine and halothane. Biopsy testing has since become accepted as the current method for the diagnosis of MH susceptibility.[3] Dantrolene was introduced in 1975 as the first effective therapy for MH, and it remains today as the only drug specific to the treatment of MH.

In 1980, MHAUS was formed to provide a central clearinghouse to collect data and to provide education and information on MH. One of the most important features of MHAUS is an emergency hotline that is available for expert help with the diagnosis and treatment of an ongoing MH episode; call (800) 644-9737.

Pathophysiology

Malignant hyperthermia is a fulminating hypermetabolic state occurring in genetically predisposed individuals when exposed to triggering agents. It is now known that the primary defect in MH resides in the skeletal muscle at the level of calcium transfer in the muscle cell. The resultant intracellular hypercalcemia leads to hypermetabolism, which in turn results in increased sympathetic activity, increased carbon dioxide production, increased oxygen consumption, and disruption of the cell membranes.[4] Because of the inability of muscle tissue to return to a resting state in the susceptible patient, the primary signs of MH begin to appear.

Incidence and mortality

The incidence of MH is variously reported to be 1:15,000 in children and 1:50,000 in adults who receive a general anesthetic.[5] The mortality has been reduced from as high as 70% to less than 10%.[6]

Three major factors are responsible for the drop in mortality from MH. Increased awareness of the syndrome since its first description in 1960 has prompted careful questioning of patients in the preoperative interview to screen for a family history of untoward anesthesia events. Correlated with a positive family history, the current method of the caffeine-halothane contracture test is a reliable predictor of MH susceptibility. A pharmacologic basis for MH has been established so that when MH is suspected, the triggering agents can be avoided. When an unexpected or unpredictable MH syndrome manifests itself, sophisticated monitoring techniques give an early warning so diagnosis and treatment can be started immediately. The most important factor in the drop in mortality was the introduction of dantrolene as a drug specific for the treatment of MH.

Population affected

Every patient who is about to undergo general anesthesia should be screened for a family history of MH. Approximately 50% of MH-susceptible individuals have had a previous triggering anesthetic without developing MH. Malignant hyperthermia is rare in infants, and the incidence decreases after 50 years of age. Males more commonly develop MH than females. The reasons for these variations are not clearly understood.[7]

Socioeconomic factors in malignant hyperthermia

The social and financial ramifications of an MH episode cannot be overstated. Those patients who know they are susceptible to this potentially lethal syndrome must deal with terrible preoperative anxiety. They need continual reassurance that everyone is aware of the potential and that an anesthesia treatment plan has been developed to avoid an occurrence. Beyond the psychological and emotional factors, there are physical sequelae to an episode of MH, and the treatment is expensive.

Preparing the facility to deal with MH is costly and time-consuming. Dantrolene is expensive to stock, costing between $40 and $50 for a 20-mg vial. Although it has a long shelf life, the relative rarity of an MH occurrence causes dantrolene to become outdated far more often than it is used. Because dantrolene is difficult to mix, some institutions reconstitute the outdated drug in staff education sessions to give hands-on training. A well-stocked MH treatment cart may be available, and there should be evidence that all staff members have had periodic inservice education in dealing with MH. Table 1 shows suggested contents that might be contained in a dedicated MH cart.

Future implications

Research continues to reveal more information about MH. Other drugs and physiologic conditions have been known to stimulate a syndrome that closely resembles MH. Examples of drugs in question include phenothiazine and Haldol. This condition is referred to as neuroleptic malignant syndrome (NMS) and can be manifested by muscle rigidity, elevated body temperature, and elevated creatine phosphokinase (CPK). Other physiologic indicators of an MH-like syndrome may include rhabdomyolysis and myoglobinuria. Extreme stress and heat stroke also may be precipitating factors. These conditions can be as life-threatening as a confirmed MH crisis. Dantrolene sodium is effective in treating muscle-generated heat and helps lower body temperature and may be used to treat syndromes similar to confirmed MH.

II. Assessment

Standard 1: Assessment

Perioperative nurses assess, document, and report to the anesthesia provider and other team members any of the following information regarding MH.

Preoperative evaluation: Identify physiological status. Assess for risk factors:
- family history;
- previous clinical episode (eg, signs and symptoms of MH during anesthesia);
- diseases possibly related to MH;[8]
- central-core disease:
  - duchenne muscular dystrophy,
  - King-Denborough syndrome,
  - Schwartz-Jampel syndrome,
  - Fukyama type congenital muscular dystrophy, and
  - Becker muscular dystrophy;
- periodic paralysis:
  - neuroleptic malignant heat syndrome; and
- myotonia congenita:
  - sarcoplasmic reticulum adenosine triphosphate, and
  - deficiency syndrome and mitochondrial myopathy.

Table 1

SUGGESTED CONTENTS FOR A MALIGNANT HYPERTHERMIA CART

Suggested medication and equipment

36 ampules dantrolene sodium (ie, Dantrium) IV (20-mg vials)
4 500-mL bottles sterile water (preservative free)
6 50-mEq syringes sodium bicarbonate
2 50-mL syringes 50% dextrose
2 4-mL vials furosemide (10 mg/mL)
2 500-mL bottles 20% mannitol
2 prefilled syringes 2% lidocaine
6 20-mL ampules procainamide (1 g)
3 10-mL vials heparin (1,000 U)
2 semiautomatic dispensing syringes
2 stopcocks (3-way)
4 60-mL syringes

Other equipment

6 10-mL syringes
6 18-gauge needles
6 alcohol prep pads
1 4-oz bottle povidone-iodine paint
2 10-each boxes 4 x 4 sterile gauze
2 tourniquets
2 radial artery catheters
1 arterial line monitoring kit
1 central venous pressure line kit
2 sets cassette tubing for IV pumps
2 sets of IV tubing (pediatric and adult)
2 sets IV extension tubing
10 medication labels
2 wrist splints (1 each, pediatric and adult sizes)

Tubes for laboratory tests

6 5-mL heparinized blood gas syringes or ABG kits
2 urine specimen containers
1 bottle urine test strips for myoglobin
6 light blue tubes (pediatric and adult sizes)
6 lavender tubes (pediatric and adult sizes)

10 gold tubes with gel
10 red stopper tubes

Cooling equipment

2 nasogastric tubes (pediatric and adult sizes)
2 30-mL balloon, 3-way Foley catheters (several pediatric and adult sizes)
2 closed-system Foley catheter trays
2 peritoneal lavage trays
2 sets cystoscopy tubing
2 60-mL catheter tip syringes
2 5-in-1 connectors
2 Y-connectors
2 plastic buckets to hold ice
10 medium- and large-size plastic bags

Anesthesia equipment

(Have on cart or immediately available)
2 breathing circuits (pediatric and adult sizes)
2 breathing circuit adapters
2 pressure bags
2 soda lime canisters

Miscellaneous

1 sharps container
2 Ambu bags (pediatric and adult sizes)
1 MH cart medications/supplies checklist
1 MHAUS label on front of cart listing hotline telephone number (ie, [800] 644-9737; ask for Index Zero)

At the time cart is requested, add:

Refrigerated IV normal saline solution (1,000-mL bags)
Refrigerated normal saline for irrigation (3,000-mL bags)
Refrigerated regular insulin
Ice

III. Nursing Diagnosis and Identification of Outcomes

The following identify nursing diagnoses and outcomes related to the care of any patient with a potential or confirmed diagnosis of MH. These may be applied to an individual plan of care as appropriate.

Standard 2: Diagnosis

Nursing diagnosis: Risk for or actual altered body temperature:

♦ hyperthermia related to hypermetabolic crisis and muscular contraction, and
♦ hypothermia related to rigorous cooling processes used to treat hyperthermia.

Outcome: The patient maintains thermal regulation.

Nursing diagnosis: Risk for or actual impaired gas exchange related to difficult ventilation caused by muscular rigidity.

Outcome: The patient's pulmonary function is maintained.

Nursing diagnosis: Risk for or actual altered tissue perfusion related to
- intense muscular contraction,
- increased oxygen demand secondary to the hypermetabolic state,
- increased production of carbon dioxide,
- skeletal muscle breakdown resulting in anaerobic metabolism which leads to lactic acidosis, or
- alteration in renal perfusion from myoglobinuria related to skeletal muscle breakdown.

Outcome: The patient maintains adequate wound/tissue perfusion.

Nursing diagnosis: Risk for or actual decreased cardiac output related to cardiac dysrhythmias:
- tachycardia,
- acidosis,
- fever,
- accelerated oxygen consumption,
- peripheral vasoconstriction, or
- hyperkalemia.

Outcome: The patient maintains adequate cardiac status.

Nursing diagnosis: Risk for fluid volume excess related to ineffective diuresis.

Outcome: The patient's fluid and electrolyte balance is maintained.

Nursing diagnosis: Risk for pain related to continuous muscle contracture.

Outcome: The patient demonstrates adequate pain control.

Standard 3: Outcome Identification

The following outcomes (see the AORN "Patient outcomes: Standards of perioperative care") may be applicable to the potential or confirmed MH-diagnosed patient. Use as appropriate to the individual plan of care.

1.1 The patient is free from signs and symptoms of physical injury.

1.2 The patient is free from signs and symptoms of injury due to extraneous objects.

1.5 The patient is free from signs and symptoms of injury related to positioning.

1.9 The patient has safe administration of appropriate medications during the perioperative period.

3.1 The patient demonstrates knowledge of the physiological responses to the anesthetic and the operative or other invasive procedure.

3.2 The patient demonstrates knowledge of the psychological responses to the anesthetic and the operative or other invasive procedure.

3.4 The patient demonstrates knowledge of medication management.

4.1 The patient participates in decisions affecting his or her perioperative plan of care if MH susceptible.

IV. Plan, Implementation

Standard 4: Planning

The perioperative nurse develops a plan of care that prescribes interventions to attain expected outcomes. These outcome statements become a guide for the following nursing interventions necessary to achieve the desired results. The individualized plan of care reflects the perioperative assessment and a logical sequence to attain outcomes. Priorities for the provision of nursing care are established by the perioperative nurse in collaboration with the patient, significant others, and other health care providers. The flow chart on the following page can be used in the development of an individualized plan of care for a patient identified at increased risk for MH. (See Table 2.)

Standard 5: Implementation

Nursing interventions: The perioperative plan of care *may* include the following.
- Recognizes and reports deviation in diagnostic studies. (See Table 3.) Collection and reporting of laboratory studies is institution specific. The process should be determined prior to an MH episode.
- Elicits perceptions of surgery. Patient may give clues to further investigate a potential MH susceptibility.

Table 2

MALIGNANT HYPERTHERMIA FLOW CHART

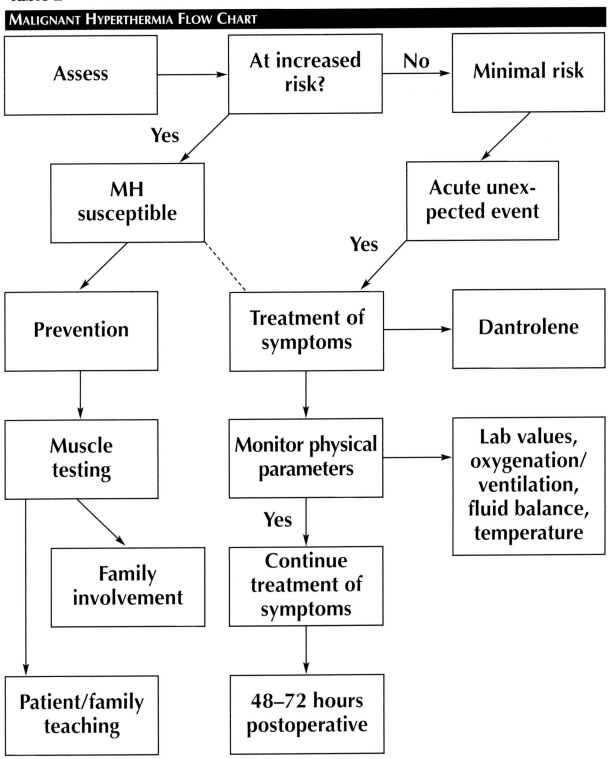

Table 3

ABG	Normal Ranges
⇓ pH	7.35–7.45
⇓ PO_2	80–100 mm Hg
⇑ PCO_2	35–45 mm Hg
Electrolytes	
⇑ K	4.0–5.4 mEq/L
⇑ Ca	4.5–5.5 mEq/L
⇑ Mg	1.8–2.4 mg/dL
⇓ Na	138–148 mEq/L
Serum	
⇑ Lactate	0.7–2.1 mmol/L
⇑ Pyruvate	0.03–0.08 mmol/L
⇑ CPK (creatine phosphokinase)	40–280 U/L
⇑ LDH (lactic dehydrogenase)	3.13–6.18 U/L
⇑ Aldolase	Age specific
⇑ Myoglobin	6–85 ng/mL
⇑ Glucose	80–120 mg/dL
⇑ Creatinine	0.5–1.4 mg/dL
⇓ PT	10–12
⇓ PTT	22–27
⇓ Platelets	50,000

♦ Provides preoperative instruction based on age and identified need.

♦ Uses supplies and equipment within safe parameters.
  - For an MH susceptible patient, assist anesthesia provider in preparation of contaminated machine (eg, removing vaporizer; flushing with oxygen at 10 L/minute for 5 minutes; replacing fresh gas outlet hose; replacing old disposable circle, reservoir bag, ventilator bellows, soda lime).[9]
  - An MH susceptible patient may be administered preoperative IV dantrolene 2.5mg/ kg before induction of anesthesia.

♦ Identifies physiological status. Identifies, as appropriate, the patient's physiological status and reports variances from norm:
  - ECG,
  - vital signs (ie, blood pressure, pulse rate, body temperature),
  - oximetry, and
  - lab values.

♦ Includes family and support persons in preoperative teaching. For an MH susceptible patient, include family/support person in preoperative instructions (eg, dantrolene, medical alert bracelet, potential for muscle testing, need for ongoing postoperative observation, familial/ genetic tendencies).

♦ Assesses skin condition. Assessment of skin color, temperature, diaphoresis.

♦ Observes characteristics of any drainage.
  - Insert 3-way Foley catheter.
  - Monitor urinary output.
  - Monitor color, amount, and consistency.
  - Monitor amount of irrigation solution used.

♦ Administers care to incision sites. Close wound as soon as MH is suspected. If wound closure is not possible, wound should be packed with saline-soaked towels or laparotomy sponges. May need to irrigate the wound with cool normal saline solution, not lactated Ringer's solution.

♦ Administers care to invasive device sites (ie, endotracheal tube, tracheostomy tube, drainage tube, percutaneous catheter, vascular access device sites). Cleanse skin, secure device, and cover as appropriate.

♦ Administers urinary drainage system care. Maintain aseptic technique during insertion, secure catheter, and place in view of anesthesia provider.

♦ Administers drainage tube system care. Maintain clean drainage device site, maintain dressings, and secure device properly.

♦ Implements aseptic technique. Initiate and complete nursing actions to maintain the condition of being free from disease-causing microorganisms.

♦ Implements protective measures to prevent skin/tissue injury due to thermal sources.
  - Administer refrigerated IV normal saline. Note: Do not use IV lactated Ringer's solution; it may contribute to the patient's acidosis.
  - Directly lavage peritoneal and/or thoracic cavity with refrigerated normal saline irrigation fluid (ie, if surgical site is open).
  - Indirectly lavage stomach (eg, connect nasogastric tube to refrigerated normal saline irrigation, not lactated Ringer's solution, with cystoscopy tubing).

– Lavage rectum (eg, connect a three-way Foley catheter with 30-mL balloon to refrigerated normal saline irrigation, not lactated Ringer's solution, with cystoscopy tubing).

– Surface cool with ice in plastic bags and hypothermia blanket to neck, axillae, and groin area.

– Discontinue cooling measure when patient's temperature reaches 38° C (100.4° F). *Note:* Care should be taken to avoid too rigorous cooling, which can result in inadvertent hypothermia.

♦ Administers prescribed medications and solutions.

– Rapidly administer IV dantrolene sodium 2–3 mg/kg initial bolus. Dantrolene should be mixed with sterile water for injection USP (without a bacteriostatic agent; 60 mL per 20-mg ampule) and shaken vigorously. Repeat dosages of dantrolene as necessary; titrate to tachycardia, hyperthermia, hypercarbia, and rigidity. Although the stated upper dosage of 10 mg/kg is suggested, more may be administered as needed.

– Administer sodium bicarbonate to correct metabolic acidosis as guided by blood gas analysis. If initial blood gas results are not available and there are dysrhythmias or cardiac arrest, consider the most likely cause is due to acidosis and/or hyperkalemia. Administer initial dose of 1 to 2 mEq/kg of bicarbonate and repeat as indicated. Thereafter, dose should be based on ABG results.

– Administer intravenous glucose and insulin (10 units regular insulin in 50 mL 50% glucose titrated to potassium level or 0.15 u/kg regular insulin in 1 cc/kg 50% glucose) to treat hyperkalemia in adults.

– Administer calcium chloride 2 to 5 mg/kg to treat life-threatening hyperkalemia.

– Administer standard anti-arrhythmic agents if dysrhythmias persist following treatment of acidosis and hyperkalemia. Life-threatening dysrhythmias should not be treated with calcium channel blocking agents.

– Avoid using potassium-containing solutions.

♦ Manages specimen handling and disposition (eg, blood and urine).

♦ Implements thermoregulation measures.

♦ Obtains consultation from the appropriate health care provider to initiate new treatments or change existing treatments. Upon suspicion and/or diagnosis of an MH crisis, notify the following personnel as appropriate:

– attending anesthesiologist,
– attending physician,
– OR charge nurse,
– anesthesia technician(s),
– postanesthesia care unit/intensive care unit,
– OR cardiopulmonary assistant(s),
– house supervisor, and
– pharmacy supervisor.

♦ Recognizes and reports deviation in diagnostic studies.

♦ Collaborates in maintenance and/or corrective therapy. Requests additional staff to assist with management of complications.

♦ Monitors physiological parameters. Assists anesthesia provider as appropriate in monitoring

– ECG,
– vital signs (ie, blood pressure, pulse rate, body temperature),
– oximetry,
– capnometry,
– arterial and venous blood gases for unexplained tachycardia,
– core temperature (esophageal, tympanic, axillary, rectal, bladder),
– serum potassium,
– calcium,
– clotting studies,
– urine color and output,
– diaphoresis,
– mottling of skin, and
– central venous pressure and arterial pressure.

♦ Administers intravenous fluid therapy. Administers refrigerated IV normal saline. *Note:* Do not use IV lactated Ringer's solution; it may contribute to the patient's acidosis.

♦ Provides postoperative instruction to patient/support person.

– Advise possible post-dantrolene therapy symptoms (ie, nausea, diarrhea, muscle weakness, double vision, dizziness or lightheadedness).

– Discuss the potential for MH susceptibility in other blood relatives.

– Inform other health care providers of the patient's known or suspected MH susceptibility.

– Give patient and family members information on the MHAUS.
♦ Develops a plan of care based on identified needs that reflect the individual's choices.

V. Evaluation of outcomes

Standard 6: Evaluation

Identify physiological status. Assess any of the following. *Note:* Not all of these signs will be present in an acute episode of MH.

♦ Masseter muscle rigidity:
– severe, sustained (ie, several minutes) contracture of the jaw muscles after administration of succinylcholine—causes difficulty in intubation;
– not relieved by further doses of succinylcholine or a nondepolarizing muscle relaxant;
– MH may follow immediately, after a delay of 20 minutes or more, or not at all.
♦ Fever:
– may see an increase of 1° C (1.8° F) every few minutes—temperatures as high as 46° C (114.8° F) have been recorded;
– palpable warmth in viscera, anesthesia tubings, soda lime canisters (with soda lime possibly turning blue).
♦ General observations:
– metabolic acidosis.
♦ Renal:
– myoglobinuria (ie, cola-colored urine);
– urinary output.
♦ Cardiovascular:
– tachycardia is often the first sign of an acute MH episode—this may be mistaken for "light anesthesia" with prompt administration of more anesthesia;
– progression of the syndrome can lead to dysrhythmias such as ventricular fibrillation and sudden cardiac arrest;
– unstable blood pressure.
♦ Laboratory test abnormalities:
– increase in creatine phosphokinase, lactate dehydrogenase, myoglobin, and carbon dioxide pressure;
– reduced pH;
– abnormal coagulation studies;
– magnesium, calcium, phosphate, and potassium imbalance.

♦ Muscle rigidity:
– most patients exhibit whole-body rigidity;
– absence of muscle rigidity does not rule out MH.
♦ Respiratory:
– tachypnea secondary to increased carbon dioxide production;
– increase in end-tidal carbon dioxide production;
– excess carbon dioxide can cause the carbon dioxide absorbent canister to become discolored and hot to the touch;
– increase in arterial carbon dioxide;
– respiratory acidosis.
♦ Skin:
– generalized erythematous flush;
– mottling of skin;
– cyanosis secondary to generalized vasoconstriction and accelerated oxygen consumption by muscles;
– diaphoresis.

Postoperative evaluation: Continue observation of patient in appropriate setting using intraoperative assessment parameters.

NOTES

1. C F Beck, "Malignant hyperthermia: Are you prepared?" *AORN Journal* 59 (February 1994) 367-390.
2. M A Denborough et al, "Anaesthetic deaths in a family," *British Journal of Anaesthesia* 34 (July 1962) 395-396.
3. P M Hopkins, P J Halsall, F R Ellis, "Diagnosing malignant hyperthermia susceptibility," *Anaesthesia* 49 (May 1994) 373-375.
4. H Rosenberg, J E Fletcher, "An update on the malignant hyperthermia syndrome," *Annals of the Academy of Medicine Singapore* 23 6 suppl (November 1994) 84-97.
5. M Golinski, "Malignant hyperthermia: A review," *Plastic Surgical Nursing* 15 (Spring 1995) 30-33, 58.
6. *Ibid*; Rosenberg, Fletcher, "An update on the malignant hyperthermia syndrome," 84.
7. R Faust et al, *Anesthesiology Review,* second ed (New York: Churchill Livingstone, 1994) 496.
8. J Camboulives, "Preventive management of malignant hyperthermia susceptible patients," in *International Congress—Malignant Hyperthermias,* ed M Aubert (Englewood, NJ: Normed Verlag 1993) 67-69.
9. *Ibid,* 68-69.

RESOURCES

Atkinson, L J; Fortunato, N H. *Berry & Kohn's Operating Room Technique,* eighth ed. St Louis, Mo: Mosby-YearBook, Inc, 1996.
Burden, N J. *Ambulatory Surgical Nursing.* Philadelphia: W B Saunders Company, 1993, 146-149.

Donnelly, A. "Malignant hyperthermia: Epidemiology, pathophysiology, treatment." *AORN Journal* 59 (February 1994) 393-405.

Golinski, J. "Malignant hyperthermia: A review." *Plastic Surgical Nursing* 15 (Spring 1995) 30-33.

Groah, L K. *Perioperative Nursing,* third ed. Stamford, Conn: Appleton & Lange, 1996.

Gruendemann, B J; Fernsebner, B. *Comprehensive Perioperative Nursing,* vol 1. Boston: Jones & Bartlett Publishers, 1995, 469-471.

Hoffer, J L. "Anesthesia." In *Alexander's Care of the Patient in Surgery,* tenth ed, M H Meeker, J C Rothrock, eds. St Louis, Mo: Mosby-YearBook, Inc, 1995, 172-174.

Larach, M G, et al. "A clinical grading scale to predict malignant hyperthermia susceptibility." *Anesthesiology* 80 (April 1994) 771-779.

Malignant Hyperthermia Association of the United States (MHAUS). *Emergency Therapy for Malignant Hyperthermia.* Sherburne, NY: MHAUS, 1995.

For more information about malignant hyperthermia, contact the Malignant Hyperthermia Association of the United States at 32 South Main Street, PO Box 1069, Sherburne, NY 13460-1069; telephone (607) 674-7901.

This malignant hyperthermia guideline was developed by the AORN Data Elements Coordinating Committee and was approved by the AORN Board of Directors in February 1997.

AORN Guidance Statement: Human and Avian Influenza and Severe Acute Respiratory Syndrome

I. Overview

A. Introduction

Assumptions

The AORN guideline on human and avian influenza and severe acute respiratory syndrome (SARS) is based on research and the experience of health care workers. It is assumed that ongoing research will result in new knowledge, procedures, and medical and nursing interventions for the treatment of patients with human and avian influenza and SARS. This guideline is designed to assist perioperative registered nurses in creating and maintaining an optimal health care environment for patients with human and avian influenza and SARS. The guideline defines the unique physical and psychosocial needs of the influenza and SARS patient populations and presents guidance for establishing a plan of care for these patients.

B. Human and Avian Influenza

During the 20th century, influenza took an enormous toll on human life. More than four pandemics occurred.

- The 1918–1919 pandemic (ie, the "Spanish flu") caused an estimated 20 to 50 million deaths worldwide. In the United States alone, there were 500,000 deaths.
- The "Asian flu" caused 60,000 deaths in the United States in 1957–1958.
- The "Hong Kong flu" pandemic of 1968–1969 caused approximately 40,000 deaths in the United States.
- The pandemic of 1977 (ie, the "Russian flu") had low mortality.[1-3]

During the last decade of the 20th century, while there were no influenza pandemics, influenza-related deaths increased to 36,000 per year in the United States. During periods of epidemics, this number increased to 40,000. Influenza continues to be the sixth leading cause of death in the United States. For those over the age of 65, it is the fifth leading cause of death.[4]

Looking at the first five years of the 21st century, it is clear that the incidence of human influenza is not declining. The emergence of avian influenza as a potential threat to humans has become significant, making the threat of a future pandemic from avian influenza very real.[1]

Definitions

For the purposes of this document, the following definitions apply.

Antigenic drift: Point mutations leading to changes in antigenicity of the major hemagglutinin (HA) and neuraminidase (NA) antigen subtypes of an influenza virus.[5]

Antigenic shift: Change in circulating major antigen (ie, HA, NA) determinants either through exchange and reassortment of genetic material or adaptation to human transmission.[5] Occasionally, the antigenic shift that occurs with the influenza A virus is an abrupt, major change in the virus.[6]

Hemagglutinin: One of the two major surface proteins of the influenza virus. Important for virus attachment to cells of the respiratory epithelium. Subtypes include H1 to H15. The only described determinants involved in sustained human-to-human transmission are H1, H2, and H3.[2]

Influenza epidemic: A seasonal outbreak of influenza viruses that are already in existence among humans.[2]

Influenza pandemic: A global outbreak of disease that occurs when a new influenza A virus emerges in the human population, causes serious illness, and then spreads easily from person to person worldwide. Influenza pandemics are caused by a new subtype or by subtypes that have never circulated among humans or that have not circulated among humans for a long period of time.[2]

Neuraminidase: One of the two major surface proteins of the influenza virus that are less important for attachment but probably are important for propagation and virulence (ie, subtypes N1 to N9).[5]

History

Hippocrates (470 BC to 410 BC) described the first case of influenza-like illness.[1] The first recorded influenza pandemic occurred in 1580 AD and spread from Europe to Asia and Africa. During the 17th century, local epidemics were reported. In the 18th century, three known pandemics occurred, in 1729–1730, 1732–1733, and 1781–1782. In the 19th century, three pandemics occurred, in 1830–1831, 1833–1834, and 1889–1890. The pandemic of 1889–1890, known as the Russian flu, killed approximately one million people. It spread throughout Europe, reaching North America in December 1889 and spreading to Latin America and Asia in 1890.[3]

The most devastating influenza pandemic in recent history (ie, the "Spanish flu") occurred in the 20th century. Worldwide, the death toll was between 20 million and 50 million people, and may have been up to 100 million globally. In the United States, the mortality rate was more than 500,000 people. The Spanish flu was caused by the influenza A (H1N1) strain. It most likely originated in the United States and spread to Europe. The Asian flu of 1957–1958 was caused by the influenza A (H2N2) strain and had a mortality rate of approximately one million people worldwide. The virus was first identified in China. In 1968–1969, the Hong Kong flu, which was caused by the influenza A (H3N2) strain, had an estimated mortality rate in the United States of 40,000. Unlike seasonal influenza, epidemics are particularly hard on people over age 65. At least initially, all three of these pandemics were characterized by a shift in age distribution of deaths to the younger population less than age 65.[3]

The influenza A strain (ie, the Russian flu) appeared in 1977. Isolated in northern China, this virus was similar to the virus that spread before 1957. Consequently, people born before 1957 generally were protected. Children and young adults born after 1957, however, were not protected because they had no prior immunity.[7]

During the 1990s and into the 2000s, avian influenza A strains H5N1 (ie, Hong Kong, China, Thailand, Vietnam), H7N2 (ie, Virginia, New York), H7N3 (ie, Canada), H7N7 (ie, Netherlands), and H9N2 (ie, China, Hong Kong) appeared, causing epidemics in the international poultry industry. With the appearance of these strains came human exposure to avian virus. Of these strains, H5N1 caused 31 deaths and H7N7 caused one death. These outbreaks demonstrated that bird-to-human transmission does occur. In the Netherlands, there were three possible H7N2 transmissions from poultry workers to family members.

Population Affected

Prevalence

In the United States, the influenza season runs from autumn to spring, with peak activity occurring from December to early March.[7,8] Five percent to 20% of the population contracts influenza every year in the United States. Of the population that contracts influenza, more than 200,000 are hospitalized from influenza complications and of these, approximately 36,000 die from influenza each year.[9] Although any person can contract this disease, some people have a higher risk of contracting influenza. This group includes those age 65 and older, children age six months to 23 months, pregnant women, and persons of any age with certain chronic medical conditions. Persons age 50–64 years also are targeted because they have an elevated prevalence of certain chronic medical conditions. Another high-risk group is those who live with or care for persons at high risk.[10]

The high-risk population described above is always at risk, particularly for the influenza A viruses that currently are circulating. History has shown that there have been influenza pandemics that were devastating to the younger population, as seen with the pandemic of 1918–1919.

Socioeconomic factors

The socioeconomic impact of influenza, whether epidemic or pandemic in nature, can be substantial. Lost productivity as a result of missed work days caused by illness or caring for a sick loved one, the cost of hospitalization, and the impact of deaths related to the disease can be devastating to the community, and indeed to the nation. In one research study, it was estimated that an influenza pandemic in the United could result in an "estimated 89,000 to 207,000 deaths; 314,000 to 734,000 hospitalizations; 18 to 42 million outpatient visits; and 20 to 47 million additional illnesses." The estimated economic impact would be $71.3 to $166.5 billion, excluding disruptions to commerce and society.[11] Clearly, preventing influenza through vaccination will reduce the incidence of the disease and its potential health effects, as well as reducing mortality, health care costs, and societal economic impact.

Epidemiology

Influenza is caused by a virus that belongs to the family of orthomyxoviridae and is classified as type A, B, or C. The key difference among type A, B, and C influenza viruses is their host range.[1]

Type A influenza viruses are the most predominate and have been isolated from humans, pigs, horses, seals, ferrets, mink, and whales. These viruses can be divided into subtypes based on their surface glycoproteins, HA, and NA.

Subtypes of HA, designated as H1 through H15, are the crucial components of influenza vaccines. "Hemagglutinin facilitates entry of viruses into host cells through its attachment to sialic acid on epithelial cell receptors, promotes membrane fusion, and elicits protective neutralizing antibody response." Hemagglutinin 1 through 3 are found in humans. Hemagglutinin 1 through 15 are found in birds.[1]

Subtypes of NA, designated as N1 through N9, are a target for antiviral agents. "Neuraminidase has enzyme activity, which cleaves sialic acid on virion proteins, facilitating the release of progeny virions from infected cells." Neuraminidase 1 through 2 are found in humans. Neuraminidase 1 through 9 are found in birds. Currently, 15 HA and nine NA glycoproteins have been identified.[1]

Many combinations of HA and NA are possible. Currently, influenza A subtypes H1N1 and H3N2 are circulating worldwide. In 2001, influenza A (H1N2) emerged after genetic reassortment between human A (H1N1) and A (H3N2).[12]

Influenza B viruses usually are found in humans, but have been isolated from seals and pigs.[1] These viruses do not cause pandemics, although they can cause epidemics. The influenza B viruses are not classified according to subtypes. Influenza C viruses cause mild illness in humans and do not cause epidemics or pandemics. Like B viruses, influenza C viruses are not classified according to subtypes.[6]

Another characteristic of influenza B viruses and subtypes of the influenza A virus is their ability to produce new strains. Through the process of antigenic drift, new strains of influenza viruses appear and replace older strains. Antigenic drift is the reason why a person is susceptible to seasonal outbreaks of influenza. "When a new strain of human influenza virus emerges, antibody protection that may have developed after infection or vaccination with an older strain may not provide protection against the strain. Thus, the influenza vaccine is updated on a yearly basis to keep up with the changes in influenza viruses."[6]

Occasionally, the antigenic shift that occurs with the influenza A virus is an abrupt, major change in the virus. When this occurs, the virus has a HA protein or HA and NA protein combination that has not been seen in humans for many years. This leads to a new influenza A subtype for which most people have little or no immunity. If the virus is transmitted human-to-human easily, the result may be a pandemic outbreak of influenza.[6]

Transmission of human influenza (ie, A, B, C) primarily is via virus-laden droplets that are expelled when an infected person coughs or sneezes. When a susceptible person is near by (eg, within three feet) the droplets are deposited onto the mucosal surfaces of the person's upper respiratory tract (ie, close contact). Another mode of transmission may occur from direct or indirect contact with respiratory secretions of an infected person. At this time, studies have not demonstrated transmission of human influenza via contact with environmental surfaces.[13]

Avian influenza, also known as bird flu, is caused by viruses that occur naturally among birds. These viruses, which are seen worldwide, live in the gastrointestinal tract of wild birds. The viruses usually do not cause illness in wild birds, but when transmitted to domestic flocks, particularly poultry (eg, chickens, ducks, turkeys), it can be devastating. All subtypes of the influenza A viruses can be found in birds.[14] Outbreaks of highly pathogenic avian influenza viruses have occurred recently; however, most avian strains are of low pathogenicity.[15] Avian influenza usually does not affect humans. Since 1997, however, several cases of human infection with avian influenza viruses have occurred.[14] Avian viruses cross over to humans by direct contact from infected birds, contaminated surfaces, or through an intermediate host such as a pig.[16]

Adaptation of the avian influenza virus occurs via mutation of the avian virus genome or genetic reassortment, which is the mixing of segments from a virus already adapted to humans.[1] As an example, if a pig is infected simultaneously with a human influenza A virus and an avian influenza virus, the potential for reassortment exists, which could result in a new virus. This virus would have most of the genes from the human virus, and HA protein and/or NA protein from the avian virus, creating a virus with surface glycoproteins not previously seen in humans. The new virus may then infect humans and can spread from person to person.[16]

Human reassortment also is possible. In this case, the human host would be infected with a human influenza strain and an avian influenza strain. If this were to happen, the reassortment would create a virus with HA from the avian virus and genes from the human virus, again resulting in a virus to which humans have little or no immunity. Consequences of this type of reassortment, in theory, could be sustained human-to-human transmission leading to an influenza pandemic.[16]

The 1918, 1957, and 1968 pandemics of the 20th century were caused by a novel type of influenza A virus of avian origin. Mutation of the genes of what was originally pure avian virus is the suspected cause of the catastrophic 1918 pandemic. In the 1957 and 1968 pandemics, the viruses involved "had components of previous human viruses as well as avian viruses."[15]

Clinical Signs and Symptoms of Influenza

When exposed, the average incubation period for influenza is two days, but it can range from one to four days. "Adults can be infectious from the day before symptoms begin through approximately five days after illness onset. Children can be infectious for more than 10 days, and young children can shed virus for several days before the onset of their illness. Severely immunocompromised persons can shed virus for weeks or months." Signs and symptoms for an uncomplicated illness include fever, myalgia, headache, malaise, nonproductive cough, sore throat, and rhinitis. Otitis media, nausea, and vomiting are commonly reported in children.[10]

For people with underlying medical conditions, such as pulmonary or cardiac disease, influenza can lead to "secondary bacterial pneumonia or primary viral influenza, or occur as part of a coinfection with other viral or bacteria pathogens." Young children can have initial symptoms mimicking bacterial sepsis with high fevers. More than 20% of children hospitalized with influenza can have febrile seizures. "Influenza ... has also been associated with encephalopathy, transverse myelitis, Reye syndrome, myositis, myocarditis, and pericarditis."[10]

Clinical signs and symptoms for human influenza are consistently predictable. With the recent outbreak of avian influenza A (H5N1 strain) in Vietnam during 2004 that affected 10 people and then 18 people in Hong Kong during 1997, however, differences in patient response became evident. Nine of the people in Vietnam had direct contact with infected chickens. None of these patients had preexisting conditions. Their ages ranged from five to 24, with the median age being 13.7 years. After exposure, the median time of incubation was three days. The range of incubation was two to four days. Similar to human influenza, the patients presented with fever and cough. They also had diarrhea, pronounced lympopenia, and radiographic abnormalities. The mortality rate was significant, with eight patients dying after 10 days. These patients experienced liver dysfunction, renal failure, coagulopathy, and pancytopenia. The 1997 Hong Kong outbreak had the same clinical signs and symptoms as the Vietnam outbreak. Additionally, rhabdomyolysis was seen in this patient population. Of the 18 people infected, six died; all were healthy young adults.[1] Although a localized incident, this outbreak nevertheless demonstrates that if human-to-human transmission was efficient, the result could have been a devastating pandemic, particularly for the young, which was also the case for the pandemic of 1918.

Developing a Program

Health care facilities should have a plan for handling influenza epidemics, as well as for future pandemics that many health care planners believe are inevitable.

Operational planning

Impact of influenza on the health care workplace
Unvaccinated health care workers can be a primary cause of influenza outbreaks in health care settings. Throughout the influenza season, health care workers encounter high-risk patients in medical practices, hospitals, home-care sites, long-term care and rehabilitation facilities, and other health care settings.[17] In addition to spreading influenza to patients, health care workers who contract influenza will be unable to provide the necessary care to their patients.

The National Foundation for Infectious Diseases reports that 23% of the staff members in an internal medicine ward became ill with influenza, resulting in 14 person-days of sick leave, postponement of eight scheduled admissions, and suspension of emergency admissions for 11 days. The average additional cost per patient was $3,798. The total cost of the outbreak was $34,179.[17]

When an influenza outbreak occurs in a health care setting, peers often have to work extended shifts. Extended shifts increase overtime costs, and studies show that attention lags after about 12 hours. In many cases, pool or temporary workers must replace health care workers who do not report to work due to illness. Additionally, regular staff members are less prone to patient-care errors than pool or temporary workers such as agency.[17]

Risk to the health care worker

An unvaccinated health care worker is an at-risk health care worker. This, of course, assumes that vaccination effectively protects against the current circulating strain of influenza causing the outbreak. If a strain of influenza rapidly appears in which effective vaccination has not been developed, or health care workers have not developed immunity from previous exposure to the circulating virus, health care workers will be at significant risk because of exposure to patients, family members, and those in the general population who have the disease.

Vaccination

Vaccination is the key to preventing influenza and its severe complications. It reduces "influenza-related respiratory illness and physician visits among all age groups, hospitalization and death among persons at high risk, otitis media among children, and work absenteeism among adults." The Advisory Committee on Immunization Practices of the Centers for Disease Control and Prevention (CDC) recommends annual vaccination for the following groups of people:

- ◆ adults 65 years of age and older;
- ◆ residents of nursing homes and other chronic-care facilities;
- ◆ adults and children with chronic pulmonary or cardiovascular disorders;
- ◆ adults and children who have required regular medical follow-up or hospitalization during the preceding year because of chronic metabolic diseases, renal dysfunction, hemoglobinopathies, or immunosuppression;
- ◆ adults and children who have conditions that can compromise respiratory function or the handling of respiratory secretions or that can increase the risk for aspiration (eg, cognitive dysfunction, spinal cord injuries, seizure disorders, other neuromuscular disorders);
- ◆ pregnant women;
- ◆ persons with chronic medical conditions;
- ◆ adults aged 50 to 64 years because of elevated prevalence of certain chronic medical conditions;
- ◆ children and adolescents aged six months to 18 years receiving long-term aspirin therapy who might be at risk for Reye syndrome after influenza infections;

- ◆ children aged six to 23 months; and
- ◆ persons who live with or care for persons at high risk, to include health care workers.[10]

Vaccination of health care workers is crucial, and all health care workers should be vaccinated against influenza. Mandatory vaccination "will protect health care workers, their patients, and communities, and will improve prevention of influenza-associated disease, patient safety, and will reduce disease burden."[10] According to the National Foundation for Infectious Diseases, 36% of health care workers receive influenza vaccinations each year. The 64% who do not get vaccinated consequently contribute to institutional outbreaks that put high-risk patients at increased risk of contracting influenza and suffering from its potentially major complications.[17]

Although vaccination is crucial in preventing influenza, there are those who should not be vaccinated. This group includes those who have

- ◆ a severe allergy to chicken eggs,
- ◆ had a severe reaction to an influenza vaccination in the past,
- ◆ developed Guillain-Barré syndrome within six weeks of getting an influenza vaccine previously, and
- ◆ children less than six months of age.

Vaccination also should be withheld from people who have a moderate or severe illness with fever. The vaccination can be administered when symptoms have lessened.[12]

Personal protective equipment and behaviors

Patients with human influenza

The primary method of transmission of human influenza is via large respiratory droplets. Consequently, standard precautions plus droplet precautions are recommended for the care of patients infected with human influenza.[18] Droplet precautions include patient placement, mask protocol, and patient transport.[19]

A patient infected with human influenza should be placed in a private room. If a private room is not available, the patient should be placed in a room with another patient who is infected with the same microorganism but not with another infection. If this is not possible, spatial separation of a least three feet should be made between infected patients and other patients and visitors.[19]

Staff members and visitors should wear masks according to protocols for droplet precautions.

Additionally, the mask should be worn when anyone is within three feet of the patient. Transporting the patient infected with human influenza should be limited and should be only for essential purposes. If transport becomes necessary, the patient should wear a mask to help minimize dispersal of respiratory droplets.[19]

Patients with avian influenza

Recent outbreaks of avian influenza in humans indicate that the risk of serious disease and increased mortality may be significantly higher than infection by human influenza viruses. Although rare, when a human is infected with avian influenza, viral adaptation can occur, which may result in easier human-to-human transmission. This in turn can possibly lead to the emergence of a pandemic strain.[18]

Avian influenza presents additional challenges to health care workers because of the uncertainty about the exact modes of transmission of avian influenza to and between humans. Additional precautions for health care workers involved in the care of patients with documented or suspected avian influenza should be implemented.[18]

Recommendations for avian influenza

Patients arriving at a health care facility with fever and respiratory symptoms should be managed according to CDC guidelines for respiratory hygiene and cough etiquette. They also should be questioned about their recent travel history. If a patient has traveled within the past 10 days to a country with avian influenza activity and is hospitalized with a severe febrile respiratory illness or is under evaluation for avian influenza, the patient should be managed using the following isolation precautions:

- ♦ standard precautions with careful attention to hand washing before and after patient contact or contact with surfaces potentially contaminated with respiratory secretions;
- ♦ eye protection within three feet of the patient;[20]
- ♦ droplet precautions and contact precautions to include patient placement, and patient transport.[20]

Should there be a suspicion of SARS, manage the patient with airborne precautions (N95 mask protocol (ie, fit tested) as well as contact precautions.[20]

Physical plant considerations

Visual alerts should be posted at facility entrances instructing patients and persons who accompany them to practice respiratory hygiene and cough etiquette (containing respiratory secretions by covering nose/mouth) if they have symptoms of a respiratory infection when they first register at the facility.[20]

During an influenza outbreak, it is best practice to provide infected patients with private rooms. If this is not possible, then semiprivate rooms should be made available. If multiple patients are admitted, and space requirements are limited, then patient care areas should be of sufficient size to maintain a distance of at least three feet between patients.[18]

Integrated services and multidisciplinary participation

Successful containment of the influenza virus requires a multidisciplinary approach. All personnel directly or indirectly involved in patient care must understand protocols for containment. All personnel should implement standard precautions and droplet precautions, and should enforce respiratory hygiene and cough etiquette for infected patients. A coordinated effort must be made to ensure that adequate procedures are in place for the disinfection of environmental surfaces, beds, bedrails, bedside equipment, and other frequently touched surfaces. Linen should be considered infectious and handled in a manner that prevents skin and mucous membrane exposures, as well as contamination of clothing.

Health care provider education and competency

Health care provider education and competency should be mandatory for all facility employees and physicians. Educational activities should include information concerning etiology of human and avian influenza, importance of vaccination, standard precautions, respiratory hygiene and cough etiquette, masking, and droplet precautions. Additionally, health care providers should be able to demonstrate behaviors that are required to successfully implement standard precautions, respiratory hygiene and cough etiquette, masking, droplet precautions, and using fit-tested respirators if SARS is suspected.

C. Severe Acute Respiratory Syndrome

During the 21st century, SARS became a global threat after making its debut in November 2002. By February 2003, the illness had spread to more than 12 countries, including Asia, North America, Europe, and South America. According to the World Health Organization (WHO), a total of 8,098 people worldwide became ill with SARS during the 2003 outbreak. Of the 8,098, 774 died. In the United States, only eight people, all of whom had traveled to global sections of world where SARS had been identified, had laboratory evidence of SARS.[21]

History

Severe acute respiratory syndrome may have originated in Guangdong Province in southern China in November 2002. A Chinese physician carried SARS to a Hong Kong hotel where several hotel guests on the same floor as the physician contracted the disease in February 2003. Airline passengers who had SARS and were traveling from Hong Kong spread the disease to Singapore, Toronto, and Hanoi. In March 2003, a diagnosis of SARS was made on the Chinese physician in Hong Kong.[22] A physician from the Hanoi, Vietnam, office of the WHO was called to investigate a patient with an atypical pneumonia from a Hanoi hospital.[23] Additional WHO officials and the CDC were called in. A global alert was issued for SARS, and infectious disease experts started studying this new infectious respiratory disease.[22]

Population Affected
Prevalence

SARS was recognized as a global threat when it spread to nearly 30 countries in Asia, North America, and Europe.[22] The first pandemic of the 21st century is attributed to SARS.[24] Transmission has occurred most often from person to person via droplet spread when an infected person coughs or sneezes. Most of the SARS outbreaks involved health care workers who were in close contact with infected patients. The 2003 global outbreak was contained, but there is still a possibility of recurrence.

Socioeconomic factors

In 2003, the SARS epidemic resulted in more than 800 deaths and other sequela. Some airports had no passengers, and stock markets lost value.[25] The SARS epidemic spread to more than 30 countries in a short time. The disease created anxiety around the world because of its capacity to spread quickly via international air travel, communicability, novelty, and the fact that a large number of health care workers were becoming infected. Nurses in Canada working with SARS patients were concerned about working conditions, staffing, employee health and safety, and wages.[26]

Epidemiology

The scientific community accepts the coronavirus (CoV) as the cause of SARS.[27,28] To stop the spread of SARS, there must be early diagnosis by virus isolation or serological testing.[29] The coronaviruses are a viral group that, when viewed under a microscope, appear to have a halo or crown-like (ie, corona) structure. These viruses commonly cause mild to moderate upper respiratory illness in humans. In animals, they are linked with respiratory, gastrointestinal, liver, and neurological disease.[30] The SARS-CoV has been found in wild civets and raccoon dogs in southeastern China, where they are considered culinary delicacies; on the other hand, domestic pigs and poultry are not hosts. Asymptomatic humans have a lag time during the incubation period; therefore, because they are still healthy, they are able to travel by air to any destination after being exposed. After the individual becomes symptomatic, SARS is most likely spread through person-to-person transmission. Health care workers are at high risk if there has been no suspicion of SARS but patients are positive for SARS.

Clinical Signs and Symptoms of SARS

Symptoms of SARS include, but are not limited to,

- ♦ fever (ie, greater than 100.4° F [38.0° C]);
- ♦ cough, shortness of breath, and dyspnea;
- ♦ headache;
- ♦ general malaise; and/or
- ♦ diarrhea (affects only a small percent of patients).[22,30]

Some of the above symptoms, and the patients' chest x-rays, initially led physicians to diagnose the disease as an atypical pneumonia.[30] Patients develop progressive respiratory compromise quickly. Symptoms usually occur in 2 to 7 days; sometimes 10 days after infection. Supportive treatment consists of antibiotics, steroids, and treatment of individual patient symptoms.[22]

Developing a Program

Health care facilities should have a written preparedness and response plan that is flexible and scalable and designed to address the variable nature of a SARS outbreak.

Operational planning

Impact of SARS on the workplace

A SARS coordinator should be appointed to serve as the point person for communicating information both internally and externally.[31] Testing the facility's response via a tabletop exercise is effective.

Staffing needs must be evaluated by health care facilities. Designated teams should be created in advance for the care of SARS patients to provide emergency and routine care. Infection control education also should be provided to these teams in advance to foster preparedness.[31] If there is a more extensive outbreak, nursing staff members may need to be relocated to other areas. Issues may occur that will exceed the scope of the health care facility. These must be addressed at community, regional, and national levels.

Psychology

During a SARS outbreak, it may be exhausting to wear full personal protective equipment (PPE) for lengthy periods of time. The focus required for donning and removing equipment also may be laborious. The health care facility should make arrangements to provide mental health professionals to assist its staff in coping with a SARS outbreak and the related stressors.[31] In 2003, the Toronto nurses and other health care workers were placed under work quarantine and required to wear a mask at all times in the presence of others. They were not allowed any physical contact with their family members. Stress and tension levels were high. Nurses mourned the loss of colleagues and worried about the effect of SARS on their families and what was yet to come.[26] SARS and other emerging infectious diseases may create a new type of workplace.

All health care workers must wear full PPE when caring for patients with SARS or suspected of having SARS. This includes eyewear, gown, gloves, and an N95 mask.

Personnel Protective Behavior: Recommendations for SARS

A comprehensive infection control program should be in place in the health care facility. Primary infection control strategies include the following.

Standard precautions—Health care workers should wear eye protection in addition to using routine standard precautions when caring for patients.[32]

Transmission-based precautions—The second tier of precautions are transmission-based precautions, which include

- *contact precautions*—health care workers should wear gowns, gloves, and eyewear when caring for patients in their environment;[32,33] and
- *airborne precautions*—health care workers should wear an N95-filtering disposable respirator during patient care. The facility should have training, fit-testing, and fit-checking in place as part of a complete respiratory program, which is required by the Occupational Safety and Health Administration.[34] Furthermore, the patient should be assigned to an isolation room with negative air pressure.[32]

Physical plant considerations

Key infection control measures for inpatient care areas include the following.

- Use negative pressure isolation rooms.
- Use private rooms with separate bathrooms if airborne precautions cannot be fully implemented. Keep doors closed.
- Assign patients with SARS or suspected of having SARS to the same unit. Keep equipment on that unit dedicated for their care.
- Use disposable equipment for patient care if available.
- Organize patient care activities. Keep only essential equipment, items, and supplies in rooms with patients who have SARS.
- Minimize patient movement or transport.
- Reduce traffic. Restrict visitors to the health care facility, patient care unit, and patient. Only essential health care workers should have access to patient rooms.[22]

If possible postpone surgery on patients with infectious diseases; if a patient who has SARS is in urgent need of a surgical procedure, the perioperative team must be prepared to follow precautions. Key infection control measures for the OR include the following.

- Schedule the procedure at the end of the day when other patients are not present and only a minimum number of staff members are present.[32]
- Place a surgical mask on the patient before transport to the OR.[33]

232

◆ Ensure that contact precautions are maintained during patient transport.

◆ Handle specimens from patients carefully. Place specimen in a leak-proof container and clean the exterior surface of the container with a chemical germicide when transferred off the surgical field.[34] Ensure that all specimen containers are labeled properly and identified as infectious material. Place the container in a biohazard bag for transport to the laboratory.

◆ Minimize the number of staff members in the OR involved in the care of the patients with SARS. Arrange for additional staff members to assist by stationing them outside the room to get needed supplies and equipment.

◆ Place isolation signage on the doors to the OR indicating that transmission-based precautions should be used.

◆ Remove unnecessary equipment from the OR. Keep supply cabinet doors closed.

◆ Request that the anesthesia care team use a smaller anesthesia cart designated for isolation patients and use single-use items if possible.

◆ Confine and contain contamination during the procedure within the immediate vicinity of the surgical field when possible.[33]

◆ Reestablish a safe and clean environment when a surgical procedure is completed on a patient who has SARS.[35]

◆ Ensure that health care workers wear full PPE as required for contact and airborne precautions to reduce the risk of exposure to bloodborne or infectious microorganisms throughout the surgical procedure, cleaning, and recovery period.

◆ Carefully handle surgical instruments, equipment, furniture, and soiled linen and trash. Clean the patient transport vehicle. Use an Environmental Protection Agency (EPA)-registered hospital disinfectant for cleaning. Discard unused disposable supplies after completion of the surgical intervention.[22]

◆ Environmental services personnel should be trained and supervised in proper cleaning and disinfection methods.

Integrated services and multidisciplinary participation

An optimum level of communication between the facility's infection control team, clinical staff members, and public health authorities should be ongoing.[22]

Nursing staff members in the facility's emergency department and clinics must be prepared to identify patients who are suspected of having SARS and know how to manage an influx of patients.[37] The infection control team should be involved with nursing staff members to provide guidance and direction in coordinating the hospital experience of patients who have SARS.

Health care facility administrators should take a proactive and multidisciplinary approach by conducting a disaster drill involving an influx of patients who have SARS to operationalize their policies and protocols, assess readiness, and evaluate plan effectiveness.[38] A coordinated multidisciplinary response is required to manage a SARS outbreak.[31] Clinical services may include, but are not limited to,

◆ emergency department (eg, entry screening and triage, isolating patients suspected of having SARS as soon as possible);

◆ engineering (eg, air handling system, maintenance of negative pressure isolation rooms);

◆ environmental services.

◆ human resources personnel;

◆ infection control team, which includes infection control practitioners and hospital epidemiologist;

◆ intensive care unit;

◆ laboratory;

◆ materials management (eg, acquisition of PPE and N95 respirators) because supplies may run short during an outbreak;

◆ medical patient care unit;

◆ medical staff members;

◆ nursing leadership;

◆ outpatient clinics;

◆ pharmacy;

◆ public relations department personnel (eg, to communicate with press and public);

◆ radiology;

◆ risk management;

◆ safety department;

◆ security department (eg, access control efforts);

◆ senior management and finance representative; and

◆ staff development and education department.

This multidisciplinary group includes patient care, administration, and support staff. A representative from the local or state health department should be involved to coordinate planning with the community.[31]

Employee education and self-protective behavior

Facility staff members from all disciplines providing care to patients with SARS should participate in a comprehensive education program. The contents of the program should have a basic component for all staff members and a discipline-specific component that is current and appropriate for the specialty. Competency in standard, contact, and airborne precautions and the use of fit-tested respirators is mandatory for the care of patients with SARS.

Staff members must exercise vigilance in their practice by following infection control policies and procedures of the health care facilities where they work. These documents need to be reviewed by the infection control committee and staff development personnel at least annually. Inservice programs should be provided for all staff members so that infection control precautions are understood and followed to prevent SARS transmission; preparation is the key.[36] Practicing self-protective behavior with staff members builds confidence.

During the inservice program, stress the importance of planning and communicating with staff members. In the perioperative arena, communication is vital among the surgical team members throughout the patient's surgical experience. Postoperative disposition of patients with SARS needs to be determined and agreed upon. Nurse managers should take the lead in planning the logistics of patient care in consultation with the infection control practitioner and the hospital epidemiologist. If the facility does not have an isolation cubicle in the postanesthesia care unit, patients with SARS may need to be directly admitted to the intensive care unit isolation room for recovery. The nurse manager must confer with the physicians and OR nurses caring for patients with SARS to implement the plan of care. It is vital to adhere to infection control precautions to limit transmission of SARS to staff members.

Physician education and self-protective behavior

Anesthesia care providers should exercise care during the induction and extubation phases of the procedure to protect members of the surgical team that are in close contact and may be exposed to exhalations from SARS patients. Using PPE, to include full-face shields, is essential, especially if a bronchoscopy is being performed. The patient should be orally suctioned in a gentle manner to prevent aerosolization when intubating. Health care providers must be careful and precise when removing and placing laryngoscope blades, endoscope, or bronchoscopes to prevent splatter and minimize the opportunity of particle aerosolization.[22] The anesthesia care provider is at risk when performing endotracheal intubation.[39] He or she should minimize touching other equipment with gloves used for intubation or extubation.[22]

Employees and physicians should understand the importance of proper hand hygiene after removing PPE. Personnel should wash hands with soap and water or use an alcohol-based waterless hand hygiene product before and after patient contact. The health care facility should require adherence and proficiency in self-protective behavior.

Precautions for Avian Influenza, Human Influenza, and SARS

Human influenza precautions include

- ◆ standard precautions (eg, careful attention to hand washing before and after patient contact or contact with surfaces potentially contaminated with respiratory secretions),[22] and
- ◆ droplet precautions (eg, surgical mask, patient placement in a private room or shared with another patient with the same epidemiology).[19]

Avian influenza precautions include

- ◆ standard precautions (eg, careful attention to hand washing before and after patient contact or contact with surfaces potentially contaminated with respiratory secretions),
- ◆ eye protection within three feet of the patient,[22] and
- ◆ droplet precautions and contact precautions (eg, patient placement, if SARS is suspected an N95 mask protocol [fit tested], patient transport).[20]

SARS precautions include

- ◆ standard precautions with careful attention to hand washing before and after patient contact or contact with surfaces potentially contaminated with respiratory secretions,[32]
- ◆ eye protection within three feet of the patient,[22]

♦ contact precautions (eg, gown, gloves, eyewear),[32,33] and

♦ airborne precautions (eg, patient is placed in a negative air pressure room, health care workers wear fit-tested N95 masks).[32]

II. Nursing Process Application

A. Perioperative Nursing Vocabulary

The perioperative nursing vocabulary is a clinically relevant and empirically validated standardized nursing language. It relates to the delivery of care in the perioperative setting. This standardized language consists of a collection of data elements (ie, the Perioperative Nursing Data Set [PNDS]), and includes perioperative nursing diagnoses, interventions, and outcomes.[40]

Care of the perioperative patient with human and avian influenza SARS, and other types of similar diseases must be individualized to each patient's needs. The perioperative nurse must bear in mind that care must be taken to protect the surgical team, other patients, and their family members because of the contagious nature of these diseases. Documentation should reflect the unique aspects of care provided using the PNDS. The examples listed below may not apply to all types of surgery for patients with human and avian influenza, SARS, and other similar diseases. Each situation must be assessed for appropriate outcomes, nursing diagnoses, and interventions.

B. Nursing Diagnoses

The perioperative nurse analyzes the assessment data to determine nursing diagnoses. Following is a partial list of nursing diagnoses that may be associated with patients who have human or avian influenza or SARS.

X28 (D2)—infection, risk for.

C. Outcome Identification

To develop a plan of care for the patient, the perioperative nurse identifies desired patient outcomes collaboratively with the patient. Following is a partial list of nursing outcomes that may be associated with patients who have human or avian influenza or SARS.

O10 (D2)—The patient is free from signs and symptoms of a surgical site infection.

D. Planning

The perioperative nurse develops a plan of care for patients who have human or avian influenza or SARS that prescribes nursing interventions to attain expected outcomes. Interventions and activities are selected according to individual patient needs and the type of procedure to be performed. Following is a partial list of interventions that may be associated with patients who have human or avian influenza or SARS.

I4   Administers care to wound sites.
I7   Administers prescribed antibiotic therapy.
I21   Assesses susceptibility for surgical site infection.
I83   Manages culture specimen collection.
I86   Monitors body temperature.
I88   Monitors for signs and symptoms of infection.
I98   Protects from cross-contamination.

III. Conclusion

This guideline is intended to be used in the event of an outbreak of human or avian influenza or SARS to promote safe care for those affected patients who may require urgent or emergent surgical intervention or other invasive procedures. Perioperative personnel should use strict infection control measures while caring for these types of infectious patients to limit transmission.

These diseases are extremely complex and require special understanding by perioperative team members to ensure optimal patient outcomes. This document addresses assumptions, definitions, history, prevalence, socioeconomic factors, epidemiology, and clinical signs and symptoms. In addition, it addresses

♦ developing a program;
♦ operational planning;
♦ impact on the workplace;
♦ risks to health care workers;
♦ vaccination;
♦ use of PPE;
♦ personal protective behaviors;
♦ physical plant considerations;
♦ integrated services, which includes a multidisciplinary approach;
♦ employee and physician education and competency; and
♦ the nursing process application regarding this patient population.[40]

Human and Avian Influenza and SARS

This guideline may require modification based on specific patient and facility needs. It is AORN's intent that practitioners will use this document in their facilities to develop policies, procedures, and protocols specific to perioperative care of patients affected by outbreaks of human and avian influenza and SARS for patients who must undergo surgical or other invasive procedures.

NOTES

1. A Trampuz, M Rajesh, T Smith, et al, "Avian influenza: A new pandemic threat?" *Mayo Clinical Procedures* 79 (2004) 523-530.

2. "Information about influenza pandemics," Department of Health and Human Services, Centers for Disease Control and Prevention, *http://www.cdc.gov/flu/avian/gen-info/pandemics.htm* (accessed 10 Aug 2005).

3. "Pandemic influenza, academic health center—University of Minnesota," Center for Infectious Disease Research and Policy (CIDRAP), *http://www.cidrap.umn.edu/cidrap/content/ influenza/panflu/biofacts/panflu.htm* (accessed 7 Oct 2005) 3.

4. R K Zimmerman; "Recent changes in influenza epidemiology and vaccination recommendations," *The Journal of Family Practice* 54 (January 2005) S1.

5. Appendix 2, "Glossary of terms, influenza pandemic contingency plan," *Health Protection Agency,* Version 7.0 (February 2005) 47.

6. "Influenza viruses," Department of Health and Human Services, Centers for Disease Control and Prevention, *http://www.cdc.gov/flu/avian/gen-info/flu-viruses.htm* (accessed 10 Aug 2005) 1-2.

7. "Focus on the flu," National Institute of Allergy and Infectious Diseases, National Institutes of Health, *http://www3.niaid.nih.gov/new/focuson/flu/illustrations/timeline/timeline.htm* (accessed 15 Aug 2005).

8. "Information about influenza and its prevention, Influenza Dot Com, *http://www.influenza.com/Index.cfm?FA=HOME* (accessed 17 Aug 2005).

9. "Influenza (flu) fact sheet—Key facts about influenza and influenza vaccine, Centers for Disease Control and Prevention, *http://www.cdc.gov/flu/keyfacts.pdf* (accessed 17 August 2005) 1.

10. S Harper, K Fukuda, T Uyeki, et al, "Prevention and control of influenza—Recommendations of the Advisory Committee on Immunization Practices (ACIP)," *Morbidity and Mortality Weekly Report* 54 no RR-8 (July 29, 2005) 1.

11. M Meltzer, N Cox, K Fukuda, "The economic impact of pandemic influenza in the United States: Priorities for intervention," *Emerging Infectious Diseases* 5 (September–October 1999).

12. "Background on influenza," Department of Health and Human Services, Centers for Disease Control and Prevention, *http://www.cdc.gov/flu/protect/keyfacts.htm* (accessed September 4, 2005) 3.

13. "Updated infection control measures for the prevention and control of influenza in health-care facilities," Department of Health and Human Services, Centers for Disease Control and Prevention, *http://www.cdc.gov/professionals/ infectioncontrol/healthcarefacilities.htm* (accessed 20 Jan 2005).

14. A Monto, "The threat of an avian influenza pandemic," *The New England Journal of Medicine* 352 (January 2005) 323.

15. "Key facts about avian influenza (bird flu) and avian influenza A (H5N1) virus," Department of Health and Human Services, Centers for Disease Control and Prevention, *http://www.cdc.gov/flu/avian/gen-info/facts.htm* (accessed 10 August 2005).

16. "Transmission of influenza A viruses between animals and people," Department of Health and Human Services, Centers for Disease Control and Prevention, *http://www.cdc.gov/avian/gen-info/transmission.htm* (accessed 10 Aug 2005)

17. "Call to action: Influenza immunization among health care workers," National Foundation for Infectious Diseases, *http://www.nfid.org/publications/calltoaction.pdf* (accessed 9 Oct 2005).

18. "Interim recommendations for infection control in health-care facilities caring for patients with known or suspected avian influenza," (May 21, 2004) Department of Health and Human Services, Centers for Disease Control and Prevention, *http://www.cdc.gov/flu/avian/professional /infect-control.htm* (accessed 9 Oct 2005).

19. "Droplet precautions," Department of Health and Human Services, Centers for Disease Control and Prevention, *http://www.cdc.gov/ncidod/hip/ISOLAT/droplet_prec_excerpt_print.htm* (accessed 9 Oct 2005).

20. "Respiratory hygiene/cough etiquette in health-care settings," (Dec 17, 2003) Department of Health and Human Services, Centers for Disease Control and Prevention, *http://www.cdc.gov/flu/professionals /infection-control/resphygiene.htm* (accessed 9 Oct 2005).

21. "Severe acute respiratory syndrome (SARS): What everyone should know about SARS," (May 3, 2005) Department of Health and Human Services, Centers for Disease Control and Prevention, *http://www.cdc.gov/ncidod/sars/basics.htm* (accessed 9 Oct 2005).

22. M Farley, L M Socha, "Severe acute respiratory syndrome and its effects on health care," *SSM* 9 (October 2003) 20-25.

23. B Reilly et al, "SARS and Carlo Urbani," *The New England Journal of Medicine* 348 (May 15, 2003) 1951.

24. J S M Peiris et al," The severe acute respiratory syndrome," *The New England Journal of Medicine* 349 (December 18, 2003) 2431-2441.

25. J M Drazen, "SARS—Looking back over the first 100 days," *The New England Journal of Medicine* 349 (July 24, 2003) 319-320.

26. J Howard-Ruben, "SARS unmasked: Canadian nurses tell of hardship, loss," *Nursing Spectrum* 15 (October 20, 2003) 32-34.

27. J Gerberding, "Faster ... but fast enough? Responding to the epidemic of severe acute respiratory syndrome," *The New England Journal of Medicine* 348 (May15, 2003) 2030-2031.

28. K V Holmes, "SARS-associated coronavirus," *The New England Journal of Medicine* 348 (May 15, 2003) 1948-1951.

29. B Tomlinson, C Cockram, "Experience at Prince of Wales Hospital, Hong Kong," *The Lancet* 361 (May 3, 2003) 1486-1487.

30. D Tilton, "Severe acute respiratory syndrome," *Managing Infection Control* 3 (2003) 14-22.

31. A Srinivasan et al, "Foundations of the severe acute respiratory syndrome preparedness and response plan for healthcare facilities," *Infection Control and Hospital Epidemiology* 25 (2004) 1020-1025.

32. J E Williamson, "SARS Update: CDC finds new coronavirus may cause illness," *OR Today* 3 (2003) 8-9.

33. "Recommended practices for standard and transmission-based precautions in the perioperative practice setting," in *Standards, Recommended Practices, and Guidelines* (Denver: AORN, Inc, 2005) 447-451.

34. K M Pyrek, "Is a global flu pandemic imminent?" *Infection Control Today* 9 (March 2005) 34-42.

35. "Recommended practices for environmental cleaning in the surgical practice setting," in *Standards, Recommended Practices, and Guidelines* (Denver: AORN, Inc, 2005) 361-366.

36. "Canadian warning: ORs should prepare for SARS," *Same-Day Surgery* (March 2004) 30-31.

37. M Fishman et al, "Patient safety tools: SARS, smallpox, monkeypox, and avian flu," *Disaster Management & Response* 3 (July–September 2005) 86-90.

38. "Are you ready for an influx of SARS patients?" *ED Accreditation Update* (November 2004) 1-3.

39. R A Fowler et al, "Transmission of severe acute respiratory syndrome during intubation and mechanical ventilation," *American Journal of Respiratory and Critical Care Medicine* 169 (2004) 1198-1202.

40. Beyea, S, ed, *Perioperative Nursing Data Set: The Perioperative Nursing Vocabulary*, second ed (Denver: AORN, Inc, 2002) 83.

RESOURCES

"AORN guidance statement: Safe on-call practices in perioperative settings," in *Standards, Recommended Practices, and Guidelines* (Denver: AORN, Inc. 2005) 193-195.

Chan, S. "Nurses fighting against severe acute respiratory syndrome (SARS) in Hong Kong," *Journal of Nursing Scholarship* 35 (2003) 209.

Esswein, E J, et al. "Environmental and occupational health response to SARS, Taiwan, 2003," *Emerging Infectious Diseases* 10 (July 2004) 1187-1194.

Fenwick, A. "On the front line of SARS," *American Journal of Nursing* 103 (2003) 118-119.

Maunder, R, et al. "The immediate psychological and occupational impact of the 2003 SARS outbreak in a teaching hospital," *Canadian Medical Association Journal* 168 (May 13, 2003) 1245-1251.

McGillis Hall, L, et al. "Media portrayal of nurses' perspectives and concerns in the SARS crisis in Toronto," *Journal of Nursing Scholarship* 35(2003) 211-215.

Moore, D, et al. "Protecting health care workers from SARS and other respiratory pathogens: Organizational and individual factors that affect adherence to infection control guidelines," *American Journal of Infection Control* 33 (March 2005)

Patrick, D M. "The race to outpace severe acute respiratory syndrome (SARS)," *Canadian Medical Association Journal* 168 (May 13, 2003) 1265-1266.

"Recommended practices for cleaning, handling, and processing anesthesia equipment," in *Standards, Recommended Practices, and Guidelines* (Denver: AORN, Inc, 2005) 289-298.

"Recommended practices for traffic patterns in the perioperative setting," in *Standards, Recommended Practices, and Guidelines* (Denver: AORN, Inc., 2005) 483-485.

Tan, Y M, et al. "Management of inpatients exposed to an outbreak of severe acute respiratory syndrome (SARS)," *Journal of Hospital Infection* 58 (2004) 210-215.

Tsang, K W, et al. "A cluster of cases of severe acute respiratory syndrome in Hong Kong," *The New England Journal of Medicine* 348 (May 15, 2003) 1977-1985.

Approved by the AORN Board of Directors, November 2005. Scheduled for publication in the *AORN Journal* in 2006.

AORN Guidance Statement: "Do-Not-Use" Abbreviations, Acronyms, Dosage Designations, and Symbols

Preamble

Confusing or easily misinterpreted abbreviations, acronyms, or symbols put caregivers at risk for making errors and compromising patient safety. Unintentional as an error may be, a misplaced decimal point, a "U" interpreted as a "0" (zero), QOD confused for QID, or AS misinterpreted as OS puts patients at risk for medical error with potential catastrophic results (eg, overdose, inadequate dose, omission due to laterality error, wrong medication administered, error in frequency of administration). Improving communication through reducing and standardizing abbreviations, acronyms, and symbols is a significant step toward reducing the occurrence of errors related to the inability to accurately read and interpret written medical orders and transcribed verbal orders.

The purpose of this guidance statement is to heighten the awareness of perioperative registered nurses concerning the dangers associated with the use of abbreviations, acronyms, and symbols, with the goal of eliminating their use in health care documentation. All perioperative settings should address the issue of error-prone abbreviations. These practice settings include, but are not limited to, hospital operating rooms, ambulatory surgery centers, preanesthesia and postanesthesia care units, cardiac catheterization departments, endoscopy suites, radiology departments, and all other areas where operative and other invasive procedures may be performed. Patient safety in the perioperative setting may be improved by focusing on communication among caregivers through the creation of a standardized list of "do-not-use" abbreviations, acronyms, and symbols.

Effective Jan 1, 2004, the Joint Commission on Accreditation of Healthcare Organizations (JCAHO) developed a list of dangerous abbreviations, acronyms, and symbols that are not to be used within accredited health care facilities (Table 1). This requirement is intended as a means to improve communication among caregivers (see National Patient Safety Goal #2).[1] The Joint Commission's minimal list of required do-not-use abbreviations, acronyms, and symbols is the beginning of a process to assist organizations with the expansion of their error-prevention programs to improve safety for patients. The Joint Commission recommends that organizations limit the use of abbreviations initially by eliminating nine specific error-prone abbreviations from health care documentation. Seven additional error-prone abbreviations, acronyms, or symbols will be reviewed on an annual basis for inclusion on the official do-not-use

Table 1

JCAHO's Required List of "Do-Not-Use" Abbreviations, Acronyms, and Symbols[1]		
Do Not Use	**Potential Problem**	**Use Instead**
U (for unit)	Mistaken for "0" (zero), the number "4" (four), or "cc."	Write "unit"
IU (for international unit)	Mistaken for IV (intravenous) or the number 10 (ten).	Write "International Unit"
Q.D., QD, q.d., qd (daily) Q.O.D., QOD, q.o.d, qod (every other day)	Mistaken for each other. The period after the Q can be mistaken for "I" and the "O" mistaken for "I."	Write "daily" Write "every other day"
Trailing zero (X.0 mg)* Lack of leading zero (.X mg)	Decimal point is missed.	Write X mg Write 0.X mg
MS MSO4 and MgSO4	Can mean morphine sulfate or magnesium sulfate; confused for one another.	Write "morphine sulfate" or "magnesium sulfate."

1. *Applies to all orders and all medication-related documentation that is handwritten (including free-textcomputer entry) or on preprinted forms.*

Exception: *A "trailing zero" may be used only where required to demonstrate the level of precision of the value being reported, such as for laboratory results, imaging studies that report size of lesions, or catheter/tube sizes. It may not be used in medication orders or other medication-related documentation.*

Reprinted with permission from Joint Commission on Accreditation of Healthcare Organizations, http://www.jcaho.org /accredited+organizations/patient+safety/06_dnu_list.pdf *(accessed 31 Jan 2006).*

Table 2

POTENTIAL ADDITIONAL "DO-NOT-USE" ABBREVIATIONS, ACRONYMS, AND SYMBOLS[1]		
Do Not Use	Potential Problem	Use Instead
> (greater than) < (less than)	Misinterpreted as the number "7" (seven) or the letter "L." Confused for one another.	Write "greater than" Write "less than"
Abbreviations for drug names	Misinterpreted due to similar abbreviations for multiple drugs	Write drug names in full
Apothecary units	Unfamiliar to many practitioners. Confused with metric units.	Use metric units
@	Mistaken for the number "2" (two).	Write "at"
cc	Mistaken for U (units) when poorly written.	Write "mL" or "milliliters"
μg	Mistaken for mg (milligrams), resulting in one thousand-fold overdose.	Write "mcg" or "micrograms"

Reprinted with permission from Joint Commission on Accreditation of Healthcare Organizations, http://www.jcaho.org/accredited+organizations/patient+safety/06_dnu_list.pdf *(accessed 31 Jan 2006).*

list. Implementing this change in practice keeps an organization on a trajectory focused on patient safety as a number-one priority.

Guidance Statement

AORN recommends that all perioperative settings implement the Joint Commission's National Patient Safety Goal #2, adopt the minimum required list of do-not-use abbreviations, educate perioperative registered nurses regarding the removal of these items from all health care documentation, and monitor compliance with this activity. Table 1 represents the Joint Commission's official list of do-not-use abbreviations, acronyms, and symbols, published Jan 1, 2004.

The minimum required list is the first step in fulfilling JCAHO's National Patient Safety Goal #2. With the goal of eliminating all abbreviations from the health care setting, the Joint Commission is encouraging, but not mandating, each organization to voluntarily expand the above list with the addition of the do-not-use abbreviations, acronyms, and symbols identified as possible future inclusions to the "Official 'do not use' abbreviations list." Items in Table 2 have been identified by the Joint Commission, in concert with the Institute for Safe Medication Practice (ISMP), United States Pharmacopecia (USP), and the National Coordinating Council for Medication Error Reporting and Prevention

(NCCMERP), to be considered annually as potential error-prone abbreviations to be included on the official do-not-use list.

Furthermore, AORN strongly recommends consideration be given to the selection of problem-prone, high-risk, high-volume abbreviations, acronyms, and symbols unique to the perioperative practice setting when augmenting the minimally required list of do-not-use items. At a minimum, abbreviations related to laterality should be eliminated from all documentation within the perioperative setting (Table 3).

Further sources of information to help guide in the selection of do-not-use items may be derived from a review of problem-prone, high-risk, high-volume abbreviations, acronyms, and symbols found within handwritten, preprinted, and electronic forms of perioperative communication, such as
- ◆ surgical procedure list,
- ◆ surgeon preference or procedure cards,
- ◆ perioperative documentation (ie, preoperative, intraoperative, postoperative),
- ◆ progress notes,
- ◆ specimen labeling,
- ◆ consent,
- ◆ history and physical,
- ◆ surgical schedules,
- ◆ staff orientation and competency materials, and
- ◆ patient teaching materials.

Table 3

AORN RECOMMENDATIONS		
Error-Prone Abbreviation	**Potential Problem**	**Preferred Term**
L, R, Bil	Illegibility leads to confusion related to correct identification of laterality	Write out "left," "right," and "bilateral"

Another strategy to improve communication among caregivers is a process to ensure that the signatures of the provider initiating the medical order and the caregiver transcribing the verbal order are legible. AORN suggests that all health care providers use block print and sign their names to all written and verbal orders. The extra step of block-printing the name affords the caregiver an opportunity to contact the provider if a question, concern, or issue were to arise related to the written order. If the caregiver is unable to read the written order, confusion or misinterpretation could result and lead to an adverse patient event.

This guidance statement reflects suggested minimal requirements to promote safety in patient care. It is not to be considered an all-inclusive listing of error-prone abbreviations, acronyms, dosage designations, or symbols. It is the responsibility of the health care practitioner, in concert with the patient care organization, to ensure that documentation clearly and unambiguously reflects the individualized treatment of the patient.

NOTES

1. "National patient safety goals," Joint Commission on Accreditation of Healthcare Organizations, *http://www.jcaho.org/general+public/patient+safety/04_npsg.htm* (2004) and *http://www.jcaho.org/accredited+organizations/patient+safety/npsg.htm* (2005–2006) (accessed 7 Sept 2005).

2. "Official 'do not use' list," Joint Commission on Accreditation of Healthcare Organizations, *http://www.jcaho.org/accredited+organizations/patient+safety/dnu.htm* (accessed 7 Sept 2005).

RESOURCES

Abbreviations Lists

Hicks, R W; Cousins, D D; Williams, R L. *Summary of Information Submitted to MEDMARX in the Year 2002: The Quest for Quality* (Rockville, Md: US Pharmacopecia Center for the Advancement of Patient Safety, 2003) 41-44.

Institute for Safe Medication Practices. "ISMP's list of error-prone abbreviations, symbols, and dose designations,"

ISMP Medication Safety Alert 8 (Nov 27, 2003). Also available at *http://www.ismp.org/PDF/ISMPAbbreviations.pdf* or *http://www.ismp.org/PDF/ErrorProne.pdf* (accessed 8 Sept 2005).

Joint Commission on Accreditation of Healthcare Organizations. "Medication errors related to potentially dangerous abbreviations," *Sentinel Event Alert* 23 (September 2001). Also available at *http://www.jcaho.org/about+us/news+letters/sentinel+event+alert/sea_23.htm* (accessed 8 Sept 2005).

"New Joint Commission 'do not use' list: Abbreviations, acronyms, and symbols," American Academy of Physical Medicine and Rehabilitation, *http://www.aapmr.org/hpl/pracguide/jcahosymbols.htm* (accessed 7 Sept 2005).

"Recommendations to enhance accuracy of prescription writing," (adopted Sept 4, 1996, revised June 2, 2005) National Coordinating Council for Medication Error Reporting and Prevention (NCCMERP), *http://www.nccmerp.org/council/council1996-09-04.html* (accessed 8 Sept 2005).

Implementation/Staff Education

Beyea, S C. "Best practices for abbreviation use," *AORN Journal* 79 (March 2004) 641-642.

"Five dangerous medical abbreviations," Ohioans First, *http://www.ohioansfirst.org/abbreviations/abbrev.htm* (accessed 7 Sept 2005).

"Implementation tips for eliminating dangerous abbreviations," Joint Commission on Accreditation of Healthcare Organizations, *http://www.jcaho.org/accredited+organizations/patient+safety/05+npsg/tips.htm* (accessed 8 Sept 2005).

"Maximizing patient safety in the medication use process: Practice guidelines and best demonstrated practices," Wisconsin Patient Safety Institute, *http://www.wpsi.org/media/documents/pdf/Max_Pat_Saft_2002.pdf* (accessed 31 Jan 2006).

"Patient safety program," US Department of Defense, *https://patientsafety.satx.disa.mil* (accessed 7 Sept 2005).

"Preventing medical errors: More on dangerous abbreviations," *Patient Safety News,* Show #25, March 2004, US Food and Drug Administration, *http://www.accessdata.fda.gov/scripts/cdrh/cfdocs/psn/transcript.cfm?show=25* (accessed 31 Jan 2006).

Regional Medication Safety Program for Hospitals: Health Care Improvement Foundation. *Medication Safety Solutions Kit,* information available from Delaware Valley Healthcare Council, *http://www.dvhc.org/safety/program/details.asp?ID=CQe3RU219Ngec94UQJ3g.* Also available from ECRI, *http://www.ecri.org /products_and_services/products/medication_safety/medsafety brochure.pdf* (accessed 7 Sept 2005).

Approved by the AORN Board of Directors, November 2005. Scheduled for publication in the *AORN Journal* in 2006.

AORN Guidance Statement: Environmental Responsibility

Introduction

This document is intended to guide perioperative registered nurses in the development of environmentally responsible practices. This document may be used by health care organizations to provide direction for the creation of environmentally responsible policies and procedures. This guidance document addresses

- infectious and noninfectious waste management,
- recycling practices,
- resource conservation,
- supply conservation and management practices,
- reprocessing, reuse, repair and refurbishing,
- sterilization and disinfection, and
- construction for efficiency and conservation.

It is recognized that not all portions of this document may be usable by all health care organizations because of the varying standards and regulations set forth in various geographic locations. It also is recognized that the perioperative setting is varied and includes hospitals, obstetrical surgical suites, ambulatory facilities, physicians' offices, specialty centers for invasive procedures (eg, cardiac catheterization laboratories, radiology departments, endoscopy suites), and other areas where invasive procedures or interventions are performed

Background

Nurses comprise a large single group of health care providers and are in a position to influence environmental management practices. Nurses have long played a role in the protection of the environment. In the 1800s, Florence Nightingale was one of the first nurses to advocate for a healthy environment.[1] Nurses have an ethical responsibility to actively promote and participate in resource conservation and to protect the environment.

US health care organizations generate in excess of two million tons of waste annually.[2] Approximately 85% of this waste is noninfectious, with a large amount being generated in the operating room.[3] Inpatient facilities spend more than five billion dollars a year on energy consumption. Health care energy consumption is increasing to support new and existing technology.[4] Sterilizing, heating and cooling processes, and hand sanitization contribute to use of water, a limited natural resource.

In addition to waste generation, energy and water consumption has a significant negative impact on the environment.

Guidance Statement

The perioperative registered nurse should serve as a steward of the environment by being knowledgeable about perioperative practices that negatively affect the environment. Perioperative registered nurses should actively promote and participate in resource conservation. Effective resource conservation leads to an improvement of environmental health. The perioperative registered nurse should strive to understand the political, economic, and public health components of environmental responsibility.[5] The following strategies provide a framework on which to build an environmentally responsible practice.

Infectious and Noninfectious Tissue and Waste Management

More than four million tons[2] of general waste are produced annually by US health care facilities.[6] Waste materials can be classified as potentially infectious or noninfectious. Waste management is a major expenditure for health care organizations. Infectious waste management alone can consume as much as 20% of a hospital's annual budget for environmental services.[7]

Waste generated from the operating room includes potentially infectious and noninfectious waste as well as material that requires special disposal (eg, liquid chemicals, hazardous materials). Mercury-based products and dioxin generated by incineration of polyvinylchloride (PVC) are hazardous chemicals. Mercury, a heavy metal and neurotoxin, is a frequent contaminant found in medical waste. Dioxin, a known human carcinogen, has been implicated in cancer of the lung, thyroid, hematopoietic system, and liver as well as soft tissue sarcoma.[8] Polyvinylchloride is found in many medical supplies, packaging, and building materials. The resulting air pollutants from medical waste incineration not only affect the local community, but also can migrate to pollute distant environments and populations.[8] Disposal of mercury and medical waste are subject to regulation by local, state, or federal governmental agencies. Health care organizations must comply with the regulations.[9]

Perioperative nurses can significantly affect waste management practices by encouraging and implementing strategies that promote a safe and healthy environment. These strategies should be cost effective and conserve resources. Strategies that should be considered include, but are not limited to, the following.

♦ Conduct a survey to assess types of waste generated in perioperative practice settings.

♦ Conduct a cost analysis of waste management considering
  – the volume of noninfectious waste, and
  – the weight of potentially infectious waste generated and treatment technology available.[7]

♦ Define potentially infectious waste according to local, state, and federal regulations.

♦ Provide education to all health care workers, to include, but not limited to,
  – the definition of potentially infectious waste,
  – the importance of and process for segregation of potentially infectious waste from noninfectious waste,
  – the costs of waste management,
  – the environmental impact of waste disposal,[10] and
  – state and federal guidelines and regulations for disposal of waste.

♦ Review and update organization-wide waste management policies.

♦ Limit contents of biohazardous waste containers (eg, red bags) to potentially infectious waste.

♦ Explore methods of waste segregation, which may include
  – placing noninfectious waste and biohazard containers side by side in a convenient location, and
  – using a bag-in-bag collection system (ie, clear bag inserted inside red bag for collection of waste used to set up for a procedure; clear bag is removed from bag holder but left in room before start of procedure when infectious waste may be generated).[7] Consider risks to health care workers when using this system.

♦ Eliminate use of mercury-based products—ie, inventory, remove, and replace mercury-containing devices with nonmercury-containing devices (eg, digital thermometers, sphygmomanometers, batteries, bougies, cantor tubes, fluorescent lights).[3]

♦ Work with waste management services to explore alternatives to incineration, including, but not limited to,
  – microwaving,
  – autoclaving,
  – radiowaving, and
  – electrotechnologies.[11]

♦ Explore recycling programs for noninfectious waste (eg, paper, irrigation bottles, sterilization wraps and other plastics).

♦ Evaluate the environmental impact of reusable, reposable, and disposable products.

♦ Develop an ongoing performance improvement program for waste management.

♦ Dispose of chemicals in accordance with state and local regulations, including, but not limited to,
  – dilution,
  – inactivation of solution before release, and
  – consideration of a program of controlled release.[12]

♦ Consider membership in Healthy Hospitals for the Environment (H2E), located online at *http://www.H2E-online.org* (accessed 23 Jan 2006); and Health Care Without Harm (HCWH), located online at *http://www.noharm.org* (accessed 23 Jan 2006).[8]

Recycling Practices

A significant amount of hospital waste is composed of noninfectious material, much of which may be recyclable.[13,14] Recyclable items found in the perioperative environment include, but are not limited to, plastic bottles, sterilization wrap, peel packs, glass, paper, aluminum and metal cans, and corrugated cardboard.[15,16] Only items that are clean and noninfectious, as defined by local, state, and federal regulations, should be recycled.[3] Recycling noninfectious waste materials has environmental and financial benefits that may include[17]

♦ providing materials for remanufacture,
♦ preserving resources for future generations,
♦ decreasing air and water pollution,
♦ conserving energy, and
♦ limiting the expansion of landfills and incinerator use.

Health care facilities should modify purchasing and waste disposal practices to favor recycling.[14,16] Perioperative nurses can significantly affect waste management practices by encouraging and implementing recycling strategies that promote a safe and healthy environment. These strategies should be cost effective and conserve resources. Strategies that should be considered include, but are not limited to, the following.

♦ Perform a waste assessment to identify items appropriate for recycling.

♦ Investigate available community recycling programs to determine feasibility of participation.

♦ Obtain recycling containers from local waste management systems.[18]

♦ Begin with simple items (eg, paper, cardboard, plastics).

♦ Contact manufacturers regarding recycling programs.

♦ Identify waste versus recycling receptacles with distinguishing features:
  – use color-coded receptacles (eg, green for paper, silver for metal, blue for plastic); and
  – use a slotted top for paper, a round top for cans.

♦ Provide receptacles in areas where the waste is generated.

♦ Provide education to all health care workers regarding recycling practices, including separation procedures.[18]

♦ Implement a process improvement program to demonstrate changes and to identify additional recycling opportunities.

♦ Give feedback to healthcare workers related to the results of the waste management efforts to reinforce this behavior.

Resource Conservation

Health care organizations should conserve finite natural resources such as water, electricity, and natural gas. The average water consumption by US hospitals is 139,214 gallons per day.[19] Health care organizations use 62 billion kilowatt hours of electricity annually, with a higher intensity than other commercial buildings (ie, 26.5 kWh per square foot).[20] The average per square foot consumption of electricity in health care organizations is $1.67, compared to $0.99 per square foot in commercial buildings, and inpatient facilities use more electricity than outpatient facilities.[20] Conserving electricity minimizes air pollution caused by electrical generation and reduces costs.[20]

Heath care organizations also consume large quantities of natural gas (252 billion cubic feet

annually) and have a much higher natural gas intensity than the average commercial building (143.0 cubic feet per square foot).[21] The average per square foot consumption of natural gas is $0.48 per square foot compared, to $0.24 per square foot in commercial buildings.[21]

Perioperative registered nurses should actively promote and participate in resource conservation measures for water, electricity, and natural gas. Conservation strategies should be incorporated into daily practice, including, but not limited to, the following.

♦ Conduct a resource utilization assessment.

♦ Provide education to health care workers about the importance and benefits of resource conservation.[19,22]

♦ Create resource conservation suggestion boxes and place in prominent areas.[23,24]

♦ Install signs encouraging resource conservation.[23,24]

♦ Develop a team of health care workers (eg, "green team") to evaluate resource conservation opportunities and effectiveness.[16,24]

♦ To conserve electricity,
  – install occupancy sensors in certain areas of the practice setting to control lighting based on the presence or absence of personnel and patients;[25]
  – turn off lights when rooms are not in use;[26]
  – turn off equipment when not in use;[24]
  – install and use energy-efficient electrical equipment, lights, and appliances;
  – reduce flow to surgical vacuum pumps to minimum acceptable level and maintain proper operation;[23,27] and
  – insulate hot water pipes.[28]

♦ To conserve natural gas,
  – insulate hot water pipes,[28] and
  – shut off natural gas to equipment and areas that are not in current use.[28]

♦ To conserve water,
  – ensure the return of sterilizer steam condensate to the boiler tank for reuse;[19,27,28,29]
  – eliminate use of city water for cooling sterilizer condensate, possibly by using holding tanks as an alternative;[23,27,30]
  – establish a preventive maintenance program for the evaluation and replacement of faulty steam traps on sterilizers;[19,23,24,28,31]
  – recirculate noncontact sterilizer cooling water;[30]

- install flow control fixtures on all faucets;[27,28,31]
- install scrub sinks with timers and foot or knee controlled turnoff valves;
- install an on-demand water heater near sinks to avoid running water while waiting for hot water;[31]
- turn off water while scrubbing until needed for wetting or rinsing hands;
- evaluate the use of waterless surgical scrub products;
- evaluate the use of microfiber mops for cleaning;[32]
- install high-pressure, low-volume nozzles on scrub sinks and showers;[29]
- recycle and reduce water use whenever possible;[24]
- operate washers, disinfectors, and steam sterilizers only when full, if possible;[19,23,24,27-29]
- avoid flash sterilization of single items or small loads when possible;[31]
- repair leaks in water lines and faucets;[19,23,31] and
- replace older equipment (eg, sterilizers, ice machines, automated endoscope reprocessors, disinfectors) with water-efficient models.[19,22,29,31]

Supply Conservation and Management Practices

Supply management is essential to ensure that the correct products are available when needed.[33] Cost containment measures that minimize waste production provide economic benefits without compromising quality of care. Effective supply chain management will offer opportunities to minimize process inefficiencies and product waste.

Perioperative nurses can significantly affect supply management practices by encouraging and implementing strategies that promote a safe and healthy environment. The strategies should be cost effective and conserve resources. Strategies that should be considered include, but are not limited to, the following.

- Standardize products, devices, and equipment.[34]
- Collaborate with other health care organizations to purchase partial quantities of infrequently used supplies.
- Preference cards and pick-lists should list the minimum number of items to be routinely opened and specify items to be available but unopened.[33,35]

- Open implantable devices only when the desired specifications are known and confirmed by the surgeon.[35]
- Identify processes or practices that increase efficiency or reduce cost, to include
  - monitoring preference card/pick-list supply utilization and remove items not used;
  - reducing excess supply inventory and returning slow-moving inventory;
  - rotating stock with expiration dates to use oldest inventory first;[36] and
  - evaluating excess supplies from customized packs.
- Evaluate implementation of a value analysis and product standardization program for supply purchase and selection.
- Consider natural resource requirements specific to item (eg, clean water availability).[36,37]
- Consider the impact of the item on the waste stream when purchasing supplies and equipment.[3,16]
- Collaborate with vendors to return unopened, expired items or donate items to charities or nonprofit organizations.[38]
- Purchase items made from recycled products.[39]
- Use double-sided photocopies.[39]
- Use reusable totes and pallets instead of cardboard boxes or wooden pallets for transport of goods.[39]

Reprocessing

Reprocessing single-use devices can potentially reduce the amount of waste entering the waste stream.[39,40,41] A recent estimate shows that facilities with 250 beds or more rely on reprocessing to extend their budgets and reduce waste.[40] In 2004, reprocessing was estimated to have reduced the waste generated by health care organizations by more than 449 tons destined for landfills.[40]

If a health care organization chooses to practice reprocessing of single-use devices as a means of decreasing the amount of waste entering the waste stream, the perioperative registered nurse should investigate and evaluate the environmental impact of reprocessing on the organization's waste stream as well as the total environmental impact. Refer to the AORN guidance statement on the reuse of single-use devices for more tools to use for evaluation of reprocessing[42] and adherence to the US Food and Drug Administration regulations controlling reprocessing of single-use devices.

Reuse, Repair, and Refurbishing

Reuse of medical equipment demonstrates the health care organization's commitment to supply conservation and fiscal responsibility through

- conservation of resources and energy,
- optimization of resources, and
- reduction of the pollution that occurs with waste disposal in the environment.[43] (Pollution is reduced because the final disposal of the item is delayed.[38])

Reuse includes the repair, refurbishing, washing, or recovery of worn or used items.[38] Strategies the perioperative nurse should consider when deciding to purchase reusable items or repair and refurbish an item include, but are not limited to, the following.

- Identify factors affecting the longevity of instruments and equipment, such as
  - adequate inventory to reduce frequency of reprocessing and wear;
  - education of health care workers who use and reprocess instruments;
  - education of health care workers who operate and maintain equipment; and
  - adequate storage facilities to protect the instruments and equipment from damage.[44]
- Implement proactive maintenance, repair, or restoration programs for instruments and equipment to prevent malfunction and maintain integrity.
- Consider purchasing reusable medical equipment, instruments, and supplies.
- Educate health care workers regarding their practice accountability for
  - safe care and handling of instruments and equipment,
  - environmental and workplace practices supporting care and handling of instruments and equipment, and
  - repair and refurbishing initiatives of the health care institution.
- Consider projected life span when purchasing instruments and equipment.
- Consider reuse of clean items internally (eg, corrugated boxes, packaging materials, interoffice envelopes, furniture).

Sterilization and Disinfection

Various sterilization and disinfection technologies that affect the environment are used in health care settings. Sterilization technologies in current use include steam, dry heat, ethylene oxide gas, hydrogen peroxide gas plasma, and ozone.[45] High-level disinfectants commonly used include liquid chemicals such as peracetic acid, glutaraldehyde, and orthophthalaldehyde. Steam and dry heat are not known to generate by-products harmful to the environment, but these methods of sterilization do consume natural resources (ie, water, electricity, or natural gas).[20] Ethylene oxide gas sterilization and liquid chemical disinfectants can result in harm to the environment if used irresponsibly or contrary to existing local, state, and federal regulations.[46] Ethylene oxide gas, for example, is an air pollutant, a known carcinogen, a potential reproductive hazard, an allergic sensitizer, and a potent neurotoxin.[47] When choosing a sterilizing or disinfecting method or product, the effect on the environment should be considered.

Perioperative nurses can significantly affect the environment by encouraging and implementing strategies that are cost effective and/or conserve resources. Strategies that should be considered include, but are not limited to, the following.

- Develop a program for monitoring the environmental effects of sterilization and disinfection products on the environment.
- Ensure that the necessary equipment and supplies are available to deal with spillage of sterilizing or disinfecting chemicals.
- Use, maintain, and monitor sterilizers according to the manufacturers' written instructions.[45]
- Establish, ensure, and maintain proper safety measures for handling hazardous materials (eg, monitoring compliance with emission control regulations for ethylene oxide sterilizers, glutaraldehyde disposal).
- Provide education for health care workers regarding the environmental impact of the sterilant or disinfectant being used and appropriate safety measures.
- Use and dispose of liquid chemicals employed in sterilization or disinfection in accordance with manufacturers' written instructions and local, state, and federal governmental agency requirements.
- When possible, purchase items for which the sterilization or disinfection process has the least potential for harm to the environment.[3]
- Additional glutaraldehyde precautions include
  - using fume cabinets,[48]

– considering cold sterilization alternatives to glutaraldehyde,[45] and

– limiting areas in the facility where glutaraldehyde is used and stored.

Construction for Efficiency and Conservation

Building design, construction, and materials significantly affect the natural environment and health outcomes of patients, staff, and community.[49] Although such a discussion is beyond the scope of this document, perioperative registered nurses involved in the planning, design, and construction of health care facilities should incorporate the principles of "green" building design—ie, designs that are energy efficient and water conserving, among other qualities—wherever possible. Nurses interested in green building codes should refer to Healthy Hospitals for the Environment (H2E), located online at *http://www.H2E-online.org;* Health Care Without Harm (HCWH), located online at *http://www.noharm.org;* or the US Green Building Council, located online at *http://www.usgbc.org* (accessed 23 Jan 2006).[50]

Summary

This document has provided strategies for perioperative registered nurses to use in becoming effective stewards of the environment, addressing

♦ infectious and noninfectious waste management;

♦ recycling practices;

♦ resource conservation;

♦ supply conservation and management practices;

♦ reprocessing, reuse, repair, and refurbishing,

♦ sterilization and disinfection, and

♦ construction for efficiency and conservation.

Glossary

Green building codes: Codes used during building design that require the building to be energy efficient and water conserving, have low environmental impact, and have high indoor air quality, among other requirements.[49,50]

Noninfectious waste: Materials with no inherent hazards or infectious potential (eg, packaging materials, paper).[7]

Potentially infectious waste: The definitions of potentially infectious waste vary from state to state, but for the purposes of this document, potentially infectious waste is waste (eg, blood, body fluids, sharps) that is capable of producing infectious diseases.[7]

Reprocessing of single-use devices: Includes all operations necessary to render a contaminated reusable or single-use device patient-ready. Single-use devices to be reprocessed may be either used or unused. Reprocessing steps include disassembling for cleaning, decontamination, inspecting, packaging, relabeling, sterilization, testing, and tracking.[41]

Reuse: The repeated or multiple use of any medical device, whether marketed as reusable or single use. Repeated/multiple use may be on the same patient or on different patients with applicable reprocessing of the device between uses.[41]

Waste: Waste can be classified as potentially infectious and noninfectious materials. In this document, waste refers to the combination of potentially infectious and noninfectious waste.

NOTES

1. "Nurses can make a difference: Environmentally responsive health care," The Nightingale Institute for Health and the Environment, *http://www.nihe.org* (accessed 8 Oct 2005).

2. "Medical waste: The issue," Health Care Without Harm, *http://www.noharm.org/us/medicalWaste/issue* (accessed 8 Oct 2005).

3. A Melamed, "Environmental accountability in perioperative settings," *AORN Journal* 77 (June 2003) 1157-1168.

4. B Scrantom, "Health care: New paths to energy savings," *Building Operating Management* (January 2003), *http://www.facilitiesnet.com/bom/article.asp?id=1522* (accessed 8 Oct 2005).

5. B Sattler, "Pioneering the environmental health frontier," Maryland Nurses Association Newsletter, *http://www.oarm.org/details.cfm?type=news&ID=91* (accessed 14 May 2005).

6. B K Lee, M J Ellenbecker, R Moure-Ersaso, "Alternatives for treatment and disposal cost reduction of regulated medical wastes," *Waste Management* 24 no 2 (2004) 143-151.

7. R Garcia, "Effective cost-reduction strategies in the management of regulated medical waste," *American Journal of Infection Control* 27 (April 1999) 165-175.

8. B Sattler, "The greening of health care: Environmental policy and advocacy in the health care industry," *Policy, Politics & Nursing Practice* 4 (Feb 2003) 6-13.

9. J Andrews, "New diet of products can help hospitals watch their 'waste' lines" *Healthcare Purchasing News* (June 2003) 14-19.

10. C Schierhorn, "Haste makes (infectious) waste: Saving money by segregating hospital refuse," *Health Facilities Management* 15 (Sept 2002) 34-37.

11. M Cox, C Rhett, A Gudmundsen, "Environmental protection through waste management: Implications for staff development," *Journal of Nursing Staff Development* 13 (March–April 1997) 67-72.

12. B Jolibois, M Guerbet, S Vassal, "Glutaraldehyde in hospital wastewater," *Archives of Environmental Contamination and Toxicology* 42 (February 2002) 137-144.

13. F D Daschner, M Dettenkofer, "Protecting the patient and the environment—New aspects and challenges in hospital infection control," *Journal of Hospital Infection* 36 (May 1997) 7-15.

14. Walsh Integrated Environmental Systems, "Environmental impact," *http://www.walsh environmental .com/products/ben_environmentalimpact.htm* (accessed 9 Oct 2005).

15. "Recycling fact sheet," Health Care Without Harm, *http://www.noharm.org/details.cfm?type=document &id=599* (accessed 9 Oct 2005).

16. "Waste minimization, segregation, and recycling in hospitals," Health Care Without Harm, *http://www .noharm.org/library/docs/Going_Green_4-1_Waste _Minimization _Segregation.pdf* (accessed 9 Oct 2005).

17. "Reduce, reuse, and recycle," US Environmental Protection Agency, *http://www.epa.gov/epaoswer/non-hw /muncpl/reduce.htm* (accessed 9 Oct 2005).

18. "Hospitals and health care institutions," Recycling Works Tipsheet, Pennsylvania Department of Environmental Protection, *http://www.dep.state.pa.us/dep/deputate /airwaste/wm/recycle/tips/hospitals.htm* (accessed 9 Oct 2005).

19. "Water conservation at work,"Southwest Florida Water Management District, *http://www.swfwmd.state.fl.us /conservation/waterwork/checkhospital.htm* (accessed 9 Oct 2005).

20. "A look at health care buildings—How do they use electricity?" Energy Information Administration, *http://www.eia.doe.gov/emeu/consumptionbriefs/cbecs /pbawebsite/health/health_howuseelec.htm* (accessed 9 Oct 2005).

21. "A look at health care buildings—How do they use natural gas?" Energy Information Administration, *http://www.eia.doe.gov/emeu/consumptionbriefs/cbecs /pbawebsite/health/health_howuseng.htm* (accessed 9 Oct 2005).

22. "Green tips," Ontario Ministry of the Environment, *http://www.ene.gov.on.ca/cons/3781-e.htm* (accessed 9 Oct 2005).

23. "Water conservation checklist: Hospitals/medical facilities—Every drop counts!" North Carolina Department of Environment and Natural Resources, Division of Pollution and Environmental Assistance, *http://64.233.161.104/ search?q=cache:7jnhCXPu4ulJ:www.p2pays.org/ref/23 /22006.pdf+water+use* (accessed 9 Oct 2005).

24. "Water conservation @ hospitals," City of Greeley Water Conservation, *http://www.ci.greeley.co.us/cog /PageX.asp?fkOrgId=44&PageURL=Hospitals* (accessed 9 Oct 2005).

25. US Environmental Protection Agency, *Light Brief* (Washington, DC: US Environmental Protection Agency, June 1992) 7000.

26. R Reeves, "Energy conservation important to MHCP," *Entre Nous* (Winter 2004) 8.

27. "Water efficiency and management for hospitals," North Carolina Department of Environment and Natural Resources, Division of Pollution and Environmental Assistance, *http://www.p2pays.org/ref/14/13679.htm* (accessed 9 Oct 2005).

28. "Water conservation ideas for health care facilities," Pennsylvania Department of Environmental Protection, *http://www.dep.state.pa.us/dep/subject/hotopics/drought /facts/health.htm* (accessed 9 Oct 2005).

29. "Water efficiency practices for health care facilities," New Hampshire Department of Environmental Services, *http://www.des.state.nh.us/factsheets/ws/ws-26-14 .htm* (accessed 9 Oct 2005).

30. "Hospital cost reduction case study: Norwood Hospital," Massachusetts Water Resources Authority, *http://www.mwra.state.ma.us/04water/html/bullet1.htm* (accessed 23 Jan 2006).

31. "Water efficiency in hospitals (small to medium), extended care homes, and laundries," Association of Manitoba Municipalities, *http://www.amm.mb.ca/images /resources/waterefficiency/extcare.pdf* (accessed 26 June 2005).

32. "Using microfiber mops in hospitals," US Environmental Protection Agency, *http://www.epa.gov/region09 /cross_pr/p2/projects/hospital/mops.pdf* (accessed 9 Oct 2005).

33. P Camp, "Controlling costs while maintaining quality care," *Surgical Services Management* 8 (Dec 2002) 24-30.

34. D Karr, "Standardization and cost savings," *Surgical Services Management* 5 (April 1999) 32-38.

35. N Phillips, ed, "Coordinated roles of scrub person and circulator," in *Berry & Kohn's Operating Room Technique,* tenth ed (St Louis: Mosby, 2004).

36. Baker, D; Hale, D. "Potential cost savings opportunities: The supply chain," *SSM* 9 (April 2003) 33-38.

37. "Value analysis helps to tighten surgical products supply chain," *OR Manager* 18 (May 2002) 1, 14-16.

38. *Pollution Prevention Guide for Hospitals,* US Environmental Protection Agency, *http://www.dtsc.ca.gov/Pollution Prevention/p2-hospital-guide.pdf* (accessed 9 Oct 2005).

39. "Green purchasing," Health Care Without Harm, *http://www.noharm.org/greenPurchasing/issue* (accessed 9 Oct 2005).

40. J E Williamson, "Great expectations: Hospitals find FDA regs build stronger case for reprocessing," *Healthcare Purchasing News* (June 2005) 28-32.

41. D Dunn, "Reprocessing single-use devices: The equipment connection," *AORN Journal* 75 (June 2002) 1143.

42. "AORN guidance statement: Reuse of single-use devices," in *Standards, Recommended Practices, and Guidelines* (Denver: AORN, Inc, 2005) 185-191.

43. M Szczepanski, "The nursing process: A tool for healing the environment," *Nursing Management* 24 (Oct 1993) 56-58.

44. "Recommended practices for cleaning and caring for surgical instruments and powered equipment," in *Standards, Recommended Practices, and Guidelines* (Denver: AORN, Inc, 2005) 395-403.

45. "Recommended practices for sterilization in perioperative practice settings," in *Standards, Recommended Practices and Guidelines* (Denver: AORN, Inc, 2005) 459-469.

46. "Ethylene oxide: Hazard summary," US Environmental Protection Agency, *http://www.epa.gov/ttnatw01/hlthef/ethylene.html* (accessed 9 Oct 2005).

47. A D LaMontagne, K T Kelsey, "Evaluating OSHA's ethylene oxide standard: Exposure determinants in Massachusetts hospitals," *American Journal of Public Health* 91 (March 2001) 412-417.

48. M Jim, "Instrument reprocessing in theatres: Drivers for change," *British Journal of Perioperative Nursing* 12 (January 2002) 34-38.

49. G Vittori, *Green and Healthy Buildings for the Health Care Industry* (Austin, Tex: Center for Maximum Potential Building Systems, 2002).

50. "Is green building budding?" in *The Washington Post* (April 16, 2005), USGBC in the News, *http://www.usgbc.org/News/usgbcinthenews_details.asp?ID=1485& CMSPageID=159* (accessed 9 Oct 2005).

RESOURCES

Almuneef, M; Memish, Z A. "Effective medical waste management: It can be done," *American Journal of Infection Control* 31 (May 2003) 188-192

Alt, S. "Think of environment when choosing supplies," *Hospital Materials Management* 26 (Sept 2001) 11.

Association for the Advancement of Medical Instrumentation (AAMI). *AAMI Standards and Recommended Practices: Sterilization, Part 3—Industrial Process Control* (Arlington, Va: AAMI, 1999).

Bultitude, M F, et al. "Prolonging the life of the flexible ureterorenoscope," *International Journal of Clinical Practice* 58 (August 2004) 756-757.

Burdick, J S; Hambrick, D. "Endoscope reprocessing and repair costs," *Gastrointestinal Endoscopy Clinics of North America* 14 (October 2004) 717-724.

"CDC issues new environmental guidelines," *OR Manager* 19 (August 2003) 20, 22.

Cohoon, B D. "Reprocessing single-use medical devices," *AORN Journal* 75 (March 2002) 557-567.

Cys, J. "Speaking of reuse," *Materials Management in Health Care* 12 (June 2003) 26-28.

"FDA wants to know more about reuse of opened-but-unused items," *OR Manager* 18 (September 2002) 1, 7.

"Good manufacturing practices (GMP)/Quality system (QS) regulation," US Food and Drug Administration, *http://www.fda.gov/cdrh/devadvice/32.html* (accessed 9 Oct 2005).

Hensley, S. "More hospitals buy into device recycling," *Modern Healthcare* 29 (February 1999) 88.

"Integrating green purchasing into your environmental management system (EMS), US Environmental Protection Agency, *http://www.epa.gov/epp/ems.htm* (accessed 9 Oct 2005).

International Association of Health Care Central Service Material Management. "IAHCSMM position statement on the reuse of single-use medical devices," presented at the AAMI/FDA Conference on Reuse of Single-Use Devices: Practice, Patient Safety, and Regulation, Washington, DC, May 5, 1999.

Kleinbeck, S V M; English, N L; Hueschen, J H. "Reprocessing and reusing surgical products labeled for single use," *Surgical Services Management* 4 (January 1998) 21-24.

Lewis, C. "Reusing medical devices: Ensuring safety the second time around," *FDA Consumer* 34 (September/October 2000) 8-9.

"New FDA regulations may force hospitals to abandon reprocessing," *Infection Control and Prevention Report* 5 (Sept 2000) 133-136.

Pope, A M; Snyder, M A; Mood, L H. *Nursing, Health, and the Environment: Strengthening the Relationship to Improve the Public's Health* (Washington, DC: National Academy Press, 1995).

"Reuse of single-use devices," (Clinical Issues) *AORN Journal* 73 (May 2001) 957-964.

Schultz, J. *Clinical Study Guide: Minimizing Potential for Endoscope Contamination* (Denver: Healthstream, 2005).

Schultz, J. "Reusing single-use medical devices," *Surgical Services Management* 4 (July 1998) 11-13.

Schroer, P. "Reuse of single-use devices," *Medical Device Technology* 11 (December 2000) 44, 48-53.

Selvey, D. "Medical device reprocessing: Is it good for your organization?" *Infection Control Today*, *http://www.infectioncontroltoday.com/articles/111feat1.html?wts=20051009035349&hc=44&req=Selvey%2c+and+Don* (accessed 9 Oct 2005).

Spry, C; Leiner, D C. "Rigid endoscopes—Ensuring quality before use and after repair," *AORN Journal* 80 (July 2004) 103-109.

"Survey: One-fourth of operating rooms resterilize opened-but-unused medical devices," *OR Manager* 19 (November 2002).

"Survey: ORs are split on reuse of single-use items," *OR Manager* 15 (September 1999) 1, 11, 14-16.

Thomas, L A. "Endoscope precleaning," *Gastroenterology Nursing* 28 (July/Aug 2005) 334-335.

Thomas, L A. "Endoscope staging," *Gastroenterology Nursing* 28 (May/June 2005) 243-245.

Thomas, L A. "Transporting the endoscope," *Gastroenterology Nursing* 29 (March/April 2005) 145-146.

US Food and Drug Administration. "Medical devices; current good manufacturing practice (CGMP) final rule; quality system regulation," *Federal Register* 61 (Oct 7, 1996). Also available at *http://www.fda.gov/OHRMS/DOCKETS/98fr/61FR52654100796.htm* (accessed 9 Oct 2005).

Whelan, C. "Stats: Reprocessing growth," *Materials Management in Health Care* 13 (May 2004) 41-42.

Zafar, A B; Butler, R C. "Effect of a comprehensive program to reduce infectious waste," *American Journal of Infectious Waste* 28 (February 2000) 51-53.

Approved by the AORN Board of Directors, November 2005. Scheduled for publication in the *AORN Journal* in 2006.

AORN Guidance Statement: Fire Prevention in the Operating Room

Introduction

AORN recognizes that fire is an inherent risk in ORs. Fire is an ever-present danger and poses a real hazard to patient and health care worker safety. In 2003, the Joint Commission on Accreditation of Healthcare Organizations (JCAHO) issued a sentinel event alert related to fires that occur during operative and invasive procedures. The bulletin raised the level of awareness about the dangers of surgical fires. The Joint Commission recommends that health care organizations prevent surgical fires by providing education and training for perioperative practitioners.[1] In July 2004, surgical fire prevention was added to the 2005 National Patient Safety Goals for ambulatory and office-based surgical facilities.[2]

The approach to developing policies and procedures to reduce fire risk should be multidisciplinary and involve all professionals who provide patient care. Facilities are encouraged to report surgical fires to JCAHO, ECRI, or the US Food and Drug Administration (FDA). Systematic reporting of fires can help educate care providers about how and why fires occur and can help prevent fires in the future.[1]

Background

Fires involving surgical patients have been reported by hospitals and ambulatory surgical centers; some medical device manufacturers, and other experts, such as ECRI, for many years. There is no centralized database being collected by any agency at present on the total number of surgical fires;[3] however, data from ECRI and the FDA estimate that approximately 100 surgical fires occur each year, resulting in approximately 20 patient injuries that are serious, with one to two deaths per year.[1,4] The overriding consideration with surgical fires is that they are 100% preventable.[1,4]

Fires occur when the elements that support combustion—an ignition source, a fuel source, and an oxidizer—come together. These three elements are referred to as the "fire triangle." All three elements are present in abundance during operative and invasive procedures[4] (Tables 1-3). Operating rooms in hospitals and ambulatory surgery suites, physicians' offices, and endoscopy suites are some of the critical areas where fires occur, and they contain all the elements that support combustion.

Ignition sources are anything that produces heat; the two most common sources are the electrosurgical unit (ESU) and the laser. Other equipment that produces heat includes, but may not be limited to, fiber-optic light cables and light source boxes; drills, saws, and burrs; hand-held electrocautery devices; argon beam coagulators; and defibrillators.[4]

Almost everything in the perioperative arena can be a fuel source, especially when an accelerant, such as oxygen, is present. The items used to set up the sterile field and protect the patient (eg, linens, drapes, gowns, supplies, preps, gauzes, clothes) should all be considered fuel sources. The patient's body hair and body gases also can be fuel sources.[5]

The primary oxidizers in the surgical environment are oxygen and nitrous oxide. Fires can occur when the oxygen level in the atmosphere rises above the level of ambient air (ie, 21%). Oxygen can escape into the air when patients are given mask or nasal oxygen. A level above 21% should be treated as an oxygen-enriched environment.[6]

Guideline

Education

Education and training in fire risk reduction strategies for perioperative RNs, surgical technologists, anesthesia care providers, surgeons, and other personnel is essential to promote and maintain a fire-safe perioperative environment. Health care industry representatives and students should be included in fire drill education. Each perioperative team member is responsible for promoting a culture of fire safety. Preparation is the key to ensuring readiness for preventing fires in the OR. Recommendations from ECRI include that

- perioperative team members participate in fire drills;
- team members receive training on the use of fire fighting equipment, rescue methods, and evacuation;
- staff members know where medical gas panels and ventilation and electrical systems are located, which personnel are permitted to shut them off, and when;
- staff members in the perioperative care setting be shown how to initiate a "Code Red" or fire alarm at their facility;
- staff members know specific protocols to contact the local fire department;[4]
- students rotating through the perioperative area are included in fire education and training; and
- health care industry representatives are educated on fire safety hazards in the perioperative area during their credentialing process.

Table 1

FIRE RISK—IGNITION	
Ignition sources	**Strategies to manage**
Electrosurgical unit (ESU)	■ Use the lowest possible power setting.
	■ Place the patient return electrode on a large muscle mass close to the surgical site.
	■ Large reusable return electrodes should be used according to the manufacturer's instructions.
	■ Always use a safety holster.
	■ Do not coil active electrode cords.
	■ Inspect the active electrode to ensure integrity.
	■ Do not use ESU in the presence of flammable solutions.
	■ Ensure that cords and plugs are not frayed or broken.
	■ Do not place fluids on top of the ESU.
	■ Do not use the ESU near oxygen or nitrous oxide.
	■ Ensure that the ESU active electrode tip fits securely into the active electrode hand piece.
	■ Ensure that any connectors and adaptors used are intended to connect to the ESU and fit securely.
	■ Do not bypass ESU safety features.
	■ Ensure that the alarm tone is always audible.
	■ Remove any contaminated or unused active accessories from the sterile field.
	■ Keep the active electrode tip clean.
	■ Use wet sponges or towels to help retard fire potential.
	■ Never alter a medical device.[1]
	■ Do not use rubber catheters or protective covers as insulators on the active electrode tip.[2]
	■ Use cut or blend instead of coagulation when possible.
	■ Do not open the circuit to activate the ESU.
	■ Ensure that the active electrode is not activated in close proximity to another metal object that could conduct heat or cause arcing.[3]
	■ After prepping, allow prep to dry and fumes to evaporate. Wet prep and fumes trapped beneath drapes can ignite.[4]
	■ Provide multidisciplinary inservice programs on the safe use of ESUs based on the manufacturer's instructions.
Argon beam coagulator	■ Argon beam coagulators combine the ESU spark with argon gas to concentrate and focus the ESU spark. Argon gas is inert and nonflammable, but because it is used with an ESU, the same precautions as with an ESU should be taken.
	■ Always use a safety holster.
	■ Ensure that the active electrode is not activated in close proximity to another metal object that could conduct heat or cause arcing.[1]
Lasers	■ Use a laser-specific endotracheal tube (ie, a tube that has laser-resistant coating or contains no material that will ignite) if head, neck, lung, or airway surgery is anticipated.[5]
	■ Wet sponges around the tube cuffs may provide extra protection to help retard fire potential. Moist towels around the surgical site also may retard fires.
	■ Do not use liquids or ointments that may be combustible.
	■ Inflate cuffed tube bladders with tinted saline (eg, methylene blue) so that inadvertent rupture may be detected during chest or upper airway surgery.
	■ Do not use uncuffed, standard endotracheal tubes in the presence of a laser or the ESU.
	■ If an endotracheal tube fire occurs, oxygen administration should be stopped, and all burning or melted tubes should be removed from the patient immediately.
	■ Prevent pooling of skin prep solutions.

Table 1, continued

FIRE RISK—IGNITION	
Ignition sources	**Strategies to manage** (continued)
	▪ Drapes that will resist ignition should be used close to the area being lased.
	▪ Have water and the correct fire extinguisher type available in case of a laser fire.[6]
Fiber optic light sources	▪ Ensure that the light source is in good working order.
Fiber optic light cables	▪ Place the light source in standby, or turn it off when the cable is not connected.
	▪ Place the light source away from items that are flammable.
	▪ Do not place a light cable that is connected to a light source on drapes, sponges, or anything else that is flammable.
	▪ Do not allow cables that are connected to hang over the side of the sterile field if the light source is on.
	▪ Ensure that light cables are in good working order and do not have broken light fibers.[7]
Power tools/drills/burrs	▪ Instruments/equipment that move rapidly during use generate heat. Always ensure that they are in good working order.
	▪ A slow drip of saline on a moving drill/burr helps to reduce heat buildup.
	▪ Do not place drills, burrs, or saws on the patient when they are not in use.
	▪ Remove instruments/equipment from the sterile field when not in use.[8]
Defibrillator paddles	▪ Select paddles that are the correct size for the patient (eg, pediatric paddles on a child).
	▪ Ensure that the gel recommended by the paddle manufacturer is used.
	▪ Adhere to appropriate site selection for paddle placement.
	▪ Contact between the paddles and the patient should be optimal and no gaps should be present before activating the defibrillator.[9]
Electrical equipment	▪ Ensure that all equipment is periodically inspected by biomedical personnel for proper function.
	▪ Check biomedical inspection stickers on the equipment; they should be current.
	▪ Do not use equipment with frayed or damaged cords or plugs.
	▪ Remove any equipment that emits smoke during use.[10]

NOTES

1. "Recommended practices for electrosurgery," in Standards, Recommended Practices, and Guidelines (Denver: AORN, Inc, 2004) 245-259.

2. "A clinician's guide to surgical fires: How they occur, how to prevent them, how to put them out," Health Devices 32 (January 2003) 1-24.

3. Fire Safety Self Study Guide (Denver: HealthStream, 2004).

4. "Recommended practices for skin preparation of patients," in Standards, Recommended Practices, and Guidelines (Denver: AORN, Inc, 2004) 357-360.

5. K A Ball, Lasers: The Perioperative Challenge (Denver: AORN, Inc, 2004) 145.

6. "Recommended practices for laser safety in practice settings," in Standards, Recommended Practices, and Guidelines (Denver: AORN, Inc, 2004) 319-324.

7. "Recommended practices for endoscopic minimally invasive surgery," in Standards, Recommended Practices, and Guidelines (Denver: AORN, Inc, 2004) 267-271.

8. ECRI, "The patient is on fire! A surgical fire primer," Medical Device Safety Reports 21 (January 1992) 19-34. Also available at http://www.mdsr.ecri.org/summary/detail.aspx?doc_id=8197&q=%22The+patient+is+on+fire%22 (accessed 12 Jan 2005).

9. ECRI, "Fires from defibrillation during oxygen administration," Health Devices 23 (July 1994) 307-308. Also available at http://www.mdsr.ecri.org/summary/detail.aspx?doc_id=8128&q=%22Fires+from+Defibrillation%22 (accessed 12 Jan 2005).

10. "Recommended practices for safe care through identification of potential hazards in the surgical environment," in Standards, Recommended Practices, and Guidelines (Denver: AORN, Inc, 2004) 301-307.

Table 2

FIRE RISK—FUEL	
Fuel sources	**Strategies to manage**

Patient and staff linens
   Drapes
   Gowns
   Towels
   Lap pads
   Sponges
   Dressings
   Tapes
   Bed linens
   Caps/hats
   Shoe covers
	▦ Assess the flammability of all materials used in, on, or around the patient. Linens and drapes are made of synthetic or natural fibers. They may burn or melt depending on the fiber content.[1]
	▦ Do not allow drapes or linens to come in contact with activated ignition sources (eg, laser, electrosurgical unit [ESU], light sources).[2-4]
	▦ Do not trap volatile chemicals or chemical fumes beneath drapes.[5]
	▦ Moisten drapes, towels, and sponges that will be in close proximity to ignition sources (eg, laser, ESU).[2,3]
	▦ Ensure that oxygen does not accumulate beneath drapes.
	▦ If drapes or linens ignite, pat out small fires with a wet sponge or towel. Remove burning material from the patient.
	▦ Extinguish any burning material with the appropriate fire extinguisher or water, if appropriate.[6]

Prep solutions	▦ Use flammable prep solutions with caution. ▦ Do not allow prep solutions to pool on, around, or beneath the patient. ▦ After prepping, allow prep to dry and fumes to evaporate. Wet prep and fumes trapped beneath drapes can ignite. ▦ Do not activate ignition sources in the presence of flammable prep solutions. ▦ Do not allow drapes that will remain in contact with the patient to absorb flammable prep solutions.[5]
Skin degreasers, tinctures, aerosols	▦ These products may be used before skin prep to degrease or clean the skin or as part of the dressing. These products may contain chemicals that are flammable (eg, ether in collodian). Allow all fumes to evaporate before surgery. The laser or ESU should not be used after the dressing is in place.[3]
Body tissue and patient hair	▦ The patient's own body can be a fuel source. Coat any body hair that is in close proximity to an ignition source with a water-based jelly to retard ignition.[4] ▦ Ensure that surgical smoke from burning patient tissue is properly evacuated. Surgical smoke can support combustion if allowed to accumulate in a small or enclosed space (eg, the back of the throat).[3]
Intestinal gases	▦ Patient intestinal gases are flammable. Electrosurgery or laser should be used with caution whenever intestinal gases are present. Do not open the bowel with the laser or ESU when it appears gas is present. ▦ Use suction during rectal surgery to remove any intestinal gases that may be present.[3]

NOTES

1. "Recommended practices for product selection in perioperative practice settings," in Standards, Recommended Practices, and Guidelines (Denver: AORN, Inc, 2004) 347-350.

2. "Recommended practices for laser safety in practice settings," in Standards, Recommended Practices, and Guidelines (Denver: AORN, Inc, 2004) 319-324.

3. "Recommended practices for electrosurgery," in Standards, Recommended Practices, and Guidelines (Denver: AORN, Inc, 2004) 245-259.

4. "Recommended practices for endoscopic minimally invasive surgery," in Standards, Recommended Practices, and Guidelines (Denver: AORN, Inc, 2004) 267-271.

5. "Recommended practices for skin preparation of patients," in Standards, Recommended Practices, and Guidelines (Denver: AORN, Inc, 2004) 357-360.

6. "A clinician's guide to surgical fires: How they occur, how to prevent them, how to put them out," Health Devices 32 (January 2003) 1-24.

Table 3

FIRE RISK—OXIDIZERS	
Oxidizers	Strategies to manage
Oxygen (O₂)	■ Oxygen should be used with caution in the presence of ignition sources. Oxygen is an oxidizer and is capable of supporting combustion.[1] ■ Ensure that anesthesia circuits are free of leaks. ■ Pack wet sponges around the back of the throat to help retard oxygen leaks. ■ Inflate cuffed tube bladders with tinted saline (eg, methylene blue) so that inadvertent ruptures can be detected. ■ Use suction to help evacuate any accumulation of O₂ in body cavities, such as the mouth or chest cavity. ■ Do not use the laser or electrosurgical unit (ESU) near where O₂ is flowing. ■ Use a pulse oximeter to determine the patient's oxygenation level and the need for oxygen. ■ Allow O₂ fumes to evaporate before using the laser or ESU. ■ When using mask or nasal O₂, ensure that fumes do not accumulate under the drapes. ■ Ensure that drapes are tented to help prevent oxygen accumulation when mask or nasal O₂ is used.[2-4]
Nitrous oxide	■ The strategies to manage O₂ also should be used to manage risks associated with nitrous oxide.[2-4]
Sevoflurane	■ Temperatures greater than 200° F (99.33° C) may result from the degeneration of sevoflurane by desiccated absorbents (eg, soda lime). This can result in a fire in the anesthetic circuit. Scheduled replacement of the absorbent or pouring water into the absorbent may prevent temperature buildup. Oxygen left running at the end of the procedure dries out the absorbent. Remind the anesthesia care provider to turn off the O₂ at the end of each procedure.[5]

NOTES

1. "A clinician's guide to surgical fires: How they occur, how to prevent them, how to put them out," Health Devices 32 (January 2003) 1-24.

2. "Recommended practices for electrosurgery," in Standards, Recommended Practices, and Guidelines (Denver: AORN, Inc, 2004) 245-259.

3. "Recommended practices for laser safety in practice settings," in Standards, Recommended Practices, and Guidelines (Denver: AORN, Inc, 2004) 319-324.

4. "Recommended practices for endoscopic minimally invasive surgery," in Standards, Recommended Practices, and Guidelines (Denver: AORN, Inc, 2004) 267-271.

5. M Laster, P Roth, E I Eger, "Fires from the interaction of anesthetics with desiccated absorbent," (Technology, Computing, and Simulation) Anesthesia and Analgesia 99 (September 2004) 769-774.

A health care facility's fire plan should be reviewed and actively discussed, and the use of fire extinguishers should be demonstrated when staff members are hired and at least annually. Perioperative clinical leaders must take additional action to keep patients and staff members safe. Fire drills should be conducted regularly based on local, state, and JCAHO guidelines. Fire drills should include the following.

♦ Use of the acronym **RACE** as the response component of the fire safety plan:
  - **R**—Rescue the individual that is involved in the fire.
  - **A**—Alarm should be sounded as soon as possible.
  - **C**—Confine the fire.
  - **E**—Extinguish the fire and evacuate if required.[5]

Fire Prevention

- Use of National Fire Protection Association (NFPA) standards for classification of the different types of fire extinguishers, including
  - Class A: for use on wood, paper, cloth, and most plastics (eg, combustible materials);
  - Class B: for use on flammable liquids or grease; and
  - Class C: for use on energized electrical equipment.[4]
- The acronym **PASS** should be reviewed to operate the fire extinguisher.
  - **P**—Pull the pin.
  - **A**—Aim nozzle at the base of the fire.
  - **S**—Squeeze the handle.
  - **S**—Sweep the stream over the base of the fire.[7]

To enhance user skill and confidence, allow every staff member time to practice handling the fire extinguisher. Teach staff members to use the fire extinguisher with their back toward an escape exit for easier access. Labels on the fire extinguisher should be checked for color, size, and shape of the extinguisher to prevent personnel assisting in extinguishing fires from using the wrong extinguisher (eg, water on an electrical fire). The following information will help staff members become more competent.

- Staff members should be shown where fire extinguishers are located in the perioperative setting.
- Operating room doors should be able to open completely without equipment blocking them.
- Staff members should know the location of all fire exits and ensure that these exits are clear and accessible at all times.
- Surgical team members should know where the medical gas shutoff valves are and their facility's policy on who should turn them off and when.
- Review roles of every staff member at the point of the fire's origin and away from the immediate area.
- Take staff members through evacuation routes, both primary and secondary, to an evacuation location point beyond a firewall.[4]

Depending on the size of the perioperative setting, planning for an initial fire drill may take up to three months.[5] Key points in planning a fire drill include

- choosing a date and time;
- developing a well-thought-out scenario(s);
- obtaining the facility fire drill evaluation form, and modifying it where necessary;
- completing a fire drill record, and noting all participants and pertinent details;
- identifying observers and their locations;
- designating surgical team members who will participate in the event and briefing them on the scenario;
- reviewing fire safety/drill policy and procedures and their roles with staff members;
- notifying facility administrators of the upcoming fire drill and posting signs;
- including the facility safety officer as a resource and advisor;
- discussing the drill in a debriefing session;
- evaluating the effectiveness of the staff members and equipment used; and
- identifying areas for improvement and areas of strength.[8]

Every fire drill should be considered a forum for learning. Perioperative staff member preparedness will ensure an effective and efficient response to a fire in a smooth and coordinated manner (Sample Forms 1 and 2).

Evacuation plan

All perioperative departments should develop and implement a well-rehearsed and well-thought-out fire evacuation plan. Evacuation plans help ensure that all staff members are familiar with the proper evacuation routes and equipment that may be used before or during an evacuation. In the event a fire occurs in the perioperative area, personnel should follow the standard fire emergency response procedure and activate RACE.

Surgical team duties in a fire evacuation. Each surgical suite should have designated fire responder teams with defined responsibilities to take if a fire occurs in the surgical suite. There should be a chain of command that includes an authority who has jurisdiction to manage the incident. If the OR must be evacuated, several steps should be taken by personnel responsible for the care of the patient in the OR. First, surgical team members should become oriented in relation to where they are located, the proximity of the nearest exit, and how to safely evacuate to that destination. The roles of the surgical team may be as follows.

Sample Form 1

PERIOPERATIVE SERVICES OR CODE RED FIRE DRILL EVALUATION FORM			

Fire drill date: _____   Designated observer: _____

Criteria:	Yes	No	Comments
▪ Evacuation plan is posted.			
▪ Randomly chosen staff member(s)			
¡ describes evacuation routes,			
¡ knows how to report a fire, and			
¡ knows location of extinguisher.			
▪ Fire extinguishers			
¡ in place, seal intact, charged, properly mounted;			
¡ labeled as to type and class of fire;			
¡ serviced within past 12 months;			
¡ checked monthly; and			
¡ staff member describes how to operate fire extinguisher by using PASS method.			
▪ Fire exits			
¡ free and unobstructed, and			
¡ marked with working illuminated signs.			
▪ Corridors of egress are free of equipment/obstructions.			
▪ Fire/smoke barrier doors closed during activation of pull station.			
▪ Staff members activated RACE, the standard fire emergency response procedure.			
▪ Staff members use proper body mechanics to transport patients.			
▪ Staff members close all doors.			
▪ Nursing leader/designee shuts off medical gases.			
▪ All patients are accounted for with medical records intact.			
Response evaluated:			
▪ Did staff members act in a calm and organized manner?			
▪ Did staff members perform as a cohesive team?			

Opportunities for improvement:

_____
_____
_____

Staff member (observer) signature: _____

- ◆ The perioperative registered nurse in charge/designee should
  - notify the safety officer, telephone operator, or designated person of a fire and its location;
  - document the time the fire started;
  - establish how many people are in the department;
  - set up a communication point and identify a person to staff it;
  - determine the state of ongoing surgery/procedures in each area;
  - consult with the anesthesia care provider in charge on how to handle each patient;
  - assign personnel to assist where needed;
  - ask visitors to leave if necessary; and
  - evacuate patients who may need to be moved immediately.
- ◆ The perioperative RN circulating should
  - ensure the patient's safety by remaining with him or her and comforting him or her;
  - activate the fire alarm system and call the fire code to alert all necessary personnel;
  - extinguish small fires or douse them with liquid if appropriate;
  - remove any burning material from the patient or sterile field, and extinguish it on the floor;

Sample Form 2

PERIOPERATIVE SERVICES OR CODE RED FIRE DRILL RECORD

Fire drill date: _____   Shift: _____

Fire drill start time: _____   Finish time: _____

Designated observers:
_____
_____
_____

List fire drill participants and titles:

Participant	*Title*

Planned scenario: _____
_____
_____
_____

Time and individual who pulled fire alarm: _____

Patient evacuation times: _____

Other remarkable events: _____
_____
_____
_____

Individual completing form: _____

- prevent fire from spreading to shoes or surgical clothing by not stepping on it;
- provide the scrub person and anesthesia care provider with needed supplies;
- collaborate with the anesthesia care provider on the need to turn off the medical gas shutoff valves;
- carefully unplug all equipment if the fire is electrical;
- be aware of the safest route for escape;
- obtain a transport stretcher if necessary;
- remove IV solutions from poles and place them with the patient for transporting out of the OR;
- help the anesthesia care provider disconnect any leads, lines, or other equipment that may be needed for transporting the patient; and
- not delay leaving the OR suite.
♦ The scrub person should
  - remove from the patient materials that may be on fire and help put out the fire,
  - obtain sterile towels or covers for the surgical site and instruments,
  - gather a minimal number of instruments onto a tray or basin and place them with the patient for transport, and
  - assist with patient transfer from the OR table to a stretcher/bed for transport out of the OR.

♦ The surgeon should
  - remove from the patient materials that may be on fire and help put out the fire;
  - control bleeding and prepare the patient for evacuation;
  - place sterile towels or covers over the surgical site;
  - conclude the procedure as soon as possible, if the patient is not in immediate danger; and
  - help move the patient if necessary.
♦ The anesthesia care provider should
  - shut off the flow of oxygen/nitrous oxide to the patient or field and maintain breathing for the patient with a valve mask respirator (ie, ambu bag);
  - collaborate with the circulating nurse on the need to turn off the medical gas shutoff valves;
  - disconnect all electrically powered equipment on the anesthesia machine;
  - disconnect any leads, lines, or other equipment that may be anchoring the patient to the area;
  - maintain the patient's anesthetic state and collect the necessary medications to continue anesthesia during transport; and
  - place additional IV fluids on the bed for transport with the patient, if time permits.
♦ Ancillary personnel should
  - help clear corridors for evacuation,
  - secure equipment for transporting the patient as directed by the circulating nurse,
  - follow instructions for evacuating the patient if needed, and
  - assist where directed.

Patients should be evacuated horizontally to a safe area on the same floor. It is very important to maintain an accurate count of all patients and staff members during the evacuation. After evacuation of the room, the last person to leave the room should close the doors and place a wet towel at the base of them. After the fire, everything should be left in place so the safety officer and the fire department can conduct a thorough investigation of the cause of the fire.[9]

Risk reduction strategies

Risk reduction strategies involve educating surgical team members about the components of the fire triangle and developing policies and procedures that will prevent surgical fires. Fuel sources must be managed in a way that will prevent fires, ignition sources must be controlled so that they do not come in contact with fuels, and oxidizers must be contained or properly vented so that they do not come in contact with fuels or ignition sources. Keeping the sides of the fire triangle apart is critical.

Notes
1. "Preventing surgical fires," *Sentinel Event Alert* 29 (June 24, 2003). Also available at *http://www.jcaho .org/about+us/news+letters/sentinel+event+alert/print /sea_29.htm* (accessed 12 Jan 2005).
2. "2005 Ambulatory care National Patient Safety Goals," Joint Commission on Accreditation of Healthcare Organization, *http://jcaho.org/accredited+organizations/ patient+safety/05+npsg/05_npsg_amb.htm* (accessed 12 Jan 2005).
3. ECRI, "Surgical fires," *Operating Room Risk Management* 2 (November 2004) 6.
4. "A clinician's guide to surgical fires: How they occur, how to prevent them, how to put them out," *Health Devices* 32 (January 2003) 1-24.
5. ECRI, "The patient is on fire! A surgical fire primer," *Medical Device Safety Reports* 21 (January 1992) 19-34. Also available at *http://www.mdsr.ecri.org/summary/ detail.aspx?doc_id=8197&q=%22The+patient+is+on+fire %22* (accessed 12 Jan 2005).
6. C Smith, "Surgical fires: Learn not to burn," *AORN Journal* 80 (July 2004) 25-26.
7. L Salmon, "Fire in the OR: Prevention and preparedness," *AORN Journal* 80 (July 2004) 42-54.
8. D Stewart, "Fire and life safety for surgical services: What's new and what to review," *SSM* 9 (April 2003) 26-31.
9. P M McCarthy, K A Gaucher, "Fire in the OR: Developing a fire safety plan," *AORN Journal* 79 (March 2004) 588-600.

Originallly published May 2005, *AORN Journal.*

AORN Guidance Statement: The Role of the Health Care Industry Representative in the Perioperative Setting

Introduction

The purpose of this statement is to provide general guidelines to assist the individual facility in developing policies relating to the role of the heath care industry representative in the perioperative setting. The term health care industry representative refers to all health care industry employees who provide services in the perioperative setting (eg, clinical consultants, sales representatives, technicians, repair/maintenance personnel). A systematic method of providing education, training, and instruction related to new technology, equipment, techniques, and procedures is essential for perioperative staff to provide safe patient care. The health care industry representative who possesses the requisite education, knowledge, and expertise can play a vital role in providing technical assistance, instruction, and training to perioperative team members.

Background

It may be hazardous to both patients and perioperative team members when clinicians use equipment with which they are unfamiliar. Misuse of complex technology can cause patient injury and even death. Incidents involving new technology and the presence of the health care industry representative in the perioperative setting have been highly publicized, especially when the end result is patient injury or death.[1] Hospitals have been cited and fined for allowing the use of surgical equipment not approved by the hospital; not providing formal training to physicians, nurses, and other perioperative team members on the proper use of the equipment; and permitting an unauthorized person from the medical device company to participate in a procedure.[2]

Tragic incidents have drawn attention to the need for individual facility policies to address formal instruction of physicians, nurses, and other members of the perioperative team on the operation of new medical devices before their use. Policies and procedures should be in place to authorize the introduction of new equipment and the admittance of nonmedical professionals into the room where the surgical or other invasive procedure will be performed. These policies and procedures should delineate acceptable activities and

conduct of the health care industry representative in the perioperative setting. The role of the health care industry representative is to provide essential technical training and assistance related to the device for the safe care of the patient. The health care industry representative should not be considered part of the clinical team and should not be requested to perform tasks outside his or her approved role.[1]

All perioperative team members are responsible for acquiring instruction on new procedures, techniques, technology, and equipment with which they are not familiar, before their use in a surgical procedure. The health care industry representative, who has completed specialized training to provide technical instruction and support to the perioperative surgical team expedites the procedure and facilitates desired safe patient outcomes. Health care industry representatives have a valid, but restricted, role in the perioperative setting.[3]

Guidance Statement

A health care industry representative may be present during a surgical procedure under conditions prescribed by the health care organization, in accordance with accreditation requirements, and in compliance with local, state, and federal regulations. In consideration of patient safety and confidentiality, AORN recommends the following precepts to guide policy development.

Perioperative team members are responsible for acquiring instruction on new procedures, techniques, technology, and equipment before their use in a surgical procedure. This instruction may be provided by a health care industry representative and may take place in a formal inservice program or as one-on-one instruction. The facility should maintain evidence of documented competencies for perioperative team members, especially when introducing new procedures, techniques, technology, and equipment.[4]

As the patient's advocate, the RN responsible for the patient's care during the procedure is accountable for maintaining the patient's safety, privacy, dignity, and confidentiality. The RN should monitor the health care industry representative's activities whenever possible and facilitate the representative's service to the perioperative team during the procedure. The RN should monitor and limit the movement and number of people in the operating room during the procedure to prevent increased airborne contamination.[5] The RN should be informed before the procedure that a health care industry representative will be present during a specific procedure as well as the purpose for being in attendance.

Policies should be developed in collaboration with the facility's risk manager and/or legal counsel to ensure compliance with applicable local, state, and federal laws.[2]

Conditions should be specified under which the health care industry representative may be present during a surgical or other invasive procedure.

Each facility should develop a system that clearly delineates limits on the health care industry representative's activities in the room where the surgical or other invasive procedure is performed based on community standards, accreditation requirements, and local, state, and federal regulations.

The role of the health care industry representative is to provide technical support, as opposed to direct patient care; the representative should never function as a member of the scrubbed team. The health care industry representative with specialized training and facility approval may perform calibration to adjust devices to the surgeon's specification (eg, pacemakers and lasers)

The health care industry representative with previous perioperative experience (eg, RN, surgical technologist) should be held to the same rules and restrictions as all other health care industry representatives.

Each facility should develop a system that addresses informed patient consent regarding the presence and role of the health care industry representative during an operative or other invasive procedure in both routine and emergency situations. This system should include the name of the representative and documentation of consent in the patient's medical record.[5,6]

Each facility should develop a system which documents that the health care industry representative has completed instruction in the principles of asepsis, fire and safety protocols, infection control practices, bloodborne pathogens, and patients' rights. Based on community standards, this may range from maintaining up-to-date documentation supplied by the representative's employing company to providing facility-specific instruction and training.

The health care industry representative must be aware of and follow the regulations of the federal Health Insurance Portability and Accountability Act[7] and the Bloodborne Pathogens Standard.[8]

The health care industry representative's presence and purpose should be authorized by the designated department administrator and the surgeon in accordance the facility policy.

While in the facility, the health care industry representative should wear identification, preferably a photo identification badge, and be appropriately attired, including personal protective equipment as described in the "Recommended practices for surgical attire" and the "Recommended practices for standard and transmission based precautions in the perioperative practice setting" in the AORN *Standards, Recommended Practices and Guidelines.*

Experienced health care industry representatives who are accompanied by persons in training from their own organization for the purposes of orientation should make prior arrangements with the health care organization and comply with accreditation requirements, and local, state, and federal regulations.

The guidelines of the Association for the Advancement of Medical Instrumentation state: "Medical equipment and other complex devices must be reviewed and approved prior to their use by the facility's service provider."[9] The term *service provider* is defined as an entity with the responsibility to provide inspection and/or other maintenance services on a specific piece of equipment. A service provider may be a department within the health care organization or a contracted provider.[9]

A clearly defined mechanism should exist to address departures from established policy.

NOTES

1. E Murphy, "The presence of sales representatives in the OR," *AORN Journal* 73 (April 2001) 822-824.

2. "New York incident underscores need for policy on sales reps in OR," *Operating Room Risk Management* (December 1998).

3. P Lebowitz, M Hart Yeary, "Allowing sales representatives in the OR creates new liability issues," *News & Business* (Nov/Dec 2001).

4. Joint Commission on Accreditation of Healthcare Organizations, *Comprehensive Accreditation Manual for Hospitals: The Official Handbook* (Oakbrook Terrace, Ill: Joint Commission on Accreditation of Healthcare Organizations, 2005).

5. "Recommended practices for traffic patterns in the perioperative practice setting," *Standards, Recommended Practices and Guidelines* (Denver: AORN Inc, 2006) 659-662

6. "Standards for privacy of individually identifiable health information; final rule," 45 CFR Parts 160 and 164, Centers for Medicare and Medicaid Services, *http://www.cms.hhs.gov/hipaa/hipaa2/regulations/privacy/finalrule/PvcFR01.pdf* (accessed 4 Oct 2005).

7. "Administrative simplification in the health care industry," US Department of Health and Human Services, *http://aspe.os.dhhs.gov/admnsimp/index.shtml* (accessed 4 Oct 2005).

8. "Bloodborne pathogens and needlestick prevention," Occupational Safety and Health Administration, *http://www.osha.gov/SLTC/bloodbornepathogens/index.html* (accessed 4 Oct 2005).

9. Association for the Advancement of Medical Instrumentation, "Recommended practice for a medical equipment management program," ANSI/AAMI EQ56:1999/(R)2004 (Arlington, Va: Association for the Advancement of Medical Instrumentation, 1999) 4.1.2.1.

RESOURCES

"AORN OR protocol," Healthstream, *http://www.healthstream.com/Products/STS/RepDirect/orProtocol.htm* (accessed 4 Oct 2005).

Approved by the AORN Board of Directors, November 2005. Scheduled for publication in the *AORN Journal* in 2006.

AORN Guidance Statement: Care of the Perioperative Patient With an Implanted Electronic Device

Introduction

This document is intended to serve as a guide for perioperative nurses involved in the care of surgical patients with implanted electronic devices (IEDs) who are undergoing surgical and other invasive procedures. This document does not address care of patients undergoing surgery for implantation of an electronic device; it covers only issues surrounding the care of patients with existing electronic implants. Because of the rapid advancement of science and medical technology, this document does not presume to address every IED. Manufacturers' written directions for specific devices should be followed. This document is intended to help perioperative nurses provide safe care for patients with IEDs because these patients require extraordinary safety precautions in the surgical environment.

Implanted electronic devices provide a vast number of options in the treatment of many disease processes that cannot be managed with medications alone. Common examples of IEDs include permanent pacemakers, which are used to treat profound bradycardia; implantable cardioverter defibrillators (ICDs), which are used to treat sustained ventricular tachycardia (VT); deep brain stimulators (DBSs), which are used to treat tremors and Parkinson's disease; and spinal cord stimulators (SCSs), which are used to deliver low-voltage stimulation to the spinal cord to block the sensation of pain and to stimulate the sacral nerve for treatment of neurogenic bladder and tremors. Sudden failure of these implanted devices can result in patient injury or sudden cardiac death (SCD).[1] When precautions are implemented, patient risk for injury can be minimized.

The goal of every surgical intervention is to provide optimal patient outcomes while maintaining a safe environment. Some medical equipment devices necessary for performing surgical and other invasive procedures may interfere with the functioning of IEDs. Manufacturers of IEDs recommend precautions for and/or avoiding certain devices that create electromagnetic fields.[2] Because of the potential for interference, patients with IEDs require special safety precautions when undergoing a surgical procedure. The perioperative registered nurse should be knowledgeable about the specific IED and associated precautions that should be implemented to protect the patient from injury.

Implanted electronic devices are widely used in a number of diverse medical applications, ranging from the familiar cardiac pacemaker to the less frequently encountered cochlear implant. The perioperative nurse should be aware that these devices require that special precautions be taken. One predominantly important precaution is managing the sources of inherent electromagnetic interference (EMI) in the perioperative patient care environment. Cardiac patients are particularly at risk because they may be dependent on the proper function of an IED to sustain their lives. Understanding what types of IEDs exist, how they function, and the precautions that must be taken when caring for patients with IEDs is critical for every perioperative nurse because patients with these devices may be encountered in any perioperative environment. The history, application, function, and safety issues of the different types of IEDs will be addressed in this document.

Definitions

For the purposes of this document, the following definitions apply.

Conducted EMI: Occurs when an electromagnetic source comes in direct contact with the body. Can be generated by electrosurgery and defibrillation.[3]

Direct coupling: The contact of an energized metal active electrode tip with another metal instrument or object within the surgical field.

Electromagnetic: Magnetism that is induced by an electric current.[4]

Electromagnetic interference (EMI): Any electromagnetic disturbance that interrupts, obstructs, or otherwise degrades or limits the effective performance of electronics/electrical equipment. *Synonym:* radio frequency interference.[5]

Implanted electronic devices (IEDs): Electronic medical devices that have been implanted in a patient to treat a physiological defect or to replace a sensory function.

Microwave: A short electromagnetic wave between about 1 mm and 1 m in length.

Radiated EMI: Occurs when the body is placed within an electromagnetic field; no contact with the source is necessary. Can be generated by magnetic resonance imaging (MRI), positron emission tomography (PET), and radiation therapy.[3]

Shortwave: A radio wave with a wavelength between 10 m and 100 m.

General Safety Issues and Concerns

Electronic devices implanted in a patient may be affected by other IEDs or medical equipment that a patient may come in contact with in a health care facility. These devices may include

- cardiac pacemakers or ICDs,
- electrosurgical devices,
- ultrasound equipment, or
- MRI equipment.

All of these devices have the potential to adversely affect an IED.[6] Perioperative registered nurses should be aware of potential patient safety hazards associated with specific IEDs and the appropriate patient care interventions required to protect patients from injury. (See Exhibit A, at the end of this document, for a summary of potential patient safety hazards.)

Exposure to shortwave and microwave diathermy should be avoided if an implanted device has metallic leads, even if the implanted device is not turned on. The energy from diathermy can cause tissue heating at the site surrounding the implant and has the potential to cause tissue injury. *Note:* As used here, the term "diathermy" does not include electrocautery and electrosurgical devices or ultrasonic imaging devices.[7] Examples of implants with metallic leads include cardiac pacemakers and defibrillators, cochlear implants, bone growth stimulators, deep brain stimulators, spinal cord stimulators, and other nerve stimulators.[7,8]

General Patient Management

Preoperative

- The perioperative registered nurse should routinely assess patients for the presence of any IEDs.[9] Patient education occurring at the time of the implant surgery should include instructions to the patient to always report the presence of the implant to health care providers, especially when a surgical procedure is necessary.[10] A patient who has an IED should have been given a product identification card at the time of implantation; the patient may have the card with him or her, or the medical record may contain a copy of the card.[10]
- The perioperative registered nurse may contact the patient's implanting surgeon to inform him or her that the patient is scheduled for surgery and ask the implanting physician to send the following IED information to the preoperative assessment nurse, the operating surgeon, and the operative suite:[10,11]

- manufacturer and model of IED,
- location of the device,
- when the device was last evaluated,
- if the device can be turned off before or during surgery,
- what settings should be reprogrammed into the device immediately postprocedure,
- whether the implanting physician wishes to be contacted when the patient enters the postanesthesia care unit (PACU), and
- whether the patient needs to schedule an appointment with the implanting physician.[12]
- The information above should be documented on the medical record before surgery.
- Determine whether electrosurgery and/or defibrillation are necessary for the procedure.
- Contact the appropriate health care industry representative and arrange for his or her presence before, during, and after the surgery, if requested by the physician.[13]
- Notify the anesthesia care provider of the presence of the IED.

Intraoperative

- Notify all perioperative team members that the patient has an IED in place, and review potential safety concerns and equipment conflicts.[11,14]
- The programming device and personnel who are qualified to program the IED should be in the OR before the start of the procedure.[3]
- When electrosurgery is necessary, bipolar electrosurgery should be used.[14]
- If the use of monopolar electrosurgery is required, the current pathway should be perpendicular to the IED's lead system. This can be achieved by manipulating the placement of the patient return electrode; however, a perpendicular pathway is not always a realistic possibility. If monopolar electrosurgery must be used, the active electrode and the dispersive electrode should be located as close together as possible.[3] A reusable, capacitive-coupled return electrode may be used if the perpendicular current pathway does not pass through the IED or the IED lead system.[15]
- Place the active electrode and the dispersive electrode as far from the IED generator and wires as possible.[16]
- The current path from the active electrode to the dispersive electrode should not pass through the area containing the IED or the electrodes.[16]

- Avoid placing the dispersive electrode directly over the site of a metal implant.[15] The dispersive electrode should be placed in such a way that the current will flow away from the IED. The distance between the dispersive electrode and the active electrode should be as small as possible.[17]
- To prevent EMI, care should be taken not to arc current between the active electrode and another surgical instrument. The instrument and active electrode should be in direct contact before activation.
- If the IED appears to have been inadvertently reprogrammed by the use of electrosurgery, it is advisable to return the device to the appropriate mode before continuing the procedure.[3]
- The humidity and temperature in the OR should be maintained within recommended ranges to reduce the possibility of creating static electricity in the environment. The OR temperature should be between 20° C and 24° C (68° F and 76° F) and humidity should be between 50% and 60%.[18(p147)]
- For patients who have pacemakers and other IEDs in the chest area and who require defibrillation, anterior-posterior-type paddles should be used. The anterior paddle should be placed as far from the pulse generator as possible. This should allow the current to flow away from the IED. The lowest possible defibrillator current setting should be used. Inability to defibrillate at low current settings will necessitate an increase in power, and damage to the IED may be unavoidable.[3]

Postoperative

- If necessary, notify the implanting physician and/or the health care industry representative that electrosurgery or defibrillation was used during surgery. An evaluation of IED function similar to that performed before surgery should be done early in the postoperative period.[3,16]
- Continue to monitor the patient closely during the postoperative period for signs of complications and IED malfunction.

Cardiac IEDs

Implanted electronic devices provide a vast array of treatments for patients with cardiac dysfunctions. The ability to electrically stimulate the chambers of the heart with an implanted device has helped many patients who have cardiac dysfunction and limited options for treating their disease with medications. For this reason, IEDs are popular treatment modalities. Pacemakers, ICDs, and ventricular assist devices (VADs) are three examples of IEDs used today to treat cardiac dysfunction. Specifically, pacemakers are used to treat patients with compromised cardiac output caused by profound bradycardia.[1] Implantable cardioverter defibrillators treat patients with a known risk for SCD caused by ventricular fibrillation (VF).[1] Ventricular assist devices are implantable pumps used for circulatory support in patients with congestive heart failure.[3]

History and Current Application

Pacemakers
Cardiac pacemakers first were introduced in 1954.[19] Pacemakers consist of a power source that delivers an electric impulse that travels along leads that have contact with the heart. Early pacemakers fired at a fixed rate and did not have the ability to sense the patient's heartbeat.[1] As technology improved, pacemakers with the ability to sense the patient's heart rate were introduced, helping to eliminate the hazard of the pacemaker competing with the intrinsic heartbeat and potentially creating a ventricular dysrhythmia.[1] The development of the sensing demand pacemaker in the 1960s brought with it the problem of interference.[3] Specifically, sensing pacemakers were able to sense and react to the changing needs of the heart, but they also could sense and react to electromagnetic signals that were not cardiac in origin.[3] Pacemakers have evolved from the limited capability of stimulating only one chamber of the heart to those capable of stimulating both atrial and ventricular chambers, adjusting rates to physiologic demands, providing telemetric information and autoprogramming and reprogramming functions, and providing antitachycardia functions.[20] The transvenous route performed with fluoroscopy is the most common insertion method.[1]

Implanted cardioverter defibrillators
Implanted cardioverter defibrillators are similar to pacemakers in that they have a power source and leads that attach to the heart and sense the patient's heartbeat. Early ICDs consisted of defibrillating patches placed via thoracotomy on the ventricular epicardium and connected to an internal defibrillator that discharged when it sensed VT or VF.[1] Lowe

and Wharton (1955) report that the development of nonthoracotomy lead systems inserted transvenously has made epicardial patch systems rare.[21] The greatest challenge in treating patients with spontaneous VF is that electrical counter shock is the only treatment for patients at risk for SCD caused by VF;[1] therefore, patients may be totally dependent on the ICD to save their lives. Realizing that patients often died of VT or VF because the necessary equipment and personnel to defibrillate patients were unavailable, Mirowski and his associates (1980) conceived of an implantable device that could sense the dysrythmia and deliver a counter shock to terminate the life-threatening disorder.[22] In 1980, the first device of this kind was implanted at Johns Hopkins Hospital in Baltimore.[1]

Ventricular assist devices

A VAD is a type of mechanical heart that is surgically implanted in the patient's chest during open-heart surgery[20] and that is used to treat patients with end-stage heart failure. Blood fills the device through a cannulation site in the ventricle or atrium. Within the device, a diaphragm is actuated pneumatically, electrically, or magnetically, and it pumps blood into the aorta or pulmonary artery.[18] After the pump is implanted, it needs power to operate. The driveline passes through the skin and attaches to the power base unit, which consists of a system controller and batteries. The power source is worn externally in a holster or waist pack.[19] Government-funded research and development work in cardiac support systems began in 1966. Clinical trials of an air-driven left ventricular assist system started in 1986, and an electric system was tested in 1991. The device has been used in patients aged 11 to 78 years, with an average age of 50 years, and in as many as 4,000 patients in the United States and elsewhere.[19]

Ventricular assist devices initially were used as "bridges to transplantation," helping people survive as they waited for a heart transplant. Today, VADs play another role; they allow disease-weakened hearts to recover. In patients not eligible for heart transplantation, VADs offer permanent support, which is called destination therapy.[19] Clinical trials have demonstrated that destination therapy doubles the one-year survival rate of patients with end-stage heart failure as compared to treatment with medication.[20]

Safety Concerns

Pacemakers, ICDs, and VADs are IEDs that rely on sensing capability for proper function of the device and appropriate treatment being delivered to the patient. Electromagnetic interference is the most common safety issue noted when caring for patients with existing cardiac IEDs, mostly because EMI can alter what the device is sensing. This potentially could change the rhythm or, in some cases, render the device incapable of delivering appropriate treatment.

Electromagnetic interference occurs in two forms: conducted and radiated. Conducted EMI occurs when an electromagnetic source comes in direct contact with the body. This type of EMI can be generated by electrosurgery and defibrillation. Radiated EMI occurs when the body is placed within an electromagnetic field; no contact with the source is necessary. This type of EMI can be generated by MRI, PET, and radiation therapy.[3]

The electrosurgical unit (ESU) is a commonly used device that cuts and coagulates tissue with high-voltage, high-frequency (ie, 10,000 Hz) current.[3(p640)] Practically every surgical intervention requires some form of electrosurgery to help facilitate hemostasis. Some surgical procedures would be nearly impossible to perform without electrosurgery. There are two types of electrosurgical current: monopolar and bipolar. Monopolar current begins at the tip of the instrument, travels through the body, and returns to the generator through a dispersing ground pad. When monopolar electrosurgery is used, surgeons may use the active electrode to pass current through other surgical instruments. If the ESU is activated before the active electrode is in contact with the instrument, the current can arc through the air toward the instrument and demodulate the signal to the IED. If allowed to demodulate, the signal can dip well into the frequency range that pacemakers and ICDs are designed to sense. The result is that the IED might interpret the current as cardiac in origin and respond inappropriately or not respond at all.[3]

Ventricular assist devices also are affected by EMI generated by electrosurgery. Theoretically, the timing circuit of one model can be disrupted, but this rarely is reported. Ventricular assist devices that are run by electricity may exhibit an erratic pattern of current output during electrosurgery use. This results in a significant decrease in device output.[3]

Bipolar electrosurgery does not require a patient-return electrode because the current flows between the two tips of a bipolar forceps that is positioned around tissue to create a surgical effect. Current passes from the active electrode of one tip of the forceps through the patient's tissue to the dispersive electrode of the other forceps tip, thus completing the circuit without entering another part of the patient's body. This means that the current flows only through the area of tissue that is in direct contact with the instrument.[17] Using bipolar electrosurgery rather than monopolar electrosurgery may be advantageous when trying to avoid possible arcing that could demodulate; however, bipolar electrosurgery is much less powerful than monopolar electrosurgery and may be inappropriate for many surgical procedures.

Other dangers inherent to monopolar electrosurgery include burns, triggering ventricular or atrial fibrillation, and loss of battery output. A continuous train of electrical impulses conducted down the lead can induce ventricular or atrial fibrillation, cause thermal burns at the lead-tissue interface, and pass from the leads to the pulse generator and cause irreversible loss of battery output.[3]

Some surgeries and emergency situations employ the use of defibrillation as part of the surgical procedure. Patients with existing pacemakers and ICDs may experience permanent damage to the pulse generator, particularly after repeated attempts at defibrillation. In addition, the current shunted away from the pacemaker or ICD can lead to myocardial burns at the lead-tissue interface.[3]

Patient Management

Preoperative
- If the IED was not evaluated within the previous six months, it should be evaluated for programming, telemetry, thresholds, and battery status.
- If the make and model of the IED is unavailable, a chest x-ray may be helpful in identifying the pacemaker or ICD. Each device has a serial number and a unique silhouette that can be used for device identification.[3] Modern pacemakers employ a variety of different pacing modes, so it is important to be familiar with the North American Society of Pacing and Electrophysiology/British Pacing and Electrophysiology Group (NBG) generic pacemaker codes. The first

three letters of the code describe the basic antibradycardia functions, and the last two letters describe the programmability and antitachycardia functions.[3] Similar coding also is found on ICDs. This code, which is located on the device, also can be identified via chest x-ray.
- For a pacemaker-dependent patient, it is advised that the device be reprogrammed to an asynchronous mode if EMI is likely to cause significant malfunction (eg, monopolar electrosurgery for surgical procedures involving the upper abdomen or chest wall).
- For patients with adaptive-rate devices, including ICDs, this feature should be programmed off during surgery because exposure to other EMI might cause a device malfunction.[23] Magnet-activated testing should be programmed off.[20]
- For patients with an ICD, tachycardia sensing should be programmed off.[23]
- Patients with a VAD should be evaluated in a similar manner. Most surgical procedures involving patients with VADs take place at institutions that can provide technical and surgical support for these devices.[3]

Intraoperative
- If monopolar electrosurgery must be used, the current pathway should be perpendicular to the pacemaker's lead system when possible. This is done by manipulating the placement of the dispersive electrode; however, a perpendicular pathway is not always a realistic possibility, especially when the IED has a dual lead system.
- If it is impossible to place the pacemaker in a triggered or asynchronous mode and it becomes apparent that the ESU is adversely affecting the pacemaker, the electrosurgery current should be activated for no more than one second at a time, allowing at least 10 seconds for the device to function properly. This will permit the pacemaker enough time to maintain cardiac output. It is widely assumed that placing a magnet over any pacemaker pulse generator will invariably cause asynchronous pacing as long as the magnet remains in place; however, in some pacemakers, the magnet response may have been programmed off. In others, a variety of magnet responses may have been programmed, some of which do not provide immunity to EMI sensing. In still other pacemakers, the device will con-

tinue to pace asynchronously or pacing will cease after a programmed number of intervals.[24] If possible, one should determine before EMI exposure what type of pulse generator is present and what must be done to provide protection. If this is not possible, one can observe the magnet response during EMI to ascertain whether there is protection from EMI sensing. During electrosurgery, for example, if the active electrode triggers rapid pacing or inhibits pacing stimuli in a pacemaker-dependent patient despite magnet application, then activation of the ESU should be limited to short bursts.[23]

■ The use of electrosurgery also may interfere with the ability of the electrocardiogram (ECG) to monitor the heart, so heart rate and blood pressure should be monitored using an arterial line. When the ESU is not in use, the ECG should be checked for arrhythmias or alterations in pacemaker function.

■ Patients with VADs that require the use of electrosurgery should have the device placed in the fixed rate mode for the duration of the surgery. Adequate pumping is not possible during electrosurgery, so the ESU should be activated for no more than one second at a time, allowing 10 seconds for the VAD to function properly. Cardiac output should be monitored. It may be necessary for an external hand pump to be available in the OR during surgery.[3]

■ Patients with VADs who require defibrillation may need to have the timing circuit disconnected from the external controller before defibrillation. This may require the use of a fixed rate mode, depending on the type of VAD, during the period of defibrillation, but it will eliminate the possibility of damage to the circuit. During this time, a pneumatic or manually run pump will be needed.[3]

■ In patients with pacemakers and ICDs who require defibrillation, anterior-posterior-type paddles should be used. The anterior paddle should be placed as far from the pulse generator as possible. This should allow the current to flow away from the generator. If the anterior type of paddles must be used, the paddles should be placed along a line perpendicular to the lead(s). This may be difficult if the patient has a dual-lead system. The lowest possible defibrillator current setting should be used. Inability to defibrillate at low current settings will necessitate an increase in power, and damage to the pulse generator may be unavoidable. For these reasons, a temporary pacing system should be available.[3]

Postoperative

■ Inform the cardiologist, cardiothoracic surgeon, and/or the health care industry representative that electrosurgery or defibrillation was used during surgery. An evaluation of pacemaker and ICD function similar to that performed before surgery should be done in the early postoperative period and again 24 to 48 hours later. This is necessary because failure of the device to capture due to damage at the lead-tissue interface may not be apparent until 24 to 48 hours after surgery. If any of the postoperative measurements of the demand or magnet rates vary from those obtained before surgery, one must suspect that the pacemaker has been reprogrammed inadvertently during surgery or has sustained permanent damage.[3]

■ Alteration of the VAD motor current occurs only during exposure to electrosurgery and has no permanent effect on the device. Defibrillation, however, can damage the timing circuit, depending on the model and if the timing circuit is left connected during surgery. The surgeon or cardiologist responsible for the care of the patient should be informed if the circuit is damaged during surgery because repair or replacement should be considered.[3]

Neurostimulators

Deep brain stimulators, SCSs, vagal nerve stimulators (VNSs), and programmable ventricular shunts all are examples of neurological IEDs. Neurological IEDs are devices that help to restore functionality to people who have neurological or sensory impairments. This is accomplished by electrically stimulating the nervous system. Electrodes are placed in specific regions of the nervous system with regard to the patient's pathology. Neurostimulation used to treat movement disorders, such as those caused by Parkinson's disease, involves implanting leads in specific regions of the brain (ie, DBS) that then are connected to a programmable pulse generator. Electrodes may be implanted in the spine (ie, SCS) to control intractable pain, and they also may be used for sacral nerve stimulation to alleviate urinary incontinence and on the left vagus nerve (ie, VNS) to treat intractable seizures.[25]

History and Current Application

In 1964, E. A. Spiegel, MD, and H. T. Wycis, MD, along with their team members at Temple University Hospital, created the first neurological IED.[26] The physicians, however, were reluctant to use a new device, so their first device was never implanted. C. Norman Shealy, MD, is credited with implanting the first neurological IED spinal cord stimulator in 1967.[26] For the past three decades, neurological IEDs have continued to evolve. Thorough patient selection and screening, combined with physician experience, has resulted in a 50% to 60% good long-term results. More than 20,000 DBSs,[27(p76)] 130,000 SCSs,[27(p76)] and 15,000 VNSs have been implanted.[28 (p1,662)]

Deep brain stimulators

The first IED to treat tremors associated with Parkinson's disease was approved by the US Food and Drug Administration (FDA) in August 1997.[29] Deep brain stimulators consist of four electrodes that are placed in the ventricle. These electrodes then are connected to a pulse generator. The pulse generator usually is placed in the subcutaneous tissues in the chest, similar to the cardiac pacemaker.[29] The electrical stimulation blocks the abnormal brain signal that induces tremors. These devices can be turned off and adjusted from high to low frequency settings.

Spinal cord stimulators

The use of electrical stimulation for patient with spinal cord injuries was first attempted in the 1960s.[30] Spinal cord stimulators have been used to stimulate phrenic nerves and the diaphragm to permit a patient freedom from a respirator and to promote easier mobility. Spinal cord stimulators also are used in the treatment of intractable pain. An SCS is used to reduce pain, not eliminate it. Spinal cord stimulator studies have shown a 50% reduction in pain, increased activity levels, and a decreased reliance on narcotic medications.[31(p3)] Spinal cord stimulators have helped patients with chronic pain lead more comfortable and productive lives.

Patients with implanted cardiac pacemakers or defibrillators should not use spinal stimulators. Use of a transcutaneous electrical nerve stimulator unit is acceptable.[32]

Vagal nerve stimulators

In 1985, Zabara[27] developed the concept of vagal stimulation to control seizures; however, it was not until 1997 that the FDA approved the use of VNSs.[27]

Vagal nerve stimulators are composed of implantable (eg, generator, leads) and external (eg, computer, software, programming wands) components. The generator or stimulator, which is the main component, is very similar to a cardiac pacemaker. It is a pulse generator that is programmed by a computer, and it runs on battery power. The pulse generator is implanted on the left side of the upper chest just under the skin. The lead is a flexible tube that is attached to the left vagus nerve on the left side of the neck.[33] The pulse generator has a life span of approximately 16 years. The battery life span ranges from six to 10 years.[33(p4)] Vagal nerve stimulators operate by sending electrical signals through the implanted leads via the left vagus nerve to the brain. This signal stimulates the brain to reduce the frequency and duration of seizures.

Programmable ventricular shunts

Ventricular shunts are used to treat patients with hydrocephalus. Shunts are long tubes that draw cerebrospinal fluid (CSF) away from the brain and into a body cavity, such as the chest or abdomen.[34] One of the major setbacks in ventricular shunts is shunt failure. This leads to repeated surgeries to adjust the shunt to drain the CSF. In September 1999, the FDA approved the first programmable shunt.[34] Programmable shunts allow surgeons to adjust the settings on the shunt from outside the body, thereby decreasing the need for repeated surgeries.

Neurostimulators or neurological IEDs are similar to cardiac pacemakers in design. They deliver electrical stimulation to targeted structures in the appropriate area of the nervous system. After it is programmed, a neurological IED can be turned on and off by a patient or clinician using a magnet or a patient-therapy controller. In the OR, because the neurological IED generates electrical impulses, it may be affected by or have an adverse effect on medical equipment (eg, cardiac pacemakers, cardioverters/defibrillators, external defibrillators, ultrasonic equipment, ESU) or procedures (eg, radiation therapy, some MRI procedures).[25]

Safety Concerns

Neurological IEDs, like implantable cardiac devices, generate electrical impulses and have the potential for interference from other medical devices with electromagnetic forces. Electromagnetic interference is the primary concern. In the perioperative setting, many procedures and devices have the potential to cause interference with IEDs, including electrosurgery, defibrillation, MRI, ultrasonic equipment, and other IEDs.[35]

More than 177,000 neurological IEDs have been implanted,[27(p76)] so perioperative team members must be aware of and understand potential complications before patients with IEDs enter the OR. This knowledge can help team members deal with potential complications and possibly prevent patient injury.[3]

Devices and procedures that may cause damage to or interfere with the function of the neurological IED or harm to the patient include defibrillators, cardioverters, electrosurgery, and MRI. If a patient is in ventricular or atrial fibrillation, patient survival always should be the first consideration. Steps should be taken to minimize the electrical circuit flowing through the neurological IED during defibrillation. These steps include

- positioning paddles as far from the neurological IED as possible,
- positioning paddles perpendicular to the neurological IED,
- using the lowest clinically appropriate output settings, and
- having perioperative team members confirm that the neurological IED is functioning properly after defibrillation.

Use of monopolar electrosurgery may cause the tissue around the leads to be damaged. In addition, the insulation on the leads may be damaged, which could cause device failure or shock the patient.[35] Damage to the neurological IED itself also may occur, and this could cause changes in stimulation settings, changes in parameters, or complete device failure. These are potentially serious risks, so the use of the ultrasonic scalpel is being investigated as an alternative to monopolar electrosurgery. Ultrasonic scalpels do not emit electromagnetic impulses.[3] If electrosurgery is deemed necessary, bipolar electrosurgery is recommended. If bipolar electrosurgery is not a suitable option and monopolar electrosurgery is necessary, the following precautions should be taken.

- The neurological IED should be turned off. If this cannot be accomplished by the patient, a staff member, or the physician, the appropriate health care industry representative may need to be notified.
- Use only a low voltage mode/setting.
- Keep the grounding pad as far from the neurological IED as possible.

- After using the ESU, perioperative team members should confirm that the neurological IED is functioning properly.

With the increasing popularity of intraoperative MRI, perioperative team members should be aware of MRI safety issues. Magnetic resonance imaging is not recommended for patients who have a neurological IED. It may cause heating at the lead site, resulting in tissue damage. Magnetic resonance imaging also may cause damage to the neurological IED itself, resulting in patient injury or device failure.[36]

The following devices used in the perioperative setting are unlikely to cause interference with neurological IEDs; however, special precautions should be taken when using them.[36]

- Keep the external magnetic coils of neurological IEDs a minimum of 18 inches (45 cm) away from bone growth stimulators.
- Turn the neurological IED off when dental drills, ultrasonic probes, diagnostic ultrasound, electrolysis, and lasers are used. Keep the device six inches (15 cm) away from the neurological IED. Keep the laser directed away from the neurological IED.
- For questions about precautions when other IEDs are present, contact the manufacturer of the other IED and notify the physicians involved in both therapies.

Patient Management

Preoperative

■ Vagus nerve stimulators can pose a serious risk to a patient's respiratory status. Patients with VNSs may have increased swallowing difficulties, so the risk of aspiration is increased.[33] The perioperative nurse and anesthesia care provider should be aware of the risk of spontaneous airway obstruction.[28]

Intraoperative

■ The patient, physician, a staff member, or the appropriate representative should turn off the IED.

Implantable Hearing Devices

Four types of implantable electronic hearing devices are used today. These devices are cochlear implants, implanted bone conduction stimulators, implantable and semi-implantable hearing aids, and auditory brainstem implants.

History and Current Application

Cochlear implants

Cochlear implants are used for people with sensorineural hearing loss. The first cochlear implant procedures on humans were done in 1961.[37] Graeme Clark and colleagues in Australia began research into cochlear implants in the late 1960s and implanted a multichannel device into the world's first cochlear implant recipient in 1978.[38] Cochlear implants now are the standard treatment for individuals whose ability to hear, even with hearing aids, is so poor that their ability to effectively communicate through speech is affected.[39] Statistics from 2003 indicate that approximately 60,000 people worldwide have received a cochlear implant since 1983.[39(p1)] Cochlear implants are seen more commonly than the other types of implantable hearing devices described here.

Cochlear implants consist of an implant system and an external component. After being implanted, these components work together to allow a patient with sensorineural hearing loss to hear by converting mechanical sound energy into electrical impulses that are transmitted directly to the acoustic nerve.[37] Cochlear implants consist of internal and external parts. The external parts, which consist of a receiver, speech processor, and transmitting coil, may be removed from the patient at any time. The internal receiver/stimulator is surgically implanted into the patient's inner ear and into the bone behind the ear.[38] The external receiver is worn near the ear and is used to pick up sound.

The external speech processor usually is clipped to the wearer's clothing, or for children, it may be kept in a special backpack. The external transmitting coil is surrounded by the transmitting antenna. This transmitting coil is held in place by two magnets of opposite polarity—one in the transmitting coil and the other implanted within the internal receiver/stimulator. The internal receiver/stimulator is surgically implanted and, in addition to the previously mentioned magnet, contains a multi-channeled electrode. A cochleostomy is made, and the electrode is placed into the cochlea. After all parts are connected, electromagnetic induction will cause stimulation of the cochlear nerve, which allows the patient to perceive sound.[10]

Implantable and semi-implantable hearing aids

Implanted bone conduction stimulators, which also are known as temporal bone stimulators,[40] typically are used for people with a conductive hearing loss.[41]

Implantable and semi-implantable hearing aids are implanted in the middle ear[42] or directly stimulate the inner ear.[38] The various designs are categorized by the type of output transducer used. Electromagnetic stimulation of the middle ear was first done in 1957. One of the earliest types used was piezoelectric crystal, which first was used in Japan in about 1978.[40]

The semi-implantable hearing aid allows sound to be produced through direct stimulation of the ossicles.[41] The components of this device include a microphone speech processor, which is connected to a transmitter. This transmitter has an external coil that transcutaneously transmits electrical energy to the internal device. The internal device has an internal receiving coil, which is implanted in the temporal bone. The internal receiving coil is connected to a receiver that provides electrical energy to the mechanical driver. The mechanical driver is attached to the incus. This results in vibration of the ossicles, which allows the patient to hear.[42]

Bone-conduction stimulators

One of the first bone-anchored hearing devices (ie, a temporal bone stimulator) was developed in Sweden in 1977. One brand currently is approved by the FDA.[40] A transcutaneous bone-conduction device was developed in 1986. This device has an external unit and an internal unit. The external unit is composed of a microphone and a sound processor system worn on the user's body and held in place with an implanted magnet assembly behind the user's ear. The internal unit is implanted into the temporal bone.[40] These devices are used in the treatment of severe conductive hearing loss, in patients with mixed hearing loss, and sometimes for patients with sensorineural hearing loss in one ear.[43]

Bone-conduction devices have an external processor, which consists of a microphone, amplifier, and a transducer, a device that connects the bone-anchored implant to the external processor. Both the fixture placed in the mastoid bone and the coupling devices are made of titanium.[42]

Auditory brainstem implants

Auditory brainstem implants are used to restore auditory sensation for patients who are totally deaf. The deafness is due to bilateral eighth cranial nerve lesions or neurofibromatosis Type 2. These patients have undergone surgical removal of a tumor and do not plan to undergo radiation treatment.[44]

One auditory brainstem implant system was approved by the FDA in October 2000.[45] The FDA New Device Approvals notice stated that pre-approval testing involved implantation of this auditory brainstem implant system in 90 patients.[45(p1)] The auditory brainstem implant consists of an implantable receiver/stimulator package, an electrode lead, and an electrode array. The receiver/stimulator comes with a magnet that can be removed via a small incision with local anesthesia if the patient is required to undergo MRI.[43]

Safety Issues and Concerns

Studies have been conducted to determine the compatibility of MRI and cochlear implants.[41] In at least one study, MRI was not an absolute contraindication for these patients. Another study determined that MRI should be done only if there is a strong medical indication for the test.[37] Currently, patients with cochlear implants should avoid undergoing MRI unless it is absolutely necessary because of the possibility that the implant can become inactivated.[46]

Roberts et al studied the effects of EMI on cochlear implants using common dental office equipment. This equipment included a bipolar and monopolar ESU. The ESU was tested using cut level 1 and various coagulation settings.[37] The study concluded that bipolar electrosurgery was safe, but monopolar electrosurgery may present a hazard to the cochlear implant device itself and has the potential to cause tissue damage that would prevent further reimplantation.[37]

Patients with cochlear implants are educated about the importance of avoiding contact with static electricity. A sudden shock from walking across a carpeted room in the wintertime has been known to inactivate an implant.[10] Static electricity can damage the components of an auditory brainstem implant.[47] The speech processor and headset should be removed when the potential for static electricity generation exists.[47]

Patient Management

Preoperative
■ The patient should not have an MRI scan because the strong magnetic field can inactivate the implant.
■ Computed tomography (CT) scans are acceptable for patients with cochlear implants.[10]

Intraoperative
■ External devices can be removed before the beginning of the surgical procedure, so they should be removed after induction of anesthesia, as would be done with other devices that assist with communication, such as hearing aids or eyeglasses.
■ The internal receiver/stimulator will be damaged by monopolar electrosurgery. Only bipolar electrosurgery should be used after the internal receiver/stimulator is implanted.[10] The radio frequency current of ESUs can damage the electrodes implanted in the cochlea or the surrounding tissue. Current leakage and direct coupling when an energized metal active electrode tip comes in contact with another metal instrument or object potentially can damage or cause injury to the device or tissues.[15] Monopolar electrosurgery should not be used in the head and neck area of a patient with a cochlear implant.[1,10,45,48]
■ Some models of cochlear implants have extracochlear reference electrodes, and some do not. If an implant has extracochlear reference electrodes, bipolar electrosurgical instruments may be used if the electrosurgical device is kept more than 10 cm from the extracochlear electrodes.[35]
■ Bipolar electrosurgery may be used on patients with auditory brainstem implants when the following precautions are observed.
    ▪ The electrosurgical electrode must not come in contact with the implant.
    ▪ The electrosurgical electrode should be kept more than 1 cm from the ground electrodes of the auditory brainstem implants.[47]
■ An isolated electrosurgical generator should be used. This can significantly decrease the risk of electrosurgical current traveling an alternate pathway to ground.[48]
■ Avoid using ionizing radiation therapy directly over the site of the implant. Ionizing radiation can damage the implant.[47]
■ Magnetic resonance imaging must be avoided with auditory brainstem implants unless the removable magnet is surgically removed before this test. The external speech processor and headset must be removed before the patient enters the scanner room.[47]

Postoperative
■ External devices may be replaced as soon as the surgical procedure has been completed.

■ Testing should be done to be sure the device continues to function.

Implantable Infusion Pumps

There are a number of implantable medication devices available for patients with a variety of therapeutic needs. These needs include chronic pain management, administration of chemotherapeutic medications, and administration of insulin. The devices specifically covered in this document include venous access devices (eg, subcutaneous infusion ports, implantable infusion pumps) and insulin pumps. Some devices are used for intraventricular administration of chemotherapy.[49]

History and Current Application

Intra-arterial medication infusion pumps became widely used in the early 1980s. One common use is hepatic artery medication infusion for the prevention or treatment of metastases from a colon cancer into the liver or for the treatment of hepatocellular carcinoma. This involves inserting a cannula into an artery that provides the blood supply to an area of a tumor. The cannula is connected to a pump device that is placed in the subcutaneous tissue.[49]

Venous access devices include subcutaneous infusion ports and implantable infusion pumps.[50] Subcutaneous infusion ports are implanted in the subcutaneous tissue for administration of medications into a central vein, hepatic artery, the epidural space, or the peritoneal cavity. These usually have a silicone or plastic port with a stainless steel or plastic reservoir. The ports are used for intermittent infusions of medications administered via a special Huber needle to access the port. During the intermittent infusion, the medication is infused and then flushed with a heparinized solution until the next infusion is ordered.[50]

Implantable infusion pumps also are placed into a vein or artery, the spine, a body space, or a ventricle in the brain. These devices can be used to deliver anticoagulants to control thromboembolic disease; insulin to control diabetes; morphine to treat pain from malignancy; or chemotherapy to a localized area for treatment of tumors, such as tumors in the liver or brain.[50] They also can be used to treat locally recurrent ovarian or colon cancer by delivering chemotherapy into the peritoneal space.[49] The implantable infusion pump also may be implanted in an area of subcutaneous tissue as close as is reasonable to the area of the tumor. The pumps usually are made of titanium, stainless steel, and silicone rubber. The pump steadily delivers medication using a bellows device or through radio signals.[50] The prevalence of individuals with an implantable medication delivery system is 0.05 people per 100,000 in Europe, North America, Australia, and Japan.[50(p904)]

One type of insulin pump consists of a pump reservoir connected to a small battery-operated pump via a subcutaneously-implanted infusion set.[51] The infusion set includes a cannula, which is inserted just under the skin and is changed every few days.[52] Other than the need to be aware of the presence of this device and monitor the patient's blood glucose, this type of insulin pump presents no major concern for perioperative nurses because the patient can remove the monitor for the duration of the surgical procedure. This device currently is available in European Union countries and is available only for investigational use in the United States.[53]

Safety Issues and Concerns

Magnetic resonance imaging can affect the function of implantable and programmable medication delivery systems. There has been a report of the pump motor stalling and stopping delivery of the medication when it is exposed to the magnetic field. The pump resumed normal medication delivery after it was removed from the magnetic field. No damage to the mechanical or electrical components of the pump occurred; however, the authors of the report recommend that medication be removed from the pump before MRI tests. Following the procedure, the pump should be refilled and the medication delivery system tested.[51]

If a patient will be undergoing an x-ray, CT scan, MRI scan, or any other type of radiation therapy, patient instructions from an implantable insulin pump manufacturer recommend removing the external pump and remote control from the patient's body and the treatment area. In addition, avoid close exposure to medical imaging equipment. The patient should avoid using the monitor near other strong electromagnetic sources, such as television and radio transmitters and high-voltage power lines.[53]

Patient Management

Refer to General Patient Management (pp 154-155).

Sacral Nerve Stimulators

Two treatment modalities currently are available for patients with dysfunction of the lower urinary tract.[54] Used only after more conservative therapies fail to produce positive results, a surgically implanted neurostimulator or sacral nerve stimulator may be a patient's last resort. Patients with spinal cord injuries have been treated successfully with posterior sacral nerve rhizotomies and placement of a nerve stimulator on the anterior sacral nerve roots.[54] Patients with chronic problems, such as urinary urge incontinence, nonobstructive urinary retention, urgency-frequency problems, problems with micturition, and neurogenic bladder, also have benefited from these devices.[54-56]

History and Current Applications

A device called the Finetech-Brindley bladder system was introduced and tested in baboons between 1969 and 1977.[27] This device provided intradural stimulation of the anterior sacral roots, which assisted with emptying the bladder.[54,56] The first human implantation occurred in 1976, but it was not until two years later that additional patients were successfully treated with nerve stimulation.[27]

Sacral nerve stimulation for treatment of overactive bladder conditions initially was developed in the late 1980s by Schmidt and Tanagho. The first of these implants were done in 1981.[27] The model used now was approved by the FDA in 1997.[55]

Currently, two devices are used to treat neurogenic bladder dysfunction.[27] One involves use of "mild electrical stimulation of the sacral nerve that influences the behavior of the bladder, sphincter, and pelvic floor muscles."[57] This device is used to treat urinary retention and to alleviate urinary urge incontinence and urgency-frequency symptoms of overactive bladder.[55] The second device works by initiating a contraction of the detrusor muscle.

Sacral nerve stimulators as therapy for urinary retention and urinary urge incontinence have been placed in about 10,000 patients. Sacral nerve stimulators that facilitate bladder emptying are less frequently implanted, totaling approximately 2,500 systems.[27(p76)]

These systems basically consist of three components. The first component is the pulse generator, which is battery-powered or controlled by an external portable control unit and programmed by a clinician.[56] The second component consists of electrodes placed intradurally or extradurally. The third component consists of the cables used to connect the pulse generator to the electrodes.[27]

Patient Management

Preoperative

◼ The perioperative nurse should follow the instructions of the neurostimulator's manufacturer. To prevent potential injury to the patient, it is important to determine exactly how the device producing the electrical stimulation works and how it may function during a surgical procedure to determine whether the device should be turned off during that time.[17]

Intraoperative

◼ Large, reusable, capacitive coupled return electrode systems should not be used.[17]

◼ The active electrode should be kept at least six inches from the implanted components of the device. This includes any cables, metallic electrodes, or leads, as well as the electrical components.[17]

Osteogenic Stimulators

Osteogenic (ie, bone-growth) stimulators are used to stimulate bone growth in patients with fresh fractures, to assist in healing postosteotomy, to stimulate grafted bone to vertebrae in spinal fusions, and for treatment of delayed fracture healing or nonunion following a fracture.[57] Implanted osteogenic stimulators deliver electrical impulses directly to the site where bone regrowth needs to occur. Types of bone-growth stimulators currently used include electrical, electromagnetic, and ultrasonic. These devices can be used invasively or noninvasively.

History and Current Application

In 1971, successful healing of a nonunion fracture with electrical stimulation was reported. The female patient had a nonhealing fracture of the medial malleolus for more than two years before it was healed successfully with direct current electrical stimulation.[58] Within the next five years, numerous investigators reposted the benefits of various types of electrical energy on bone growth in humans.[58] In 1979, the FDA approved the use of three types of electrical stimulation devices for treatment of long bone nonunion.[58]

The first clinical study on the benefits of electrical stimulation in lumbar spinal fusion was reported in 1974. During the next few years, implantable electrical stimulation devices were used with much success on both anterior and posterior spinal fusions and spinal fractures with nonunion.[58] The FDA approved use of electrical stimulators to be used as an adjunct treatment to spinal fusion in 1987.[59]

Electromagnetic fields typically are used as a noninvasive technique, and direct current electrical stimulation is used when invasive electrical stimulation is indicated.[60] Direct current stimulation involves surgical implantation of electrodes at the desired site for bone growth.[58,61] The negative electrode is placed at the site where bone repair is desired, and the positive electrode is place in nearby soft tissue. A generator is placed in nearby subcutaneous tissue or in an intermuscular plane.

Other techniques of electrical stimulation involve capacitive coupling and inductive coupling pulsed electromagnetic stimulation. These devices either are totally external devices or have a combination of implanted components and external components.[61]

Capacitive coupling for bone growth stimulation is delivered through two charged metal devices attached to a source of voltage that produces an electric field. This form of stimulation is delivered through external electrodes.[58,60]

Inductive coupling involves using single or double coils that deliver an electrical current from an external generator.[60,61] One inductive coupling bone healing system was introduced in 1979, and 300,000 patients have been treated using this system.[62]

Pulsing electromagnetic field therapy involves the use of time-varying current applied to metallic coils. These are applied to the desired treatment area and can be applied externally.[58]

Ultrasonic bone growth stimulators are external devices that apply pulsed ultrasound to the skin over the site of a fracture. This is the newest noninvasive technique and has the advantage that the treatment time may be as short as 20 to 30 minutes per day.

The electrodes and generator of a totally implantable device are made primarily of medical grade titanium containing a lithium battery.[58,63] A portion of one type of a spinal fusion system has a platinum coating.[63] These devices can produce continuous electrical stimulation for about six months.[63] The prevalence of spinal fusion systems is five people per 100,000 in Europe, North America, Australia, and Japan.[64(p904)]

Safety Issues and Concerns

One study measured temperature increases in the area of spinal fusion stimulators when MRI was performed. It was discovered that if a broken lead was present, the temperature was considerably higher than the temperature near an intact lead. This led to the recommendation that before MRI scanning is performed on a patient with a spinal fusion stimulator, it is important to make sure all spinal fusion stimulator leads are intact.[64]

Diathermy used over an area with an implanted bone growth stimulator can cause damage to the tissues surrounding the device or to the electronics of the device itself.[32] The magnetic external coils of a neurological IED should be kept to a minimum of 18 inches (45 cm) from bone growth stimulators.[36]

Patient Management

Preoperative

▪ Externally worn spine stimulators should be removed before the surgical procedure.

Intraoperative

▪ Electrosurgery should be avoided. Electrosurgical devices can produce radio frequency currents strong enough to cause direct coupling.[32] Direct coupling is the contact of an energized metal active electrode tip with another metal instrument or object within the surgical field.[16] When direct coupling occurs, the active electrode directly touches or comes very close to the implanted device, allowing the implanted device to become energized. This energy will seek a pathway to the return electrode. This could cause injury to the patient or damage to the implanted device.[32]

▪ An ultrasonic scalpel is considered safe to use.[14]

▪ Specific instructions on the totally implantable bone growth stimulation system specify when electrosurgery is necessary. Following implantation of this device, the electrode (ie, cathode-negative electrode) should remain connected,

Care of the patient must be individualized and appropriate to the specific device involved. Documentation should reflect the unique aspects of each patient's care. The PNDS provides a common language for perioperative nursing documentation. The examples listed below may not apply to all of the various IEDs. Each patient and device must be assessed for appropriate outcomes, nursing diagnoses, and interventions.

Domains

The following is a list of domains that may be associated with the patient undergoing surgical or other invasive procedures with an IED:

- D1—safety,
- D2—physiological responses, and
- D3-B—behavioral responses—patient and family: rights/ethics.[70]

Outcomes

The following is a partial list of nursing outcomes that may be associated with the patient undergoing surgical or other invasive procedures with an IED.

- O2—The patient is free from signs and symptoms of injury caused by extraneous objects.
- O4—The patient is free from signs and symptoms of electrical injury.
- O14—The patient's respiratory status is consistent with or improved from baseline levels established preoperatively.
- O15—The patient's cardiac status is consistent with or improved from baseline levels established preoperatively.
- O30—The patient's neurological status is consistent with or improved from baseline levels established preoperatively.
- O23—The patient participates in decision making affecting the perioperative plan of care.
- O24—The patient's care is consistent with the perioperative plan of care.[70]

Nursing Diagnoses

The following is a partial list of nursing diagnoses that may be associated with the patient undergoing surgical or other invasive procedures with an IED:

- X4—Anxiety;
- X28—Infection, risk for;
- X29—Injury, risk of;
- X30—Knowledge, deficient;
- X47—Sensory perception, disturbed;

- X56—Surgical recovery, delayed;
- X62—Urinary elimination, impaired;
- X64—Verbal communication, impaired;
- X72—Intracranial adaptive capacity, decreased; and
- X74—Pain, chronic.[70]

Interventions

The following is a partial list of nursing interventions that may be associated with the patient undergoing surgical or other invasive procedures with an IED.

- I3—Administers care to invasive device sites.
- I11—Applies safety devices.
- I30—Develops individualized plan of care.
- I37—Evaluates for signs and symptoms of electrical injury.
- I38—Evaluates for signs and symptoms of injury as a result of positioning.
- I44—Evaluates postoperative cardiac status.
- I45—Evaluates postoperative respiratory status.
- I46—Evaluates postoperative tissue perfusion.
- I47—Evaluates physiological response to plan of care.
- I54—Evaluates response to pain management interventions.
- I58—Identifies and reports the presence of implantable cardiac devices.
- I72—Implements protective measures to prevent injury due to electrical sources.
- I92—Obtains consultation from the appropriate health care providers to initiate new treatments or change existing treatments.
- I122—Uses supplies and equipment within safe parameters.
- I127—Verifies presence of prosthetics or corrective devices.
- I138—Implements protective measures prior to operative or invasive procedure.
- I145—Implements protective measures during neurosurgical procedures.
- I152—Evaluates for signs and symptoms of physical injury to skin and tissue.[70]

Conclusion

This guideline is intended to promote safe care for patients with IEDs who undergo surgical and other invasive procedures. Perioperative registered nurses should be aware of potential patient safety hazards

and the generator should be removed from the tissues and placed outside of the body until the procedure is completed. The generator should be replaced in the subcutaneous tissue at the end of the procedure.[65]

Gastric Electronic Stimulation

Electronic stimulation applied to appropriate areas in the body is beneficial in treating some disease processes that otherwise are difficult or impossible to treat with medication. Gastroparesis is an example of one such disease. Gastroparesis is characterized by delayed gastric emptying of solids without evidence of mechanical obstruction; it presents with nausea and early satiety in mild cases and chronic vomiting, dehydration, and weight loss in severe cases.[66] Gastric motility is controlled by myoelectric activity of the stomach, so abnormalities in gastric myoelectrical activity may result in gastric motility disorders, such as gastroparesis.[67]

Application of pacing techniques to the gastrointestinal tract is an attractive idea because the stomach, like the heart, has a natural pacemaker, and the myoelectric activity it generates may be entrained by electrical pacing.[67] In 1963, Bilgutay proposed the feasibility of using electrical stimulation in the gastrointestinal tract to treat paralytic ileus.[68] Using transluminal electrical stimulation via a nasogastric tube, researchers observed under fluoroscopy augmented gastric contractions and gastric emptying.[68] By the late 1960s and early 1970s, researchers conducted experiments that studied gastrointestinal myoelectric activity and its relationship with contractile activity. The results of these experiments, coupled with new techniques of recording myoelectric activity, gave rise to further research in gastrointestinal pacing.[68] Scientists today study the effects of varying the parameters of electrical stimulation applied to the wall of the stomach by an implanted device.

One IED derived from the research is the gastric electrical stimulation system. This type of therapy is indicated for the treatment of chronic nausea and vomiting associated with gastroparesis when conventional medication therapies are not providing adequate relief of symptoms for diabetic or idiopathic patients.[69] The components of a gastric electrical stimulation system include

- ♦ an implanted neurostimulator, usually surgically placed in the upper abdominal region;
- ♦ two intramuscular leads with electrodes that are implanted in the muscle wall of the stomach; and
- ♦ a programming device that the physician uses to control and adjust the settings of the neurostimulator.[69]

Patient management

Preoperative
▪ The perioperative team should be aware of the manufacturer's written warnings and precautions. The system can affect cardiac pacemakers, cardioverters/defibrillators, external defibrillators, MRI, ultrasonic equipment, electrosurgery, and radiation therapy.[69]

Nursing Process Application

The perioperative nursing vocabulary is a clinically relevant and empirically validated standardized nursing language. It relates to the delivery of care in the perioperative setting. This standardized language consists of a collection of data elements (ie, the Perioperative Nursing Data Set [PNDS]) and includes perioperative nursing diagnoses, interventions, and outcomes.[70] In 1999, the PNDS was recognized by the American Nurses Association committee on nursing practice information infrastructure as a data set useful in the practice of nursing. The perioperative patient focused model provides the conceptual framework for the PNDS and the model for perioperative nursing practice. The patient and his or her family members are at the core of the model. The model depicts perioperative nursing in four domains and illustrates the relationship between the patient, family members, and the care provided by the perioperative professional nurse.

Each data element in the PNDS is represented by a unique identifier. The domains are represented by the letter "D," followed by numbers one to four to indicate the particular domain being addressed. Nursing diagnoses are represented by the letter "X" and a number unique to the diagnosis. Interventions are represented by the letter "I" and a unique number, and outcomes are represented by the letter "O" and a unique number. These designations are used in this document as appropriate.

associated with specific IEDs and the appropriate patient care interventions and resources required to protect patients from injury.

Perioperative registered nurses should be knowledgeable about the types of IEDs that may be encountered in the practice setting, how they function, and the precautions that must be taken when caring for patients with these devices. Competency related to specific devices should be measured and documented according to individual facility policy. It is AORN's intent that perioperative registered nurses use this document to assist in the development and implementation of policies and procedures for caring for patients with IEDs who are undergoing surgical and other invasive procedures.

NOTES

1. P Seifert, "Surgical interventions," in *Cardiac Surgery: Perioperative Patient Care* (St Louis: Mosby, Inc, 2002) 508-526.

2. "Sources of electromagnetic interference (EMI) for pacemakers, implantable cardioverter defibrillators (ICDs), and heart failure devices," Guidant, Inc, *http://www.guidant.com/patient/living/* (accessed 14 Jan 2005).

3. J D Madigan et al, "Surgical management of the patient with an implanted cardiac device: Implications of electromagnetic interference," *Annals of Surgery* 230 (November 1999) 639-647.

4. *Mosby's Medical, Nursing & Allied Health Dictionary*, fifth ed (St Louis: Mosby-Year Book, Inc, 1998) 545.

5. "Electromagnetic interference (EMI)," Institute for Telecommunication Sciences, *http://www.its.bldrdoc.gov/fs-1037/dir-013/_1935.htm* (accessed 12 Nov 2004).

6. "InterStim therapy for urinary control: Product technical manual must be reviewed prior to use for detailed disclosure," Medtronic, Inc, *http://www.medtronic.com/neuro/ interstim/interstim_warning.html* (accessed 12 Nov 2004).

7. "Safety alert (May 16, 2001)," Medtronic, Inc, *http://www.medtronic.com/neuro/diathermy_alert/alert_physicians.html* (accessed 12 Nov 2004).

8. D W Fiegal, Jr, "FDA public health notification: Diathermy interactions with implanted leads and implanted systems with leads," US Food and Drug Administration, *http://www.fda.gov/cdrh/safety/121902.pdf* (accessed 14 Jan 2005).

9. "Competency statements in perioperative nursing," in *Standards, Recommended Practices and Guidelines* (Denver: AORN, Inc, 2004) 19-21.

10. C J Linstrom, "Cochlear implantation: Practical information for the generalist," *Primary Care; Clinics in Office Practice* 25 (September 1998) 583-617.

11. "Perioperative management of implanted medical devices—Draft 2" (Williamsport, Pa: Susquehanna Health System, May 2004).

12. "Preadmission testing pacemaker or ICD letter" (Williamsport, Pa: Susquehanna Health System).

13. "AORN statement on the role of the health care industry representative in the operating room," in *Standards, Recommended Practices, and Guidelines* (Denver: AORN, Inc, 2004) 153-154.

14. "Electrosurgical precautions," in *University of Iowa Hospitals and Clinics Policy and Procedure Manual* (Iowa City: University of Iowa HealthCare, February 2004).

15. "MEGA 2000 and patients with pacemakers" (Draper, Utah: Megadyne Medical Products, Inc, 2004).

16. "Recommended practices for electrosurgery," in *Standards, Recommended Practices, and Guidelines* (Denver: AORN, Inc, 2004) 245-259.

17. C Peterson, "Rectifying counts; neurostimulators; double gloving; reprocessing single-use devices; simultaneous counting," (Clinical Issues) *AORN Journal* 76 (September 2002) 510-512.

18. L Rhyne, B C Ulmer, L Revell, "Monitoring and controlling the environment," in *Patient Care During Operative and Other Invasive Procedures*, ed M L Phippen, M P Wells (Philadelphia: W B Saunders Co, 2000) 147.

19. "HeartMate® destination therapy," Hearthope.com, *http://www.hearthope.com/1.html* (accessed 14 Jan 2005).

20. "Ventricular assist device," HeartCenterOnline for Patients, *http://heartcenteronline.com/myheartdr/common/articles.cfm?ARTID-340* (accessed 30 July 2004).

21. J E Lowe, J M Wharton, "Cardiac pacemakers and implantable cardioverter-defibrillators," in *Surgery of the Chest*, sixth ed, D C Sabiston, Jr, F C Spencer, eds (Philadelphia: W B Saunders Co, 1995).

22. M Mirowski et al, "Termination of malignant ventricular arrhythmias with an implanted automatic defibrillator in human beings," *The New England Journal of Medicine* 303 (Aug 7, 1980) 322-324.

23. J L Atlee, A D Bernstein, "Cardiac rhythm management devices (Part II): Perioperative management," *Anesthesiology* 95 (December 2001) 1492-1506.

24. S P Kutalek et al, "Approach to generator change," in *Clinical Cardiac Pacing and Defibrillation*, second ed, K A Ellenbogen, G N Kay, B L Wilkoff, eds (Philadelphia: W B Saunders Co, 2000) 645-668.

25. C M Bernards, "An unusual cause of airway obstruction during general anesthesia with a laryngeal mask airway," *Anesthesiology* 100 (April 2004) 1017-1018.

26. "History of neurostimulation: Part II: Implanted neuroaugmentive devices," The Burton Report, *http://www.burtonreport.com/InfSpine/NSHistNeurostimPartII_ImpNeuroAugmenDevices.htm* (accessed 12 Nov 2004).

27. N J M Rijkhoff, "Neuroprostheses to treat neurogenic bladder dysfunction: Current status and future perspectives," *Childs Nervous System* 20 no 2 (2004) 75-86.

28. H W Roberts, "The effect of electrical dental equipment on a vagus nerve stimulator's function," *Journal of the American Dental Association* 133 (December 2002) 1657-1664.

29. J Weaver, S J Kim, A Torres, "Cutaneous electrosurgery in a patient with a deep brain stimulator," *Dermatologic Surgery* 25 (May 1999) 415-417.

30. "Electrical stimulation in spinal cord injury," International Functional Electrical Stimulation Society, *http://www.ifess.org/Services/Consumer_Ed/SCI.htm* (accessed 14 Jan 2005).

31. "Introduction to neurostimulation," Medtronic, *http://www.medtronic.com/neuro/paintherapies/pain_treatment_ladder/neurostimulation/neuroneurostimulation.html* (accessed 16 Aug 2004).

32. "Bone growth stimulation: Questions and answers," Spine Universe.com, *http://www.spineuniverse.com/displayaritcle.php/article1555.html* (accessed 13 Aug 2004).

33. *Patient's Manual for Vagus Nerve Stimulation with the VNS Therapy™ System* (Houston: Cyberonics, Inc, 2002).

34. C A Liberante, "New relief for constant condition," York Neurosurgical Associates, *http://www.yna.org/new%20pages/ YDRhydro.html* (accessed 12 Nov 2004).

35. E Eisenberg, H Waisbrod, "Spinal cord stimulator activation by an antitheft device: Case report," *Journal of Neurosurgery* 87 (December 1997) 961-962.

36. *Deep Brain Stimulation MRI Guidelines* (Minneapolis: Medtronic, April 2002) 1-14.

37. S Roberts et al, "Impact of dental devices on cochlear implants," *Journal of Endodontics* 28 (January 2002) 40.

38. "Cochlear implants: Wiring for sound," Australian Academy of Science, *http://www.science.org.au/nova/029/029key.htm* (accessed 14 Jan 2005).

39. G A Gates, R T Miyamoto, "Cochlear implants," *The New England Journal of Medicine* 349 (July 31, 2003) 421-423.

40. A J Maniglia, "State of the art on the development of the implantable hearing device for partial hearing loss," *Otolaryngologic Clinics of North America* 29 (April 1996) 225-243.

41. J M Black, J Hokanson-Hawks, A Keene, "Assist hearing in profound deafness," in *Medical-Surgical Nursing*, sixth ed (Philadelphia: W B Saunders Co, 2001) 1840-1841.

42. D R McEwen, "Otologic surgery," in *Alexander's Care of the Patient in Surgery*, 12th ed, J C Rothrock, ed (St Louis: Mosby, 2003) 717-749.

43. "Bone-anchored hearing aid," Hear-it, *http://hear-it.org/printpage.dsp?printable=yes&page=2020* (accessed 14 Jan 2005).

44. M Kalamarides et al, "Hearing restoration with auditory brainstem implants after radiosurgery for neurofibromatosis Type 2," *Journal of Neurosurgery* 95 (December 2001) 1028-1033.

45. "New device approvals—Nucleus 24 auditory brainstem implant system," US Food and Drug Administration, Center for Devices and Radiological Health, *http://www. fda.gov/cdrh/pdf/p000015.html* (accessed 22 Aug 2004).

46. S C Smeltzer, B G Bare, "Sensorineural function," in *Brunner and Suddarth's Textbook of Medical Surgical Nursing* (Philadelphia: Lippincott, Williams and Wilkins, 2004) 1744.

47. "Proposed package insert," US Food and Drug Administration, Center for Devices and Radiological Health, *http://www.fda.gov/cdrh/pdf/p000015.html* (accessed 22 Aug 2004).

48. "Is electrosurgery safe for patients with internal or external electronic devices?" *Clinical Information Hotline News* 6 (December 2001) 1-2. Also available at *http://www.valleylab.com/displaynews.cfm?articlepageid=380&menu* (accessed 12 Nov 2004).

49. M Goodman "Chemotherapy: Principles of administration," in *Cancer Nursing*, fifth ed, C H Yarbro et al, ed (Boston: Jones and Bartlett Publishers, 2000) 407-408.

50. N H Fortunato, ed, *Berry & Kohn's Operating Room Technique*, 10th ed (St. Louis: Mosby, Inc, 2004) 114-116.

51. "The Medtronic Mini-Med 2007 implantable insulin pump system," Medtronic, *http://www.minimed.com/patientfam/pf_products_implantpump_noneu.shtml* (accessed 12 Nov 2004).

52. "How pump therapy works," Medtronic, *http://www.minimed.com/patientfam/pf_ipt_ptov_howtherapyworks.shtml* (accessed 12 Nov 2004).

53. "Safety information: Medtronic MiniMed," Medtronic, *http://www.minimed.com/common/safety.html* (accessed 12 Nov 2004).

54. P E V van Kerrebroeck, "The role of electrical stimulation in voiding dysfunction," *European Urology* 34 suppl (1998) 27-30.

55. "InterStim therapy for urinary control: Product technical manual must be reviewed prior to use for detailed disclosure," Medtronic, Inc, *http://www.medtronic.com/neuro/interstim/interstim_warning.html* (accessed 12 Nov 2004).

56. J R Vignes et al, "Dorsal rhizotomy with anterior sacral root stimulation for neurogenic bladder," *Stereotactic and Functional Neurosurgery* 76 no 3-4 (2001) 243-245.

57. "The challenge: Treating selected bladder control problems and improving outcomes," Medtronic, *http://www.medtronic.com/neuro/interstim/solution.html* (accessed 12 Nov 2004).

58. M Oishi, S T Onesti, "Electrical bone graft stimulation for spinal fusion: A review," *Neurosurgery* 47 (November 2000) 1041-1055.

59. J Soyhan et al, "Demography, clinical characteristics, psychological and abuse profiles, treatment, and long-term follow-up of patients with gastroparesis," *Digestive Diseases and Sciences* 43 (November 1998) 2398-2404.

60. J T Ryaby, "Clinical effects of electromagnetic and electric fields on fracture healing," *Clinical Orthopedics and Related Research* 355 suppl (October 1998) S205-S215.

61. R K Aaron, D M Ciombor, B J Simon, "Treatment of nonunions with electric and electromagnetic fields," *Clinical Orthopedics* 419 (February 2004) 21-29.

62. "Frequently asked questions," EBI Medical, *http://www.ebimedical.com/patients/faq.cfm* (accessed 12 Nov 2004).

63. "Products: Spine systems—Spine fusion stimulators," EBI Medical, *http://www.ebimedical.com/products/index.cfm?s=0E* (accessed 12 Nov 2004).

64. W Kainz et al, "Electromagnetic compatibility of electronic implants—Review of the literature," *Wiener Klinische Wochenschrift* 113 (Dec 17, 2001) 903-914.

65. "EBI Bone Healing System," EBI Medical, *http://www.ebimedical.com/products/detail.cfm?p=0C* (accessed 12 Nov 2004).

66. K Hornbuckle, J L Barnett, "The diagnosis and work-up of the patient with gastroparesis," *Journal of Clinical Gastroenterology* 30 (March 2000) 117-124.

67. Z Lin et al, "Treatment of gastroparesis with electrical stimulation," *Digestive Diseases and Sciences* 48 (May 2003) 837-848.

68. A M Bilgutay et al, "Gastro-intestinal pacing: A new concept in the treatment of ileus," *Annals of Surgery* 158 (September 1963) 338-348.

69. "Safety information on Enterra therapy," Medtronic, *http://www.medtronic.com/neuro/gastro/indications use.html#enterra* (14 Jan 2005).

70. S Beyea, ed, *Perioperative Nursing Data Set*, second ed (Denver: AORN, Inc, 2002).

Originally published July 2005, *AORN Journal.*

Exhibit A: Care of the Patient With an Implanted Electronic Device

IMPLANTED DEVICE	SAFETY CONCERN	PREOPERATIVE PATIENT MANAGEMENT	INTRAOPERATIVE PATIENT MANAGEMENT	POSTOPERATIVE PATIENT MANAGEMENT
All implanted devices				
	Electrosurgery	Assess patients for the presence of any implanted electronic device (IED). Check for a product identification card if an IED is present. Contact the implanting surgeon to inform him or her that the patient is scheduled for surgery. Obtain and document ♦ manufacturer and model of IED, ♦ location of the device, ♦ when the device was last evaluated, ♦ if the device can be turned off before or during surgery, ♦ settings that should be reprogrammed into the device immediately after the procedure, ♦ if the implanting physician wants to be contacted when the patient enters the postanesthesia care unit, and ♦ if the patient needs to schedule an appointment with the implanting physician. Determine if electrosurgery and/or defibrillation is necessary Contact the appropriate health care industry representative and arrange for his or her presence before, during, and after the surgery if requested by the physician. Notify the anesthesia care provider that an IED is present.	Notify all perioperative team members the patient has an IED in place and review safety concerns and equipment conflicts. Be sure the programming device and qualified programming personnel are in the OR before starting the procedure. Suggest the use of a bipolar electrosurgical unit (ESU). Place the dispersive electrode as far from the IED as possible, maintaining a perpendicular pathway for the current to travel and making sure it is not over an implant and the current does not go through the IED. Do not arc current between the active electrode and another surgical instrument. If the IED has been reprogrammed by electrosurgery, stop the procedure and reprogram the device. Maintain the OR temperature between 20° C and 24° C (68° F and 76° F) and humidity between 50% and 60%.	If necessary, notify the implanting physician and/or the health care industry representative that electrosurgery or defibrillation was used during surgery. Early in the postoperative period, do an evaluation of IED function similar to that performed before surgery. Postoperatively, monitor the patient closely for signs of complications and IED malfunction.
	Defibrillation		For patients with IEDs in the chest area who require defibrillation, use anterior-posterior-type paddles. Place the anterior paddle as far from the pulse generator as possible. Use the lowest defibrillator current setting possible.	

Care of the Patient With an IED

Implanted Device	Safety Concern	Preoperative Patient Management	Intraoperative Patient Management	Postoperative Patient Management
Cardiac				
Pacemakers Implantable cardioverter defibrillators (ICDs)	Electrosurgery	1. If the IED has not been evaluated during the previous 6 months, it should be tested for programming, telemetry, thresholds, and battery status. 2. If the make and model of IED is not known, a chest x-ray may be helpful in identifying it. 3. The device should be reprogrammed to an asynchronous mode. 4. Adaptive-rate device features should be programmed off. 5. Magnet-activated testing should be programmed off.	1. The current pathway should be perpendicular to the pacemaker's lead system when possible. 2. The ESU may interfere with electrocardiogram (ECG) monitoring of the heart, so the heart rate and blood pressure (BP) should be monitored through an arterial line. When the ESU is not in use, the ECG should be checked for arrhythmias or alterations in pacemaker function. 3. If it is impossible to place the device in an asynchronous mode, and the ESU is adversely affecting the pacemaker, the ESU current should only be activated for 1 second at a time. Ten seconds should elapse between 1-second activations. 4. Bipolar ESU is recommended. 5. Tachycardia sensing should be programmed off.	1. Inform the patient's cardiologist or cardiothoracic surgeon that ESU or defibrillation was used during surgery. 2. An evaluation of the pacemaker and ICD function should be done in the early postoperative period and again at 24 and 48 hours.
	Defibrillation		1. Position paddles at least 6 inches from the device. 2. Place paddles in the anterior and posterior position. 3. The lowest defibrillator current settings should be used. 4. Have a temporary pacing system available in case of pulse generator damage.	

IMPLANTED DEVICE	SAFETY CONCERN	PREOPERATIVE PATIENT MANAGEMENT	INTRAOPERATIVE PATIENT MANAGEMENT	POSTOPERATIVE PATIENT MANAGEMENT
Cardiac, continued				
Ventricular assist device (VAD)	Electrosurgery	1. If IED has not been evaluated within the previous 6 months, it should be tested for programming, telemetry, thresholds, and battery status. 2. If the make and model of the IED is not known, a chest x-ray may be helpful in identifying it.	1. The ESU may interfere with ECG monitoring of the heart, so the heart rate and BP should be monitored through an arterial line. When the ESU is not in use, the ECG should be checked for arrhythmias or alterations in pacemaker function. 2. The device should be placed in the fixed rate mode for the duration of the surgery. 3. The ESU current should only be activated for 1 second at a time. Ten seconds should elapse between 1-second activations. 4. Cardiac output should be monitored. 5. Have an external hand pump available in the OR.	1. Inform the patient's cardiologist or cardiothoracic surgeon that ESU or defibrillation was used during surgery. 2. The surgeon or cardiologist responsible for the care of the patient should be informed if the circuit is damaged during surgery. Repair or replacement should be considered.
	Defibrillation		1. Disconnect the timing circuit from the external controller before defibrillation 2. Depending on the type of VAD, a fixed rate mode may be required during defibrillation.	
Neurological				
Deep brain stimulators Programmable ventricular shunts Spinal cord stimulators Vagal nerve stimulators	Electrosurgery	1. Magnetic resonance imaging is not recommended.	1. Bipolar ESU is recommended. 2. The device should be turned off. Notify the appropriate vendor representative. 3. Use only low voltage mode/setting. 4. Keep the grounding pad as far away from the device as possible.	1. Perioperative team members should confirm that the device is functioning properly.
	Defibrillation		1. Position paddles as far away from the IED as possible. 2. Position paddles perpendicular to the IED. 3. Use the lowest output settings.	
	Magnetic resonance imaging (MRI)		1. Magnetic resonance imaging is not recommended.	
	Bone growth stimulator		1. Keep magnetic external coils of a neurological IED a minimum of 18 inches (45 cm) away from bone growth stimulators.	
	Dental drills Ultrasonic probes Diagnostic ultrasound Electrolysis		1. Turn the device off. 2. Keep 6 inches away from device.	

IMPLANTED DEVICE	SAFETY CONCERN	PREOPERATIVE PATIENT MANAGEMENT	INTRAOPERATIVE PATIENT MANAGEMENT	POSTOPERATIVE PATIENT MANAGEMENT
Neurological, continued				
	Lasers		1. Turn the device off. 2. Keep lasers directed away from the device.	
Implantable hearing devices				
Cochlear implants Auditory brainstem implant (ABI) Bone-conduction stimulators	Static electricity	1. Educate patients and staff members that a static electric shock has been known to inactivate cochlear implants.	1. Educate patients and staff members that a static electric shock has been known to inactivate cochlear implants.	1. Perioperative team members should confirm that the device is functioning properly.
	Electrosurgery		1. Bipolar ESU is recommended. 2. Bipolar instruments should be kept more than 10 cm from extracochlear electrodes. 3. Monopolar ESU should not be used in the head and neck area. 4. For patients with ABIs, the bipolar electrode should be kept 1 cm from the ground electrodes of the ABI.	
	MRI	1. Magnetic resonance imaging is not recommended and should only be done if it is a medical necessity.	1. Magnetic resonance imaging is not recommended and should only be done if it is a medical necessity.	
	Miscellaneous		1. Remove external devices after induction of anesthesia. 2. Avoid using ionizing radiation directly over the site of the implant.	
Implantable infusion pumps				
	MRI	1. Magnetic resonance imaging may cause the device to malfunction. 2. Remove the external pump and remote control from the patient's body and the treatment area. 3. Avoid exposure to medical imaging equipment.	1. Remove the external pump and remote control from the patient's body and the treatment area. 2. Avoid exposure to medical imaging equipment.	
	X-ray	1. Remove the external pump and remote control from the patient's body and the treatment area.		

IMPLANTED DEVICE	SAFETY CONCERN	PREOPERATIVE PATIENT MANAGEMENT	INTRAOPERATIVE PATIENT MANAGEMENT	POSTOPERATIVE PATIENT MANAGEMENT
Sacral nerve stimulators				
	Miscellaneous	1. Determine how the device functions and whether it can be turned off.	1. The ESU active electrode should be kept 6 inches from the implanted device.	
Osteogenic (bone-growth) stimulators				
	MRI	1. Before imaging, the stimulator should be tested to make sure all leads are intact.		
	Miscellaneous	1. Externally worn stimulators should be removed before the surgical procedure.		
	Electrocautery		1. Monopolar ESU is not recommended. 2. Ultrasonic scalpel is considered safe. 3. Electrodes should remain connected. 4. The generator should be removed from subcutaneous tissues and placed outside of the body until the procedure is complete.	
Gastric electronic stimulation				
	Miscellaneous	1. Review manufacturers' written warnings and precautions. 2. Devices can affect other IEDs. 3. Device is affected by MRI, ultrasonic equipment, ESU, and radiation therapy.		

AORN Guidance Statement: Creating a Patient Safety Culture

Introduction

The purpose of this guidance statement is to assist managers and clinicians in developing policies and procedures related to creating a patient safety culture.

Since the Institute of Medicine (IOM) report released in 1999, the vast majority of patient safety initiatives have focused on micro issues, such as medication errors and wrong-site surgery, with little emphasis on the macro issue of culture. Edgar Schien, professor of management at the Sloan School of Management, Massachusetts Institute of Technology, defines *culture* as the set of shared, implicit assumptions that a group holds and that determines how it perceives, thinks about, and reacts to its various environments.[1] In broader terms, culture is a mindset centering on shared values, attitudes, or beliefs within an organization. As defined in the health care literature, a safety culture is an environment that encourages reporting,[2] ends blame,[3] involves senior leadership,[4] and focuses on systems.[5]

Lucian Leape, adjunct professor of health policy, Harvard School of Public Health, Harvard University, Boston, has stated the single greatest impediment to error prevention is that "we punish people for making mistakes."[6] Medical errors are grossly unreported across the country; only 2% to 3% of major errors are reported,[6] and when reported, they don't create stories or generate action.[7] Analytical methods such as root cause analysis (RCA) and the failure mode and effects analysis (FMEA) will not work in detecting the causes or errors if health care workers are bound by a "code of silence," fear retribution, or are uncomfortable revealing imperfection in a process for which they are responsible.[8]

To date, most of the work in patient safety has been reactive. As the culture matures with increased information and trust, the emphasis will switch to a more proactive or generative approach.

Background

In review of the literature, few hospitals have assessed their organizations' safety culture, nor have many actually measured the impact of interventions. One study, conducted in April 2001, reported that 15 California hospitals conducted a safety culture survey with two objectives: (1) measure attitudes toward patient safety and organizational culture; and (2) determine how the culture of safety varied among the hospitals and between the various types of health care workers.[9] The majority of the participants in the study responded in ways that indicated a positive safety culture; however, senior leadership gave fewer problematic responses than frontline workers, and clinicians—in particular nurses—were more pessimistic.[10]

Johns Hopkins Hospital conducted a systematic assessment on safety and developed a strategic plan to improve safety.[11] Its study revealed a comparable culture of safety as compared to the airline industry, but identified several areas for improvement. Key messages identified were that senior leaders need to be more visible to frontline caregivers when addressing safety; safety planning must be proactive; physicians are less aware of safety initiatives than nurses; and physicians must actively participate in the education process.[11]

Preamble

The intention of this guidance statement is to provide a framework from which perioperative teams can foster a patient-centric safety culture and assist with the development of policies and procedures that will support that culture. A patient-centric safety culture consists of five major subcultures: reporting, flexible, just, learning,[5] and wary[2] (Figure 1).

Reporting Culture

A reporting culture is a culture in which all members of the perioperative team readily report errors and near misses. A reporting culture can be assessed by the types of errors reported by staff. As the safety culture matures, there is increased risk-taking associated with errors reported. In a true reporting culture, individuals report events to allow all staff in the organization to learn from the experience.

Suggested strategies[5-7]
- Focus on both actual events and near misses.
- Use FMEA proactively to anticipate and prevent potential error.
- Discuss close calls, "good catches," and how harm to the patient was avoided or minimized.
- Develop a documentation system that is easy to use.
- Develop a reporting system that focuses on storytelling and knowledge-sharing.

Figure 1

PATIENT-CENTRIC SAFETY CULTURE

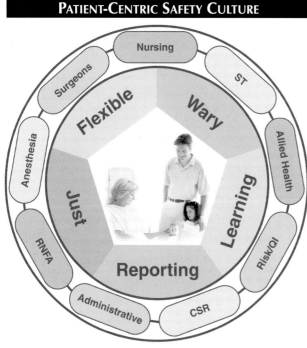

© Kate A. O'Toole. Used with permission.

- Focus on individual cases that provide learning opportunities.
- Identify ways to circulate stories and lessons learned throughout the facility.
- Provide feedback to the staff on all issues reported.
- Develop metrics for success (eg, increase number of reports).
- Prioritize improvement initiatives based on themes discovered and potential risks revealed.
- Use a process that emphasizes quality improvement (eg, Plan, Do, Check, Act).

Flexible Culture

A flexible culture is a culture that is nimble enough to keep pace with the rapid changes in health care.

Suggested strategies[7,9-11]
- Identify model for improvement programs that focuses on rapid cycle change.
- Develop processes that ensure shared leadership.
- Shared leadership is a hallmark of the organization.
- An environment of respect, collaboration, and trust exists between all team members and leadership.

Learning Culture

A learning culture is a culture that is capable and ready to gain knowledge from experiences and data, and that is willing to implement major changes as indicated from safety information systems. A learning culture is informed and learns from incidents and near misses.[8]

Suggested strategies
- Foster learning opportunities through open communication.
- Develop the ability to adapt to the changing health care environment and be receptive to change.
- Frontline staff is engaged to use initiative to problem-solve unique situations.
- Individual performance is linked to team performance.

Wary Culture

A wary culture is a culture in which the all members of the perioperative team are continually aware of the unexpected. Being vigilant is a healthy state that is a combination of being informed and aware that, at any given moment, an untoward event can occur. Healthy reporting, learning, and flexible cultures will facilitate a wary culture.

Suggested strategies[5,7,12,13]
- Go "looking for trouble"; conduct executive walk-arounds in all perioperative areas.
- Become preoccupied with opportunities for improvement.
- Be willing to challenge assumptions.
- How can we "stop the line" and still stay efficient?
- How can we get better when we know we are the best?

Just Culture

A just culture is a culture that provides an environment of trust where all members of the perioperative team are encouraged to provide safety-related data and are acutely aware of the distinction between acceptable and unacceptable behavior. Errors and mistakes must be evaluated in a manner such that contributing factors are reviewed first, and then accountability is determined in relation to actions. A just culture is not a nonpunitive (ie, blame-free) environment, but rather an environment where actions are analyzed to ensure that individual accountability is established and appropriate actions are taken.[12]

Health care organizations must adopt a disciplinary system theory approach in promoting a just culture that freely reports errors. To understand the interrelationship between discipline and patient safety, four behavioral concepts are examined: human error, negligence, intentional rule violations, and reckless conduct.[7]

When evaluating an adverse event, care must be taken to determine whether human error or misconduct has occurred. Historically, most disciplinary actions are based upon the outcome of the mishap; if a patient is harmed, then that health care worker is considered blameworthy. By assigning blame, the health care organization stands to lose an opportunity to learn from the error and the error may reoccur. Disciplinary policies must balance the benefits of a learning culture with the need to retain personal accountability and discipline.[12] Adverse event investigation tools may be created to augment the use of the suggested strategy identified below.

Suggested strategy
James Reason, professor of psychology, University of Manchester, United Kingdom, created a model to assist managers to determine culpability after an untoward event has occurred.[13] (Figure 2 is an adaptation of the Reason model applied to the perioperative setting.) Perioperative leadership should apply this model when investigating incidences to determine whether disciplinary action is warranted. Six basic steps are used. It is important to focus on the error and not the outcome.

Step 1. The first line of questioning is to establish intent. Was this action or omission deliberate? If there was deliberate intent, the action or omission is culpable.

Step 2. If no intent is established, then determine whether substance use or abuse was involved. If abuse is determined, culpability is established. If the health care worker is taking a medication for medical reasons and is aware that he or she could be impaired, culpability is present; however, it is not as egregious as abuse.

Step 3. If the health care worker is not under the influence of drugs or alcohol, the next determinant is whether he or she knowingly violated safe operating procedures. This aids in determining reckless behavior. The threshold for reckless behavior is met when procedures are available, correct, and workable, but still are violated by the health care worker. If there are no adequate procedures in place, a systems error has occurred. When evaluating the situation, care must be taken to determine whether "normalization of deviance" is taking place—that is, whether there is a policy or procedure in place, but it not widely followed.

Step 4. If a policy or procedure is violated, a substitution test is conducted. Peers are asked how they would behave in a similar situation. If the peers respond the same as in the error in question, a systems-induced error is established. If they respond differently, possible negligence should be considered.

Step 5. The next question is whether the health care worker has a history of unsafe acts. If the questions in steps 1 through 4 are unsubstantiated, and there is no history of unsafe acts, then it is human error with no culpability. If the health care worker does have a history of unsafe acts, this particular incident may not be culpable; however, the organization should review the record for trends and may consider moving the health care worker to a lower-risk environment.

Step 6. The last question and assessment is where the possibility of mitigating circumstances is examined. Possible factors include stressors (eg, anger, fear, personal issues), distractions, and interruptions (eg, pagers, music, environmental temperature, extraneous conversation, overhead paging). Environmental influences include but are not limited to, physical plant and wrong size room for operative and other invasive procedures (eg, overcrowded, not ergonomic).

It is important to note that the accountability model does not evaluate or determine the proof legally required to prove reckless behavior or criminal negligence. This model should not be used for performance rating of surgical team members. It should be utilized by leadership after all the facts have been gathered, but as soon after the event as possible. If more than one person is involved, the model should be applied separately for each person.

Figure 2

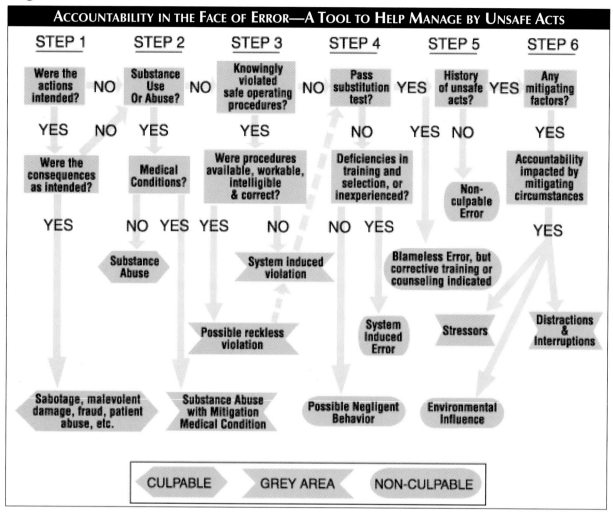

Summary

AORN believes all health care organizations must strive to create a culture of safety. Such a culture will provide an atmosphere where all members of the perioperative team can openly discuss errors, process improvements, or system issues without fear of reprisal. A culture of safety places an emphasis on flexibility and learning as a means of improving safety and reducing errors. Characteristics of a culture of safety include the following:

♦ communication is open and honest;
♦ the emphasis is on the team rather than the individual;
♦ standards and practices are developed in a multidisciplinary framework;
♦ staff members are helpful and supportive of each other;

♦ staff members trust each other;
♦ surgical team members have a friendly, open relationship emphasizing credibility and attentiveness;
♦ the environment is resilient, encourages creativity, and is patient outcomes-driven;
♦ the focus is on work flow and process; and
♦ these attributes are supported by an informed culture that learns from incidents and near misses.

A commitment to safety must be articulated at all levels of the organization. Safety must be valued as the top priority, even at the expense of efficiency. Health care organizations must allocate an appropriate amount of resources and provide the necessary incentives or rewards to promote a robust patient safety culture. AORN recognizes that most patient safety initiatives will fail in the absence of a viable safety culture.

Glossary

Accountable: Responsible for one's actions or conduct.

Adverse event: Experiencing harm from error.

Culture: The shared norms, values, and practices associated with a nation, organization, or profession.[14]

Error: Failure of a planned action to be completed as intended, or the use of a wrong plan to achieve an outcome.

Failure mode and effects analysis (FMEA): A proactive tool used to anticipate and prevent the potential for product or process failure.

Just culture: An environment where actions are analyzed to ensure that individual accountability is established and appropriate actions are taken.[15]

Medical error: An adverse event or near miss that is preventable with the current state of medical knowledge.[16]

Near miss: An event or situation that could have resulted in an accident, injury, or illness, but did not, either by chance or timely intervention.[17]

Negligence: Failure to use such care as a reasonable prudent and careful person would use under similar circumstances.[17]

Root cause analysis (RCA): A process for identifying the basic or causal factor(s) that underlie variation in performance, including the occurrence or possible occurrence of a sentinel event.[18]

Safety: Freedom from accidental injury.

Safety culture: An environment that encourages reporting,[2] ends blame,[3] involves senior leadership,[4] and focuses on systems.[5]

NOTES

1. E H Schein, *Organizational Culture and Leadership,* second ed (San Francisco: Jossey-Bass, 1992).

2. P Hudson, "Applying the lessons of high-risk industries to health care," *Quality and Safety in Health Care* 12 Suppl 1 (December 2003) i7-i12.

3. L Larson, "Ending the culture of blame: A look at why medical errors happen-and what needs to change," *Trustee* 53 (February 2000) 6-10.

4. H S Ruchlin et al, "The role of leadership in instilling a culture of safety: Lessons from the literature," *Journal of Healthcare Management* 49 (January/February 2004) 47-59.

5. J M Krumberger, "Building a culture of safety," *RN* 64 (January 2001) 32ac2-32ac3.

6. J Reason, *Human Error* (New York: Cambridge University Press, 1990).

7. D Marx, "Patient safety and the 'Just Culture': A primer for health care executives," Medical Event Reporting System for Transfusion Medicine, *http://www.mers-tm.net/support/Marx_Primer.pdf* (accessed 2 Dec 2005).

8. "The IOM medical errors report: 5 years later, the journey continues," *The Quality Letter for Healthcare Leaders* 17 (January 2005) 2-10.

9. V F Nieva, J Sorra, "Safety culture assessment: A tool for improving patient safety in healthcare organizations," *Quality and Safety in Health Care* 12 suppl 2 (December 2003) ii17-23.

10. S J Singer et al, "The culture of safety: Results of an organization-wide survey in 15 California hospitals," *Quality and Safety in Health Care* 12 (April 2003) 112-118.

11. P J Pronovost et al, "Evaluation of the culture of safety: Survey of clinicians and managers in an academic medical center," *Quality and Safety in Health Care* 12 (December 2003) 405-410.

12. "Just culture toolkit," The Risk Management and Patient Safety Institute, *http://www.rmpsi.com/education/liveprograms/JustCultureToolkit.pdf* (accessed 2 Dec 2005).

13. J Reason, *Engineering a Safety Culture* (London: Ashgate Publishing, 1997) 209.

14. R L Helmreich, A C Merritt, *Culture at Work in Aviation and Medicine: National, Organizational, and Professional Influences* (Brookfield, Vt: Ashgate, 1998).

15. R H Kilmann, M J Sexton, R A Serpa, eds, "Five key issues in understanding and changing culture," in *Gaining Control of the Corporate Culture* (San Francisco: Jossey-Bass, 1985), 1-17.

16. "Glossary of terms," in *Doing What Counts for Patient Safety: Federal Actions to Reduce Medical Errors and Their Impact,* Quality Interagency Coordination Task Force, *http://www.quic.gov/report%2Dbackup/mederr8.htm#terms* (accessed 2 Dec 2005).

17. "Sentinel event glossary of terms," Joint Commission on Accreditation of Healthcare Organizations, *http://www.jcaho.org/accredited+organizations/sentinel+event/glossary.htm* (2 Dec 2005).

18. D E Broadbent, *Third Report: Organising for Safety* (London: Health and Safety Commission, 1993).

RESOURCES

Carroll, J S; Quijada, M A. "Redirecting traditional professional values to support safety: Changing organisational culture in health care," *Quality and Safety in Health Care* 13 suppl 2 (December 2004) ii16-21.

Davies, H T; Nutley, S M; Mannion, R. "Organisational culture and quality of health care," *Quality in Health Care* 9 (June 2000) 111-119.

Hofstede, G H; Hofstede, G J. *Cultures and Organizations: Software of the Mind,* second ed (New York: McGraw Hill, 2005).

Kowalczyk, L. "Hospitals study when to apologize to patients," *Boston Globe,* July 24, 2005. Available at *http://www.boston.com/tools/archives* (fee required).

Barach, P; Small, S D. "Reporting and preventing medical mishaps: Lessons from non-medical near miss reporting systems," *BMJ* 320 (March 18, 2000) 759-763.

"Safety climate survey (IHI tool)," Institute for Healthcare Improvement, *http://www.ihi.org/IHI/Topics/Patient Safety/SafetyGeneral/Tools/Safety+Climate+Survey +%28IHI+Tool%29.htm* (accessed 2 Dec 2005).

Schein, E H. "Culture: The missing concept in organization studies," *Administrative Science Quarterly* 41 no 2 (June 1996) 229-240.

Schein, E H. "Three cultures of management: The key to organizational learning," *MIT Sloan Management Review* 38 (Fall 1996) 9-20. Also available at *http:// sloanreview.mit.edu/smr/issue/1996/fall/1* (accessed 2 Dec 2005).

Wachter, R M; Shojania, K G. *Internal Bleeding: The Truth Behind America's Terrifying Epidemic of Medical Mistakes,* second ed (New York: Rugged Land, 2005).

Approved by the AORN Board of Directors, November 2005. Scheduled for publication in the *AORN Journal* in 2006.

AORN Guidance Statement: Postoperative Patient Care in the Ambulatory Surgery Setting

Introduction

This guidance statement provides a framework for health care practitioners to use when developing and implementing policies and procedures for postoperative patient care in the ambulatory surgery setting. AORN defines *postoperative* as "the time [that] begins with admission to the postanesthesia care area and ends with a resolution of surgical sequelae."[1(p31)] This includes the postanesthesia phases I, II, and III. These phases are defined by the American Society of PeriAnesthesia Nurses' (ASPAN's) *Standards of Perianesthesia Nursing Practice* as follows.[2]

Phase I focuses on providing a transition from a totally anesthetized state to one requiring less acute interventions. Recovery occurs in the postanesthesia care unit (PACU). The purpose of this phase is for patients to regain physiological homeostasis and receive appropriate nursing intervention as needed.

Phase II focuses on preparing the patient for self-care, care by family members, or care in an extended care environment. The patient is discharged to phase II recovery when intensive nursing care no longer is needed. In the phase II area, sometimes referred to as the step-down or discharge area, the patient becomes more alert and functional.

Phase III focuses on providing ongoing care for patients who require extended observation or intervention after transfer from phase I or phase II. Interventions are directed toward preparing the patient for self-care or care by family members. Phase III is designed for patients who are unable to meet the criteria for discharge from phase II and the ambulatory unit. These patients may need alternative care, such as home health care or a stay in an overnight short-stay hospital unit or recovery center.

This guidance statement is directed specifically to ambulatory surgery centers (ASCs). It also may be used in other ambulatory settings that perform surgery or other invasive procedures. The ambulatory surgery setting is defined as an area where outpatient surgery or other invasive procedures are performed, including, but not limited to, freestanding surgery centers, hospital-based ambulatory surgical units, physicians' offices, cardiac catheterization suites, endoscopy units, and radiology departments.

Perioperative nurses have limited contact with patients before surgery, which may lead to an increased risk for adverse patient outcomes. Ambulatory surgery centers must have consistent approaches to postoperative patient care to ensure patient safety. This guidance statement is intended to promote patient safety in the ambulatory surgery setting.

Guidance Statement

Ambulatory surgery centers should develop written policies and procedures for postoperative patient care. Policies and procedures should include, but not be limited to, the following elements:

- staffing,
- supplies and equipment,
- postanesthesia care,
- fast tracking of patients,
- pain management,
- documentation,
- discharge criteria,
- discharge instructions, and
- monitoring of outcomes.

The criteria in this guidance statement represent the minimum levels of care.

Perioperative Nursing Data Set

The Perioperative Nursing Data Set (PNDS) is a clinically relevant and empirically validated standardized nursing vocabulary describing perioperative nursing. It relates to the delivery of care in all perioperative settings. This standardized language consists of a collection of data elements and includes perioperative nursing diagnoses, interventions, and outcomes. The PNDS should be used to develop ambulatory surgery patient plans of care and to standardize nursing documentation. In addition, PNDS outcomes, as well as outcome indicators, interventions, and nursing diagnoses, can be

- incorporated into competencies, policies and procedures, job descriptions, pathways, guidelines, and care plans;
- linked to the electronic health record;
- used as a tool for teaching new nurses about perioperative nursing; and
- applied in performance improvement projects and benchmarking.

Each data element in the PNDS corresponds to a unique identifier. The domains are represented by the letter "D" followed by numbers 1 to 3 to indicate the particular domain being addressed. Nursing diagnoses are represented by the letter "X" and a number unique to the diagnosis. Interventions are represented by the letter "I" and a unique number, and outcomes are represented by the letter "O" and a unique number. These designations are identified in this document with unique identifiers noted in parentheses. A list of outcomes, interventions, and nursing diagnoses specific to each domain is printed in an appendix of the PNDS reference book.[3]

The PNDS is conceptualized by the perioperative patient focused model. The patient and his or her family members are at the center of the model's framework. The model depicts perioperative nursing in four domains and illustrates the relationship between the patient, family members, and the care provided by the perioperative RN. The patient-centered domains are

- D1—patient safety;
- D2—physiological responses to surgery; and
- D3—patient and family member behavioral responses to surgery, including
  - behavior responses—knowledge, and
  - behavior responses—rights and ethics.[3]

Nursing Care Policies

Perianesthesia nursing care policies and procedures should be available in the PACU and all areas where other postoperative care (phase I, II, or III) is delivered.[4] At a minimum, each nurse should review the policies and procedures periodically, and the review process should be documented. Specific criteria for postanesthesia care policies and procedures should include

- assessment of data elements;
- supplies and equipment required for each phase of recovery;
- postoperative patient care;
- emergency medications[5] and equipment;
- patient classification;
- infection control (O10);
- pain management (O20), patient knowledge of pain (O29), and pain control;
- documentation of patient care;
- patient transfer; and
- care of patients receiving moderate sedation.[6]

Staffing

A staffing plan should be developed and used to provide an adequate number and mix of personnel to meet patient care needs.[7,8] The staffing plan should include criteria regarding the number of patients, number of ORs and procedure rooms, average patient length of stay, and intensity of care.[6] An operational patient classification system may help in determining and allocating nursing personnel.[9] The ASPAN "Recommended staffing guidelines" should be used as a guide to calculate requirements for postanesthesia staffing needs (Table 1).

Staffing for an ASC PACU should conform to national and state guidelines and regulations for safe postanesthesia nursing care.[4] Additional practice standards that apply to postanesthesia care also should be followed and should include personnel competency requirements that meet state licensure guidelines, organizational guidelines, accreditation and professional standards, procedure-specific training, and professional experience.[10,11] Personnel should be trained in the use of emergency equipment and cardiopulmonary resuscitation for both adult and pediatric patients if pediatric care is provided.[12] Advanced cardiac life support and pediatric advanced life support training, if pediatric care is provided, is recommended for all PACU nurses. All staff members should undergo a comprehensive orientation program, and competencies should be documented.

Supplies and Equipment

A checklist of required supplies and equipment for PACU phase I and PACU phase II should be developed.[13] A method should be in place to ensure all equipment is maintained according to manufacturers' specifications.[14] Equipment must be available to

- administer oxygen (I87);
- provide suction (I87);
- maintain IV access (I34); and
- monitor postoperative cardiac status (I44) (I120)
  - blood pressure,
  - heart rhythm and rate, and
  - oxygen saturation.[15]

Emergency equipment, an emergency communication system, and knowledgeable emergency assistive personnel should be readily available.[14,16] Emergency equipment and supplies should include a defibrillator, medications, oxygen, a positive-pressure breathing device, suction equipment, and appropriate nasal and oral airways.[17,18]

Table 1

Recommended Staffing Guidelines*

Phase I level of care

Class 1:2

One nurse to two patients who are
- One unconscious, stable, without artificial airway, and older than the age of 8; and one conscious, stable, and free of complications
- Two conscious, stable, and free of complications
- Two conscious, stable, 8 years of age and younger, with family or competent support staff present

Class 1:1

One nurse to one patient
- At the time of admission, until the critical elements are met
- Requiring mechanical life support and/or artificial airway
- Any unconscious patient 8 years of age and younger
- A second nurse must be available to assist as necessary

Class 2:1

Two nurses to one patient
- One critically ill, unstable, complicated patient

Two licensed nurses, one of whom is an RN competent in Phase I postanesthesia nursing, are present** whenever a patient is receiving Phase I level of care.

Phase II level of care

Class 1:3

One nurse to three patients
- Older than 8 years of age
- 8 years of age and younger with family present

Class 1:2

One nurse to two patients
- 8 years of age and younger without family or support staff present
- Initial admission of patient postprocedure

Class 1:1

One nurse to one patient
- Unstable patient of any age requiring transfer.

Two competent personnel, one of whom is an RN competent in Phase II postanesthesia nursing, are present** whenever a patient is receiving Phase II level of care. An RN must be present at all times during Phase II.

Phase III level of care

Class 1:3/5

One nurse to three to five patients
- Examples include, but are not limited to,
  - patients awaiting transportation home,
  - patients with no caregiver,
  - patients who have had procedures requiring extended observation/intervention (ie, potential risk for bleeding, pain management, postoperative nausea, vomiting).

Phase III staffing is dictated by patient acuity and intensity of nursing care. Care is managed by an RN competent in the Phase III level of care. The nurse:patient ratio is not to exceed one nurse to five patients.

* Adapted with permission from the American Society of PeriAnesthesia Nurses.
** The American Society of PeriAnesthesia Nurses defines "present" as being in the particular place where the patient is receiving care.

Postanesthesia Care

A postanesthesia care policy and procedure should be written for transporting, monitoring, and evaluating patients in the PACU.[19] Patients should have a complete systems assessment during the first few minutes of PACU care.[4] This assessment should include, but not be limited to,

- vital signs (I59) (I128) (I16);
- respiratory adequacy (I45);
- postoperative cardiac status (I59);
- peripheral circulation (ie, postoperative tissue perfusion) (I46);
- postoperative neurological status (I146);
- level of consciousness (I144) (I146);
- alertness (I144) (I146);
- lucidity (I144) (I146);
- orientation (I144) (I146);
- IV patency (I34);
- allergies and sensitivities (I123);
- pain management (I16);
- motor abilities (I146);
- return of sensory and motor control in areas affected by local or regional anesthetics (I146);[4]
- skin integrity (I38) (I46);[3,4]
- temperature regulation (I78);
- positioning (I38);
- surgical wound site (I4) (I130);
- nausea and vomiting (I128) (I153); and
- fluid and electrolyte balance (I132).

The postanesthesia nurse should provide ongoing assessments and re-evaluations concurrently with nursing interventions.[4,20]

A nursing care plan should be based on the initial patient assessment and documented appropriately. The perioperative nurse analyzes the assessment data to determine nursing diagnoses. Following is a partial list of nursing diagnoses that may be associated with patients undergoing ambulatory surgery:

- X38 (D2)—pain, acute;
- X73 (D2)—nausea;
- X28 (D2)—infection, risk for;
- X26 (D2)—hypothermia; and
- X21 (D2)—gas exchange, impaired.[3]

Postoperative Patient Outcomes

Nursing interventions are initiated to achieve a desired conclusion and/or to reduce the probability of undesired outcomes.[3,21] Following is a partial list of patient outcomes that may be associated with a patient's postoperative experience:

- (O14)—the patient's respiratory status is consistent with or improved from baseline levels established preoperatively;
- (O25)—the patient's right to privacy is maintained;
- (O30)—the patient's neurologic status is consistent with or improved from baseline levels established preoperatively;
- (O19)—the patient demonstrates knowledge of medication management.[3]

Fast Tracking of Patients

Fast tracking is defined as transferring a patient directly from the OR to PACU phase II, bypassing PACU phase I. Policy and procedures should be developed before initiating a patient fast-tracking process.[22-25] Patient education concerning fast tracking begins during the preoperative assessment.

Wherever fast tracking is practiced, a collaborative plan of care should be developed by anesthesia care providers and perianesthesia nurses.[22] The plan should include

- written guidelines addressing patient selection,[26]
- preoperative patient education,
- selection and management of anesthetic agents,
- assessment criteria,
- discharge criteria, and
- monitoring and reporting of patient outcomes.

Pain Management

Policies and procedures for treatment of pain, nausea, and vomiting in the PACU should be written.[27,28] Every patient should receive an initial and ongoing evaluation and assessment of pain. Assessment of pain, the fifth vital sign, includes pain intensity, location, quality, duration, onset, and treatment effectiveness.[20,27] Each facility should adopt a consistent pain management scale for assessing pain, including scales for special patient populations. Separate documentation should be maintained for each pain site.[27,29]

A policy and procedure that specifies that anesthesia orders take precedence over surgeon's orders for immediate postoperative treatment in the PACU should be developed.[27] Anesthesia orders should be documented and include preferred medications to be used for treating the patient.[27]

Documentation

A comprehensive system for documenting patient events, assessments, and treatments to prevent duplication and provide for a smooth progression of care should be established.[5,30] The PNDS should be incorporated into the nursing documentation.[3] The PACU record should allow for checklist documentation of routine care rather than narrative documentation. Descriptive notes should focus on deviations from expected outcomes and individual patient responses to treatment and interventions.[4]

Postoperative documentation should include the patient's assessment, treatment, and reactions to treatment.[30] Specific documentation should include, but not be limited to,

- ♦ respiratory status (I87);
- ♦ cardiac status (I44);
- ♦ peripheral circulation (I46);
- ♦ neurological status (I146);[30]
- ♦ pain (I16) (I51), nausea, or vomiting (I128) (I153);
- ♦ condition of the surgical site (I130) or bleeding (I132);
- ♦ temperature (I86) (I131) (I55);
- ♦ chills or shivering (I78) (I89);
- ♦ urinary status (I23) (I89) (I153);
- ♦ administration of fluids or electrolytes (I5) (I153);
- ♦ administration of medication and responses (I8) (I51);[30]
- ♦ administration of antibiotics (I7) (I51);
- ♦ emotional status (I68) (I137) (I147);[3] and
- ♦ unusual events or postoperative complications (I92) (I111).[30]

Discharge Criteria

Discharge policies and procedures should be written and implemented.[31] Discharge criteria should be based on standards or general guidelines for discharging patients established by accrediting organizations and anesthesia and postanesthesia provider associations.[6] The patient's postprocedure status should be assessed before he or she is discharged from the postsedation or postanesthesia recovery room.[20]

The discharge policy should clearly specify who is responsible for discharging the patient from PACU phase I, II, and III.[15] Written criteria should include specific guidelines patients must meet before being discharged to the next level of care or discharged directly home.[28,32] These criteria should include a numeric scoring system to evaluate the patient's condition.[4,31]

Discharge criteria should include an evaluation of the patient for nausea, vomiting, pain, chills, shivering, the surgical site condition, and bleeding. The patient's emotional status, fluid and urinary status, cognitive abilities, peripheral circulation, and temperature also should be evaluated.[4]

Patient Transfer

Whenever a patient is transferred from one level of care to another level of care, the perioperative RN should communicate all pertinent information to the next caregiver. After the perioperative RN completes the final assessment before patient discharge, the perioperative RN will provide a transfer report.[2] Communication between caregivers is essential for patient safety and appropriate and consistent nursing care. Items in the transfer report should include, but are not limited to,

- ♦ vital signs (O15) and airway patency (O14);
- ♦ level of consciousness (O30);
- ♦ muscular strength (O30);[33]
- ♦ allergies;
- ♦ condition of operative site/dressing (O11);
- ♦ location and patency of tubes and/or drains;
- ♦ medications given and response to those medications (O9);
- ♦ intake and output (eg, IV, estimated blood loss) (O13);[33]
- ♦ tests ordered with pertinent results, if available;
- ♦ pain level (O29);
- ♦ nausea and vomiting (O13);[2]
- ♦ psychosocial status (O28) (O31); and
- ♦ discharge orders.

An emergency care and transfer plan should be in place, including a formal policy and procedure for hospital admission.[28] Personnel should be familiar with the process for transporting patients according to the plan. A policy for handling patients who leave the facility against medical advice also should be written.[31]

Discharge Instructions

Written postoperative and follow-up care instructions should be provided to each patient and should reflect the patient's individual informational needs specific to home care, response to unexpected events,[8,15,34] and follow-up by the physician.[16] Discharge instructions should be reviewed with the patient and a responsible adult before discharge.[15,31,35] Discharge information should include medication use, side effects, signs and symptoms to report, and when to contact the health care provider for additional assistance.[27,36]

Monitoring of Outcomes

Policies and procedures for completing discharge follow-up with the patient to assess and evaluate the patient's status should be written.[36-39] Discharge follow-up should include ongoing pain assessment and determination of the efficacy of the prescribed pain medication.[27,40] If a staff member other than a professional nurse conducts the follow-up telephone call, the protocol should include a decision tree with a branch identifying professional nurse interventions for any unexpected outcome. Results of patient follow-up telephone calls should be documented.

The facility should collect data to monitor its performance.[41] Data collected should include patients' perceptions of care, treatment, and provision of services, including specific individual needs and expectations, how well the facility met these needs, surgical site infections, how the facility can improve patient safety, and the effectiveness of pain management, when applicable.[41]

NOTES

1. "Competency statements in perioperative nursing," in *Standards, Guidelines, and Recommended Practices* (Denver: AORN, Inc, 2004) 19-31.

2. *Standards of Perianesthesia Nursing Practice* (Cherry Hill, NJ: American Society of PeriAnesthesia Nurses, 2002) 4-5.

3. *Perioperative Nursing Data Set: The Perioperative Nursing Vocabulary*, second ed, S Beyea ed (Denver: AORN, Inc, 2002) 97.

4. R Ferrara-Love, "Immediate postanesthesia care," in *Ambulatory Surgical Nursing*, second ed, N Burden, ed (Philadelphia: WB Saunders Co, 2000) 409-476.

5. S Smith, "Progressive postanesthesia care: Phase II recovery," in *Ambulatory Surgical Nursing*, second ed, N Burden, ed (Philadelphia: WB Saunders Co, 2000) 477-503.

6. D Geuder, "Postoperative patient care," in *Ambulatory Surgery Principles and Practices*, third ed, N J Vinson, ed (Denver: AORN Inc, 2003) 133-144.

7. "Standard III: Staffing and personnel management," in *Standards of Perianesthesia Nursing Practice* (Cherry Hill, NJ: American Society of PeriAnesthesia Nurses, 2002) 14.

8. "Surgical and related services," in *Accreditation Guidebook for Office Based Surgery* (Wilmette, Ill: Accreditation Association for Ambulatory Health Care, 2004) 47-52.

9. J A Kusler-Jensen, "A patient classification system for ambulatory surgery centers," *AORN Journal* 64 (August 1996) 273-277.

10. "Standards for postanesthesia care," in *ASA Standards, Guidelines and Statements* (Park Ridge, Ill: American Society of Anesthesiologists, 2002) 7.

11. "Quality of care provided," in *Accreditation Guidebook for Office Based Surgery* (Wilmette, Ill: Accreditation Association for Ambulatory Health Care, 2004) 19-21.

12. "Management of human resources," in *2004 Comprehensive Accreditation Manual for Ambulatory Care* (Oakbrook Terrace, Ill: Joint Commission on Accreditation of Healthcare Organizations, 2004) HR1-HR12.

13. "Resource 5: Equipment for preanesthesia phase, PACU phase I, phase II, and phase III," in *Standards of Perianesthesia Nursing Practice* (Cherry Hill, NJ: American Society of PeriAnesthesia Nurses, 2002) 32-35.

14. "Facilities and environment," in *Accreditation Guidebook for Office Based Surgery* (Wilmette, Ill: Accreditation Association for Ambulatory Health Care, 2004) 35-38.

15. "Guidelines for ambulatory anesthesia and surgery," American Society of Anesthesiologists, *http://www.asahq.org/publicationsAndServices/standards/04.pdf* (accessed 9 April 2004).

16. D O'Brien, V A Walter, N Burden, "Special procedures in the ambulatory setting," in *Ambulatory Surgical Nursing*, second ed, N Burden, ed (Philadelphia: WB Saunders Co, 2000) 817-842.

17. J Odom, "Conscious sedation/analgesia," in *Ambulatory Surgical Nursing*, second ed, N Burden, ed (Philadelphia: WB Saunders Co, 2000) 309-330.

18. "Resource 6: Emergency drugs and equipment," in *Standards of Perianesthesia Nursing Practice* (Cherry Hill, NJ: American Society of PeriAnesthesia Nurses, 2002) 36-37.

19. "Practice guidelines for postanesthesia care," American Society of Anesthesiologists, *http://www.asahq.org/publicationsAndServices/postanes.pdf* (accessed 29 Sept 2004).

20. "Provision of care, treatment, and services," in *2004 Comprehensive Accreditation Manual for Ambulatory Care* (Oakbrook Terrace, Ill: Joint Commission on Accreditation of Healthcare Organizations, 2004) PC1-PC50.

21. J C Rothrock, *Perioperative Nursing Care Planning* (St Louis: Mosby, Inc, 1990) 497.

22. "A position statement on fast tracking," in *Standards of Perianesthesia Nursing Practice* (Cherry Hill, NJ: American Society of PeriAnesthesia Nurses, 2002) 73.

23. M Mamaril, "Fast-tracking the postanesthesia patient: The pros and cons," *Journal of Perianesthesia Nursing* 15 (April 2000) 89-93.

24. A C Watkins, P F White, "Fast-tracking after ambulatory surgery," *Journal of PeriAnesthesia Nursing* 16 (December 2001) 379-87.

25. P F White et al, "PACU fast-tracking: An alternative to 'bypassing' the PACU for facilitating the recovery process after ambulatory surgery," *Journal of PeriAnesthesia Nursing* 18 (August 2003) 247-253.

26. R I Patel et al, "Fast-tracking children after ambulatory surgery," *Anesthesia and Analgesia* 92 (April 2001) 918-922.

27. K Cunningham, "Pain management," in *Ambulatory Surgery Principles and Practices*, third ed, N J Vinson, ed (Denver: AORN Inc, 2003) 145-149.

28. "Anesthesia services," in *Accreditation Guidebook for Office Based Surgery* (Wilmette, Ill: Accreditation Association for Ambulatory Health Care, 2004) 41-45.

29. D A Krenzischek, L Wilson, "An introduction to the ASPAN pain and comfort clinical guideline," *Journal of PeriAnesthesia Nursing* 18 (August 2003) 232-236.

30. "Management of information," in *2004 Comprehensive Accreditation Manual for Ambulatory Care* (Oakbrook Terrace, Ill: Joint Commission on Accreditation of Healthcare Organizations, 2004) IM1-IM20.

31. R A Marley, B M Moline, "Patient discharge issues," in *Ambulatory Surgical Nursing*, second ed, N Burden, ed (Philadelphia: WB Saunders Co, 2000) 504-526.

32. "Surgical care," in *Guidelines for Optimal Ambulatory Surgical Care and Office-Based Surgery* (Chicago: American College of Surgeons, 2000) 14-20.

33. "Criteria for initial, ongoing, and discharge assessment and management," in *Standards of PeriAnesthesia Nursing Practice* (Cherry Hill, NJ: American Society of PeriAnesthesia Nurses, 2004) 27-31.

34. R A Marley, J Swanson, "Patient care after discharge from the ambulatory surgical center," *Journal of Perianesthesia Nursing* 16 (December 2001) 399-417.

35. R M Tappen, J Muzic, P Kennedy, "Preoperative assessment and discharge planning for older adults undergoing ambulatory surgery," *AORN Journal* 73 (February 2001) 464-474.

36. "Resource 4: Criteria for initial, ongoing, and discharge assessment and management," in *Standards of Perianesthesia Nursing Practice* (Cherry Hill, NJ: American Society for PeriAnesthesia Nurses, 2002) 27-30.

37. "The postop phone call: An effective tool?" *OR Manager* 19 (January 2003) 25-27.

38. K Heseltine, F Edlington, "A day surgery post-operative telephone call line," *Nursing Standard* 13 (November 1998) 39-43.

39. S Barnes, "Not a social event: The follow-up phone call," *Journal of Perianesthesia Nursing* 15 (August 2000) 253-255.

40. M C Redmond, "Extensions of care: Phase III recovery," in *Ambulatory Surgical Nursing*, second ed, N Burden, ed (Philadelphia: WB Saunders Co, 2000) 527-249.

41. "Improving Organizational Performance," in *2004 Comprehensive Accreditation Manual for Ambulatory Care* (Oakbrook Terrace, Ill: Joint Commission on Accreditation of Healthcare Organizations, 2004) P16.

Originally published April 2005, *AORN Journal.*

AORN Guidance Statement: Preoperative Patient Care in the Ambulatory Surgery Setting

Introduction

The purpose of this guidance statement is to provide a framework that health care practitioners can use to develop and implement policies and procedures for preoperative patient care in the ambulatory surgery setting. This guidance statement is directed specifically to ambulatory surgery centers (ASCs). It also may be used in other ambulatory settings that perform surgery or other invasive procedures. The ambulatory surgical setting is defined as an area in which outpatient surgery or other invasive procedures are performed, including, but not limited to, freestanding surgery centers, hospital-based ambulatory surgery units, physicians' offices, cardiac catheterization suites, endoscopy units, and radiology departments.

Perioperative nurses have limited contact with patients before surgery, which may lead to an increased risk for adverse patient outcomes. Ambulatory surgery centers must have consistent approaches to preoperative patient care to ensure patient safety. This guidance statement is intended to promote patient safety in the ambulatory surgery setting.

Guidance Statement

Ambulatory surgery centers should develop written policies and procedures for preoperative patient care. Policies and procedures should include, but not be limited to, the following elements:

- staffing,
- preadmission assessment,
- preadmission testing,
- anesthesia evaluation,
- preoperative teaching,
- preoperative nursing assessment,
- documentation of the preoperative nursing assessment,
- fast tracking of patients,
- prevention of postoperative infections, and
- monitoring of outcomes.

The criteria in this guidance statement represent the minimum levels of care.

Perioperative Nursing Data Set

The Perioperative Nursing Data Set (PNDS) is a clinically relevant and empirically validated standardized nursing vocabulary describing periopera- tive nursing. It relates to the delivery of care in all perioperative settings. This standardized language consists of a collection of data elements and includes perioperative nursing diagnoses, interventions, and outcomes. The PNDS should be used to develop ambulatory surgery patient plans of care and to standardize nursing documentation. In addition, PNDS outcomes, as well as outcome indicators, interventions, and nursing diagnoses, can be

- incorporated into competencies, policies and procedures, job descriptions, pathways, guidelines, and care plans;
- linked to the electronic health record;
- used as a tool for teaching new nurses about perioperative nursing; and
- applied in performance improvement projects and benchmarking.

Each data element in the PNDS corresponds to a unique identifier. The domains are represented by the letter "D," followed by numbers 1 to 3 to indicate the particular domain being addressed. Nursing diagnoses are represented by the letter "X" and a number unique to the diagnosis. Interventions are represented by the letter "I" and a unique number, and outcomes are represented by the letter "O" and a unique number. These designations are identified in this document with unique identifiers noted in parentheses. A list of outcomes, interventions, and nursing diagnoses specific to each domain is printed in an appendix of the PNDS reference book.[1]

The PNDS is conceptualized by the perioperative patient focused model. The patient and his or her family members are at the center of the model's framework. The model depicts perioperative nursing in four domains and illustrates the relationship between the patient, family members, and the care provided by the perioperative RN. The patient-centered domains are

- D1—patient safety;
- D2—physiological responses to surgery; and
- D3—patient and family member behavioral responses to surgery, including
  - behavior responses—knowledge, and
  - behavior responses—rights and ethics.[1]

Nursing Care Policies

Preoperative nursing care policies and procedures should be available in the preoperative care unit.[2] At a minimum, each nurse should review these policies and procedures periodically, and the review process should be documented. Specific criteria for the preoperative care policies and procedures should include

- assessment of data elements;
- preoperative patient care;
- supplies and equipment;
- emergency medications[3] and equipment;
- fast tracking of perioperative patients;
- infection control (O10);
- pain management (O29), patient knowledge of pain, and pain control (O20); and
- documentation of care.

Staffing

A staffing plan should be developed and used to provide an adequate number and mix of personnel to meet patient care needs.[4-6] An adequate number of RNs should be available to provide patient assessments. The staffing plan for the preoperative area should include criteria regarding the number of patients; number of ORs and procedure rooms; types of procedures scheduled; medications to be administered; types of patients (eg, elderly, pediatric); average patient preparation time; preoperative procedures (eg, insertion of invasive lines, radiological studies, regional blocks); patient acuity; and intensity of care.[4,7] Licensed practical nurses (LPNs) and unlicensed assistive personnel (UAP) may be included in preoperative staffing plans. Unlicensed assistive personnel may be assigned to assist with delegated patient care tasks as determined by the RN and according to federal, state, and local regulations.[8] All personnel should be qualified and competent according to state licensure requirements, accreditation and professional standards, procedure-specific training, and experience.[5,9] Personnel should be trained in the use of emergency equipment and cardiopulmonary resuscitation for both adult and pediatric patients if pediatric care is provided.[5] Basic life support training is recommended for all nurses in the preoperative care unit. All staff members should undergo a comprehensive orientation program, and competencies should be documented.

Preadmission Assessment

Specific admission criteria and guidelines should be identified for all perianesthesia care settings, and patients should meet the admission criteria.[10] The perioperative RN should ensure all admissions are identified as appropriate and evaluated based on written guidelines for preadmission.[10-13]

Preadmission telephone calls or face-to-face interviews should be conducted by a professional RN.[13,14] Pre-established admission criteria should be used to identify patients who need a face-to-face interview versus those who can be interviewed by telephone.

Preadmission nursing assessment criteria should determine preoperative status.[13] The assessment should include, but should not be limited to, the following:

- appropriate baseline physical assessment (I59) (I144);
- allergies and sensitivities (I123);
- signs of abuse or neglect (I113);[15]
- cultural, emotional, and socioeconomic assessment (I57) (I68);
- comprehensive pain assessment (I16) (I17);
- medication history, including nonprescription medications, illicit drugs, and herbal medications and supplements (I30);[16,17]
- anesthetic history;[18]
- results of radiological examinations and other preoperative testing (I30) (I111);
- discharge planning (I30) (I80);
- referrals (I63) (I92);
- identification of physical alterations that require additional equipment or supplies (I64);
- preoperative patient teaching (I135) (eg, medications to be taken or held before surgery, preoperative shower, NPO requirements [I107]);[13,19]
- informed consent and/or knowledge of planned procedure (I32);
- advance directive review (I97) (I103);[20]
- development of a care plan (I30); and
- documentation and communication of all information per facility policy (I27) (I92).[6,12]

Preoperative Testing

Policies and procedures that include criteria for preoperative testing should be developed by each ASC and approved by the appropriate medical staff members. The requested preoperative tests should be based on the patient's clinical conditions.[18,21] The criteria also should identify requirements for medical history and physical examination and documentation of such.[16]

A medical history and physical examination should be conducted before a surgical or invasive procedure and documented on the patient's medical record.[6] The history and physical should be reviewed immediately before surgery, and any changes to the patient's condition should be documented. Facility policy should be congruent with regulation and accreditation agency requirements.

Diagnostic testing to determine the patient's health care needs should be performed in a timely manner as defined by the health care organization.[10] Special screening may be needed for high-risk patients with certain conditions (eg, cardiac disease, obesity, sleep apnea).[22] Specific studies may be conducted for special categories of surgical procedures or type of anesthesia. Findings from the history, physical examination, and designated studies must be documented in the patient's medical record before anesthesia is administered or surgery is performed.[22,23]

Anesthesia Evaluation

An appropriate preanesthesia evaluation and assessment should be conducted by an anesthesia care provider before induction of anesthesia and surgery for patients receiving any type or level of anesthesia.[16,18,24] A preanesthesia assessment must be conducted for each patient to determine whether he or she is an appropriate candidate for moderate or deep sedation or anesthesia. A preanesthesia evaluation may not be required when the patient is only receiving local anesthesia. A patient receiving only local anesthesia may require a preanesthesia evaluation if the patient has significant comorbidities (eg, morbid obesity).

The assessment should include past and present medical and medication history, previous anesthesia experiences, evidence of a patient physical status assessment, American Society of Anesthesiologists physical status classification, results of relevant diagnostic studies, and the planned choice of anesthesia.[16] An anesthesia plan should be developed based on this information.[18]

Preoperative Teaching

A preoperative teaching plan should be developed for each patient. The teaching plan should include preoperative instructions[18] and patient preparation. The plan should address acceptable NPO require-

ments before surgery; preoperative showers or medications, when ordered; and physical, emotional, social, and procedural issues.[13,19,25,26] The teaching plan should describe perioperative routine care (I56), as well as the preparation phase; length of time in each phase of the perioperative period; other care providers; use of preoperative medications; management of postoperative pain and nausea; fast tracking, if applicable; discharge criteria; and continuum of care services.[13,27] Preoperative teaching should include the patient's family members or guardian (I79).

Preoperative Nursing Assessment

A perioperative RN should conduct a preoperative nursing assessment on the day of surgery. Perioperative nurses assess, document, and communicate patient status to all members of the health care team. Data collection involves the patient and his or her significant others or guardians. On the day of surgery, the perioperative RN should verify the information obtained during the preadmission assessment. The RN is responsible for ensuring that the preoperative assessment is complete and the patient's emotional needs are met.[13] Assessments for special populations, such as pediatric patients, older adult patients,[27] high-risk patients,[22] and patients with special needs,[13] may require additional preparation.

A preoperative assessment should be completed on admission. Interventions relating to the assessment may include, but are not limited to,
- verification of the patient's identity using two identifiers (I26) (eg, patient's name, date of birth, social security number, an assigned identification number)—neither identifier should be the patient's location or diagnosis.[28]
- review of preadmission assessment;
- appropriate baseline physical assessment (I59) (I144) (I60) (I64) (I66);
- review of preoperative status (I27) (I66);
- review of medications, including nonprescription medications, illicit drugs, and herbal medications and supplements (I30);
- allergies and sensitivities (I123);
- NPO status (I107);[22]
- hypothermia assessment and management (I131);[29]
- pain scale assessment (I16);[30,31]

♦ relevant preoperative needs of the patient and family members (I57) (I63) (I79);

♦ advance directives (I103) (I97);

♦ identification of planned procedure by the patient or his or her significant other or guardian (I32);

♦ verification of surgical site, side, or level, as applicable (I143);[6,17,32]

♦ prescribed surgical preparation (eg, preoperative shower, enema, medication) (I30);

♦ prosthetic devices (eg, dentures, hearing aids, contact lenses, glasses) (I90) (I127);

♦ implantable electronic devices (eg, pacemakers [I58], brain stimulators, pain pumps);

♦ availability of safe transportation home and aftercare (I35);

♦ contact information for the patient's support person (I109);

♦ understanding of preoperative teaching and discharge planning (I135) (I136) (I137) (I62);[16] and

♦ documentation of information per facility policy (I27) (I92).

A nursing care plan should be based on the patient assessment and documented appropriately. The perioperative RN analyzes the assessment data to determine nursing diagnoses. Following is a partial list of nursing diagnoses that may be associated with patients undergoing ambulatory surgery.

♦ X30 (D3)—knowledge deficit;

♦ X34 (D1)—physical mobility, impaired;

♦ X4 (D3)—anxiety;

♦ X28 (D2)—infection, risk for;

♦ X20 (D2)—fluid volume, risk for imbalance—related to altered nutritional state; and

♦ X26 (D2)—hypothermia.[1]

Preoperative Patient Outcomes

Nursing interventions are initiated to achieve a desired conclusion and/or to reduce the probability of undesired outcomes.[1,33] Following is a partial list of patient outcomes that may be associated with a patient's perioperative experience:

♦ (O22)—the patient demonstrates knowledge of wound healing;

♦ (O25)—the patient's right to privacy is maintained;

♦ (O20)—the patient demonstrates knowledge of pain management.[1]

Communication of the Preoperative Nursing Assessment

Policies and procedures should be written for communicating to the appropriate surgical team members any changes in the patient's status noted during the preadmission interview and assessment. A process should be developed for reporting and acting on abnormal findings (I27) (I30).

Prevention of Postoperative Infections

Prevention of postoperative infection begins in the preoperative period. Outcome O10 states, "the patient is free from signs and symptoms of infection."[1] Policies and procedures for reducing the risk of postoperative infection should be written and followed.[34,35] Prophylactic antibiotics should be considered and used according to the published guidelines, which include, at a minimum, the following elements (I10):[36]

♦ surgical procedures for which prophylactic antibiotics are recommended;

♦ the selection of appropriate medications;

♦ the timing of administering medications;

♦ the route of administration; and

♦ the personnel responsible for procuring, preparing, and administering the medication.[37]

Depending on the type of prophylactic medication used, administration should occur between 30 minutes and one hour before incision.[37,38]

Body temperature should be monitored and maintained as close to normothermia as possible during the preoperative period (I86) (I78) (I55).[39] Hypothermia may delay healing and predispose patients to wound infections.[40]

Documentation

Policies and procedures for documenting preoperative patient information should be established. Nursing documentation should incorporate the PNDS.[1] A preadmission checklist should be implemented to ensure all required patient-specific information is documented properly. Documentation requirements include, but are not limited to,

♦ a preadmission patient survey;

♦ a preoperative nursing assessment;

♦ signed consents for surgery and anesthesia (I124);

◆ written permission to leave postoperative follow-up telephone messages by voice mail or with a designated individual in keeping with the Health Insurance Portability and Accountability Act privacy guidelines (I151);

◆ history and physical in the patient's medical record;

◆ test results;

◆ preanesthesia assessment;

◆ pain scale assessment (I16);[30,31]

◆ identified possible risks, such as the potential for malignant hyperthermia or latex allergy (I123);[13]

◆ surgical procedure and site verification (I26) (I143);[32]

◆ advance directives (I103); and

◆ documentation of education and instructions provided (O31) (I27).

Monitoring of Outcomes

The facility should collect data to monitor its performance.[41] Data collected should include patients' perceptions of care, treatment, and provision of services, including specific individual needs and expectations, how well the facility met those needs, surgical site infections, how the facility can improve patient safety, and the effectiveness of pain management, when applicable.[41]

NOTES

1. *Perioperative Nursing Data Set: The Perioperative Nursing Vocabulary*, second ed, S Beyea, ed (Denver: AORN, Inc, 2002).

2. R Ferrara-Love, "Immediate postanesthesia care," in *Ambulatory Surgical Nursing*, second ed, N Burden, ed (Philadelphia: WB Saunders Co, 2000) 409-476.

3. S Smith, "Progressive postanesthesia care: Phase II recovery," in *Ambulatory Surgical Nursing*, second ed, N Burden, ed (Philadelphia: WB Saunders Co, 2000) 477-503.

4. "Standard III: Staffing and personnel management," in *Standards of Perianesthesia Nursing Practice* (Cherry Hill, NJ: American Society of PeriAnesthesia Nurses, 2004) 14.

5. "Management of human resources," in *2004 Comprehensive Accreditation Manual for Ambulatory Care* (Oakbrook Terrace, Ill: Joint Commission on Accreditation of Healthcare Organizations, 2004) HR1-HR12.

6. "Surgical and related services," in *Accreditation Guidebook for Office Based Surgery* (Wilmette, Ill: Accreditation Association for Ambulatory Health Care, 2004) 47-52.

7. "Resource 3, patient classification/recommended staffing guidelines," in *Standards of Perianesthesia Nursing Practice* (Cherry Hill, NJ: American Society of PeriAnesthesia Nurses, 2004) 25-26.

8. "AORN official statement on unlicensed assistive personnel," in *Standards, Recommended Practices, and Guidelines* (Denver: AORN, Inc, 2004) 167-168.

9. "Quality of care provided," in *Accreditation Guidebook for Office Based Surgery* (Wilmette, Ill: Accreditation Association for Ambulatory Health Care, 2004) 19-21.

10. "Provision of care, treatment, and services," in *2004 Comprehensive Accreditation Manual for Ambulatory Care* (Oakbrook Terrace, Ill: Joint Commission on Accreditation of Healthcare Organizations, 2004) PC1-PC50.

11. "Standard VI: Assessment," in *Standards of Perianesthesia Nursing Practice* (Cherry Hill, NJ: American Society of PeriAnesthesia Nurses, 2002) 17.

12. "Resource 4: Criteria for initial, ongoing, and discharge assessment and management," in *Standards of Perianesthesia Nursing Practice* (Cherry Hill, NJ: American Society for PeriAnesthesia Nurses, 2002) 27-30.

13. G D Williams, "Preoperative preparation of the ambulatory surgery patient," in *Ambulatory Surgical Nursing*, second ed, N Burden, ed (Philadelphia: WB Saunders Co, 2000) 346-362.

14. D Dunn, "Preoperative assessment criteria and patient teaching for ambulatory surgery patients," *Journal of PeriAnesthesia Nursing* 13 (October 1998) 274-291.

15. "Provision of care, treatment, and services," in *2004 Comprehensive Accreditation Manual for Ambulatory Care* (Oakbrook Terrace, Ill: Joint Commission on Accreditation of Healthcare Organizations, 2004) PC.3.10.

16. R E Grundman, "Preoperative patient care," in *Ambulatory Surgery Principles and Practices*, third ed, N J Vinson, ed (Denver: AORN, Inc, 2003) 109-124.

17. "What's being done to make ambulatory surgery safer?" *OR Manager* 19 (March 2003) 30-35.

18. "Guidelines for ambulatory anesthesia and surgery," American Society of Anesthesiology, *http://www.asahq.org/publicationsAndServices/standards/04.pdf* (accessed 29 Sept 2004).

19. P Patterson, "NPO status: Have ASCs changed policies?" *OR Manager* 17 (March 2001) 25-27.

20. "Be proactive on advance directives," *OR Manager* 17 (June 2001) 25-26.

21. J M Mathias, "Assess first, test later, centers say," *OR Manager* 17 (May 2001) 26-28.

22. B A Scales, "Screening high-risk patients for the ambulatory setting," *Journal of Perianesthesia Nursing* 18 (October 2003) 307-316.

23. "Clinical records and health information," in *Accreditation Guidebook for Office Based Surgery* (Wilmette, Ill: Accreditation Association for Ambulatory Health Care, 2004) 29-31.

24. "Anesthesia services," in *Accreditation Guidebook for Office Based Surgery* (Wilmette, Ill: Accreditation Association for Ambulatory Health Care, 2004) 41-45.

25. M J Bernier et al, "Preoperative teaching received and valued in a day surgery setting," *AORN Journal* 77 (March 2003) 563-582.

26. "Practice guidelines for preoperative fasting and the use of pharmacologic agents to reduce the risk of pulmonary aspiration: Application to healthy patients undergoing elective procedures," American Society of

Anesthesiologists, *http://www.asahq.org/publications AndServices/NPO.pdf* (accessed 16 April 2004).

27. R M Tappen, J Muzic, P Kennedy, "Preoperative assessment and discharge planning for older adults undergoing ambulatory surgery," (Elder Care) *AORN Journal* 73 (February 2001) 464-474.

28. "2005 National Patient Safety Goals FAQs," Joint Commission on Accreditation of Healthcare Organizations, *http://www.jcaho.org/accredited+organizations/ patient+safety/05+npsg/05_npsg_faqs.htm* (accessed 1 Jan 2005)

29. M C Karlet, "Malignant hyperthermia: Considerations for ambulatory surgery," *Journal of PeriAnesthesia Nursing* 13 (October 1998) 304-312.

30. K Cunningham, "Pain management," in *Ambulatory Surgery Principles and Practices*, third ed, N J Vinson, ed (Denver: AORN, Inc, 2003) 145-149.

31. D A Krenzischek, L Wilson, "An introduction to the ASPAN pain and comfort clinical guideline," *Journal of PeriAnesthesia Nursing* 18 (August 2003) 228-236.

32. "Correct site surgery toolkit" (Denver: AORN, Inc, 2004).

33. J C Rothrock, *Perioperative Nursing Care Planning* (St Louis: Mosby, 1990) 497.

34. "Surveillance, prevention, and control of infection," in *2004 Comprehensive Accreditation Manual for Ambulatory Care* (Oakbrook Terrace, Ill: Joint Commission on Accreditation of Healthcare Organizations, 2004) IC1-IC24.

35. "Facilities and environment," in *Accreditation Guidebook for Office Based Surgery* (Wilmette, Ill: Accreditation Association for Ambulatory Health Care, 2004) 35-38.

36. "Antimicrobial prophylaxis in surgery," *The Medical Letter on Drugs and Therapeutics* 39 (Oct 24, 1997) 97-101.

37. "ASHP therapeutic guidelines on antimicrobial prophylaxis in surgery," American Society of Health-System Pharmacists, *http://www.medqic.org/cms-service/stream/ asset/TK8_tagged.pdf?asset_id=847853* (accessed 29 Sept 2004).

38. "Suggested recommendations and guidelines for surgical prophylaxis," Medical College of Wisconsin, *http:// www.intmed.mcw.edu/drug/SurgProph.html* (accessed 29 Sept 2004).

39. "Recommended practices for safe care through identification of potential hazards in the surgical environment," in *Standards, Recommended Practices, and Guidelines* (Denver: AORN, Inc, 2004) 301-307.

40. A Kurz, D I Sessler, R Lenhardt, "Perioperative normothermia to reduce the incidence of surgical-wound infection and shorten hospitalization," *The New England Journal of Medicine* 334 (May 9, 1996) 1209-1215.

41. "Improving organizational performance," in *2004 Comprehensive Accreditation Manual for Ambulatory Care* (Oakbrook Terrace, Ill: Joint Commission on Accreditation of Healthcare Organizations, 2004) PI6.

Originally published April 2005, *AORN Journal*.

AORN Guidance Statement: Reuse of Single-Use Devices

Introduction

Today's economic environment has compelled health care organizations to explore methods to reduce health care costs. One prospective approach to controlling rising costs is to reprocess single-use medical devices. Reprocessing is rigorously regulated by the US Food and Drug Administration (FDA). AORN, the Association of periOperative Registered Nurses, recognizes the need for each health care facility to provide safe, cost-effective, quality care to patients and realizes that many facilities in today's marketplace are reprocessing and reusing devices labeled for single use. These devices are reprocessed either within the facility or by an external third party contracted to provide the reprocessing service.

Background

As surgery evolved and increased in complexity, the number of single-use devices utilized during surgery increased and continues to rise. In response to this trend, the practice of reprocessing and reusing single-use medical devices began during the 1970s.[1] As technology led to a wide variety of materials used in device manufacture and devices became more complex, concern for patient safety, informed consent, and ethical practice intensified. In the late 1990s, the FDA determined that increased regulation of reprocessing was needed to promote safe practice and protect the public's safety. Although original equipment manufacturers have been regulated for many years, the FDA determined that they, along with third-party reprocessors and hospital reprocessors, should be regulated uniformly according to the Food, Drug, and Cosmetic Act. The FDA sought the expertise of manufacturers, reprocessors, hospitals, users, and other interested parties in developing a regulatory document, and in August 2000, it published its rule governing the reprocessing/reusing of devices labeled for single-use only. The document is applicable to both hospitals and third-party reprocessors.

Reprocessing of single-use devices (SUDs) is additionally addressed in the Medical Device User Fee and Modernization Act of 2002 (MDUFMA), which establishes new statutory requirements for SUDs, including labeling to identify the devices as reprocessed, submission of validation data for many reprocessed SUDs, and submission of premarket notification (510[k]) with validation data for some SUDs that previously were exempt from 510(k) submission requirements. Firms and hospitals that are reprocessing are considered by the FDA as manufacturers and therefore must comply with statutory and regulatory requirements.[2] In addition, the FDA has published an approved list of single-use devices that are acceptable for reprocessing and a list of items that may not be reprocessed. In essence, the regulations regard reprocessors in the same way as original equipment manufacturers.[3,4]

Guidance Statement

Reprocessing single-use medical devices is chosen by some health care facilities as a cost containment effort and to reduce the amount of waste generated. It is the role and responsibility of each health care facility to determine whether and to what extent it will engage in such practice. As licensed professionals, perioperative nurses must demonstrate accountability to the nursing profession, to other members of the health care team, and to the public they serve.[5] AORN, the professional organization of and for perioperative nurses, believes certain basic tenets must underpin any reprocessing program. The foremost concern is for the patient's safety. Therefore,

- if a device cannot be cleaned, it cannot be reprocessed and reused;
- if sterility of a post-processed device cannot be demonstrated, the device cannot be reprocessed and reused;
- if the integrity and functionality of a reprocessed SUD cannot be demonstrated and documented as safe for patient care and/or equal to the original device specifications, the device cannot be reprocessed and reused; and
- if anything is opened it needs to be decontaminated before reprocessing.

Per requirements of the MDUFMA regulation, the FDA has published a list of reprocessed SUDs that have 510(k) approval/clearance; whose manufacturers have provided supplemental data on functionality, cleaning, and sterility; and which now are on the published list of devices that are acceptable for reprocessing.[2]

Although some operational savings may be realized by reusing certain devices, any cost-benefit analysis would necessarily include labor costs;

program costs, including quality system requirements such as sterility and post-processing device testing (see section on quality system requirements); documentation costs; and the potential cost of device failure. Using the results of a thorough cost-benefit analysis, each provider facility must make an informed choice as to whether it wishes to invest the necessary resources to develop a safe reprocessing system within the facility. Use of an external reprocessor presents a different, but related, set of factors for consideration. When a decision is made in favor of using an external reprocessing company, it is the user facility's responsibility to assess the quality of services provided under the contractual arrangement.[6] The user facility should review the processes used by the contracted agent and determine whether correct procedures are being followed.[7] Regardless of whether an internal reprocessing program is developed or an external reprocessing company is selected, the user facility should be aware that the FDA views any reprocessor as a manufacturer and, as such, subject to federal regulations.[3,8,9]

Federal Regulatory Requirements

In August 2000, the FDA issued guidance on the practice of reprocessing and reusing medical devices intended to be used only once. The FDA's goal in issuing this regulation was to ensure a reprocessing and reuse regulatory program that is based on good science and protects the public health. At the same time, the FDA intended to ensure equitable regulatory requirements for all parties engaged in reprocessing. In the guidance document,[10] the FDA indicates that hospitals and third parties that reprocess SUDs are subject to the same regulations as the original equipment manufacturers. The MDUFMA also addressed reprocessing of SUDs by amending the federal Food, Drug and Cosmetic Act (the Act) and establishing new statutory requirements applicable to reprocessed SUDs, including requirements for

- ◆ quality system regulations,
- ◆ medical device reporting,
- ◆ registration and listing,
- ◆ labeling,
- ◆ premarket approval and premarket notification,
- ◆ medical device corrections and removals, and
- ◆ medical device tracking.[2]

Quality System Regulation

All manufacturers, including hospital and third-party reprocessors, are subject to the FDA Good Manufacturing Practices (GMP) requirements. These requirements are presented in the quality system regulation that governs the methods, facilities, and controls used for designing, manufacturing, packaging, labeling, storing, installing, and servicing medical devices.[3] Quality system refers to the organizational structure, responsibilities, procedures, processes, and resources for implementing quality management. For device manufacturers, including reprocessors, this system is required in addition to any quality improvement program that may be in place as required by other regulatory bodies. The quality system regulation addresses the areas shown in Table 1.[11]

Medical Device Reporting (MDR)

Under MEDWATCH, the FDA's medical device reporting program resulting from the Safe Medical Devices Act of 1990 (Public Law 101-629),[12] both manufacturers and users are required to report deaths or serious injuries to the FDA if it can be reasonably determined that a medical device may have caused or contributed to the incident. Manufacturers also must report certain device malfunctions.[13] Because the FDA considers reprocessors to be manufacturers when they reprocess an SUD,[9] hospital reprocessors have dual reporting responsibility. They are subject to manufacturer's reporting requirements (21 CFR, Part 803 Subpart E)[14] as well as those for the device user facility (21 CFR, Part 803, Subparts A and C).[15,16] Although user facilities must report only deaths or serious injury, manufacturers' reporting requirements are more extensive and require additional supplemental information. Manufacturers (reprocessors) also must report any event that requires the manufacturer (reprocessor) to take immediate remedial action. The Jan 26, 2000, issue of the *Federal Register* contains the most recent MDR requirements. Hospitals that reprocess SUDs are subject to both user facility reporting and the more comprehensive manufacturer reporting requirements.[17]

Registration and Listing

All persons or entities owning or operating establishments that manufacture, prepare, or process devices must register with the FDA. The FDA uses

Table 1

QUALITY SYSTEM REGULATION[1]	
Area Addressed	**Code of Federal Regulations**
Management responsibility	21 CFR, Part 820.20, 22, 25
Design controls	21 CFR, Part 820.30
Document controls	21 CFR, Part 820.40
Purchasing controls	21 CFR, Part 820.50
Product identification and traceability	21 CFR, Part 820.60, 65
Production and process validation	21 CFR, Part 820.70, 72, 75
Acceptance activities such as inspections, tests, or other verification activities	21 CFR, Part 820.80, 86
Nonconforming product control	21 CFR, Part 820.90
Corrective and preventive action	21 CFR, Part 820.100
Labeling and packaging controls	21 CFR, Part 820.120, 130
Handling, storage, distribution, and installation controls	21 CFR, Part 820.120, 140, 150, 160
Records including device master record, device history record, quality system record, and complaint files controls	21 CFR, Part 820.180, 181, 184, 186, 198
Servicing controls	21 CFR, Part 820.200
Use of statistical techniques to establish, control, and verify the acceptability of process capability and product characteristics	21 CFR, Part 820.250

1. *"Quality system regulation,"* CFR 21 Part 820, US Food and Drug Administration, http://www.accessdata.fda.gov/scripts/cdrh/cfdocs/cfCFR/CFRSearch.cfm?CFRPart=820 *(accessed 3 Oct 2005).*

this information to identify and locate establishments that it is required to inspect. When registering, the following information must be provided:
- name and address,
- business names used,
- business name of owner or operator, and
- establishment type.

When registering for the first time, a specific FDA form is required. An additional registration form must be submitted annually thereafter. In addition to registering with the FDA, each reprocessing entity must provide a list of the devices it intends to reprocess. A separate listing form must be submitted for each device to be reprocessed. Devices are listed by category. The following information is required:

- FDA classification name,
- FDA product code,
- brand name, and
- common or usual name.

Additional information about registration and listing is available in the *Code of Federal Regulations* (21 CFR, Part 807).[18] The necessary forms can be obtained from the Office of Compliance, Center for Devices and Radiologic Health (HFZ-307), US Food and Drug Administration, 2094 Gaither Road, Rockville, MD 20850. The Center for Devices and Radiologic Health (CDRH) offers an additional document, *CDRH Guidance for Industry: Instructions for Completion of Medical Device Registration and Listing Forms FDA 2891, 2891a, and 2892.* This document can be obtained from the

Division of Small Manufacturers Assistance (DMSA) at telephone number 800-638-2041 or 301-638-2041; e-mail *DMSA@CDRH.fda.gov.*

Labeling

The FDA directions for labeling can be found in 21 CFR, Part 801.[19] The term *labeling* includes package inserts as well as the information printed on the actual label of the package. Labeling requirements include the name and location of the manufacturer (reprocessor) and adequate direction for the device's intended use. If the manufacturer (reprocessor) knows of uses other than the intended use of the device, FDA requires the manufacturer (reprocessor) to provide adequate labeling for alternate uses of the device as are known. In addition, MDUFMA added new labeling requirement for reprocessed SUDs (Section 502[v] of the Act). Beginning after January 26, 2004, reprocessed SUDs that are introduced into interstate commerce must prominently and conspicuously bear the statement "Reprocessed device for single use. Reprocessed by [insert the name of the manufacturer that reprocessed the device]."[2] For additional information about labeling requirements, obtain a copy of the FDA guidance document *Labeling Regulatory Requirements for Medical Devices* from *http://www.fda.gov/cdrh/dsma/470.pdf* or contact the Division of Small Manufacturers Assistance (DSMA) by phone at 800-638-2041 or 301-638-2041; e-mail *DMSA@CDRH.fda.gov.*

Premarket Approval and Premarket Notification

After registering with the FDA and submitting a list of devices to be manufactured (reprocessed) and distributed for use, the registered entity must meet premarket submission requirements for each listed device. Certain devices may be exempt from the premarket submission requirement. If exempt, the device need only be listed with the FDA. Additional information about exemptions can be found in 21 CFR, Part 807.75.[20] The FDA has defined a phase-in period for premarket submissions to accommodate entities that are presently engaged in reprocessing. Following the phase-in period, a premarket submission must be submitted for any new device to be manufactured (reprocessed) at least 90 days before beginning distribution of the device.

There are two types of premarket submissions: a premarket notification, or 510(k), and a premarket approval (PMA) application. The type of submission required is based on the device classification, as defined in 21 CFR, Part 814.[21] Unless specifically exempted, a premarket notification (510[k]) is required for all Class I and Class II devices. A premarket notification (510[k]) submission must contain enough information for the FDA to determine whether the particular device is "substantially equivalent" to another device that has been previously judged to be safe and effective and has been cleared for marketing/reprocessing. The predicate device selected must have the same intended use as the device for which the 510(k) is submitted. The predicate device may be the original SUD of the original equipment manufacturer (OEM) provided that the 510(k) compares the unique characteristics of the submitted device to those of the predicate device so the FDA can determine equivalency with respect to safety and effectiveness. The following information is required for a premarket notification (510[k]) submission:

♦ device trade name, proprietary name, usual name, or classification name;

♦ entity registration number;

♦ device classification;

♦ action taken to determine device performance standards;

♦ proposed labels, labeling, and advertisements to describe the device, its intended use, and the directions for its use, including photos and/or engineering drawings if appropriate;

♦ appropriate data to show that the registered entity has considered the consequences and effects any changes or modifications in the device might have on the safety and effectiveness of the device;

♦ 510(k) summary or 510(k) statement as defined in 21 CFR, Part 807.92, 93;[22]

♦ financial disclosure statement;[9]

♦ statement certifying truth, accuracy, and completeness of material submitted; and

♦ any other information requested by the FDA.

For specific guidance on preparing 510(k) submissions, consult *Regulatory Requirements for Medical Devices,* available at *http://www.fda.gov/cdrh/manual/510kprt1.html,* or contact the Division of Small Manufacturers Assistance. Locate other relevant guidelines at *http://www.accessdata.fda.gov/scripts/cdrh/cfdocs/cfGGPSearch.CFM.*

All Class III devices require a PMA. A PMA application must include valid scientific evidence demonstrating the safety and effectiveness of the original and/or reprocessed device. Each PMA application should evaluate the unique characteristics of the submitted device. Clinical data (eg, results of clinical trials) may be required. Some clinical trials require FDA approval of an investigational device exemption (IDE) application for the device(s) to be studied. For additional information, consult the following sources:

- 21 CFR, Part 814.20;[21]
- 21 CFR, Part 812;[22]
- *Device Advice: Premarket Approval (PMA)*, available at *http://www.fda.gov/cdrh/devadvice/pma* (accessed 3 Oct 2005);
- *Guidance for Institutional Review Boards and Clinical Investigators*, "Significant risk and nonsignificant risk medical device studies," available at *http://www.fda.gov/oc/ohrt/irbs/devices.html* (accessed 3 Oct 2005); and
- *Device Advice: Clinical Trials and Investigational Device Exemption (IDE)*, available at *http://www.fda.gov/cdrh/devadvice/ide/application.shtml* (accessed 3 Oct 2005).

The FDA also requires a satisfactory inspection of the manufacturing (reprocessing) facilities before approving a PMA application. The application should include a comprehensive manufacturing (reprocessing) section that clearly identifies all manufacturing (reprocessing) controls. Under MDUFMA, some SUDs that previously were exempt from 510(k) submission requirements under Sections 510(l) or (m) of the Act are no longer exempt and are required under Section 510(o)(2) of the Act to submit 510(k) notifications that include validation data. Validation data also was required for some reprocessed SUDs that already had been cleared under 510(k). Under Section 510(o) of the Act, reprocessors that either did not submit validation data for those reprocessed SUDs within specified time frames or received "not substantially equivalent letters" from the FDA can no longer legally market those reprocessed devices. Finally, under Section 515(c)(2) of the Act, reprocessors of Class III SUDs are required to submit premarket reports instead of premarket approval applications.[2]

Medical Device Corrections and Removals

Device correction and/or removal from the point of use must be promptly reported to the FDA when the correction or removal is initiated by the manufacturer (reprocessor) to reduce a health risk to the user or to correct a violation of the Food, Drug, and Cosmetic Act. For example, if a facility reprocessed an SUD that resulted in a patient's adverse reaction and the hospital chose to remove the remainder of the lot of those reprocessed SUDs from circulation to decrease the possibility of other patients having adverse reactions, that action would be a removal and the facility would be required to report the removal to the FDA. Corrections are defined as

the repair, modification, adjustment, relabeling, destruction, or inspection of a device without its physical removal from its point of use.[23]

Removal is defined as

the physical removal of a device from its point of use to some other location for repair, modification, adjustment, relabeling, destruction, or inspection.[23]

Distributed devices withdrawn from the marketplace due to a minor violation of the Food, Drug, and Cosmetic Act or as a matter of stock rotation need not be reported. Stock recoveries need not be reported, nor should devices removed for routine servicing. The term *stock recoveries* refers to devices that have been prepared for use, but have not left the physical premises and jurisdiction of the manufacturer (reprocessor)—eg, devices that have not left the reprocessing area. However, each correction and/or removal must be documented regardless of whether it is reported to the FDA.

When a report must be filed with the FDA, the report must be filed within 10 days of the correction/removal action. The report should include the following information:

- registration number of the entity manufacturing/reprocessing the device;
- date of the report;
- sequence number of the report from that entity;
- name, address, and telephone number of the reporting entity;
- name, title, address, and telephone number of individual responsible for the correction/removal action;
- brand name, classification name, and common name of the device and its intended use;
- marketing status of the device;
- model, catalog, and code number of the device and the manufacturer's (reprocessor's) lot, serial, or other identification number for the device;

♦ description of event leading to correction/removal action;

♦ any injuries resulting from device use;

♦ total number of devices manufactured (reprocessed) subject to the correction/removal action;

♦ date of manufacture/distribution/reprocessing and expected shelf life of the device;

♦ name, address, telephone number of all to whom the device has been distributed and the number of devices distributed to each; and

♦ copies of all communication regarding the correction/removal action and the names and address of all recipients of the communication.

For additional information about correction and removal requirements, consult 21 CFR, Part 806.

Medical Device Tracking

Medical device tracking is intended to ensure that manufacturers (reprocessors) of certain devices can locate those devices should corrective action and/or notification about such devices become necessary. Original equipment manufacturers are subject to the medical device tracking regulation only when the FDA issues a tracking order for a device manufactured by the OEM. Reprocessors are subject to the medical device tracking regulation only when the FDA issues an order for the specific device(s) being reprocessed. For additional information on device tracking, including the types of devices currently subject to tracking orders, consult *Guidance on Medical Device Tracking,* available at *http://www.fda.gov/cerh/modact/tracking/pdf* or from the Center for Devices and Radiologic Health (CDRH) at 301-827-0111. Request document number 169.

Definitions

Class I medical device: A medical device for which general controls provide reasonable assurance of the safety and effectiveness of the device or, if there is insufficient evidence to reasonably ensure safety and effectiveness, the device is not life-supporting or life-sustaining, its use is not substantially important in preventing impairment of human health, and/or its use "does not present a potential unreasonable risk of illness or injury."[23]

Class II medical device: A medical device for which general controls alone do not provide reason-

able assurance of device safety and effectiveness but for which there is sufficient information to establish special controls (eg, performance standards, guidelines, patient registries, postmarket surveillance) to provide that assurance.[23]

Class III medical device: A medical device for which neither general controls nor special controls provide reasonable assurance of device safety and effectiveness and the device is life-supporting or life sustaining or its use "is of substantial importance in preventing impairment of human health" or "presents a potential risk of illness or injury."[23]

Opened-but-unused device: A device whose sterility is compromised before being introduced onto the sterile field and which is not contaminated with blood and/or other potentially infectious materials (OPIM) external to the sterile field.[24]

Reprocessing: Includes all operations to render a contaminated reusable or single-use device patient ready. Single-use devices to be reprocessed may be either used or unused. Reprocessing steps include cleaning, decontamination, and sterilization/disinfection.[9]

Resterilization: The repeated application of a process intended to remove or destroy all viable forms of microbial life, including bacterial spores.[9] Because sterility is not an absolute, the accepted sterility assurance level (SAL) is usually defined as 10^{-6}.

Reuse: The repeated or multiple uses of any medical device whether marketed as reusable or single-use. Repeated/multiple use may be on the same patient or on different patients with applicable reprocessing of the device between uses.[25]

Single-use device (SUD): A device intended by the manufacturer to be used on one patient during one procedure. The device is not intended for reprocessing and/or use on another patient or on the same patient at another time. Device labeling may or may not identify the device as single-use or disposable, but manufacturer instructions for reprocessing are absent.[9]

Third-party reprocessor: A business establishment, separate from the user facility and the device manufacturer, one of whose primary businesses is to reprocess single-use/disposable medical devices.

NOTES

1. "Reuse of single-use devices," *AORN Journal* 73 (May 2001) 957-966.

2. "Medical Device User Fee and Modernization Act (MDUFMA) of 2002," PL 107-250, 107th Congress, *http://www.fda.gov/cdrh/mdufma* (accessed 3 Oct 2005).

3. "Guidance for industry and for FDA staff: Enforcement priorities for single-use devices reprocessed by third parties and hospitals," (Aug 14, 2000) US Food and Drug Administration, *http://www.fda.gov/cdrh/reuse/1168.html* (accessed 3 Oct 2005).

4. "Medical devices; reprocessed single-use devices; termination of exemptions from premarket notification; requirement for submission of validation data," US Food and Drug Administration, *http://www.fda.gov/OHRMS /DOCKETS/98fr/03-16109.html* (accessed 3 Oct 2005).

5. "AORN explications for perioperative nursing," in *Standards, Recommended Practices, and Guidelines* (Denver: AORN, Inc, 2005) 86-115.

6. Joint Commission on Accreditation of Healthcare Organizations, "Standard LD.3.50: Services provided by consultation, contractual agreements, or other agreements are provided safely and effectively," in *Comprehensive Accreditation Manual for Hospitals* (Oakbrook Terrace, Ill: Joint Commission on Accreditation of Healthcare Organizations, 2005) LD 13.

7. "Letter re: Reusable medical devices rented or leased from third parties," US Food and Drug Administration, *http://www.fda.gov/cdrh/comp/rentleasethird.html* (accessed 23 Aug 2005).

8. "Quality system regulation, Definitions," CFR 21, Part 820.3, US Food and Drug Administration, *http:// www.accessdata.fda.gov/scripts/cdrh/cfdocs/cfCFR /CFRSearch.cfm?fr=820.3* (accessed 3 Oct 2005).

9. "Letter to American College of Healthcare Executives: Reuse of single-use or disposable medical devices," US Food and Drug Administration, *http:// www.fda.gov/cdrh/comp/policymayaply.html* (accessed 3 Oct 2005).

10. Center for Devices and Radiological Health, US Food and Drug Administration, US Department of Health and Human Services, *Enforcement Priorities for Single-Use Devices Reprocessed by Third Parties and Hospitals* (Washington, DC: US Government Printing Office, Aug 14, 2000).

11. "Quality system regulation," CFR 21, Part 820, US Food and Drug Administration, *http://www.accessdata .fda.gov/scripts/cdrh/cfdocs/cfCFR/CFRSearch.cfm?CFR Part=820* (accessed 3 Oct 2005).

12. "Safe Medical Devices Act of 1990," Public Law 101-629, *http://thomas.loc.gov/cgi-bin/query/C?c101:./temp /~c101exlXhd* (accessed 23 Aug 2005).

13. "Medical device reporting: General provisions," CFR 21, Part 803.1, US Food and Drug Administration, *http://www.accessdata.fda.gov/scripts/cdrh/cfdocs/cfcfr /CFRSearch.cfm?fr=803.1* (accessed 3 Oct 2005).

14. "Manufacturer reporting requirements," CFR 21, Part 803, Subpart E, US Food and Drug Administration, *http://www.accessdata.fda.gov/scripts/cdrh/cfdocs/cfcfr /CFRSearch.cfm?CFRPart=803* (accessed 23 Aug 2005).

15. "Medical device reporting: General provisions," CFR 21, Part 803, Subpart A, US Food and Drug Adminis-

tration, *http://www.accessdata.fda.gov/scripts/cdrh /cfdocs/cfcfr/CFRSearch.cfm?CFRPart=803* (accessed 23 Aug 2005).

16. "User facility reporting requirements," CFR 21, Part 803, Subpart C, US Food and Drug Administration, *http://www.accessdata.fda.gov/scripts/cdrh/cfdocs/cfcfr /CFRSearch.cfm?CFRPart=803* (accessed 23 Aug 2005).

17. US Department of Health and Human Services, "Medical device reporting: Manufacturer reporting, importer reporting, user facility reporting, distributor reporting," *Federal Register* 65 (Jan 26, 2000) 4112-4121.

18. "Establishment regulation and device listing for manufacturers and initial importers of devices," CFR 21, Part 807, US Food and Drug Administration, *http://www .accessdata.fda.gov/scripts/cdrh/cfdocs/cfcfr/CFR Search.cfm?CFRPart=807* (accessed 23 Aug 2005).

19. "Labeling," CFR 21, Part 801, US Food and Drug Administration, *http://www.accessdata.fda.gov/scripts /cdrh/cfdocs/cfcfr/CFRSearch.cfm?CFRPart=801* (accessed 23 Aug 2005).

20. "Exemption from premarket notification," CFR 21, Part 807.65, US Food and Drug Administration, *http://www .accessdata.fda.gov/scripts/cdrh/cfdocs/cfcfr/CFRSearch.cfm ?fr=807.65* (accessed 23 Aug 2005).

21. "Premarket approval of medical devices," CFR 21, Part 814, US Food and Drug Administration, *http://www .accessdata.fda.gov/scripts/cdrh/cfdocs/cfcfr/CFRSearch.cfm ?CFRPart=814* (accessed 23 Aug 2005).

22. "Investigational device exemptions," CFR 21, Part 812, US Food and Drug Administration, *http://www.access data.fda.gov/scripts/cdrh/cfdocs/cfcfr/CFRSearch.cfm?CFR Part=812* (accessed 3 Oct 2005).

23. "Medical devices: Reports of corrections and removals, definitions," CFR 21, Part 806.2, US Food and Drug Administration, *http://www.accessdata.fda.gov/scripts /cdrh/cfdocs/cfcfr/CFRSearch.cfm* (accessed 3 Oct 2005).

24. "Guidance for industry and for FDA staff: Enforcement priorities for single-use devices reprocessed by third parties and hospitals," US Food and Drug Administration, *http://www.fda.gov/cdrh/reuse/1168.html#_Toc492780057* (accessed 2 Feb 2006).

25. Center for Devices and Radiological Health, US Food and Drug Administration, US Department of Health and Human Services, "FDA's proposed strategy on reuse of single-use devices, docket no 99N-4491," *Federal Register* 64 (Nov 3, 1999) 59782-59783.

RESOURCES

Medical Device Quality Systems Manual: A Small Entity Compliance Guidance, US Food and Drug Administration, *http://www.fda.gov/CDRH/DSMA/GMP MAN.HTML* (accessed 3 Oct 2005).

Scheduled for publication in the *AORN Journal* in 2006.

AORN Guidance Statement: Safe On-Call Practices in Perioperative Practice Settings

Introduction

The purpose of this guidance statement is to assist managers and clinicians in developing policies and procedures related to safe call practices for perioperative personnel. Providing care for patients requiring urgent or emergent surgery after regular hours of operation is a reality for perioperative nurses. Perioperative personnel are assigned designated times to be available for unplanned, urgent, or emergent procedures or to provide care for patients whose procedures run over the scheduled time. These assignments are referred to as "call."

Many perioperative nurses take call after scheduled hours, on weekends, and on holidays in addition to their daily shift assignments. Call hours vary, but generally are eight to 16 hours on weekdays, 48 to 64 hours on weekends, and 72 hours or more for extended holiday weekends. Actual hours worked during the call period are unpredictable and can range from 30 minutes to the entire length of the call period. Covering call may strain existing resources, create stress for perioperative staff members, affect safe patient care, and increase the potential for occupational injury due to prolonged work hours.

Background

Traditionally, perioperative nurses have worked eight-hour shifts; however, several new trends in perioperative staffing patterns include fewer, but longer, work days in addition to a call schedule. The expansion of work hour flexibility enhances individual nurse satisfaction and accommodates the organization's objectives.[1] Although the call schedule may be assigned on a rotating basis according to patient population, organizational needs, and demographic challenges, perioperative nurses may take extra call to increase compensation (eg, elective overtime). Perioperative nurses also may be mandated to work beyond their scheduled work/call shift to augment staffing requirements, meet unexpected patient needs, or satisfy organizational expectations (eg, mandatory overtime). These new trends in staffing and call hours have converged to create potentially hazardous conditions for patient and employee safety. There is a lack of current research in trending the number of hours worked per day by nurses. Anecdotal reports suggest that perioperative staff nurses are working longer hours with fewer breaks and often have inadequate time for rest between shifts.[2] Twenty-four hour call shifts are becoming more common.[3]

Long hours and prolonged periods of wakefulness are among working conditions that may have a negative effect on human performance.[4-6] It has been reported that 17 hours without sleep can have an adverse affect on performance equivalent to a blood alcohol concentration of 0.05%.[1] At 24 hours without sleep, performance degradation is equivalent to a blood alcohol concentration of 0.10.[7]

Fatigue resulting from working long hours can have a detrimental effect on patient care. Work by Rogers et al demonstrates a link between working long hours and medical errors; the possibility of an error triples after 12.5 hours of work.[3,5] Moreover, this research identified that medication errors, procedural errors, documentation, and transcription errors occur more frequently as work hours increase.[7,8] Studies suggest a correlation between sleep deprivation and negative effects on memory, language/numeric skills, visual attention and concentration.[9-11] In addition to creating a risk to patient safety, research indicates that sleep-deprived and fatigued nurses are at increased risk for personal injury on duty and when driving home after an extended work day.[5,12,13]

The existing nursing shortage is contributing to extended work hours and call shifts for perioperative nurses. It is predicted the number of RNs will fall to 20% below the demand by 2010.[2] More than 126,000 nursing positions currently are estimated to be unfilled.[1] This increases the burden of perioperative nurse fatigue with longer working hours and extended call requirements.

Guidance Statement

Recognizing that long work hours are a growing concern among nursing organizations, regulatory agencies, patient safety organizations, and perioperative nurses, this document offers a framework from which managers and clinicians can develop and implement methodologies to safely establish a call schedule. The call staffing plan retains the perioperative RN as circulator and is consistent with established AORN recommendations for nurse:patient ratios. The call staffing plan should minimize long work hours and allow for adequate recuperation between shifts. This guidance statement may be adapted to any setting in which call schedules are required.

Ultimately, health care organizations are responsible for developing and implementing staffing policies and procedures relevant to individual practice settings. Perioperative nurse leaders should be knowledgeable about emerging research and incorporate new evidence into the development, evaluation, and revision of policies for safe staffing and on-call practices.[6] Health care facilities should develop an organizational culture that promotes and provides safeguards to protect staff members and patients from potential errors and workplace injuries.

Individual facility policy should focus on creating call schedules that consider the effect of working long hours on patient safety as well as on perioperative staff members' well-being.[5,6,14] Safe call practices should be based on the following considerations:

- the type of facility (eg, trauma center, ambulatory surgery center), patient needs, procedure mix, demographics (eg, large metropolitan, rural), and organization structure;
- staff experience, competencies, skill mix; and
- staffing minimums as defined by state regulation, accrediting organization standards, professional organization recommendations, and patient safety requirements.

Suggested Strategies

■ Address staffing limitations in facility-specific policy and procedures based on relevant fatigue-related outcomes studies.

■ Establish a guideline to promote patient and worker safety in relation to the number of hours worked in a 24-hour, seven-day period based on current research. All worked hours should be included. For example, a facility may limit all scheduled and call back hours to 60 hours in a seven-day work week.[6,7]

■ Implement recuperation periods between shifts and establish limits for perioperative call schedules within designated time frames.[5,6]
  ▪ Budget enough full-time equivalents (FTEs) to allow for safe staffing levels.
  ▪ The budget should include adequate replacement staff members to allow rest periods for personnel who have worked long hours.

■ Establish the number of allowed consecutive hours that may be worked. Identify when the next scheduled work shift may begin. Work hour limitations should be determined in accordance with state regulation, accrediting organization standards, professional organization recommendations, and patient safety requirements.

■ Provide education to increase awareness of perioperative staff members' personal responsibility to arrive at work fully rested.[6,7]

■ Consider call requirements for perioperative staff members based on research indicating a correlation between adverse effects of sleep deprivation and aging.[15]

■ Reduce the amount and frequency of unscheduled overtime or last-minute call assignments.

■ Evaluate economic implications of unsafe call practices in relation to workplace injuries and adverse patient outcomes.

■ Develop performance improvement activities to determine if there is a correlation between workplace injuries, errors, adverse patient outcomes, and the number of hours worked during call.

■ Involve perioperative nurses in developing call schedules and work processes.

■ Develop competency-based orientation programs for new perioperative staff members, including skill acquisition to manage urgent and emergent patient care. The orientation time frame should be determined based on the type of procedures performed and experience of perioperative staff members.

■ Establish a staffing plan to recognize and retain staff members with extended tenure.
  ▪ Develop guidelines for self-assignment of call. Management should review the call schedule before posting it to ensure appropriate coverage for patient safety.
  ▪ Explore fiscal and operational benefits of establishing a dedicated call team.
  ▪ Consider providing sleep rooms to allow perioperative staff members the option to stay at the facility during the call shift to alleviate the potential of sleep deprivation and fatigue. A sleep room also would allow for timely response to urgent and emergent cases.

Summary

Call staffing and the associated long work hours can be challenging for both perioperative staff members and the health care organization. A change in culture is needed to recognize exhaustion as an unacceptable risk to patients and perioperative personnel safety. Perioperative health care providers have a personal responsibility to arrive at work fully rested. Health care organizations have a responsibility to create work and call schedules that consider the effect of long work hours on patient safety as well as perioperative staff members' welfare. The development of standardized safe work hours and call practices should reflect current recommendations emerging from authoritative sources, legislation, and empirical data. Prolonged work periods without adequate rest may contribute to diminished performance by perioperative personnel, placing both patients and workers at risk. This guidance statement may assist managers and clinicians in developing policies and procedures for safe call practices.

NOTES

1. "Keeping patients safe: Transforming the work environment of nurses," National Academies Press, http://www.nap.edu/openbook/0309090679/html/1.html (accessed 13 Dec 2004).
2. A Page, "Appendix C: Work hour regulation in safety-sensitive industries," in Keeping Patients Safe: Transforming the Work Environment of Nurses (Washington, DC: National Academies Press, 2004) 384-435.
3. A E Rogers et al, "The working hours of hospital staff nurses and patient safety," Health Affairs 23 (July/August 2004) 202-212.
4. "The effect of health care working conditions on patient safety," Evidence Report: Technology Assessment 74 (March 2003) 1-3.
5. M R Rosekind et al, "Managing fatigue in operational settings 1: Physiological considerations and countermeasures," Hospital Topics 75 (Summer 1997) 23-30.
6. M Rosekind et al, "Managing fatigue in operational settings 2: An integrated approach," Hospital Topics 75 (Summer 1997) 31-35.
7. D M Gaba, S K Howard, "Patient safety: Fatigue among clinicians and the safety of patients," The New England Journal of Medicine 347 (Oct 17, 2002) 1249-1255.

8. Long Working Hours for Nurses Lead to Medical Errors (news release, Bethesda, Md: Health Affairs, July 7, 2004) 1. Also available at http://www.rwjf.org/news/newsRelease070604.pdf (accessed 13 Dec 2004).
9. R P Hart et al, "Effect of sleep deprivation on first-year residents' response times, memory, and mood," Journal of Medical Education 62 (November 1987) 940-942.
10. R Rubin et al, "Neurobehavioral effects of the on-call experience in housestaff physicians," Journal of Occupational Medicine 33 (January 1991) 13-18.
11. J Robbins, F Gottlieb, "Sleep deprivation and cognitive testing in internal medicine house staff," Western Journal of Medicine 152 (January 1990) 82-86.
12. A Gurjala et al "Petition to the Occupational Safety and Health Administration requesting that limits be placed on hours worked by medical residents (HRG publication #1570)," (30 April 2001) Public Citizen, http://www.citizen.org/publications/release.cfm?ID=6771 (accessed 10 Dec 2004).
13. R G Hughes, A E Rogers, "Are you tired?" American Journal of Nursing 104 (March 2004) 36-38.
14. M L Parsons, J Stonestreet, "Staff nurse retention: Laying the groundwork by listening," Nursing Leadership Forum 8 (Spring 2004) 107-113.
15. K Reid, D Dawson, "Comparing performance on a simulated 12 hour shift rotation in young and older subjects," Occupational and Environmental Medicine 58 (January 2001) 58-62.

RESOURCES

Beck, S M; Wood, D S. "Helping OR staff members cope with the anxiety of being on call," Surgical Services Management 3 (November 1997) 39-42.
Dexter, F; O'Neal, L. "Weekend operating room on call staffing requirements," AORN Journal 74 (November 2001) 664-671.
Lamberg, L. "Impact of long working hours explored," JAMA 292 (July 7, 2004) 25-26.
Lucas, C E, et al. "Mathematical modeling to define optimum operating room staffing needs for trauma centers," JAMA 192 (May 2001) 559-565.
Tucker, J B, et al. "Using queuing theory to determine operating room staffing needs," Trauma Injury, Infection, and Critical Care 46 (January 1999) 71-79.
Tucker, P. "The impact of rest breaks upon accident risk, fatigue and performance: a review," Work and Stress 17 (April 2003) 123-137.

Originally published May 2005, AORN Journal.

AORN Guidance Statement: Safe Medication Practices in Perioperative Settings Across the Life Span

Introduction

This guidance statement provides a framework for perioperative registered nurses to develop, implement, and evaluate safe medication management practices specific to the perioperative setting. This evidenced-based framework may be used to facilitate policy development and provide a foundation for the creation of quality improvement (QI)/process improvement (PI) monitors. It is the responsibility of individual health care organizations to develop a culture of medication safety. Proactively reviewing medication errors from the viewpoint of "systems failures" and "systems solutions" will help encourage a culture free from shame and blame.

Perioperative practice settings addressed by this document include traditional operating rooms, ambulatory surgery units, physicians' offices, cardiac catheterization suites, endoscopy suites, radiology departments, and all other areas where operative and invasive procedures may be performed. For the purpose of this document, the term *OR* is inclusive of all perioperative practice environments.

First published in May 2002, the current guidance statement has been reviewed and updated by AORN's Presidential Commission on Patient Safety, in collaboration with the United States Pharmacopeia (USP), to reflect current safe medication practices.

Background

The National Institute of Medicine report *To Err Is Human: Building a Better Health System* increased awareness of medication errors. The report noted that "medication errors account for one out of 131 outpatient deaths and one out of 854 inpatient deaths."[1] Medication errors can originate at any point in the medication use process and affect patients of all ages. Medication error poses a substantial threat to patients. The perioperative setting creates additional challenges for safe medication administration practices. Related factors affecting the medication process in the perioperative environment include

- the aseptic dispensing of medications onto the sterile field,
- an intermediary to receive and transfer dispensed medications to the scrubbed licensed practitioner (eg, surgeon),
- time-sensitive conditions, and
- sensory distractions intrinsic to the environment.

Specific concerns associated with medication errors in the perioperative setting include, but are not limited to,

- inconsistent practices to communicate current and previous medication regimes (ie, medication reconciliation);
- verbal orders delivered through surgical masks may be muffled and contribute to confusion in the medication order (eg, name, strength, and/or dose);
- incomplete, ambiguous, incorrect, or illegibly written or spoken orders;
- inaccurate, illegible, or outdated surgical preference cards;
- removal of the contents from the original manufacturer's packaging to aseptically deliver contents onto the sterile field;
- limited knowledge of medications by scrubbed allied heath professionals receiving medications onto the sterile field;
- inconsistent labeling of medications on and off the sterile field;
- medication dispensed to the sterile field may be handled by multiple individuals before reaching the licensed individual administering the medication;
- high-alert medications available in multiple dose forms and concentrations;
- look-alike and sound-alike medications stored in close proximity;
- patient care complexity requiring rapid perioperative interventions;
- extended work hours leading to health care worker fatigue;
- care provided by multiple health care providers simultaneously; and
- multiple patient handoffs between care providers.

The following guidance is offered to support perioperative registered nurses in the provision of safe perioperative patient care.

Guidance Statement

Health care organizations should identify in policy which people and/or job categories may participate in medication management and administration. Facility policy for safe medication practice should be based on the five "rights" of medication administration:

- the right patient,
- the right medication,
- the right dose,
- the right time, and
- the right route.

The five rights of safe medication practices should be a final check before the administration of any medication.

Health care organizations should develop standardized procedures for safe medication practices in the OR designed to include, but not limited to, the following.

- Ensure proper patient identification.
- Document all patient medications.
- Assess for medication(s) contraindications.
- Confirm weight-based dosing before administration.
- Establish dose limits.
- Minimize use of verbal orders to the extent possible.
- Manage medications off the sterile field.
- Deliver medications to the sterile field.
- Manage medications on the sterile field.
- Document all intraoperative medications.
- Monitor and document patient for effects of medications.
- Preserve all original medication/solution containers and delivery devices until the conclusion of the procedure.
- Continually evaluate the medication delivery process for patients within the surgical setting.
- Define procedures for the questioning of any medication order thought to be unclear or inappropriate.[2]

General Risk Reduction Strategies

The following risk reduction strategies offer guidance for the development of policies, procedures, and associated QI and PI monitoring tools and reporting processes related to safe medication handling in the OR. The goal should be to meet or exceed the expectations for safe medication practice as outlined by published national patient safety initiatives (eg, the National Patient Safety Goals of the Joint Commission on Accreditation of Healthcare Organizations [JCAHO], guidelines of the Institute for Safe Medication Practices [ISMP] and USP).

Patient Identification

Minimize the potential for medication error related to incorrect identification of the patient through the establishment of standardized identification processes. Documentation of these processes may provide the necessary data to monitor outcomes for improvement.

- Consider the preoperative checklist as a permanent part of the patient care record.
- Perform patient identification using at least two patient identifiers, neither of which are to be the patient's room number.[3]
- Verification of patient identification should include information from the patient's identification (ID) band(s) or identification record when an ID band is not appropriate.
- Consider using the patient's date of birth as one means of identification (eg, pediatric population).
- Ensure that the contents of patient charts are verified for correct patient information.
- Imprints of patient information (eg, Addressograph stamp) on documents should be legible.
- Standardized forms should have patient identification in the same place on every page; duplexed pages should be identified on both sides in the same place.
- Identify in facility policy which people and/or job categories may participate in medication management and administration.

Accurate Medication List

Provider access to patient-specific information facilitates continuity of care and ensures that essential components for patient care decisions related to the medication management process are available. Readily accessible information should aid in the identification of risk related to medication allergy interaction, contraindication, and medication-medication or herbal-medication interaction. Documentation of this activity is an essential component of outcomes management in regard to patient safety.[4]

- Develop a consistent multidisciplinary approach for documenting the patient's medications using a standardized reconciliation sheet that is readily available for review before the procedure.[3]
- Actively involve the patient or authorized representative in the process of obtaining a complete list of the patient's current medications.[3]

Medication Contraindications

Whenever possible, written medication orders should be reviewed for appropriateness by a pharmacist before dispensing the medication. Concerns and issues related to medication, dose, frequency, route of administration, therapeutic duplication of the medication, its therapeutic class or chemical family, allergies, potential interactions, and contraindications are all elements of the review process.[4,5]

- Existing medication allergy information for each patient must be readily available and communicated to all members of the perioperative team.
- Allergy information may be obtained from patients, family members, legal guardians, and/or prior medical records.
- Health care organizations should provide readily available resources for perioperative personnel to identify medication class, nutrition and herbal supplement interactions (eg, calcium channel blockers and grapefruit) and associated medication class allergies (eg, amoxicillin and keflex).
- An organization-wide process should be in place to cross-reference patient drug allergy interactions, contraindication, and medication-medication/herbal-medication interaction potentials.[3]
  - Patient medications should be validated and cross-referenced during the medication-ordering phase of the medication delivery process.
  - Reference tools such as computer programs or charts should be used.

Accurate Dose Calculation

The patient's weight should be documented in both pounds and kilograms. Both mathematical formats provide a visual cue to eliminate discrepancies and to alert health care personnel to the proper numerical value used in weight calculations. Accurate weight measurement is critical for accurate dose calculation.[4] The medication dose calculation process should include, but is not limited to, the following.

- Accurately obtain weights on all patients before surgery.
- A facility-approved weight conversion chart (ie, pounds to kilograms) should be available for quick reference.

- Redesign patient care forms to clearly reflect weight in both pounds and kilograms.
- If there are discrepancies in weight or dose calculations, the patient should be reevaluated and the weight and dose recalculated.
- Medications ordered using weight-based dose schedules should be independently calculated and verified by two licensed individuals.
- Automate medication dosage calculations whenever possible.

Dose Limits

Health care organizations should identify high-risk and high-alert medications within the organization and develop processes to safeguard against error. Medications with narrow therapeutic ranges are considered at risk for error. Creating conversion charts targeting dose limits for high-risk medications will contribute to their safe use in surgery.[4]

- Dosage conversion charts or electronic aids should be used to calculate maximum dose limits, especially for high-alert medications.
- Separate weight-based conversion charts for children and adults should be developed for each of the major error-prone medications identified for that population at risk.

Verbal Orders

Verification of critical components of perioperative verbal orders, before the implementation of the order, affords an opportunity to confirm the accuracy of the verbal order.[3] Use of verbal and telephone orders should be limited.[2] When verbal orders are necessary, provide mechanisms to ensure accuracy, such as

- record the order in the patient's record according to facility policy as soon as feasible;[2,6]
- perform a "read-back" of the written order;[2,6]
- verbalize the read-back digit-by-digit (eg, say "one-two," not "twelve");[2,6] and
- allow only licensed health care providers to receive verbal orders;

Managing Medications Off the Sterile Field

Medications should be properly stored to ensure a process for safe and efficient delivery to the patient. Several key issues to consider are environmental conditions for storing medications to ensure product stability, look-alike and sound-alike medication storage, modification of the standard alphabetical medication storage system, and the care and handling of medical gases, reagents, and chemicals to eliminate catastrophic mistakes.[4]

- ♦ Standardize and limit the variation of strengths and concentrations of medications as much as possible.[3,4]
- ♦ Store medications safely with consideration given to separation of look-alikes and sound-alikes. This includes separating by generic name and packaging to the extent possible.[3,4,7]
- ♦ Limit the use of multidose vials whenever possible.[4,8,9]
- ♦ Include the facility pharmacist in formulating processes to determine when or if unused and unopened medications are allowed to be returned to the pharmacy.[4]
- ♦ Do not store medications alphabetically.[4]
- ♦ Label storage areas with both the medication's generic and brand names.
- ♦ Verify medication labels after medication retrieval and reconfirm with the written medication order.
- ♦ Label all medications, medication containers, and other solutions off the sterile field even if only one medication is involved.[3]
- ♦ At shift change or upon staff relief, all medications, medication labels, and the amount of medication administered should be verified concurrently by entering and exiting personnel.
- ♦ Discard any unlabeled solution or medication found in the OR.
- ♦ Treat medical gases, chemicals, and reagents (eg, formalin, normal saline, Lugol's solution, radiopaque dyes, glutaraldehyde) in the OR with the same care and caution as medications.

Delivering Medications to the Sterile Field

Before administering any medication, a verification process should include a review of the product label for the medication name, strength, and expiration date. This review process should be accomplished in conjunction with an examination of the written medication order to confirm that the correct medication is to be administered. A visual inspection should be made for any indication that the medication was compromised during the storage process (eg, particulates, discoloration).[4]

- ♦ Confirm all medications listed on the physician's preference list with the surgeon before delivery to the sterile field.

- ♦ Orders with abbreviations, symbols, or acronyms should be clarified with the ordering clinician to minimize confusion or misinterpretation.
- ♦ Verify medication in its original container for the correct name, strength, dosage, and route with the surgeon's preference card or documented verbal order.
- ♦ Actively communicate the medication name, strength, dosage, and expiration date as the medication is passed to the sterile field.[4]
  - – Verbally and visually confirm all medications delivered to the sterile field, including medication name, strength, dosage, and expiration date.[4]
  - – Medications should be verified concurrently by the circulating registered nurse and scrub person.
  - – If there is no designated scrub person, the circulating registered nurse should confirm the medication visually and verbally with the licensed professional performing the surgical procedure.
- ♦ Deliver one medication at a time onto the sterile field.
- ♦ Do not remove stoppers from vials for the purpose of pouring medications.
- ♦ Use commercially available sterile transfer devices when possible (eg, sterile vial spike, filter straw, plastic catheter).
- ♦ Reconfirm maximum dose limits.

Managing Medications on the Sterile Field

Communication is a vital key to the success of the medication delivery process.

- ♦ Verbally and visually confirm the medication (ie, medication name, strength, dosage, and expiration date) upon receipt from the circulating registered nurse even if only one medication is involved.[4]
- ♦ Label the medication container on the sterile field immediately before receipt of the medication. Avoid distractions and interruptions during the labeling process and while dispensing medications onto the sterile field.
- ♦ Label all medication containers and delivery devices with a minimum of the medication name, strength, and concentration when needed.[6]
- ♦ Verbally and visually confirm the medication name, strength, and dose by reading the

medication label aloud while passing a medication to the licensed professional performing the procedure.[4]

♦ When patient hand-offs (eg, personnel relief) occur, the medication verification process should take place. The medication should be confirmed for accuracy (ie, product label reviewed for the medication name, strength, and expiration date) in conjunction with a review of the written medication order to validate that the correct medication is on the field.[3]

♦ Discard any solution or medication found on or off the sterile field without an identification label.

Documenting All Intraoperative Medications

A complete and accurate accounting of the medications and solutions used during the surgical encounter is essential to address medication-related issues that may arise during all phases of perioperative care.[4]

♦ Ensure that intraoperative documentation reflects all medications (including irrigation solutions, doses, and routes of administration) administered throughout the procedure.

♦ Document medication administration per organizational policy.

♦ Documentation should incorporate the Perioperative Nursing Data Set (PNDS). The expected outcome for safe medication practices is outcome O9, "The patient receives appropriate medication(s), safely administered during the perioperative period." This outcome falls within the domain of Safety (D1). The associated nursing diagnoses may include X29, "Risk for injury." The associated interventions leading to the desired outcome include I123, "Verifies allergies"; I8, "Administers prescribed medications and solutions"; and I51, "Evaluates response to medications."[10(p103-104)]

Monitoring Patients for Effects of Medications

Assessment and documentation of the patient's response to medication administration provides vital clues related to dose effectiveness and the presence of a potential medication-related adverse effect.[4]

♦ Continually assess, monitor, and document the patient's response to medication administered.[4,10(p104)]

♦ Policies and procedures should be developed for reporting and responding to medication errors and other adverse effects.

♦ Error reporting should occur in a nonpunitive culture.[3]

Retaining All Original Medication/Solution Containers and Delivery Devices

The practice of maintaining possession of medication containers and delivery devices until the patient leaves the OR is important in the event of a medication-related error or adverse reaction. A root cause analysis should be performed following any adverse event. Maintaining possession of these containers may facilitate the analysis.

Periodic Evaluation of the Medication Management Process

An essential step in the medication management process includes ongoing review. An established QI/PI program may identify failure points contributing to medication errors and may aid in improvements in patient safety.

♦ The QI/PI program should include a routine review and update of all preprinted order sheets, and facility-approved standing orders, including
   – medication choice;
   – dose; and
   – delivery method.

♦ Eliminate or minimize the use of problem-prone abbreviations, symbols, and acronyms.[11,12,13]

Additional Strategies for Medication Safety

■ Operationalize a process for the ongoing review of key elements of the medication delivery process known to contribute to medication errors, to include
   ♦ prescribing,
   ♦ order processing,
   ♦ dispensing,
   ♦ administration, and
   ♦ monitoring.[14]

■ Provide OR personnel with appropriate and timely education related to medication safety procedures. Facilities should implement processes for validating perioperative medication competency covering all age-specific populations (eg, perioperative medication competencies in "AORN's safe medication administration tool kit").[15]

■ Use a competency checklist focused on the medication delivery process (eg, perioperative medication performance validation record in "AORN's safe medication administration tool kit").[15]

■ Establish outcomes, standards, and guidelines to monitor and manage institutional improvements in regard to medication safety, to include
  ♦ the patient receives appropriate prescribed medication(s) safely administered during the perioperative period;[10(p103)]
  ♦ the patient demonstrates knowledge of medication management;[10(p179)] and
  ♦ the patient demonstrates knowledge of pain management.[10(p179)]

■ Modify work schedule requirements in surgical settings to minimize fatigue-induced errors.

■ Provide adequate lighting in dark environments (eg, endoscopy, minimally invasive procedures, ophthalmic procedures).

■ Initiate constraints and/or forcing functions to minimize risks related to medication management and administration.
  ♦ Constraints are approaches that make a medication error difficult. Examples include dose limit protocols, automatic stop orders, triple-checking medications, and labeling all medication containers in the OR.
  ♦ Forcing functions are approaches that make a medication error impossible. Examples include removing certain medications (eg, cytotoxic agents, concentrations of saline higher than 0.9%) from the OR.[3,16]

■ Adopt guidelines for unapproved abbreviations, acronyms, and symbols outlined in national patient safety initiatives.[11,12,13]
  ♦ Care must be taken to decrease the risk for error and maximize patient safety by avoiding error-prone abbreviations and symbols known to cause confusion or lead to misinterpretation. Examples:
    – Use of the handwritten letter "U" for "units" can be mistaken for a zero.[11,12,13]
    – Zeros in combination with decimal points can lead to a 10-fold dosing error when the decimal point is not detected.[16]

♦ A supplemental list or poster placed in the workplace outlining common abbreviation mistakes may help to focus attention on high-risk avoidance.[17]

♦ Recommendations and guidance provided by the ISMP "List of error-prone abbreviations, symbols, and dose designations"; the USP "Potentially dangerous abbreviations"; and the JCAHO "Official 'do not use' list" should be considered.

■ Ensure that current and reliable medication reference materials with age-specific guidelines are readily available to the perioperative team.

■ Provide pharmacy support for consultation regarding unusual medications and dosages.

■ Standardize institutional forms to aid communication and decrease confusion while enhancing productivity between health care providers.[3]

NOTES

1. Institute of Medicine, *To Err Is Human: Building a Safer Health System,* Committee on Quality of Heath Care in America, ed L Kohn, J Corrigan, M Donaldson (Washington, DC: National Academy Press, 2000) 27.

2. "Council recommendations to reduce medication errors associated with verbal medication orders and prescriptions," (Feb 20, 2001) National Coordinating Council for Medication Error Reporting and Prevention, *http://www.nccmerp.org/council/council2001-02-20.html?USP* (accessed 23 Jan 2006).

3. "Facts about 2006 national patient safety goals," Joint Commission on Accreditation of Healthcare Organizations, *http://www.jcaho.org/accredited+organizations/patient+safety/06_npsg/06_facts.htm* (accessed 23 Jan 2006).

4. D S Rich, "New JCAHO medication management standards for 2004," *American Journal of Health-System Pharmacists* 61 (July 2004) 1349-1358.

5. "Therapeutic duplication," Administration on Aging, *http://www.homemeds.org/pdf_files/ProtocolUnnec.Therap_2.pdf* (accessed 23 Jan 2006).

6. "Joint Commission 2006 National Patient Safety Goals: Implementation expectations," Joint Commission on Accreditation of Healthcare Organizations, *http://www.jcaho.org/accredited+organizations/patient+safety/06_npsg_ie.pdf* (accessed 23 Jan 2006).

7. Joint Commission on Accreditation of Healthcare Organizations, "Look-alike, sound-alike drug names," *Sentinel Event Alert* 19 (May 2001). Also available at *http://www.jcaho.org/about+us/news+letters/sentinel+event+alert/sea_19.htm* (accessed 23 Jan 2006).

8. Institute for Safe Medication Practices, "Patient safety movement calls for reexamination of multidose vial use," *ISMP Medication Safety Alert* (June 14, 2000). Also available at *http://www.ismp.org/newsletters/acutecare/articles/20000614.asp* (accessed 23 Jan 2006).

9. Institute for Safe Medication Practices, "New official interpretation of JCAHO standard bars access to pharmacy after hours," *ISMP Medication Safety Alert* (May 30, 2001). Also available at *http://www.ismp.org/newsletters/acutecare articles/20010530.asp* (accessed 23 Jan 2006).

10. S. Beyea, ed, *Perioperative Nursing Data Set: The Perioperative Nursing Vocabulary,* second ed (Denver: AORN, Inc, 2002) 103-104, 179.

11. "The official 'do not use' list," Joint Commission on Accreditation of Healthcare Organizations, *http://www.jcaho.org/accredited+organizations/patient +safety/dnu.htm* (accessed 9 Oct 2005).

12. United States Pharmocopeia, "Abbreviations can lead to medication errors," *USP Quality Review* no 80 (July 2004). Also available at *http://www.usp.org/patient Safety/newsletters/qualityReview/qr802004-07-01.html* (accessed 23 Jan 2006).

13. "ISMP's list of error-prone abbreviations, symbols, and dose designations," Institute for Safe Medication Practices, *http://www.ismp.org/tools/errorproneabbreviations .pdf* (accessed 23 Jan 2006).

14. "Frequently asked questions," Institute for Safe Medication Practices, *http://www.ismp.org/faq.asp#Question_9* (accessed 9 Oct 2005).

15. "AORN's safe medication administration tool kit," AORN Online, *http://www.aorn.org/toolkit/safemed* (accessed 23 Jan 2006).

16. Joint Commission on Accreditation of Healthcare Organizations, "High-alert medications and patient safety," *Sentinel Event Alert* 11 (Nov 19, 1999). Also available at *http://www.jcaho.org/about+us/news+letters/sentinel +event+alert/sea_11.htm* (accessed 23 Jan 2006).

17. "Joint Commission perspectives on patient safety: Maintaining safety/reducing risk," *Joint Commission Resources* 2 (September 2002) 1-11.

RESOURCES

Agency for Healthcare Research and Quality, *http://www.ahrq.gov* (accessed 29 Oct 2003).

Institute for Safe Medication Practices, *http://www.ismp.org* (accessed 29 Oct 2003).

Institute of Medicine, *http://www.iom.edu* (accessed 29 Oct 2003).

The Leapfrog Group, *http://www.leapfroggroup.org* (accessed 29 Oct 2003).

National Patient Safety Foundation, *http://www.npsf.org* (accessed 29 Oct 2003).

The National Quality Forum, *http://www.qualityforum.org* (accessed 29 Oct 2003).

Partnership for Patient Safety, *http://www.p4ps.org* (accessed 29 Oct 2003).

United States Pharmacopeia, *http://www.usp.org* (accessed 29 Aug 2005).

Originally published May 2002, *AORN Journal.*
Revised November 2003; published March 2004, *AORN Journal.*
Revised November 2005; scheduled for publication in the *AORN Journal* in 2006.

AORN Guidance Statement: Sharps Injury Prevention in the Perioperative Setting

Introduction

The purpose of this guidance document is to assist perioperative registered nurses in the development of sharps injury prevention programs using identified best practices to reduce percutaneous injuries. It also suggests strategies to overcome obstacles to compliance with established sharps safety protocols.

The perioperative setting is a high-risk environment, and perioperative RNs are routinely faced with high risk for exposure to bloodborne pathogens from percutaneous injuries. Although the scope of the problem is not completely known, the National Institute for Occupational Safety and Health (NIOSH) estimates that 600,000 to 800,000 percutaneous injuries occur annually among heath care workers.[1] Percutaneous injuries primarily are associated with occupational transmission of the hepatitis B virus (HBV), hepatitis C virus (HCV), and HIV, but they may be implicated in the transmission of more than 20 other pathogens.[2] Understanding the etiology of percutaneous injuries in the perioperative setting is paramount to developing a safe prevention program.

Background

Percutaneous injuries occur throughout all health care facilities, and many occur in the perioperative setting.[3,4] Exposure to bloodborne pathogens occurs during all phases of the perioperative process. Research indicates that injuries from sharp devices or instruments occur in 7% to 15% of all surgical procedures. Procedures identified as posing the highest risk of injury are thoracic, trauma, burn, emergency orthopedic, major vascular, intra-abdominal, and gynecologic surgeries.[5] Risk of a sharps injury increases during more invasive, longer procedures that result in higher blood loss.[6] Fatigue resulting from working extended hours in combination with the fast pace of the perioperative environment also may contribute to increased risk of percutaneous injuries.[7-9]

Nurses comprise the largest segment of health care workers and are reported to sustain the highest number of percutaneous injuries overall.[2] Observational studies have demonstrated that perioperative personnel experience the highest percutaneous injury rates, but 70% to 96% of exposures were underreported.[5] Surgeons and first assistants have the highest risk of injury and sustain more than half (ie, 59%) of percutaneous injuries in the perioperative setting.[6] Scrub personnel experienced the second highest frequency of percutaneous injury, followed by anesthesia care providers and circulating nurses.[6]

Injuries from hollow bore needles constitute the majority of injuries and pose the highest risk of exposure to bloodborne pathogens.[10] Although the risk of injury from hollow bore needles is prevalent in the perioperative setting, the epidemiology of sharps injuries in the OR is different from that of other locations in health care. Suture needles have been identified as the most frequent mechanism of percutaneous injury in the OR; they are involved in as many as 77% of such injuries.[4,6] Scalpels are the second most frequent mechanism of injury, followed by retractors, skin or bone hooks, and sharp electrosurgical tips.[11,12]

Percutaneous injuries often are self-inflicted. Studies indicate that 6% to 16% of these injuries occur during hand-to-hand passing of sharp instruments, suture needles, and other sharp devices. The most common body part injured is the non-dominant hand. Injuries from suture needles occur most often

- when loading the needle holder or repositioning the needle;
- during hand-to-hand passing of sharp devices between scrub personnel and the surgeon;
- during suturing, particularly muscle and fascia (eg, wound closure) when the needle is being manipulated and guided with fingers;
- when retracting or stretching tissue with hands;
- when the surgeon sews toward his or her own or an assistant's hand;
- when tying suture with the needle attached;
- after the suture has just been used and remains unattended on the operative field—even if suture is unattended on the field for only a short time, the needle holder can fall off the field onto a health care worker's foot, or scrubbed personnel may reach for it in an attempt to prevent it from sliding off the field; and
- when placing the used needle in an over-filled sharps container.[3]

Injuries from scalpels most often occur

- when loading or removing a disposable scalpel blade on a reusable knife handle;

◆ during hand-to-hand passing of the scalpel;

◆ during dissection when the tissue is being retracted or spread with hands;

◆ when cutting toward the surgeon's or an assistant's fingers;

◆ immediately before or after use when the scalpel is left on the operative field unattended—even if this is for only a short time, the scalpel can fall off the field onto a health care worker's foot, or scrubbed personnel may reach for it in an attempt to prevent it from sliding off the field; and

◆ when the scalpel is placed in an over-filled or poorly located sharps container.[3]

Glove barrier failure is a common occurrence in the perioperative setting. Glove failures can be caused by punctures, tears by sharp devices, or spontaneous failures. These failures expose the wearer to bloodborne pathogens. Studies have demonstrated that glove perforations often occur after an average of 40 minutes of use during surgical procedures. When two pairs of gloves are worn (ie, double gloving), in most instances, only the outer glove is perforated when punctured by a sharp device. In addition, research demonstrates that when two pairs of gloves are worn and a puncture occurs, the volume of blood on a solid sharp device (eg, suture needle) is reduced by as much as 95%. There is evidence that double gloving can reduce the risk of exposure to blood and body fluids, if the outer glove is punctured, by as much as 87%.[6]

The Occupational Safety and Health Administration (OSHA) requires health care organizations to protect their workers and have a written exposure control plan. Protection occurs by using universal precautions, engineering controls, work practice controls, organizational controls, and communication. The standard also requires employers to maintain a log of injuries from contaminated sharps.[13]

Guidance Statement

The perioperative environment poses unique challenges for reducing the risk of injuries from sharp devices. Surgery involves precise, regimented actions that require planning, communication, and team work. These same elements can be employed to mitigate the inherent hazards associated with sharp devices encountered in the perioperative setting. Perioperative RNs should actively participate in the development and implementation of strategies to reduce the risk of sharps injuries to health care team members.

Perioperative nursing management should work with the facility risk manager or safety officer to identify the types of sharp devices and how they are used in the perioperative setting. Both perioperative nursing management and the risk manager or safety officer should have a thorough understanding of OSHA's standards.[3]

By law, an effective sharps injury and blood-borne pathogen exposure control program must be written, communicated to all workers in the perioperative setting, and uniformly supported and enforced by perioperative leadership.[2,13] A multidisciplinary team is key to the success of this process. This team, using steps consistent with the continuous quality improvement process, must conduct a baseline assessment and set priorities for developing an action plan.[2,6]

Perioperative-Specific Risk Reduction Strategies

▨ Adopt and incorporate safe habits into daily work activities when preparing and using sharp devices.

▨ Focus attention on the intent of the action when working with sharp items, and minimize rushing and distractions while applying safety techniques during critical moments.

▨ During preparation for operative or other invasive procedures:
  ▪ inspect the surgical field for adequate lighting and space to perform the procedure;
  ▪ organize the work area so that the sharps are always pointed away from staff members;
  ▪ establish a separate area to place a reusable sharp for safe handling during the procedure;
  ▪ use standardized sterile field set-ups; and
  ▪ include identification of the neutral zone in the preoperative briefing.[14]

▨ During the operative or other invasive procedure:
  ▪ wear two pairs of gloves (ie, double gloving);
  ▪ monitor gloves for punctures;
  ▪ encourage the use of blunt suture needles;
  ▪ use neutral or hands-free technique for passing sharp items whenever possible or practical, instead of passing hand-to-hand;

- give verbal notification when passing a sharp device;
- keep visual contact with the procedure site and the sharp device;
- take steps to control the location of the sharp device;
- be aware of other staff members in the area when handling a sharp device;
- keep track of and account for all sharp items throughout the procedure;
- contain used sharps on the sterile field in a designated, disposable, puncture-resistant needle container, and replace it as necessary;
- check to be sure the disposable, puncture-resistant needle container is securely closed before handing it off the field;
- load suture needles using the suture packet to assist in mounting the suture needle in the needle holder, and use the appropriate instrument to adjust and unload the needle;
- remove the needle from the suture before tying, or use "control-release" sutures that allow the needle to be removed with a straight pull on the needle holder;
- activate the safety feature of a safety engineered device immediately after use according to manufacturers' instructions;
- keep hands away from the surgical site when sharp items are in use (eg, suturing, cutting);
- use one-handed or blunt instrument-assisted suturing techniques to avoid finger contact with the suture needle or tissue being sutured;
- provide a barrier between the hands and the needle after use; and
- use gloves and an instrument to pick up sharp items (eg, suture needles, hypodermic needles, scalpel blades) that have fallen on the floor.[2,3,6,13-17]
- During postprocedure clean up:
  - inspect the surgical setup used during the procedure for sharps;
  - transport reusable sharps in a closed, secure container to the designated clean-up area;
  - inspect the sharps container for overfilling before discarding disposable sharps in it;
  - make sure the sharps container is large enough to accommodate the entire device;
  - avoid bringing hands close to the opening of a sharps container;

- do not place hands or fingers into a container to dispose of a device; and
- keep hands behind the sharp tip when disposing.[3,14,18]

Health care organizations and their employees are responsible for actively participating in strategies to reduce percutaneous injuries. The employing facility should provide an environment that reduces the risk of percutaneous injuries from contaminated sharp devices. A well-developed safety program and support from management sends a clear message to employees about the organization's commitment to preventing injuries and keeping employees safe. Fewer percutaneous injuries are reported in organizations that have a strong culture of safety. Individual health care workers have a responsibility to be educated about the prevalence and mode of transmission of bloodborne pathogens and to use measures to protect themselves.[19]

Individual Perioperative RN's Responsibilities

- Observe local, state, and federal regulations (eg, OSHA regulations).
- Comply with methods to protect yourself from disease transmission (eg, get the hepatitis B vaccination).
- Use devices with safety features that are provided by your employer.
- Prevent hollow bore percutaneous injuries during injections or bodily fluid retrieval by using
  - needleless systems or sharps with engineered sharp injury protection devices whenever possible;
  - retractable, protective sheath or self-resheathing, self-blunting, or hinged re-cap needles to administer local anesthetics and other injectable medications;
  - blunt cannulas to withdraw medications and fluids from vials; and
  - the one-handed recapping technique, only if no other alternatives exist.
- Practice using safety devices to establish familiarity and experience with them before using them in practice.
- Actively participate in the safety conversion process and help others adapt to the change.
- Use personal protective equipment.

- Use sharps receptacles that are
  - identifiable (ie, orange, orange-red), closable, and labeled with the biohazard symbol;
  - appropriately sized with a full line that is readily visible;
  - puncture resistant and leak proof;
  - located close to the point of use;
  - maintained upright when in use; and
  - routinely replaced and not allowed to overfill.
- Participate in education about bloodborne pathogens, and follow recommended infection prevention practices.
- Support and guide perioperative team members to follow these risk reduction strategies.
- Encourage perioperative staff members to proactively report hazards that pose a threat of percutaneous injury.
- Know the location in your department of the exposure control plan.
- Follow exposure control policy if injured (ie, wash site with soap and water, provide immediate care to the exposure site).[9,13]

Employer Responsibilities

- Comply with local, state, and federal regulations regarding percutaneous injury prevention.
- Create a safety-oriented culture.
- Encourage timely reporting of all percutaneous injuries by all perioperative team members.
- Analyze needle-stick and other sharps-related injuries in the perioperative setting to identify hazards and injury trends.
- Establish a communication mechanism to seek input from perioperative team members regarding risks specific to the perioperative setting.
- Provide training for all perioperative personnel that includes risk reduction strategies designed specifically to address the risks encountered in the perioperative setting.
- Evaluate and select safety devices that are acceptable to all members of the perioperative team who use them. The safety device should provide features that work effectively, are reliable, do not compromise patient or worker safety, and are ergonomically designed to the acceptable specifications of the users.
- Provide and have readily available the appropriate sharps safety devices, and provide adequate training on their use.

- Evaluate the effectiveness of established risk reduction strategies and products, provide feedback, and modify them as necessary to reduce the risk of percutaneous injuries.[7]
- Establish staffing patterns that minimize extended work hours and allow for adequate recuperation to decrease the risk of fatigue-related injuries.[20]

Overcoming Obstacles to Compliance

Psychosocial and organizational factors may impede change. An employee's risk-taking personality profile, perception that the organization is not committed to worker safety, and a perceived belief that there is a conflict between providing optimal patient care and protecting oneself from exposure contribute to an employee's resistance to changing to safer practices.[2] For example, although percutaneous injuries continue to occur in the perioperative setting, 71% of respondents in a national survey indicated that they have not evaluated blunt-tip suture needles for use in the OR, and only 2% of respondents have fully implemented blunt-tip suture needles. Only 14% of respondents had implemented safety scalpels into their ORs.[4]

Changes in attitudes about risk of exposure must occur before practice can change to comply with sharps safety protocols. It is difficult to change ingrained habits. People are most likely to change behavior when they perceive a significant personal risk. Education about the risk of contracting a bloodborne disease from a percutaneous injury with a contaminated sharp device should be presented in the early stages of a health care worker's career in order to develop safe practice habits.[5]

Surgery involves precise, regimented actions requiring planning, communication, and team work. These same elements can be employed to overcome obstacles to compliance with measures meant to mitigate the inherent hazards of sharp devices encountered in the perioperative setting. Suggested strategies to overcome obstacles to compliance include the following.

- Use frequent and multiple training methods that include audiovisual aids, articles, hands-on clinical practice, and visual reminders (eg, laminated posters).
- Develop a multidisciplinary sharps injury prevention education plan.

■ Incorporate sharps injury prevention instruction into initial nursing education to promote well-established, safe habits.

■ Include sharps injury prevention strategies during orientation of new employees.

■ Form a multidisciplinary sharps safety committee that includes, but is not limited to, perioperative RNs, surgeons, anesthesia care providers, surgical technologists, and first assistants. This team could be asked to

■ help with the selection and evaluation of acceptable safety devices (eg, scalpels that employ a one-handed technique or are totally disposable) and

■ work with physicians to explore alternative techniques, such as adhesive skin closures; alternatives for securing catheters; use of blunt suture needles, rounded scalpels, or stapling devices, when procedurally appropriate; and use of alternative methods for cutting tissue (eg, harmonic scalpel, rounded scissors, laser devices, electrosurgery active electrodes).

■ Network with other facilities to learn about their success stories.

■ Collaborate with personnel who use the device, and facilitate change instead of dictating change.

■ Inform perioperative team members about current research on disease transmission from percutaneous injuries and relate it to the individual's experience.

■ Work with resisters to gain buy-in to the sharps safety program.

■ Remove as many conventional sharp items as possible from stock.

■ Create a culture of safety in which every team member is empowered to call attention to deficiencies in sharps management.[2,9,12,13]

Selecting and Evaluating New Products

As risk reduction strategies are identified, a multidisciplinary team should evaluate and select the best products to meet the facility's needs. An ongoing review process should be developed to assess, evaluate, and modify the plan as needed. Product evaluation and selection should include the following.

■ Assemble a multidisciplinary team to develop, implement, and evaluate a process for selecting products to reduce sharps injury in the OR. Staff members who work with the product are key components of the team. A strong interdisciplinary commitment to best practices and worker safety is the optimal foundation necessary for change to occur.

■ Review the literature for research about the mechanism, frequency, time, and place of injuries, as well as the role and body part of the person sustaining the percutaneous injury to determine priority areas on which to focus.

■ Identify the products to be evaluated. Focus on their intended use in the facility and identify any special technique or design factors that will influence safety, efficiency, and user acceptability. Seek data from all sources on the safety and overall performance of the devices.

■ Ensure that participants in the evaluation represent all of the end users. To ensure a successful evaluation, users must have adequate training. Use clear, objective, consistent criteria to evaluate safety devices.

■ Continue to monitor a safety device after it has been implemented to assess performance and to identify if there is a need for additional training.[2,10]

Summary

Occupational exposure to bloodborne pathogens via percutaneous injuries is one of the most serious dangers perioperative team members face on a daily basis. The risk of sustaining a percutaneous injury can be decreased through employee education, clear communication, device engineering, and focused work practice controls. Risk reduction strategies should include specific practices aimed at reducing the unique risks of percutaneous injuries encountered in the perioperative environment. AORN recognizes the various settings in which perioperative RNs practice, and the suggested risk reduction strategies in this guidance statement are intended to be adaptable to any setting where surgical or other invasive procedures are performed.

NOTES

1. "AORN position statement on workplace safety," in *Standards, Recommended Practices, and Guidelines* (Denver: AORN, Inc, 2004) 169-171.

2. "Workbook for designing, implementing, and evaluating a sharps injury prevention program," Centers for Disease Control and Prevention, *http://www.cdc.gov/sharpssafety* (accessed 5 Jan 2005).

3. ECRI, "Sharps injuries in the operating room—A new focus for OSHA," *Operating Room Risk Management* (December 2004) 1-5.

4. J Perry, G Parker, J Jagger, "EPINet report: 2001 percutaneous injury rates," *Advances in Exposure Prevention* 6 no 3 (2003) 32-36.

5. C L Holodnick, V Barkauskas, "Reducing percutaneous injuries in the OR by educational methods," *AORN Journal* 72 (September 2000) 461-476.

6. R Berguer, P J Heller, "Preventing sharps injuries in the operating room" *Journal of the American College of Surgeons* 199 (September 2004) 462-467.

7. K Hanecke et al, "Accident risk as a function of hour at work and time of day as determined from accident data and exposure models for the German working population," *Scandinavian Journal of Work, Environment, and Health* 24 suppl (1998) 43-48.

8. T Roth, T A Roehrs, "Etiologies and sequelae of excessive daytime sleepiness," *Clinical Therapeutics* 18 (July/August 1996) 562-576.

9. Battelle Memorial Institute, JIL Information Systems, "An overview of the scientific literature concerning fatigue, sleep, and the circadian cycle," Air Line Pilots Association, *http://cf.alpa.org/internet/projects/ftdt/backgr/batelle.htm* (accessed 5 Jan 2005).

10. National Institute for Occupational Safety and Health, "Preventing needlestick injuries in health care settings," publ 2000-108 (Washington, DC: US Department of Health and Human Services, November 1999).

11. J Jagger, M Bentley, P Tereskerz, "A study of patterns and prevention of blood exposures in OR personnel," *AORN Journal* 67 (May 1998) 979-987.

12. S Wasek, "10 practical ways to implement safety devices," *Outpatient Surgery Magazine* 4 (December 2003).

13. "Regulations (Standards–29 CFR) Bloodborne pathogens 1910.1030," Occupational Safety and Health Administration, *http://www.osha.gov/pls/oshaweb/owadisp.show_document?p_table=STANDARDS&p_id=10051* (accessed 5 Jan 2005).

14. "Recommended practices for maintaining a sterile field," in *Standards, Recommended Practices, and Guidelines* (Denver: AORN, Inc, 2004) 367.

15. C Twomey, "Does double gloving double the protection?" *Infection Control Today*, *http://www.infectioncontroltoday.com/articles/051feat3.html* (accessed 5 Jan 2005).

16. "Recommended practices for sponge, sharp, and instrument counts," in *Standards, Recommended Practices, and Guidelines* (Denver: AORN, Inc, 2004) 230-231.

17. "Recommended practices for environmental cleaning in the surgical practice setting," in *Standards, Recommended Practices, and Guidelines* (Denver: AORN, Inc, 2004) 273-279.

18. "Recommended practices for standard and transmission-based precautions in the perioperative practice setting," in *Standards, Recommended Practices, and Guidelines* (Denver: AORN, Inc, 2004) 361.

19. "AORN guidance statement: Safe on-call practices in perioperative practice settings" in *Standards, Recommended Practices, and Guidelines* (Denver: AORN, Inc, 2005) 193-195.

20. K Royer, "Primer on prevention of sharps injuries" (Sharps Safety) *Outpatient Surgery Magazine* 5 (September 2004) 50.

Originally published March 2005, *AORN Journal.*

AORN Guidance Statement: Perioperative Staffing

Introduction

The purpose of this guidance statement is to provide a framework for developing a staffing plan throughout the continuum of perioperative patient care, beginning with scheduling a surgical or invasive procedure through the postoperative phase III/follow-up process. Staffing in the perioperative setting is dynamic in nature and depends on the clinical judgment, critical thinking skills, and administrative skills of nursing management in the perioperative setting. Patients undergoing surgical or invasive procedures require perioperative nursing care provided by a perioperative registered nurse, regardless of the setting. This guidance statement offers suggested staffing strategies to accommodate safe perioperative patient care while promoting a safe work environment.

Background

To provide safe and effective patient care, individual health care organizations should have staffing policies and procedures relevant to individual practice settings. The health care system is affected by increasing demand for health care, continued economic pressures, the looming nursing shortage, and financial ramifications from medico-legal issues. Patient safety is the primary focus of perioperative nurses and other health care providers. Perioperative nursing leaders need to be judicious in meeting the challenge of stretching scarce resources without compromising patient care. Perioperative department nursing leaders have an ethical responsibility to maintain staffing levels that are appropriate for providing safe patient care while they also balance shrinking budgets.

Guidance Statement

Perioperative nurse leaders should identify workforce requirements and the effect of environmental factors on staffing patterns. Surgery is performed in a wide variety of settings with uniquely different needs. Perioperative clinical staffing guidelines should be based on individual patient needs, patient acuity, technological demands, staff member competency, skill mix, practice standards, health care regulations, and accreditation requirements.[1,2] Staffing requirements are relative to department functions and assigned role expectations.

An effective staffing plan is flexible and responsive to short-term and long-term patient and organizational demands. Effective planning involves determining staffing needs, planning for the appropriate staffing mix and number of staff members, budgeting for personnel costs, and scheduling personnel. Perioperative nursing management should determine both direct and indirect patient caregivers for the unit. Additionally, productive and nonproductive time should be considered.[2] The perioperative staffing policy should state the minimum number of nursing personnel that will be provided for various types of surgical procedures. Complexity of the procedure may require more than the minimum number of nursing personnel identified. Table 1 includes recommended minimum staffing requirements.

Call

The perioperative staffing plan includes provisions for unplanned, urgent, or emergent procedures and how to provide care for patients whose procedures run over scheduled time. Call staffing plans should be based on strategies to minimize long work hours, allow for adequate recuperation, and retain the perioperative RN as circulator. Scheduling requirements for call are subject to facility type, location, nature of services provided, and patient population served. Staffing for call should be provided in accordance with standards of perioperative and perianesthesia nursing practice. Safe call practices should be based on AORN's "Guidance statement: Safe on-call practices in perioperative practice settings."[3-5]

A systematic approach based on the operational needs of the department is required to develop a staffing plan. Identifying the hours of operation defined by the department or facility, in addition to the hours needed to cover off-shift (eg, holidays, nights, weekends) emergent/urgent surgery and the number of operating/procedure rooms is the initial step in determining staffing needs.[6] Review of historical data regarding minutes/hours of service, case volumes, case mix, and technology demands and projections for the coming year are essential for staff scheduling and budgeting. The following formula provides a platform to develop an annual staffing plan and budget. The formula is flexible and can be adapted to meet the specific needs of the perioperative setting. Although the basic formula is based on 100% utilization, it can be modified to coincide with expected volume.

Table 1

MINIMUM STAFFING RECOMMENDATIONS		
Surgical phase	**Minimum requirements**	**Comments**
Scheduling	1 clerical person under the supervision of a perioperative RN	Depending on the size of the facility, this activity may be combined with other business or clerical duties. Additional staff members may be required depending on volume and the hours that the scheduling office is open.
Preplanning	1 RN[1]	Depending on the setting and level of activity, this stage may require additional RNs and ancillary support. This may include preoperative telephone calls/interviews or planning for special supplies and equipment to meet patient needs.
Registration	Clerical person	The number of clerical staff members depends on the setting, level of activity, number of patients scheduled, patient acuity, and types of procedures and may be combined with other tasks.
Day of surgery: Preoperative	1 RN[1]	The number of additional RNs should be based on the number of patients, the number of ORs/procedure rooms, patient acuity, types of procedures, complexity/intensity of patient care requirements, time required to perform tasks, a patient's age-specific needs, and the average time for individual patient preparation. Licensed practical nurses (LPNs) and unlicensed assistive personnel (UAP) may be included in preoperative staffing plans. Unlicensed assistive personnel may be assigned to help with delegated patient care tasks as determined by the RN and according to individual state boards of nursing scope of practice and other local, state, and federal regulations.[2-4]
Intraoperative	1 RN per patient per OR in the role of the circulating nurse.[5] 1 scrub person per patient per room; may be RN, surgical technologist, or LPN. In some circumstances, a scrub person may not be required.	Additional staff members, with appropriate competencies, may be used as appropriate for the following: ♦ moderate sedation—one RN dedicated to monitoring the patient and separate from the dedicated RN circulator; ♦ local anesthesia—depending on patient needs, nursing assessment, and type of procedure, an RN may be needed to monitor the patient in addition to the RN circulator; ♦ complex surgical procedures and patients with compound needs may require an additional RN circulator and scrub person; ♦ technological demands (eg, lasers, robotics, audiovisual equipment, auto transfusion device); ♦ first assist requirements. *Note:* See formula for calculating additional staffing.
Postoperative Phase I level of care	"Two licensed nurses, one of whom is a[n] RN competent in Phase I postanesthesia nursing, are present* whenever a patient is receiving Phase I level of care."[1 (p14)] Staffing will reflect the American Society of Perianesthesia Nurses' (ASPAN's) "Patient classification/ recommended staffing guidelines."	Phase I level of care** Class 1:2—One nurse to two patients who are ♦ One unconscious, stable, without artificial airway, and older than the age of 8; and one conscious, stable, and free of complications. ♦ Two conscious, stable, and free of complications. ♦ Two conscious, stable, 8 years of age and younger, with family or competent support staff member present.

Table 1, *continued*

MINIMUM STAFFING RECOMMENDATIONS

Surgical phase	Minimum requirements	Comments
		Class 1:1—One nurse to one patient ♦ At the time of admission, until the critical elements are met. ♦ Requiring mechanical life support and/or artificial airway. ♦ Any unconscious patient 8 years of age and younger. ♦ A second nurse must be available to assist as necessary. Class 2:1—Two nurses to one patient ♦ One critically ill, unstable, complicated patient.[6] Additional staff members may include support staff. Unlicensed assistive personnel may be assigned to help with delegated patient care tasks according to local, state, and federal regulations.[4]
Phase II level of care	"Two competent personnel, one of whom is a[n] RN competent in Phase II postanesthesia nursing, are present* whenever a patient is receiving Phase II level of care."[1 (p14)] Staffing will reflect ASPAN's "Patient classification/recommended staffing guidelines."	Phase II level of care** Class 1:3—One nurse to three patients ♦ Older than 8 years of age. ♦ 8 years of age and younger with family present. Class 1:2—One nurse to two patients ♦ 8 years of age and younger without family or support staff member present. ♦ Initial admission of patient postprocedure. Class 1:1—One nurse to one patient ♦ Unstable patient of any age requiring transfer.[6] Additional staff members may include support staff. Unlicensed assistive personnel may be assigned to help with delegated patient care tasks according to local, state, and federal regulations.[4]

Phase III level of care	"A[n] RN competent in Phase III postanesthesia nursing must be present* whenever a patient is receiving Phase III level of care."[1 (p14)]
	
	Staffing will reflect ASPAN's "Patient classification/recommended staffing guidelines."
		Phase III level of care**
		Class 1:3/5—One nurse to three to five patients
		♦ Examples include, but are not limited to,
		  – patients awaiting transportation home;
		  – patients with no caregiver;
		  – patients who have had procedures requiring extended observation/intervention (ie, potential risk for bleeding, pain management, postoperative nausea, vomiting).[6]
		
		Additional staff members may include support staff. Unlicensed assistive personnel may be assigned to help with delegated patient care tasks according to local, state, and federal regulations.[4]

Table 1, *continued*

MINIMUM STAFFING RECOMMENDATIONS		
Surgical phase	**Minimum requirements**	**Comments**
Discharge from service	An RN assesses the discharge readiness of the patient and confirms the order from anesthesiologist/surgeon for discharge according to facility protocol.[7]	"The perianesthesia nurse uses sound judgment in determining the appropriate method of communication and mode of transport to transfer care of the perianesthesia patient."[7] 1. "A policy exists to ensure safe transportation of patients. ◆ The professional nurse determines the mode, number, and competency level of accompanying personnel based on patient need. ◆ The professional nurse ensures the availability of appropriate transportation of the patient from the facility. ◆ An appropriate means of transportation from a freestanding facility to a full-service hospital will be used in emergency situations. 2. A professional nurse should accompany patients who ◆ require continuous cardiac monitoring. ◆ require evaluation and/or treatment during transport (ie, vasopressor infusions or pulse oximetry)."[7]
Postoperative follow-up	An RN completes discharge follow up.[8]	Ambulatory surgery patients are reassessed postoperatively. The time frames for reassessment are based on patient needs and the care, treatment, and services provided. Individual organizations should develop policies and procedures regarding the mechanism chosen (eg, postoperative telephone calls) based on the patients it serves and the services or care it provides.[9,10]

NOTES

* The American Society of Perianesthesia Nurses defines "present" as being in the particular place where the patient is receiving care.

** Adapted with permission from the American Society of PeriAnesthesia Nurses.

1. "Standard III: Staffing and personnel management," in Standards of Perianesthesia Nursing *(Cherry Hill, NJ: American Society of PeriAnesthesia Nurses, 2004) 14.*

2. "AORN official statement on unlicensed assistive personnel" in Standards, Recommended Practices, and Guidelines *(Denver: AORN, Inc, 2004) 167-168.*

3. "AORN guidance statement: Preoperative patient care in the ambulatory surgery setting," in Standards, Recommended Practices, and Guidelines *(Denver: AORN, Inc, in press).*

4 "A position statement on registered nurse utilization of unlicensed assistive personnel," in Standards of Perianesthesia Nursing *(Cherry Hill, NJ: American Society of PeriAnesthesia Nurses, 2004) 77.*

5. "AORN statement on nurse-to-patient ratios," in Standards, Recommended Practices, and Guidelines *(Denver: AORN, Inc, 2004) 157-158.*

6. "Resource 3: Patient classification/recommended staffing guidelines," in Standards of Perianesthesia Nursing *(Cherry Hill, NJ: American Society of PeriAnesthesia Nurses, 2004) 25.*

7. "Resource 11: Safe transfer of care" in Standards of Perianesthesia Nursing *(Cherry Hill, NJ: American Society of PeriAnesthesia Nurses, 2004) 49.*

8. "Resource 4: Criteria for initial, ongoing, and discharge assessment and management," in Standards of Perianesthesia Nursing *(Cherry Hill, NJ: American Society of PeriAnesthesia Nurses, 2004) 27.*

9. "Provision of care, treatment, and services," in Comprehensive Accreditation Manual for Ambulatory Care *(Oakbrook Terrace, Ill: Joint Commission on Accreditation of Healthcare Organizations, 2005) PC-1, PC-3.*

10. "Follow-up phone calls in outpatient surgery," Joint Commission on Accreditation of Healthcare Organizations, http://www.jcaho.org/accredited+organizations/ ambulatory+care/standards/faqs/provision+of+care/ anesthesia+care/followup+calls.htm *(accessed 14 Dec 2004).*

Intraoperative Staffing Formula

Direct staff patient care calculation

■ **Step 1**—Number of rooms multiplied by number of hours per day multiplied by number of days per week equals total hours to be staffed per week.

■ **Step 2**—Total hours to be staffed per week multiplied by number of people per room equals total working hours per week.

■ **Step 3**—Total working hours per week divided by 40 hours equals basic full-time equivalents (FTEs).

■ **Step 4**—Calculate benefit relief.

■ **Step 5**—Basic FTEs multiplied by benefit hours per FTEs per year divided by 2,080 hours equals relief FTEs.

■ **Step 6**—Basic FTEs added to relief FTEs equals total minimum direct care staff members.

■ **Step 7**—Calculate indirect care staff members.

■ **Step 8**—Calculate call replacement relief.

To determine the number of personnel per room:

■ Generally, there are at least two staff members for every surgical or other invasive procedure: one RN in the circulator role and one scrub person.

■ The scrub position can be filled by an RN or surgical technologist.

■ If half the procedures done in the OR require a third person for part or all of the procedure (eg, to monitor patients receiving sedation, operate complex technology, high patient acuity), use a figure of 2.5 people per room in computing staffing needs.

■ If more or less than half of the procedures done in the OR require a third person, or if a percentage of procedures require a fourth person, the number of personnel per room will need to be adjusted accordingly.

■ In the following example, a figure of 2.5 people per room is used. The following calculation can be used to determine the RN to technologist ratio of 67%:33% (2:1):

Determine the number of RNs per room by multiplying 2.5 x .67 = 1.7 RNs

Determine the number of technologists per room by multiplying 2.5 x .33 = 0.8 technologists

The above calculation can be applied to any number of total people needed per room. If an institution's FTE is greater or less than 2,080 hours per year, this also must be adjusted in the formula.

Indirect staff calculation

For the purposes of this calculation, indirect staff members include, but are not limited to, the budgeted positions of surgical services director, clinical nurse manager, charge nurse, perioperative educator, schedulers, secretaries, aids, orderlies, and housekeeping personnel as appropriate. The number of indirect care staff members will vary according to function, but a traditional compliment is one indirect caregiver to two direct caregivers.

Call hours replacement calculation

The maximum number of call hours is determined by identifying the number of shifts multiplied by the number of hours multiplied by two FTEs. The actual hours on call personnel are called in to work per year divided by 2,080 equals the replacement FTEs for call-time worked.

Relief replacement

■ Benefit hours (ie, nonproductive hours) are hours such as vacation time, holiday time, available sick time (whether paid or unpaid), education days, and any other time that personnel policies determine an employee might take off. The number of benefit hours is proportionate to the amount of vacation time and the number of long-term employees. Some organizations use an established percentage to calculate benefit hours.

■ In the OR, benefit hours also include breaks and lunches, unless the OR ceases work during those times.

■ When determining relief for lunch, it is necessary to add approximately 15 minutes to the allotted time at either end to allow for nurse-to-nurse report about what has transpired during the procedure in progress. It may take less than seven minutes for the circulating nurse to report to the relief nurse, but relief of the scrub person needs to include time needed to scrub, gown, and glove, so 15 minutes is average.

■ When computing relief for breaks and lunches, the number of minutes is multiplied by 260 days (ie, 52 weeks multiplied by five days per week).

■ Nonproductive time for orienting new staff members also needs to be included.

Example. *An OR suite has eight rooms, which are to be staffed and available as follows:*
- *8 rooms, 7 AM to 3 PM, Monday through Friday;*
- *2 rooms, 3 to 6 PM, Monday through Friday;*
- *1 room, 6 PM to 7 AM, seven days per week; and*
- *1 room, 7 AM to 6 PM, Saturday and Sunday.*

■ **Step 1**—Number of rooms multiplied by number of hours per day multiplied by number of days per week equals total hours to be staffed per week.

8 x 8 x 5 = 320
2 x 3 x 5 = 30
1 x 13 x 7 = 91
1 x 11 x 2 = 22
463 total hours staffed per week

■ **Step 2**—Total hours staffed per week multiplied by number of people per room equals total working hours per week.

463 hours x 2.5 = 1,157.5 total working hours per week

The following calculation can be used to determine the hours for a 67%:33% RN:technologist ratio.

Determine the number of RNs per room by multiplying 2.5 x .67 = 1.7 RN

Determine the number of technologists per room by multiplying 2.5 x .33 = 0.8 technologists

RNs: 1.7 x 463 hours = 787.1 total RN working hours per week

Surgical technologists: 0.8 x 463 = 370.4 total surgical technologist hours per week

Total working hours per week = 1,157.5

■ **Step 3**—Total working hours per week divided by 40 hours worked per week equals basic FTEs.

1,157.5 ÷ 40 = 28.9 basic FTEs

The following calculation can be used to determine the basic RN FTEs and surgical technologist FTEs for a 67%:33% RN:technologist ratio.

RNs: 787.1 hours ÷ 40 = 19.7 basic RN FTEs
Surgical technologists: 370.4 ÷ 40 = 9 basic surgical technologist FTEs

■ **Step 4**—Calculate benefit relief per employee.

Average vacation hours per year = 100
Holiday hours per year = 56
Available sick hours per year = 96
15 minute break x 260 days ÷ 60 minutes = 65 hours
45 minute lunch x 260 days ÷ 60 minutes = 195 hours
512 hours of benefit relief

Note: Organizations handle benefit hours differently. Benefits hours may include, but are not limited to the following.
- Vacation hours, holiday hours, and sick hours are grouped together under paid time off (PTO).
- If sick time is not established and included in the PTO, historical average sick time is used to calculate replacement FTEs.
- A percentage is used to calculate benefit hours.

■ **Step 5**—Basic FTEs multiplied by benefit hours per FTE per year divided by 2,080 hours equals relief FTEs.

28.9 x 512 hours ÷ 2,080 = 7.1 relief FTEs

The following calculation determines the RN and surgical technologist relief FTEs for a 67%:33% RN:technologist ratio.

RNs: 19.7 x 512 = 10,086.4 ÷ 2,080 = 4.8 RN relief FTEs
Surgical technologists: 9 x 512 = 4,608 ÷ 2,080 = 2.2 surgical technologist FTEs

Calculating the orientation time for new employees depends on several factors, including, but not limited to, the size and type of OR, anticipated turnover time, and increase in the number of staff due to growth of services and volume. For the purposes of the example, if four people with experience were expected to be hired for a year and each receives 12 weeks of orientation, use the following calculation:

4 staff members x 40 hours per week x 12 weeks = 1,920 hours of orientation ÷ 2,080 = 0.9 FTE for orientation

■ **Step 6**—Basic FTEs added to relief FTEs equals total minimum direct care staff members.

28.9 + 7.1 = 36 FTEs

The following calculation is used for a 67%:33% RN:technologist ratio.

RN: 19.7 basic FTEs + 4.8 benefit relief FTEs = 24.5 RN FTEs

Surgical technologist: 9 basic FTEs + 2.2 benefit relief FTEs = 11.2 surgical technologist FTEs

■ **Step 7**—Calculate indirect care staff members.

1 indirect caregiver per 2 direct caregivers = 1.25 x 463 hours per week = 578.8 ÷ 40 = 14.5 FTEs
512 benefit hours x 14.5 = 7,424 ÷ 2,080 = 3.6 relief FTEs
3.6 + 14.5 = 18.1

■ **Step 8**—Calculate call relief (see Table 2).
The total number of FTEs calculated in this example is:

Direct caregivers
RNs: 24.5 FTEs
surgical technologists: 11.2 FTEs
call replacements: 1.5 FTEs
indirect caregivers: 18.1 FTES
orientation FTEs: 0.9 FTE
Total: 56.3 FTEs

This formula is based on 100% utilization.

Post Anesthesia Care Unit (PACU) Staffing Formula

There are no standardized staffing formulas at this time for calculating perianesthesia staffing in the PACU. Neither the American Society of Perianesthesia Nurses nor AORN have a recommended staffing formula at this time. Refer to Table 1 for PACU staffing recommendations.

Summary

One of the most important responsibilities of a perioperative nursing leader is the development of an effective staffing plan relative to surgical patients' needs. AORN recognizes there are a variety of settings in which perioperative RNs practice.

Table 2

CALL RELIEF CALCULATION				
Call coverage	Maximum possible hours			Historical usage in hours
	Hours	Staff	Total	Total
260 night shifts	8 x	2 =	4,160	3,342
52 weekends	48 x	3 =	7,488	5,256
12 holidays	24 x	3 =	864	689
Total			12,512	9,287*

* The difference between the maximum possible call hours and actual usage of call hours is 3,225 hours worked. The 3,225 call hours worked per year divided by 2,080 hours (ie, one full-time equivalent [FTE]) equals 1.55 FTE replacement for call-time worked.

This guidance statement is intended to serve as a guide for perioperative nursing leaders in developing a staffing plan and is designed to be adaptable to various practice settings.

Glossary

Direct staff members: Personnel directly involved in providing care to patients undergoing surgical or other invasive procedures. These individuals provide direct patient care and include RNs, surgical technologists, nursing assistants, orderlies, RN first assistants, and surgical assistants.[2]

Indirect staff members: Personnel who support nonpatient care activities in the perioperative environment. These positions may include the director, manager, charge nurse, educator, secretaries, environmental services personnel, instrument processing personnel, materials management personnel, and clerical/business personnel. The perioperative director, management team members (eg, team leaders, charge nurse), clinical nurse specialists, and educators may be a combination of direct and indirect personnel.[2]

Productive hours: Actual hours worked; includes direct and indirect hours. Worked hours are those needed to staff the unit.[2]

Nonproductive hours: These are paid hours not worked and considered benefit hours (eg, vacation, sick time, funeral leave, holiday).[2]

Editor's note: *This staffing guidance statement was developed by the Nursing Practice Committee in December 2004. AORN would like to thank the American Society of Perianesthesia Nurses for their participation in the development of this statement.*

NOTES

1. B Fernsebner, "Key factors affecting staffing," *OR Manager* 16 (December 2000) 10-11.

2. K A Halverson Carpenter, "Staffing and scheduling," *Leadership in Action: A Managers Guide to Success* (Denver: AORN, Inc, 2004) 74.

3. "A position statement on on call/work schedule," in *Standards of Perianesthesia Nursing* (Cherry Hill, NJ: American Society of PeriAnesthesia Nurses, 2004) 79.

4. "Proposed AORN position statement for safe on-call practices," pending ratification by the 2005 House of Delegates.

5. "AORN guidance statement: Safe on-call practices in perioperative practice settings," in *Standards, Recommended Practices and Guidelines* (Denver: AORN, Inc, 2005) 193-195.

6. B Fernsebner, "Building a staffing plan based on OR's needs," (Surgical Staffing) *OR Manager* (1996).

RESOURCES

Perioperative Management Resources: Budgeting (Denver: AORN, Inc, 2004).

Originally published May 2005, *AORN Journal*.

Policy for Sunset of AORN Position Statements

All official AORN position statements and resolutions will sunset after five years unless reaffirmed by the AORN Board of Directors and/or ratified by the House of Delegates. The Board may determine that some resolutions (eg, "No smoking resolution," 1989) will become Association policy rather than remain in their original form. Courtesy resolutions will be archived after five years.

Procedure

■ Each statement/resolution will have a sunset date published along with the adoption date.

■ Staff will bring sunset statements/resolutions to the Board of Directors at the spring board meeting in the year prior to sunset.

■ The Board of Directors will determine the need to ratify, revise, or sunset statements/resolutions. The Board also may elect to take no action. All action on sunsets, reaffirmations, and proposed revisions will be reported in the Board report as part of the business conducted at that meeting in order for the membership to become aware of work in progress.

■ If the statement/resolution sunsets through archive or becoming Association policy, staff will implement and no House of Delegates action will be needed.

■ If the statement/resolution is reaffirmed with no revisions by the Board of Directors, a new sunset date will be assigned and no House of Delegates action will be needed.

■ If the statement/resolution needs revision, the Board will determine the appropriate person(s), committee, or staff to propose the revision, which will be due to the Board no later than the fall board meeting. The Board will submit the revised statement/resolution to the House of Delegates at the next Congress for ratification. Once ratified, a sunset date will be assigned.

A list of AORN archived and sunset position statements and resolutions appears on the following page.

Reference for Archived and Sunset Position Statements/Resolutions			
Title of AORN Statement/Resolution	**Origination Date**	**Sunset Date**	**Archive Date**
Resolution in Memory of Michael D. Corley	February 1989	N/A	April 1995
Resolution on Support of Vietnam Women's Memorial Project	March 1986	N/A	April 1995
Resolution on the Concern Regarding the Preparation for Entry Into the Practice of Professional Nursing	March 1975	N/A	April 1995
Resolution on Operating Room Nursing Research	January 1983	N/A	April 1995
Resolution on OR Nurse Day	March 1979	N/A	April 1995
Resolution on the Role of First Assistant	April 1983	N/A	April 1995
Resolution on Nursing Unity	February 1989	N/A	April 1995
Resolution on the Registered Care Technologist	February 1989	N/A	April 1995
Resolution on Implementation of Project Alpha	March 1981	N/A	April 1995
Resolution on the Necessity for the Registered Nurse in the Operating Room	March 1973	N/A	April 1995
Resolution on Implementation of Project Alpha— The Next Phase	November 1995	N/A	November 1996
Position Statement on the International Role of AORN	March 1995	March 2000	October 1999
Statement on Perioperative Nursing Practice in Ambulatory Surgery	March 1986	April 2000	June 1999
Statement on Protection of the Environment	November 1990	April 2000	June 1999
Regulated Medical Waste Definition and Treatment: A Collaborative Document	March 1994	March 1999	June 1999
Resolution on Necessity for Nursing Student Participation in Operating Room Nursing	March 1973	June 2004	December 2004
Official Statement on Unlicensed Assistive Personnel	March 1995	June 2006	January 2006

Copies of these Position Statements/Resolutions are available from AORN upon request.

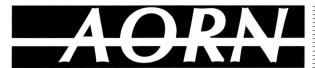

POSITION STATEMENT

Association of periOperative Registered Nurses, Inc. • 2170 South Parker Road, Suite 300 • Denver, Colorado 80231-5711 • (303) 755-6300

AORN REVISED STATEMENT ON PATIENTS AND HEALTH CARE WORKERS WITH BLOODBORNE DISEASES

PREAMBLE

Bloodborne infections, including human immunodeficiency virus (HIV), hepatitis B virus (HBV), and hepatitis C virus (HCV), pose an occupational risk to perioperative nurses. Although the precise prevalence of these diseases in the general population is not known, researchers have found that among patients seeking treatment in an emergency room, 6% were seropositive for HIV, 5% were seropositive for HBV, and 18% were seropositive for HCV.[1] The occupational risk of transmission depends on the route of exposure and concentration of infectious agent. The majority of occupational transmissions to health care workers have resulted from needle sticks and cuts with contaminated sharp items. After sustaining a needle stick by a needle contaminated with HIV, 0.3% of health care workers contracted the virus. The next highest incidence of transmission to health care workers occurred via mucous membrane splashes. After a mucous membrane splash, less than or equal to 0.1% contracted HIV. Hepatitis viruses have a higher concentration in blood; therefore, after sustaining a needle stick by a hollow-bore needle used on a patient with HBV and with no postexposure prophylaxis, 6% to 30% of health care workers contracted the disease. The risk of developing HCV after percutaneous exposure ranges from 0% to 7%, with the average being 1.8%.[2]

Federal and state regulations have been passed to reduce the risk of occupational and patient exposure to bloodborne pathogens. The Bloodborne Pathogen Standard, first published by the Occupational Safety and Health Administration (OSHA) in 1991, requires an exposure control plan, compliance with universal precautions, engineering controls, barrier protection, free HBV vaccinations, training programs, and postexposure evaluation. Since that time, changes in work practices, improved safety, and additional regulations have focused on prevention of sharps-related exposures.

Based on the Needlestick Safety and Prevention Act passed by Congress in November 2000, OSHA published revised bloodborne pathogens standards in January 2001. These revised standards add new requirements for employers, including additions to the exposure control plan, soliciting employee input, and record keeping.[3] In June 2001, the Centers for Disease Control and Prevention (CDC) published guidelines for the management of occupational exposures to HIV, HBV, and HCV. The CDC recommends postexposure prophylaxis with a combination of medications shown to be the most effective.[4] Advances also have been made to protect individuals with bloodborne infections and to provide guidance for minimizing the risk of transmission to patients. During the past two decades, much of the fear of occupational acquisition of bloodborne infections has been dispelled through education and efforts to improve the safety of workplaces.

This AORN revised position statement incorporates federal regulations and standards based on the most current scientific evidence. The AORN *Standards, Recommended Practices, and Guidelines* provide direction for many clinical issues related to prevention of occupational transmission.

TESTING FOR BLOODBORNE DISEASES

The Association supports voluntary testing after informed consent and counseling for patients and all health care workers regardless of the practice setting. In the unlikely event that a patient incurs an accidental exposure to the blood or hazardous body fluid of a health care worker, the patient should be offered voluntary, confidential testing with appropriate counseling and information to understand the implications of exposure and postexposure prophylaxis as indicated. Perioperative nurses should be aware of state laws related to consent for testing and reporting.

FACILITY RESPONSIBILITIES

The Association encourages health care facilities to support health care workers who care for patients infected with HIV, HBV, or HCV. Federal and state regulations provide the framework for developing policies, procedures, and education programs that address infection control, safety, and ethical issues related to prevention and transmission of these diseases. AORN believes that employing facilities should

- provide an environment that minimizes the risk of exposure to bloodborne pathogens,
- provide timely postexposure evaluation and prophylaxis when appropriate, and
- support seropositive health care workers' endeavors to remain employed when their health status does not impair their performance or pose risks to patients. The Americans with Disabilities Act protects employees with bloodborne infections and requires that employers provide reasonable accommodations for those individuals competent to perform the job without undue hardship to their employers.

The Association encourages facilities to have in place an exposure control plan that addresses

- vaccination of health care workers;
- availability of personal protective equipment and work practice controls;
- evaluation of safety devices with input from employees;
- education about risks and prevention of exposure, including work practice controls and use of safety devices;
- prompt reporting of exposures;
- timely postexposure follow-up and prophylaxis as appropriate;
- monitoring compliance to safety practices; and
- periodic evaluation of the effectiveness of the exposure control plan.

HEALTH CARE WORKERS' RESPONSIBILITIES

The Association recognizes that care of patients with known or unknown bloodborne infections poses an occupational risk to perioperative nurses and other health care workers. Perioperative nurses and other

health care workers should not discriminate against patients or employees with HIV, HBV, HCV, or any other bloodborne infection. Because of the occupational risk for bloodborne disease transmission, the Association believes that perioperative nurses and other health care workers should

- educate themselves about the prevalence and risk of transmission of bloodborne diseases,
- utilize measures to protect themselves and others,
- participate in the evaluation of work practice and engineering controls, and
- promptly report any exposures.

In addition, health care workers should voluntarily

- know their HIV, HBV, or HCV statuses;
- if seropositive, seek counsel from an expert panel to review and modify their practices based on the best available scientific information; and
- report their status through the appropriate facility system.

STANDARDS, EDUCATION, AND DEVELOPMENT

The Association reaffirms the ongoing commitment of its members to provide safe, equitable, competent, confidential, individualized care to all patients undergoing perioperative intervention. As a professional association, AORN promotes implementation of OSHA's "Occupational exposure to bloodborne pathogens; needlesticks and other sharps injuries; Final rule," and the "Updated US public health service guidelines for the management of occupational exposures to HBV, HCV, and HIV and recommendations for postexposure prophylaxis."[5] Further, AORN encourages continued development and implementation of national standards and guidelines governing infection control practices for invasive and exposure-prone procedures in all settings. AORN is committed to partnering between industry and health care professionals to develop improved safety devices and refine work practice controls. AORN believes in ongoing education of the public about the risk of transmission through high-risk behaviors, including unsafe sexual contact and through sharing of contaminated needles and syringes. The Association supports expenditures that focus on prevention, research, and care of patients with bloodborne diseases.

NOTES

1. G D Kelen et al, "Hepatitis B and hepatitis C in emergency department patients," *The New England Journal of Medicine* 21 (May 21, 1992) 1399.

2. Centers for Disease Control and Prevention, "Updated US public health service guidelines for the management of occupational exposures to HBV, HCV, and HIV and recommendations for postexposure prophylaxis," *Morbidity and Mortality Weekly Report* 50 (RR-11) (June 29, 2001) 3-8.

3. "29 CFR Part 1910: Occupational exposure to bloodborne pathogens; needlestick and other sharps injuries; Final rule," *Federal Register* 66 (Jan 18, 2001) 5318-5325.

4. "Updated US public health service guidelines for the management of occupational exposures to HBV, HCV, and HIV and recommendations for postexposure prophylaxis," 4-8.

5. *Ibid;* "29 CFR Part 1910: Occupational exposure to bloodborne pathogens; needlestick and other sharps injuries; Final rule," 5318-5325.

Original statement adopted by the Board of Directors July 10, 1987; ratified by the House of Delegates March 10, 1988.

Revised; ratified by the House of Delegates February 23, 1989.

Revised; approved by the Board of Directors September 29, 1991. Ratified by the House of Delegates March 19, 1992.

Revised January 1997 by Anne Uruburu, RN, MBA, CNOR, task force chair; Nancy Bjerke, RN; Cecil A. King, RN, BSN, CNOR; Jane E. Kuhn, RN, MSN, CNOR, task force members; Eileen Ullmann, RN, MHS, CNOR, staff consultant.

Approved by the Board of Directors March 1997; ratified by the House of Delegates April 10, 1997.

Revised; approved by the House of Delegates April 25, 2002.

Sunset review: March 2007

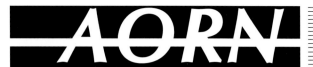

POSITION STATEMENT

Association of periOperative Registered Nurses, Inc. • 2170 South Parker Road, Suite 300 • Denver, Colorado 80231-5711 • (303) 755-6300

STATEMENT ON CORRECT SITE SURGERY

PREAMBLE

Wrong site surgery can and must be prevented.[1] Wrong site surgery is a broad term that encompasses all surgical procedures performed on the wrong patient, wrong body part, wrong side of the body, or at the wrong level of the correctly identified anatomic site.[2] The Joint Commission on Accreditation of Healthcare Organizations (JCAHO) considers all wrong site surgeries, regardless of the extent of the procedure or the outcome, to be reviewable sentinel events.

A comprehensive approach is needed in each health care delivery system to prevent wrong site surgery. Procedures and protocols should be developed collaboratively by multidisciplinary teams, including perioperative registered nurses, surgeons, anesthesia care providers, risk managers, and other health care professionals to implement the "Universal Protocol for Preventing Wrong Site, Wrong Procedure, Wrong Person Surgery."[1] As patient advocates, perioperative registered nurses should communicate with all members of the surgical team to verify the correct surgical site. Individual facility policy should clearly delineate the role and responsibility of the physician and other team members in marking and verifying the correct surgical site. Perioperative registered nurses should be key participants in multidisciplinary teams as they develop these procedures and protocols. As patient advocates, perioperative registered nurses have a duty to the public to protect the patient from injury and to safeguard the patient's health, welfare, and safety.[3] Although it is the surgeon's responsibility to diagnose a patient's need for surgery and to delineate the surgical site, verifying the correct surgical site at the time of surgery is the responsibility of perioperative registered nurses and every member of the health care team.

POSITION STATEMENT

AORN is dedicated to patient safety. Using suggested risk-prevention strategies for identification and verification of correct patient, surgical site, and procedure will reduce the risk of error. AORN endorses JCAHO's "Universal Protocol for Preventing Wrong Site, Wrong Procedure, Wrong Person Surgery"[1] (Exhibit A) and "Implementation Expectations for the Universal Protocol for Preventing Wrong Site, Wrong Procedure, and Wrong Person Surgery"[4] (Exhibit B).

Editor's note: *"Universal Protocol for Preventing Wrong Site, Wrong Procedure, Wrong Person Surgery" is a trademark of the Joint Commission on Accreditation of Healthcare Organizations, Oakbrook Terrace, Ill.*

NOTES

1. "Universal Protocol for Preventing Wrong Site, Wrong Procedure, Wrong Person Surgery," Joint Commission on Accreditation of Healthcare Organizations, *http://www.jcaho.org/accredited+organizations/patient+safety/universal+protocol/universal+protocol.pdf* (accessed 2 Feb 2006).
2. Joint Commission on Accreditation of Healthcare Organizations, "Sentinel events," in *Comprehensive Accreditation Manual for Hospitals* (Oakbrook Terrace, Ill: Joint Commission on Accreditation of Healthcare Organizations, 2004) SE-3.
3. "AORN explications for perioperative nursing" in *Standards, Recommended Practices, and Guidelines* (Denver: AORN, Inc, 2004) 53-83.
4. "Implementation Expectations for the Universal Protocol for Preventing Wrong Site, Wrong Procedure, and Wrong Person Surgery," Joint Commission on Accreditation of Healthcare Organizations, *http://www.jcaho.org/accredited+organizations/patient+safety/universal+protocol/up_guidelines.pdf* (accessed 2 Feb 2006).

Original statement adopted by the AORN Board of Directors in November 2004; ratified by the House of Delegates, New Orleans, in April 2005.
Sunset review: March 2009

EXHIBIT A: Universal Protocol for Preventing Wrong Site, Wrong Procedure, Wrong Person Surgery™

Wrong site, wrong procedure, wrong person surgery can be prevented. This Universal Protocol is intended to achieve that goal. It is based on the consensus of experts from the relevant clinical specialties and professional disciplines and is endorsed by more than 40 professional medical associations and organizations.

In developing this protocol, consensus was reached on the following principles:

- ♦ Wrong site, wrong procedure, wrong person surgery can and must be prevented.
- ♦ A robust approach-using multiple, complementary strategies-is necessary to achieve the goal of eliminating wrong site, wrong procedure, wrong person surgery.
- ♦ Active involvement and effective communication among all members of the surgical team is important for success.
- ♦ To the extent possible, the patient (or legally designated representative) should be involved in the process.
- ♦ Consistent implementation of a standardized approach using a universal, consensus-based protocol will be most effective.
- ♦ The protocol should be flexible enough to allow for implementation with appropriate adaptation when required to meet specific patient needs.
- ♦ A requirement for site marking should focus on cases involving right/left distinction, multiple structures (fingers, toes), or levels (spine).
- ♦ The Universal Protocol should be applicable or adaptable to all operative and other invasive procedures that expose patients to harm, including procedures done in settings other than the operating room.

In concert with these principles, the following steps, taken together, comprise the Universal Protocol for eliminating wrong site, wrong procedure, wrong person surgery:

- ♦ **Preoperative verification process**
  - – *Purpose:* To ensure that all of the relevant documents and studies are available prior to the start of the procedure and that they have been reviewed and are consistent with each other and with the patient's expectations and with the team's understanding of the intended patient, procedure, site, and, as applicable, any implants. Missing information or discrepancies must be addressed before starting the procedure.
  - – *Process:* An ongoing process of information gathering and verification, beginning with the determination to do the procedure, continuing through all settings and interventions involved in the preoperative preparation of the patient, up to and including the "time out" just before the start of the procedure.
- ♦ **Marking the operative site**
  - – *Purpose:* To identify unambiguously the intended site of incision or insertion.
  - – *Process:* For procedures involving right/left distinction, multiple structures (such as fingers and toes), or multiple levels (as in spinal procedures), the intended site must be marked such that the mark will be visible after the patient has been prepped and draped.
- ♦ **"Time out" immediately before starting the procedure**
  - – *Purpose:* To conduct a final verification of the correct patient, procedure, site and, as applicable, implants.*
  - – *Process:* Active communication among all members of the surgical/procedure team, consistently initiated by a designated member of the team, conducted in a "fail-safe" mode, ie, the procedure is not started until any questions or concerns are resolved.

EXHIBIT B: Implementation Expectations for the Universal Protocol for Preventing Wrong Site, Wrong Procedure, and Wrong Person Surgery™

These guidelines provide detailed implementation requirements, exemptions, and adaptations for special situations.

Preoperative verification process

- ◆ Verification of the correct person, procedure, and site should occur (as applicable):
  - At the time the surgery/procedure is scheduled.
  - At the time of admission or entry into the facility.
  - Anytime the responsibility for care of the patient is transferred to another caregiver.
  - With the patient involved, awake, and aware, if possible.
  - Before the patient leaves the preoperative area or enters the procedure/surgical room.
- ◆ A preoperative verification checklist may be helpful to ensure availability and review of the following, prior to the start of the procedure:
  - Relevant documentation (eg, history and physical, consent).
  - Relevant images, properly labeled and displayed.
  - Any required implants and special equipment.

Marking the operative site

- ◆ Make the mark at or near the incision site. Do NOT mark any nonoperative site(s) unless necessary for some other aspect of care.
- ◆ The mark must be unambiguous (eg, use initials or "YES" or a line representing the proposed incision; consider that "X" may be ambiguous).
- ◆ The mark must be positioned to be visible after the patient is prepped and draped.
- ◆ The mark must be made using a marker that is sufficiently permanent to remain visible after completion of the skin prep. Adhesive site markers should not be used as the sole means of marking the site.
- ◆ The method of marking and type of mark should be consistent throughout the organization.
- ◆ At a minimum, mark all cases involving laterality, multiple structures (fingers, toes, lesions), or multiple levels (spine). Note: In addition to preoperative skin marking of the general spinal region, special intraoperative

radiographic techniques are used for marking the exact vertebral level.

- ◆ The person performing the procedure should do the site marking.
- ◆ Marking must take place with the patient involved, awake, and aware, if possible.
- ◆ Final verification of the site mark must take place during the "time out."
- ◆ A defined procedure must be in place for patients who refuse site marking.

Exemptions

- ◆ Single organ cases (eg, Cesarean section, cardiac surgery).
- ◆ Interventional cases for which the catheter/instrument insertion site is not predetermined (eg, cardiac catheterization).
- ◆ Teeth—but, indicate operative tooth name(s) on documentation or mark the operative tooth (teeth) on the dental radiographs or dental diagram.
- ◆ Premature infants, for whom the mark may cause a permanent tattoo.

"Time out" immediately before starting the procedure

Must be conducted in the location where the procedure will be done, just before starting the procedure. It must involve the entire operative team, use active communication, be briefly documented, such as in a checklist (the organization should determine the type and amount of documentation) and must, at the least, include:

- ◆ Correct patient identity.
- ◆ Correct side and site.
- ◆ Agreement on the procedure to be done.
- ◆ Correct patient position.*
- ◆ Availability of correct implants and any special equipment or special requirements.

The organization should have processes and systems in place for reconciling differences in staff responses during the "time out."

Procedures for non-OR settings including bedside procedures

- ◆ Site marking must be done for any procedure that involves laterality, multiple structures, or levels (even if the procedure takes place outside of an OR).

♦ Verification, site marking, and "time out" procedures should be as consistent as possible throughout the organization, including the OR and other locations where invasive procedures are done.

♦ **Exception:** Cases in which the individual doing the procedure is in continuous attendance with the patient from the time of decision to do the procedure and consent from the patient through to the conduct of the procedure may be exempted from the site marking requirement. The requirement for a "time out" final verification still applies.

© Joint Commission on Accreditation of Healthcare Organizations, 2003. Reprinted with permission.

AORN has requested that JCAHO add "patient position" to the purpose statement of the "'Time out' immediately before starting the procedure." Richard Croteau, MD, executive director for strategic initiatives at JCAHO, is bringing that request forward. In the meantime, Dr Croteau clarified that "the presence of this language in the implementation guidelines for the Universal Protocol following the statement 'must, at the least, include' makes this a firm requirement of the protocol. That is, the guidelines are part of the protocol, and wherever the word 'must' is used, what follows is held by the Joint Commission to be a requirement for purposes of accreditation." In other words, the correct patient position must be verified during the time out immediately before the start of the procedure.

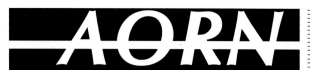

POSITION STATEMENT

Association of periOperative Registered Nurses, Inc. • 2170 South Parker Road, Suite 300 • Denver, Colorado 80231-5711 • (303) 755-6300

DEFINITION OF PERIOPERATIVE ADVANCED PRACTICE NURSE

The perioperative advanced practice nurse (APN) is a registered professional nurse who uses specialized knowledge and skills in the care of patients and families undergoing operative and other invasive procedures. The APN possesses a graduate degree in nursing that forms the foundation for an advanced practice role. The perioperative APN conducts comprehensive health assessments and demonstrates autonomy and skill in diagnosing and treating complex responses of clients (ie, patient, family, community) to actual and potential health problems that are related to the prospect or performance of operative or other invasive procedures. The perioperative APN formulates clinical decisions to manage acute and chronic illness by assessing, diagnosing, and prescribing treatment modalities, including pharmacological agents. The perioperative APN promotes wellness. The perioperative APN integrates clinical practice, education, research, management, leadership, and consultation into a single role. The perioperative APN functions in a collegial relationship with nurses, physicians, and others who influence the health environment.

RESOURCES

Coalition of Nurse Practitioners. Agenda item 12.2.5, item presented at the Coalition of Nurse Practitioners Constituent Assembly, 2-3 Dec 1993.

Mirr, M P. "Advanced clinical practice: A reconceptualized role." *AACN Clinical Issues in Critical Care Nursing* 4 November 1993) 600.

Submitted 3/1995; adopted 3/1995
House of Delegates,
Atlanta, Georgia
Reaffirmed: 6/1999, 12/2004
Sunset review: 6/2006

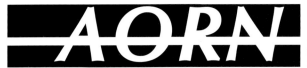

POSITION STATEMENT

Association of periOperative Registered Nurses, Inc. • 2170 South Parker Road, Suite 300 • Denver, Colorado 80231-5711 • (303) 755-6300

PERIOPERATIVE CARE OF PATIENTS WITH DO-NOT-RESUSCITATE (DNR) ORDERS

PREAMBLE

Nurses have a responsibility to uphold the rights of patients.[1] A patient with a do-not-resuscitate (DNR) order may require surgical procedures and anesthesia management. These procedures often are for palliative care, to relieve pain or distress, to facilitate care, or to improve the patient's quality of life. A DNR order should not mean that all treatment is stopped and the need for medical and nursing care is eliminated, but rather that the patient has made certain choices about end-of-life decisions.[2] A patient's rights do not stop at the entrance to the operating room.[3] Automatically suspending a DNR order during surgery undermines a patient's right to self-determination.[4] Development of a policy related to DNR orders in the operating room is supported by the Patient Self-Determination Act,[5] the Joint Commission on Accreditation of Healthcare Organizations (JCAHO), the "AORN explications for perioperative nursing,"[6] and "The patient care partnership: Understanding expectations, rights, and responsibilities."[7]

POSITION STATEMENT

■ Required reconsideration of DNR decisions with patients is an integral component of the care of patients undergoing surgery.[8]
■ Required reconsideration of DNR decisions ensures that the risks and benefits of anesthesia and surgery are discussed by health care providers and patients or patients' surrogate decision makers before surgery.

GUIDELINES

Patient autonomy must be respected as the professional responsibility of the health care team. The patient's physicians are responsible for discussing and documenting issues with the patient and/or family to determine whether the DNR order is to be maintained or completely or partially suspended during anesthesia and surgery. The discussion needs to describe poten-

tial resuscitation efforts during surgery and whether withholding resuscitation compromises the patient's basic objectives for surgery.[9] Discussion involved with the required reconsideration should include

♦ the goals of the surgical treatment,
♦ the possibility of resuscitative measures,
♦ a description of what these measures include, and
♦ possible outcomes with and without resuscitation.

If the patient has chosen to suspend the DNR order during the intraoperative period, it should be documented when the DNR order is to be reinstated.

Preoperatively, communication among the health care team, the patient, and the patient's family about DNR decisions must occur. Adequate information must be given so the surgical team supports the patient's or the patient's surrogate's right to participate in the health care decision.[10] A method of communication needs to be developed so that all health care team members are informed of the patient's decision. Following the discussion, the decision and plan must be clearly documented and communicated to all health care providers potentially involved in the perioperative care of the patient. Throughout the process, the patient has the right to modify any decision, and this also must be communicated to all involved health care providers. Patient situations that may require further ethical deliberation before surgical intervention may benefit from consultation with the hospital's ethics advisory committee.

The perioperative nurse, as a patient advocate, has a moral responsibility to the patient. If the perioperative nurse has a moral objection to the patient's decision, he or she should be allowed to make a reasonable effort to find another nurse willing to provide care to the patient. If another nurse is not available, the patient's decision will be upheld, recognizing that there are times when a patient's wishes take precedence in a clinical situation.

OPERATIONAL DEFINITIONS

The following are operational definitions of terms used in the statement.

Do-not-resuscitate (DNR) order. A specific directive, written by a physician, mandating that cardiopulmonary resuscitation should not be performed.[11]

Do-not-resuscitate (DNR) decision. The patient's or surrogate's directives regarding end-of-life choices.

Required reconsideration. An event that allows a patient or surrogate to participate in decisions about the use of cardiopulmonary resuscitation and that offers caregivers an opportunity to explain the significance of cardiac arrest and resuscitation in the perioperative setting.

Health care team. Nurses, physicians, and all others involved in clinical disciplines.

Notes

1. S Igoe, S Cascella, K Stockdale, "Ethics in the OR: DNR and patient autonomy," *Nursing Management* 24 (September 1993) 112A, 112D, 112H.

2. J M Reeder, "Do-not-resuscitate orders in the operating room," *AORN Journal* 57 (April 1993) 947-951.

3. S J Youngner, H F Cascorbi, J M Shuck, "DNR in the operating room: Not really a paradox," *Journal of the American Medical Association* 266 (November 1991) 2433-2434.

4. Igoe, Cascella, Stockdale, "Ethics in the OR: DNR and patient autonomy," 112A, 112D, 112H.

5. *Patient Self-Determination Act,* Public Law 101-508, *Federal Register* 57 (March 6, 1992).

6. "AORN explications for perioperative nursing," in *Standards, Recommended Practices, and Guidelines* (Denver: AORN, Inc, 2004) 53-83.

7. American Hospital Association, "The patient care partnership: Understanding expectations, rights, and responsibilities," *http://www.hospitalconnect.com/aha/ptcommunication/partnership/index.html* (accessed 23 November 2004).

8. C B Cohen, P J Cohen, "Required reconsideration of 'do-not-resuscitate' orders in the operating room and certain other treatment settings," *Law, Medicine & Health Care* 20 (Winter 1992) 354-363.

9. R D Truog, D B Waisel, J P Bruns, "DNR in the OR: A goal-directed approach," *Anesthesiology* 90 (January 1999) 289-295.

10. Reeder, "Do-not-resuscitate orders in the operating room," 947-951.

11. Cohen, Cohen, "Required reconsideration of 'do-not-resuscitate' orders in the operating room and certain other treatment settings," 354-363.

Resources

American College of Surgeons. "Statement of the American College of Surgeons on advance directives by patients: 'Do Not Resuscitate' in the operating room." *ACS Bulletin* 79 (September 1994) 29.

American Nurses Association. ANA Position Statement, "Nursing care and do-not-resuscitate (DNR) decisions," *http://nursingworld.org/readroom/position/ethics/etdnr.htm#DNR* (accessed 4 January 2005).

American Society of Anesthesiologists. "Ethical guidelines for the anesthesia care of patients with do-not-resuscitate orders or other directives that limit treatment," *http://www. asahq.org/publicationsAndServices/standards/09.html* (accessed 4 January 2005)

Submitted: 3/1995; Adopted: 3/1995
House of Delegates, Atlanta, Georgia
Reaffirmed: 10/1999, 12/2004
Sunset review: 12/2009

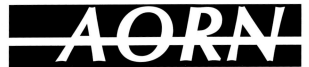 **POSITION STATEMENT**

Association of periOperative Registered Nurses, Inc. • 2170 South Parker Road, Suite 300 • Denver, Colorado 80231-5711 • (303) 755-6300

STATEMENT ON ENTRY INTO PRACTICE

AORN believes there should be one level for entry into nursing practice. AORN believes the minimal preparation for future entry into the practice of nursing should be the baccalaureate degree.

Submitted: 3/1979
Adopted: 3/5/1979, House of Delegates, St Louis
Reaffirmed: 4/1995, 6/1999, 4/2005
Sunset review: 6/2009

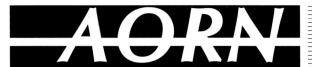

STATEMENT ON FIRE PREVENTION

PREAMBLE

AORN recognizes that fire is an inherent risk in ORs. Fire is an ever-present danger, posing a real hazard to patient and health care worker safety. In 2003, the Joint Commission on Accreditation of Healthcare Organizations (JCAHO) issued a sentinel event alert bulletin related to fires that occur during operative and invasive procedures. The bulletin raised the level of awareness of the dangers of surgical fires. The Joint Commission recommends that health care organizations prevent surgical fires by providing education and training for perioperative practitioners. The approach to developing policies and procedures to reduce fire risk should be multidisciplinary and involve all professionals who provide patient care. Facilities are encouraged to report surgical fires to JCAHO, ECRI, or the US Food and Drug Administration (FDA). Systematic reporting of fires can assist in educating care providers about how and why fires occur and help them prevent fires in the future.[1]

Fires involving surgical patients have been reported by hospitals; ambulatory surgery centers; some medical device manufacturers; and other experts, such as ECRI, for many years. Data from ECRI and the FDA estimate that about 100 surgical fires occur each year, resulting in approximately 20 patient injuries that are serious; two deaths per year have occurred. The overriding consideration with surgical fires is that they are 100% preventable; however, they still may occur.[1,2]

POSITION STATEMENT

AORN believes that fires can be prevented in the perioperative area. The perioperative registered nurse is responsible for learning about fire prevention and taking steps to minimize the risk of surgical fires. AORN believes the perioperative registered nurse should actively participate in a health care facility's fire emergency planning and preparation activities, including fire drills and evacuation planning, policy development, and education in risk reduction strategies for preventing fires.

AORN believes the following risk reduction strategies should be considered when developing a fire safety plan.

- ◆ Promote and maintain a fire-safe perioperative environment by educating and training perioperative team members in fire risk reduction strategies upon orientation and at least annually. Activities and knowledge should include
  - participation in a fire drill;
  - use of fire-fighting equipment;
  - knowledge of rescuer methods;
  - knowledge of medical gas panel and location and operation;
  - knowledge of ventilation and electrical system locations and operation, including personnel authorized to shut them off and when;
  - initiation of a fire alarm or "'Code Red'"; and
  - specific procedures for contacting the local fire department.[2]
- ◆ Each perioperative team member is responsible for promoting a culture of fire safety. Preparation is the key to ensuring readiness in preventing fires in the OR.
- ◆ All perioperative departments should develop and implement a well-rehearsed and thought-out fire evacuation plan. Evacuation plans help ensure that all staff members are familiar with the proper evacuation routes, fire exits, and equipment that may be used before or during an evacuation.
- ◆ Educate surgical team members about the components of the fire triangle.
  - Fuel sources must be managed in a way to prevent fires.
  - Ignition sources must be controlled so as not to come in contact with fuels.

– Oxidizers must be contained or properly vented to prevent contact with fuels or ignition sources.

♦ Keeping the elements of the fire triangle apart is critical.[3]

CONTRIBUTING FACTORS

Fires occur when the three elements that support combustion (ie, an ignition source, a fuel source, an oxidizer) come together. These three elements are referred to as the "fire triangle." All three elements are present in abundance during operative and invasive procedures.[2] Operating rooms in hospitals, ambulatory surgery suites, physicians' offices, and endoscopy suites are some of the critical areas where fires may take place.

Almost everything in the perioperative arena can be a fuel source, especially when an accelerant such as oxygen is present. Items used to set up the sterile field and protect patients should be considered fuel sources (eg, linens, drapes, gowns, supplies, preps, gauzes, clothes). The patient's body hair and body gases also can be fuel sources.[4]

Ignition sources are anything that produces heat; the two most common sources are the electrosurgery unit and the laser. Other equipment that produces heat includes fiber-optic light cables and light source boxes; drills, saws, and burrs; hand-held electrocautery devices; and defibrillators.[2]

The primary oxidizers in the surgical environment are oxygen and nitrous oxide. Fires can occur when the oxygen level in the atmosphere rises above 21%. Ambient air contains 21% oxygen. Anything above 21% should be treated as an oxygen-enriched environment. Oxygen can leak into the air when patients are given mask or nasal oxygen.[5]

NOTES

1. Joint Commission on Accreditation of Healthcare Organizations, "Preventing surgical fires," *Sentinel Event Alert* 29 (June 24, 2003). Also available at *http://www .jcaho.org/about+us/news+letters/sentinel+event +alert/print/sea_29.htm* (accessed 1 Dec 2004).

2. "'A clinician's guide to surgical fires. How they occur, how to prevent them, how to put them out,'" *Health Devices* 32 (January 2003) 5-24.

3. "Surgical fires," in *Operating Room Risk Management* (Plymouth Meeting, Pa: ECRI, November 2004) 1-17.

4. "The patient is on fire: A surgical fire primer," ECRI, *http://www.mdsr.ecri.org/asp/dynadoc.asp?id=113&nbr =409637&_seaech_txt=ambient+air* (accessed 1 Dec 2004).

5. C Smith, "'Surgical fires—Learn not to burn,'" *AORN Journal* 80 (July 2004) 25-26.

Original statement adopted by the AORN Board of Directors in November 2004; ratified by the House of Delegates, New Orleans, in April 2005. Sunset review: March 2009

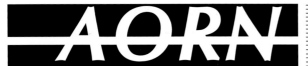 **POSITION STATEMENT**

Association of periOperative Registered Nurses, Inc. • 2170 South Parker Road, Suite 300 • Denver, Colorado 80231-5711 • (303) 755-6300

AORN STATEMENT ON THE ROLE OF THE HEALTH CARE INDUSTRY REPRESENTATIVE IN THE OPERATING ROOM

AORN recognizes the need for a structured system within the perioperative setting for education, training, and introduction of procedures, techniques, technology, and equipment to practicing health care professionals. In defined conditions, AORN believes that health care industry representatives, by virtue of their training, knowledge, and expertise, can provide technical assistance to the surgical team, which expedites the procedure and facilitates desired patient outcomes. The purpose of this statement is to affirm the valuable role health care industry representatives play in the care of surgical patients and to assist the perioperative team in maintaining the patient's safety, right to privacy, and confidentiality when a health care industry representative is present during a surgical procedure.

A health care industry representative may be present during a surgical procedure under conditions prescribed by the facility. AORN recognizes there is a wide range of geographic and regional variations regarding the activities of the health care industry representative in the operating room. This statement provides general guidelines to assist the individual facility in developing policies best suited to its community standards. Along with concerns pertinent to the facility, AORN recommends that the following precepts guide policy development:

- Policy should be developed in collaboration with the facility's risk management and/or legal counsel to ensure compliance with applicable laws.
- Each facility should develop a system that addresses informed patient consent regarding the presence and role of a health care industry representative in the operating room during a surgical procedure in both routine and emergency situations. This system should include documentation in medical records.
- As the patient's advocate, the RN responsible for the patient's care during the procedure is accountable for maintaining the patient's safety, privacy, dignity, and confidentiality. To

achieve this, the RN should monitor the health care industry representative's activities whenever possible and facilitate the representative's service to the patient and the perioperative team during the procedure. The RN should be informed prior to the procedure that a health care industry representative will be present and about his/her purpose for being there.

- Perioperative team members are responsible for acquiring instruction on new procedures, techniques, technology, and equipment with which they are not familiar prior to their use in a surgical procedure. This instruction may be provided by the health care industry representative. The facility should maintain evidence of documented competencies for health care professionals, especially when introducing new procedures, techniques, technology, and equipment as required by the Joint Commission on Accreditation of Healthcare Organizations (JCAHO).[1]
- Each facility should develop a system that documents that the health care industry representative has completed instruction in the principles of asepsis, fire and safety protocols, infection control practices, bloodborne pathogens, and patients' rights. Based on community standards, this may range from maintaining up-to-date documentation provided by the health care industry representative's employing company to providing facility-specific instruction and training.
- The health care industry representative's presence and purpose should be prescheduled with the designated operating room management authority and the surgeon in accordance with the facility policy.
- The health care industry representative should wear identification while in the facility.
- Each facility should develop a system that clearly delineates limits on the health care industry representative activities in the operating room based on community standards. The health care industry representative should not scrub in.

♦ The health care industry representative with specialized training may perform remote calibration to adjust devices to the surgeon's specification (eg, pacemakers, laser technicians).

♦ Medical equipment and other complex devices must be reviewed and approved prior to their use by the facility's service provider.[2] The term *service provider* is defined as a "group with the responsibility to provide inspection and/or other maintenance services on a specific piece of equipment. *(Note:* A service provider may be a department within the health care organization, an equipment manufacturer, an independent service organization operated by a third party, a shared service, or other similar organizations.)"[3]

♦ A clearly defined mechanism should exist to address departures from established policy.

NOTES

1. Joint Commission on Accreditation of Healthcare Organizations, *Comprehensive Accreditation Manual for Hospitals: The Official Handbook* (Oakbrook Terrace, Ill: Joint Commission on Accreditation of Healthcare Organizations, 1998) HR 4.2, EC 2.1.

2. Association for the Advancement of Medical Instrumentation, "Recommended practice for a medical equipment management program," *American National Standards Institute* (American National Standards Institute/Association for the Advancement of Medical Instrumentation, EQ56, 1999) 4.1.2.1.

3. *Ibid,* 3.1.

Original statement adopted by the Board of Directors in October 1999.
Ratified by the House of Delegates, New Orleans, La, in April 2000.
Sunset review: April 2005

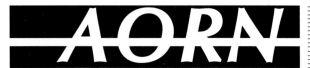 **POSITION STATEMENT**

Association of periOperative Registered Nurses, Inc. • 2170 South Parker Road, Suite 300 • Denver, Colorado 80231-5711 • (303) 755-6300

CARE OF THE PERIOPERATIVE PATIENT WITH AN IMPLANTED ELECTRONIC DEVICE

PREAMBLE

Implanted electronic devices (IEDs) are widely used in a number of diverse medical applications, ranging from the familiar cardiac pacemaker to the less frequently encountered cochlear implant. The perioperative registered nurse should be aware that these devices require special precautions. Some medical equipment devices necessary for performing surgical and other invasive procedures may interfere with the functioning of IEDs. Patients with IEDs require special safety precautions when undergoing a surgical or other invasive procedure. One predominantly important precaution is managing the sources of inherent electromagnetic interference (EMI) in the perioperative patient care environment. Cardiac patients are particularly at risk because they may be dependent on the proper function of an IED to sustain their lives.

The goal of every surgical intervention is to provide optimal patient outcomes while maintaining a safe environment. Patients with IEDs may be encountered in any perioperative environment at any time. Patients with an existing IED may require emergency surgery, and planning for their care may necessarily be abbreviated; therefore, it is critical that every perioperative registered nurse have an understanding of what types of IEDs exist, how these devices function, and precautions that must be taken.

POSITION STATEMENT

Perioperative registered nurses should be aware of potential patient safety hazards associated with specific IEDs and the appropriate patient care interventions and resources required to protect patients from injury and devices from damage.

Perioperative registered nurses should be knowledgeable about the types of IEDs, how they function, and the precautions that must be taken when caring for patients with these devices in place.

Health care facilities should provide education and training for personnel involved in the care of patients with IEDs.

All members of the surgical team have a responsibility to participate in managing the care of patients with IEDs.

The preoperative nursing assessment should include documenting the presence of any IED. Information about the specific device should be documented in the medical record before surgery. This information should include, but is not limited to,
♦ manufacturer and model of the IED,
♦ anatomic location of the device,
♦ technical considerations relative to the intraoperative phase of care, and
♦ information relative to postoperative patient education and discharge planning.

Health care facilities should have policies and procedures addressing the care and management of patients with IEDs. These should include, but are not limited to,
♦ assignment of primary responsibility for management of the IED;
♦ minimum information to be provided at the time of scheduling;
♦ a mechanism to identify and notify appropriate personnel needed in the OR to help perioperative team members deliver safe patient care; and
♦ the role, responsibilities, and limitations of health care industry representatives.

Perioperative registered nurses should refer to the AORN guidance statement "Care of the perioperative patient with an implanted electronic device" for assistance in developing and implementing policies and procedures for caring for patients with IEDs who are undergoing surgical and other invasive procedures.

DEFINITIONS

Implanted electronic device: An electronic medical device that has been implanted into a patient for the purpose of treating a physiological defect or to replace sensory function (eg, permanent pacemakers, implantable cardioverter defibrillators, deep brain stimulators, spinal cord stimulators).

Electromagnetic interference (EMI): Any electromagnetic disturbance that interrupts, obstructs, or otherwise degrades or limits the effective performance of electronics or electrical equipment. *Synonym:* Radio frequency interference.

Original statement adopted by the AORN Board of Directors in November 2004; ratified by the House of Delegates, New Orleans, in April 2005.
Sunset review: March 2009

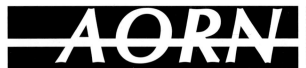

POSITION STATEMENT

Association of periOperative Registered Nurses, Inc. • 2170 South Parker Road, Suite 300 • Denver, Colorado 80231-5711 • (303) 755-6300

STATEMENT ON MANDATE FOR THE REGISTERED PROFESSIONAL NURSE IN THE PERIOPERATIVE PRACTICE SETTING

Believing it is the right of the consumer to receive the highest quality nursing care according to identified needs; and

Believing it is incumbent upon the Association to promote standards of perioperative clinical practice that provide for and/or improve the quality of nursing care delivered to patients undergoing operative and other invasive procedures, and having endorsed that belief by development of standards of perioperative clinical practice and standards of perioperative professional performance; and

Believing that the necessary nursing knowledge and skills can be acquired only in accredited nursing education programs; and

Believing that the role of the registered professional nurse in the perioperative practice setting is vital to the provision of optimal care. The unique perioperative nursing competencies include, but are not limited to:
1. Creation and maintenance of a safe and comfortable environment in which surgery can take place
2. Provision of direct and indirect patient care, which involves
   A. Use of nursing judgment, critical thinking skills, and interpersonal communication skills
   B. Knowledge of and ability to use the nursing process in assessing, diagnosing, planning, intervening, and evaluating to meet individual patient needs and to ensure positive patient outcomes

3. Supervision and education of surgical team members and education of the patient
4. Patient advocacy to help patients and families meet physical, psychosocial, and cultural needs; and

Believing that only the perioperative registered professional nurse is qualified to provide this optimum level of care in the perioperative practice setting; therefore be it

Affirmed that the perioperative registered professional nurse remain with the patient during operative and other invasive procedures; and

Affirmed that AORN will continue to support the patient's right to optimum nursing care throughout preoperative assessment and preparation, diagnosis, intraoperative intervention, and postoperative evaluation.

Submitted March 1975
Approved by the Board of Directors, March 1975
Adopted by the House of Delegates, March 27, 1975
Revised March 1997
Approved by the Board of Directors, March 1997
Approved by the House of Delegates, April 10, 1997
Reaffirmed: Board of DIrectors, October 2001
Sunset review: March 2007

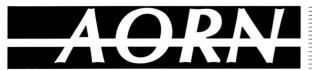

POSITION STATEMENT

Association of periOperative Registered Nurses, Inc. • 2170 South Parker Road, Suite 300 • Denver, Colorado 80231-5711 • (303) 755-6300

AORN RESOLUTION ON RESPONSIBILITY FOR MENTORING

Whereas, every patient undergoing an operative or other invasive procedure needs and deserves a perioperative registered nurse; and

Whereas, the specialty of perioperative nursing occurs within a setting characterized by rapidly changing technology and economic and cultural forces that require continuous adaptation; and

Whereas, the specialty of perioperative nursing requires the perioperative registered nurse to gain complex knowledge/skills through formal educational programs; and

Whereas, the demand for perioperative nurses currently outweighs the supply; and

Whereas, nursing school enrollments have decreased and perioperative nursing is not commonly included in core nursing curricula; and

Whereas, the aging of current perioperative nurses will have a progressive impact on the number of practicing nurses; and

Whereas, perioperative registered nurses have the opportunity to encourage interested parties to enter into nursing; and

Whereas, the Nursing, Education and Practice Improvement Act of 1998 provides federal support for nursing workforce development; and

Whereas, student nurses, as well as perioperative registered nurses entering clinical, management, and leadership roles, need a support system, role models, and guidance; and

Whereas, perioperative registered nurses are involved in life-long learning to maintain a current body of perioperative knowledge; and

Whereas, professional perioperative nursing is demonstrated by participation in professional organizations, legislative and regulatory initiatives influencing perioperative nursing practice, and active interest in international health care issues affecting the practice of perioperative nursing; and

Whereas, perioperative registered nurses have a responsibility to strengthen and advocate an environment that promotes career development and leadership;

Therefore, be it
Resolved, that perioperative registered nurses will actively seek opportunities to mentor students and other persons interested in exploring perioperative nursing as a career, novice perioperative nurses engaged in clinical practice, inexperienced perioperative nurse managers, and emerging leaders in the perioperative nursing milieu; and

Resolved, that the perioperative registered nurse mentor will model professional behavior and demonstrate a commitment to perioperative nursing by participating in professional organizations, supporting practice-related legislative and regulatory initiatives impacting perioperative nurses and nursing, and by maintaining an awareness of international health care issues affecting the practice of perioperative nursing.

Original statement adopted by Board of Directors in February 2001.
Adopted by the House of Delegates, Dallas, Texas, in March 2001.
Sunset review: March 2006

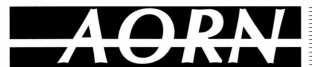

POSITION STATEMENT

Association of periOperative Registered Nurses, Inc. • 2170 South Parker Road, Suite 300 • Denver, Colorado 80231-5711 • (303) 755-6300

AORN STATEMENT ON NURSE-TO-PATIENT RATIOS

PREAMBLE

During the 1990s and the ascendence of managed care, attempts were made to control the rising cost of health care, largely as a result of recommendations to the health care community by health care consultants with expertise in accounting and business practices. New models of health care delivery were implemented that decentralized most of the diagnostic and support services, making them directly available in patient care centers. As a cost-saving measure, health care administrators reconfigured the staff to eliminate unnecessary positions. Many positions eliminated or downgraded were held by the higher paid, more experienced health care professionals, including professional registered nurses (RNs). Health care administrators directed nursing to hire and supervise assistive personnel, with less skill and requiring less pay, to assume many of the functions previously performed by RNs. At this time, the practice began of cross-training the remaining RNs to assume wider responsibilities in health care settings. Some discussion has included floating nursing staff from outside surgical services to alleviate potential shortages in the operating room. In practice, RNs have been required to float to other patient care units for which they have little or no orientation, training, experience, or support.

At the same time, the aging of the population has resulted in patients who are more acutely ill upon admission to health care centers. While numbers of professional staff and lengths of stay in acute care facilities have been ratcheted down, patients have continued to require more sophisticated care to maintain their health. This situation has been further complicated by an absence of standardized, mandatory public reporting of data that could objectively quantify the effects of altered staffing configurations.

Registered nurses are familiar with anecdotal reports of health care errors resulting in patient injuries and even death. The media has continued to fuel the health care controversy with many of these stories. In 1999, the Institute of Medicine (IOM) published its report *To Err Is Human: Building a Safer Health System,* which opened the issue of medical errors to public debate and identified national, state, and local policy directions for a safer health care system capable of reducing medical errors and improving patient safety.[1] In addition, the IOM Committee on the Adequacy of Nurse Staffing in Hospitals and Nursing Homes has begun to illustrate the relationship between nurse staffing, patient outcomes, and cost of care.[2]

Currently under review, the Code of Federal Regulations' "Conditions of Participation for Hospitals" (42 CFR §82) sets forth the only national staffing standard, and only for hospitals receiving Medicare and Medicaid:

> *The nursing service must have adequate numbers of licensed registered nurses, licensed practical (vocational) nurses, and other personnel to provide nursing care to all patients as needed.*

Prompted by the lack of federal standards, state legislatures recently have begun implementing staffing requirements ranging from minimum RN staffing in predominantly critical care settings to more general provisions for adequate number of nursing service personnel, without the definition of adequacy or specific personnel needed. In 1998, California was the first state to enact legislation that required minimum staffing levels for RNs and licensed practical nurses/ licensed vocational nurses (LPN/LVNs) for all patient care units in acute care facilities. Thus was born the public policy issue of nurse-to-patient ratios. In 1999 and 2000, state legislatures across the country have considered bills that would implement nurse-to-patient ratios or at least address sufficient nurse staffing remedies.

The American Nurses Association (ANA) has refrained from developing specific numeric recommendations for nurse staffing in hospitals, believing that a broader approach to nurse staffing in acute care settings is needed. In 1999, ANA released *Principles for Nurse Staffing* to offer nurses, administrators, legislators, and others a tool to identify appropriate nurse staffing.[3] The underlying premise is that nurse staffing can best be implemented and adjusted through the identification of nursing quality indicators and rigorous research to ascertain patient outcomes.

Like many specialty nursing associations, AORN has addressed general staffing guidelines through the "Statement on mandate for the registered professional nurse in the perioperative practice setting," last approved by the AORN House of Delegates on April 10, 1997.[4]

In consideration of the circumstances and conditions surrounding patient safety and adequate nursing staff in acute care settings, AORN upholds the following statement:

Believing that nursing is both an art and a science and that patient advocacy is the foundation of perioperative nursing practice;

Believing that perioperative nursing is dedicated to the health and safety of the surgical patient;

Believing that establishment of nurse-to-patient ratios in surgical settings must include an examination of factors such as perioperative nursing competence, patient acuity, and available resources;

Believing that scientific research and the identification of nursing quality indicators is the best means to monitor the relationship between appropriate nurse staffing and patient outcomes in the surgical setting;

Believing that an excellent practice environment will encourage perioperative nurses to continue providing good patient care in the surgical arena; and
Believing that administrative and collegial support, as well as effective relationships with physicians and surgeons, contributes to perioperative nursing's ability to provide safe patient care.

Therefore, be it
Affirmed that, wherever invasive procedures are performed, the minimum nurse-to-patient ratio is one professional perioperative registered nurse dedicated to each patient during that patient's entire intraoperative experience;

Affirmed that each patient having an invasive procedure is provided with a perioperative registered nurse in the role of circulator;

Affirmed that establishment of nurse-to-patient ratios in surgical settings must include awareness of community needs, needs of the population served, and provide for appropriate perioperative nursing staff to meet those needs. The economic situation of the provider organization should not serve as the sole basis for determining services offered. At no time should economic concerns supersede the priority for patient safety;

Affirmed that AORN advocates for state and federal legislation requiring the collection and reporting of nursing quality indicators to monitor the effects of staffing;

Affirmed that AORN works with all organizations endeavoring to reduce and eliminate health care errors and that adequate staffing is an essential element of error prevention;

Affirmed that AORN works with other specialty organizations to define nurse-to-patient ratios and safe staffing standards as used in legislation and regulations; and

Affirmed that AORN supports ongoing research to determine proper nurse staffing to sustain high quality patient outcomes.

NOTES
1. L T Kohn, J M Corrigan, M S Donaldson, eds, *To Err is Human: Building a Safer Health System* (Washington, DC: National Academy Press, 2000).
2. American Nurses Association, "2000 House of Delegates action report" (Washington DC: American Nurses Association, 2000) 3.
3. American Nurses Association, *Principles for Nurse Staffing* (Washington, DC: American Nurses Association, 1999).
4. "Statement on mandate for the registered professional nurse in the perioperative practice setting," in *Standards, Recommended Practices, and Guidelines* (Denver: AORN, Inc, 2000) 149.

Original statement adopted by the AORN Board of Directors in October 2000.
Ratified by the House of Delegates, Dallas, Texas, in March 2001.
Sunset review: March 2006

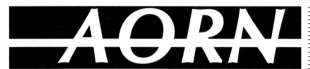

Association of periOperative Registered Nurses, Inc. • 2170 South Parker Road, Suite 300 • Denver, Colorado 80231-5711 • (303) 755-6300

INCLUSION OF PERIOPERATIVE NURSING LEARNING ACTIVITIES IN UNDERGRADUATE NURSING CURRICULA

PREAMBLE

Although the number and length of inpatient stays have decreased as health care delivery trends have increased treatment in ambulatory, home, and community settings, a large percentage of all patients still are admitted to acute care facilities to undergo surgery or other invasive procedures. An increasing number of surgical procedures are being performed on an outpatient or short-stay basis. Nurses who work in home and community settings will encounter increasing numbers of patients who are recovering at home and who require direct care as well as instruction in self-care during the recovery phase of the surgical experience. Therefore, even if they do not practice in intra-operative settings, all nurses need adequate preparation in perioperative nursing to properly assess and manage the needs of surgical patients and their families, to provide accurate and timely preoperative and postoperative teaching, to assess the readiness of patients and family members for discharge, and to provide competent guidance to patients and family members who must manage recovery at home.

Despite these trends, content and clinical activities specific to the roles of perioperative registered nurses have been gradually eliminated from most undergraduate nursing curricula over the past 30 years while the complexity of modern surgical patient care has created increased demand for perioperative nurses.[1] Recent studies predict a large shortage of nurses by 2020, which is likely to affect perioperative nursing disproportionately because the mean age of current perioperative nurses is higher than that of the general RN population.[2] As large numbers of perioperative nurses near retirement age, it will be increasingly difficult to replace them with new graduates who have had perioperative nursing learning experiences in their basic nursing curricula. Employers will need either to recruit from the ever-shrinking supply of experienced perioperative nurses or to prepare new

perioperative nurses through orientation programs. However, relying on institution-based training makes perioperative nursing more vulnerable to market forces. As long as facilities need perioperative nurses, they will support intensive orientation programs, but as soon as the supply is adequate, support for such programs disappears, and if new shortages develop, there is a time lag in getting new programs started.[3]

If vacant perioperative nursing positions cannot be filled with qualified registered nurses, it is likely that individuals who are less qualified and prepared will be asked to fill them.[4] AORN believes that every surgical patient deserves a perioperative registered nurse. The best long-term solution to a shortage of perioperative nurses is to provide basic preparation for perioperative nursing in schools of nursing. Therefore, AORN should advocate for the inclusion of perioperative nursing learning activities in all undergraduate professional nursing curricula.

The impending shortage of perioperative nurses presents career opportunities for nursing students. However, unless nursing students have clinical learning activities within perioperative settings, they will be unlikely to consider practicing in this specialty area, and they may be denied opportunities for employment in perioperative settings because they lack relevant experience. One solution to the shortage of nurses in specialties such as perioperative nursing is to change the way nurses enter specialty practice.[5] Traditionally, nurses were required to have medical-surgical nursing experience before they were given the opportunity to practice in specialty areas such as the operating room and other perioperative settings. However, new nursing graduates can be hired directly into perioperative nursing positions if they have had perioperative nursing content and clinical experiences in their basic nursing curriculum. Basing student learning activities on core competencies and standards of perioperative nursing practice would allow orientation programs for new perioperative nurses to focus on institution-specific knowledge and skills and thus be accomplished more efficiently in less time.[6]

Benefits of perioperative learning experiences to nursing students include, but are not limited to,

- learning and refining aseptic technique so that it can be applied with skill and confidence in other settings;
- applying knowledge of anatomy, physiology, and pathophysiology to understand the patient's surgical procedure, its effects on the patient, and the patient's needs for preoperative and postoperative care;
- recognition of the ethical and legal responsibilities of the professional nurse and the nurse's accountability to the patient, to the profession of nursing, and to other members of the health care team;
- developing the role of advocate for the surgical patient by identifying the patient's expressed and unexpressed needs, and responding appropriately to those needs through the action of facilitating or mediating among all providers involved in the care of the patient;
- application of nursing research findings to planning and implementing effective care for perioperative patients;
- improvement of patient assessment, communication, organization, critical-thinking, and decision-making skills in an environment where such activities must be performed quickly and accurately;
- participation as members of a multidisciplinary health care team that develops and promotes the continuity of patient care in an environment that reinforces an understanding of the professional nurse's independent and interdependent functions;
- recognition of the diverse career opportunities for professional nursing practice in perioperative settings; and
- opportunities to assess their own interest in and talents for perioperative nursing practice.

Benefits of nursing student perioperative learning experiences to schools of nursing and their faculty include, but are not limited to,

- recruitment of prospective nursing students who are interested in potential careers in perioperative nursing, including surgical technologists and other unlicensed personnel who have had work experience in the operating room;
- increased career opportunities for and marketability of graduates;
- increased student satisfaction with the nursing curriculum;
- increased variety of settings for student clinical learning activities; and
- improved level of graduates' clinical skills, such as application of aseptic technique, patient assessment, communication, organization, critical thinking, decision making, and teamwork, leading to increased graduate and employer satisfaction and improved ability to meet accreditation criteria.

Benefits of nursing student perioperative learning experiences to employers include, but are not limited to,

- larger supply of professional nurses with experience in perioperative settings from which to recruit for vacant positions;
- more efficient and cost-effective orientation of new perioperative nurses;
- improved retention of new perioperative nurses;
- improved surgical patient care in all settings; and
- increased patient satisfaction with the quality of care.

Benefits of nursing student perioperative learning experiences to patients and families include, but are not limited to,

- increased satisfaction with quality of care during the surgical experience;
- decreased preoperative and postoperative apprehension due to more effective patient and family teaching;
- reduced risk of infection due to improved aseptic technique; and
- improved ability to manage recovery from surgery at home.

In consideration of these benefits and in response to the growing need for well-prepared perioperative nurses, AORN upholds the following statement:

Believing that inclusion of perioperative nursing learning activities in basic nursing curricula offer benefits to nursing students, school of nursing faculty and administrators, employers, and patients and their families; and

Believing that professional nurses increasingly will be expected to care for surgical patients in a variety of settings; and

Believing that exposure to perioperative nursing in basic nursing curricula will stimulate interest in this specialty area of practice and provide a basis for cost-effective, efficient orientation of new perioperative nursing staff;

Therefore, be it

Affirmed that AORN strongly supports inclusion of perioperative nursing learning activities based on core competencies and standards of practice in all undergraduate nursing programs;

Affirmed that basic nursing curricula should include both didactic and clinical learning activities in preoperative, intraoperative, and postoperative phases of the perioperative continuum of care;

Affirmed that perioperative nursing content and clinical skills should be taught by faculty and cooperating agency staff who are both academically qualified and clinically experienced in perioperative nursing; and

Affirmed that AORN work with nursing faculty to develop or revise curricula to include hands-on perioperative learning activities for all nursing students.

NOTES

1. J M Beitz, P M Houck, "Advanced perioperative nursing elective for baccalaureate students," *AORN Journal* 66 (July 1997) 119-130; C Bonar, "An open letter to nursing students—Help keep perioperative nursing off the endangered species list," *AORN Journal* 65 (March 1997) 634-635; V D Wagner, C C Kee, D P Gray, "A historical decline of educational perioperative clinical experiences," *AORN Journal* 62 (November 1995) 771-782.

2. "The 'graying' of the RN workforce," *OR Manager* 13 (July 1997) 1, 8; "Study predicts large shortfall of nurses by 2020," *RN* 63 (September 2000) 14.

3. "Where will OR staff of the future come from?" *OR Manager* 13 (July 1997) 1, 8-10.

4. Bonar, "An open letter to nursing students—Help keep perioperative nursing off the endangered species list," 634-635.

5. S Trossman, "Waiting for care: Too many patients, too little staff," *The American Nurse* 32 (November/December 2000) 2.

6. M M Wells, "Determining the best length of an OR orientation program," *AORN Journal* 70 (July 1999) 72-78.

Original statement adopted by Board of Directors in February 2001.
Ratified by the House of Delegates, Dallas, Texas, in March 2001.
Sunset review: March 2006

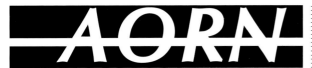

Association of periOperative Registered Nurses, Inc. • 2170 South Parker Road, Suite 300 • Denver, Colorado 80231-5711 • (303) 755-6300

ORIENTATION OF THE REGISTERED PROFESSIONAL NURSE TO THE PERIOPERATIVE SETTING

PREAMBLE

AORN has been approached many times during the past few years to provide guidelines for orientation of both novice and experienced perioperative registered nurses. We recognize that facilities come in every size and configuration, and one orientation program will not adequately address every need. We believe, however, that there are certain basic components of orientation that must be met consistently to ensure optimal patient outcomes.

AORN defines a *novice perioperative registered nurse* as any nurse who has not worked in an OR environment before. This would include a new graduate or an experienced nurse from another area of nursing. It also would include a nurse with previous OR experience who has been away from the OR for an extended period of time.

AORN defines an *experienced perioperative registered nurse* as a nurse with recent OR experience. This nurse should have at least two years of experience in a facility of similar size and patient acuity as the hiring facility. A skills assessment form should be completed to accurately assess competency levels in all specialties.

POSITION STATEMENT

AORN believes that orientation programs need to be customized to meet the individual needs of the orientee as well as the facility. Before a new nurse begins work, the nurse educator, orientation facilitator, clinical nurse specialist, and/or the nurse manager need to assess both the ability of the system to accommodate the learning experience and the orientee's baseline knowledge and preferred learning method. Orientation timelines, and therefore the impact on the budget, will vary depending on the capacity of the facility.

Scope of orientation. AORN believes that the following topics should be developed by the organization and incorporated into the orientation of perioperative registered nurses.

AORN believes that perioperative registered nurses must be oriented to both the scrub and circulating roles during the orientation period. The orientation process should include orientation to off shifts, weekends, and call situations. This should be accomplished using the preceptor system (ie, having an experienced nurse serve as an immediate resource for the orientee).

AORN supports the use of an outcome-focused orientation process that incorporates the outcomes defined in the Perioperative Nursing Data Set.[1]

Domain 1: Safety. The patient will be free of signs and symptoms of acquired physical injury. (Patient specific outcomes are in parentheses.)
- Count policy (O2)
- Culture of safety (O2 – O9)
- Electrosurgical safety (O4)
- Laser safety (O6)
- Medication safety (O9)
- Positioning (O5)
- Radiation safety (O7)
- Smoke evacuation (O6)
- Specimen handling (O2)
- Time out procedure (O2)
- Tourniquets (O2)

Domain 2: Physiologic response. The patient's physiologic responses to surgery are as expected. (Patient specific outcomes are in parentheses.)
- Assessment of patients (O24)
- Basic life support/code response (O14, O15)
- Latex allergy (O3)
- Equipment/instrumentation/supplies
  - Minimally invasive (ie, endoscopic) equipment (O2)
  - Powered equipment (O10)
  - Basic instrumentation (O10)
  - Basic OR equipment (eg, tables, lights, electrosurgical unit, suction) (O5, O2)
- Malignant hyperthermia (O12)
- Monitoring and sedation (O14, O15, O29)
- Prevention of infection

- Infection control (O10)
- Surgical attire (O10)
- Wound management (O10)
- Instrument processing (ie, care and handling) (O10)
- Sterilization/disinfection (O10)
- Skin preps (O10)
- Scrubbing, gowning, and gloving (O10)
♦ Respiratory status (O14) (eg, airway maintenance, assisting with intubation/extubation)
♦ Tissue banking (O10)

Domain 3A: Behavioral response. The patient and family are knowledgeable regarding the perioperative process.
   ♦ Advanced directives (O31)
   ♦ Informed consent (O31)
   ♦ Preoperative teaching (includes postoperative self-care) (O18 – O23)

Domain 3B: Behavioral response. The patient and his or her family member's rights and ethics are supported. (O26)
   ♦ Advocacy (O23, O24, O26)
   ♦ Age-specific policies (O21, O24)
   ♦ Cultural/population-specific policies (O23)
   ♦ Documentation (O24)
   ♦ Health Insurance Portability and Accountability Act compliance (O25)
   ♦ Patient privacy policies (O25)
   ♦ Patient self-determination act (O23)

Domain 4: Health system concerns. The perioperative nurse has knowledge regarding the health system environment.
   ♦ Career advancement
   ♦ Certification
   ♦ Code of conduct
   ♦ Committee participation
   ♦ Communication
   ♦ Critical thinking
   ♦ Disaster planning
   ♦ Employee rights

♦ Employee safety
♦ Environmental responsibility (eg, hazardous waste, recycling)
♦ Fire safety
♦ Legal issues
♦ Organizational structure
♦ Performance improvement projects
♦ Professional associations
♦ Regulatory issues
♦ Scope of practice
♦ Team roles
♦ Terminology
♦ Vendor policies

AORN believes that a basic orientation for a novice perioperative registered nurse should include every clinical specialty within the nurse's defined practice area and should be measured by successful competency assessment. The recommended exposure to a clinical specialty is at least 40 hours.

AORN believes that novice orientation should include a didactic and clinical component.

AORN believes that completion of an individualized orientation for both the novice and experienced nurse should be measured by successful competency assessment. The recommended orientation of a novice perioperative registered nurse should require at least six months and no longer than nine months. The recommended timeframe orientation of an experienced nurse should take a minimum of at least three months.

NOTES
   1. S Beyea, ed, *Perioperative Nursing Data Set: The Perioperative Vocabulary,* second ed (Denver: AORN, Inc, 2002).

Original statement adopted by the AORN Board of Directors in November 2004; ratified by the House of Delegates, New Orleans, in April 2005.
Sunset review: March 2009

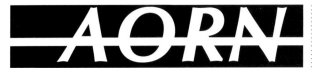

POSITION STATEMENT

Association of periOperative Registered Nurses, Inc. • 2170 South Parker Road, Suite 300 • Denver, Colorado 80231-5711 • (303) 755-6300

AORN POSITION STATEMENT ON PATIENT SAFETY

PREAMBLE

The safety of patients undergoing operative or other invasive procedures is a primary responsibility of the perioperative registered nurse.[1] Registered nurses form a professional bond with patients, who place their physical and emotional well-being in the hands of registered nurses and their surgical colleagues and who believe that the care provided will be safe and effective. The patient/caregiver bond is founded on the patient's trust in the registered nurse and the surgical team. Protecting the patient and promoting an optimal surgical outcome further strengthens that bond.

Perioperative registered nurses have created a significant literary legacy[2,3] and a strong clinical tradition of protecting patients from harm, avoiding error, and promoting safe operative practices.[4] AORN introduced its Patient Safety First initiative in 2002 to recommit the Association and its members to improving the safety of patients in surgery.[5] This initiative expands on an already substantial array of tools to assist the perioperative registered nurse in advocating for patients. AORN's *Standards, Recommended Practices, and Guidelines* reflect the perioperative registered nurse's scope of responsibility.[4] The Perioperative Nursing Data Set (PNDS) creates a common language that enables registered nurses to articulate their value, document competencies, and evaluate nursing care.[6] AORN's publications and educational offerings provide, among other things, continuing education, health policy updates, and networking opportunities. Both nursing and medical codes of ethics further promote the theme of safety and protection from error; "First, do no harm" is the universally recognized dictum of medicine's Hippocratic oath. AORN, the Association of periOperative Registered Nurses, long a proponent of patient safety, has rededicated itself to reducing error, educating registered nurses and patients about safe practices, and creating innovative and collaborative strategies to strengthen the culture of safety.

BACKGROUND

Whether the traditional operating room (OR), the ambulatory surgery center, the interventional suite, or the physician's office, the surgical setting is one of the most potentially hazardous of all the clinical environments. Infection, hemorrhage, and wrong patient/surgery/site are among the most serious potential complications. Potential hazards also include a variety of energy sources (eg, electrical, thermal, laser, radiological), chemicals (eg, medications, antiseptics, cements, intravascular dyes, irrigating solutions), biologicals (eg, bloodborne pathogens, drug resistant organisms), equipment and devices (eg, powered instruments and equipment, defibrillators, tourniquets, electrosurgical units, positioning devices), and the multiple supplies and instruments that comprise the surgical armamentarium. In addition to these technical sources of potential risk, there are human factors (eg, communication patterns, institutional culture, staffing patterns) that are increasingly recognized as a vital component in the creation of a safe, team-based OR environment. Communication between and among team members is one of the most critical according to the Joint Commission on Accreditation of Healthcare Organizations (JCAHO). A breakdown in communication was the most common reason cited by JCAHO for contributing to wrong site surgery.[7]

CONTRIBUTING FACTORS

Surgical error results from multiple factors.[8] Latent conditions created by flawed systems or processes can combine with active failures by caregivers in the clinical setting to produce accidents and errors. Among contributing factors are

- inadequate communication among team members,
- incomplete review of patient health records and diagnostic studies,
- traditional hierarchical and autocratic cultures,
- patient-related decisions made only by physicians,

- rapidly and frequently changing technology,
- intimidating management styles,
- absent or inconsistently applied policies and procedures,
- fatigue,
- multitasking,
- time pressures and constraints,
- emergency surgery,
- cultural differences between patients and staff members and among staff members,
- staffing shortages,
- a blaming culture,
- confusing packaging of medications and supplies,
- unclear instructions,
- insufficient orientation and training,
- patient characteristics requiring unusual setup or requirements, and
- failure to include the patient and family members in assessment and decision making.[9]

ERROR-REDUCTION STRATEGIES

Error reduction requires the commitment of all members of the surgical team. In addition to correcting the contributing factors identified above, individual and institutional strategies can also include the following actions.

- Reduce reliance on memory by using checklists, protocols, and computerized decision aids.
- Improve information access of patient records.
- Support contracts for new equipment and supplies that include clauses providing staff member education on the use of the equipment and supplies.
- Standardize processes as much as possible for back table/Mayo tray setups, medication doses, preoperative procedures, and other activities.
- Establish mechanisms to update procedure/preference cards.
- Participate in quality and process improvement initiatives.
- Develop policies and procedures that address unsafe practices.
- Focus on the safety aspects of products during the selection and evaluation process.
- Promote safety-related clinical competency.[10]
- Include the patient and family members (when possible) in confirming the correct patient identity, the correct surgical procedure, and the correct surgical site.

- Educate employees about the potential for errors and how to avoid them.[11]
- Encourage patients and their significant others to actively participate by partnering with the RN in the planning and implementation of the surgical experience and to question patient care activities.
- Develop a "near miss" reporting mechanism that will track trends of patient care activities that can be studied and analyzed for further error reduction.

One of the most effective team strategies is to create and nurture a culture of safety. Such a culture is founded on a sense of trust among team members and a feeling of safety when the need for change or improvement must be addressed. Establishing a culture of safety and trust is a process of changing a culture from one of blaming individuals for errors to one in which errors are treated not as personal failures but as opportunities to improve the system and prevent harm.[12] Success in the creation of a safety culture depends on the commitment of all team members to report, address, and correct system failures. Four elements are required to create such an environment:[13]

- a sense of trust among team members;
- disseminating and verifying receipt of information to all levels of staff and management;
- developing and supporting a proactive approach rather than a reactive, blaming approach; and
- making a sincere commitment to affirming safety as the first priority.

AORN'S POSITION

AORN is committed to promoting patient safety by advancing the profession through scholarly inquiry to identify, verify, and expand the body of perioperative nursing knowledge. The Association supports the establishment of an accountable, trusting, safety culture that reflects individual and collective values, beliefs, behaviors, and skills with a desire and commitment to patient safety.

AORN also is actively collaborating with the American College of Surgeons, the American Society of Anesthesiologists, JCAHO, the Center for Medicare and Medicaid Services, and other professional organizations and accrediting and regulatory agencies to foster systems and procedures that minimize surgical risk.

AORN recognizes the diverse cultural influences and human factors that can contribute to errors and unsafe work practices. The Association strives to develop programs and services that assist perioperative registered nurses in clinical, education, research, and leadership roles to create cultures of safety in their practice environments and to reduce harm to patients in all perioperative practice settings.

AORN PATIENT SAFETY RESOURCES

- AORN's Patient Safety First web site *(http://www.patientsafetyfirst.org)* provides access to numerous patient safety resources. It also is available through AORN's web site *(http://www.aorn.org).*
- AORN's Patient Safety First e-mail address *(patientsafetyfirst@aorn.org)* can be used to report safety concerns and obtain advice or referrals on safety issues.
- AORN's Patient Safety First toll-free patient safety hotline, (866) 285-5209, can be used to report safety concerns and obtain advice or referrals on safety issues.
- Safety Net, Patient Safety First's voluntary and confidential near-miss database and reporting system can be accessed at *http://www.patientsafetyfirst.org/psf_report.htm.*
- Safety-related articles and Home Studies are published in the *AORN Journal* and *AORN Connections.*
- AORN Position Statement on Correct Site Surgery
- Guideline to Eliminate Wrong Site Surgery: supported by both AORN and the American College of Surgeons
- Joint Commission on Accreditation of Healthcare Organizations, *Universal Protocol for Preventing Wrong Site, Wrong Procedure, Wrong Person Surgery.* Endorsed by AORN, the American Medical Association, American Hospital Association, American College of Physicians, American College of Surgeons, American Dental Association, and American Association of Orthopaedic Surgeons.
- *Standards, Recommended Practices, and Guidelines* (Denver: AORN, Inc, 2003). Includes competency statements and the American Nurses Association *Code of Ethics With Explications for Perioperative Nursing.*
- S C Beyea, ed, *Perioperative Nursing Data Set,* second ed (Denver: AORN, Inc, 2002). Includes registered nurse-sensitive patient outcomes and interventions.

NOTES

1. "AORN explications for perioperative nursing," in *Standards, Recommended Practices, and Guidelines* (Denver: AORN, Inc, 2004) 53-83.
2. A A Smith, *The Operating Room: A Primer for Pupil Nurses* (Philadelphia: WB Saunders, 1916) 80.
3. E L Alexander, *Operating Room Technique* (St Louis: The CV Mosby Company, 1943) 7. Currently in its 12th edition as *Alexander's Care of the Patient in Surgery,* J C Rothrock, ed (St Louis: Mosby, 2003).
4. *Standards, Recommended Practices, and Guidelines* (Denver: AORN, Inc, 2004).
5. "Safety initiative in full swing," *AORN Member News* 1 (January 2002) 8.
6. S C Beyea, ed, *Perioperative Nursing Data Set,* second ed (Denver: AORN, Inc, 2002).
7. Joint Commission on Accreditation of Healthcare Organizations, "Sentinel event alert: A follow-up review of wrong site surgery," *Joint Commission Perspectives* (January 2002) 10-11.
8. Institute of Medicine, *To Err is Human: Building a Safer Health System* (Washington, DC: National Academy Press, 1999).
9. M Leonard, C A Tarrant, "Culture, systems, and human factors—Two tales of patient safety: The KP Colorado region's experience," *The Permanente Journal* 5 (Summer 2001) 46-49.
10. J M Reeder, *Patient Safety, Competency Assessment Module* (Denver: Certification Boards, Inc, 2002).
11. S C Beyea, "Accident prevention in surgical settings—Keeping patients safe," (Research Corner) *AORN Journal* 75 (February 2002) 361-363.
12. Institute of Medicine, *Crossing the Quality Chasm: A New Health System for the 21st Century* (Washington, DC: National Academy Press, 2001) 83.
13. S C Beyea, "Creating a culture of safety," (Patient Safety First) *AORN Journal* 76 (July 2002) 163-166.

RESOURCES

Reason, J. *Managing the Risks of Organizational Accidents* (Burlington, Vt: Ashgate Publishing, 1997).

Cooper, J B; et al. "National Patient Safety Foundation agenda for research and development in patient safety," *Medscape General Medicine, Patient Safety* 2, *http://www.medscape.com/MedGenMed/PatientSafety.*

Original statement adopted by Board of Directors in November 2003.

Ratified by the House of Delegates, San Diego, in March 2004.

Sunset review: March 2009

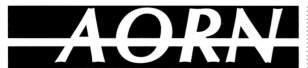

POSITION STATEMENT

Association of periOperative Registered Nurses, Inc. • 2170 South Parker Road, Suite 300 • Denver, Colorado 80231-5711 • (303) 755-6300

AORN OFFICIAL STATEMENT ON RN FIRST ASSISTANTS

PREAMBLE

Perioperative nursing practice historically has included the role of the registered professional nurse (RN) as assistant at surgery. As early as 1977, documents issued by the American College of Surgeons supported the appropriateness for qualified RNs to first assist.[1]

AORN officially recognized this role as a component of perioperative nursing in 1983 and adopted the first "Official statement on RN first assistants (RNFA)" in 1984.[2] AORN's official statement delineates the definition, scope of practice, educational requirements, and qualifications that must be met and suggests clinical privileges for the perioperative RN who practices as an RNFA. AORN supports appropriate compensation/ reimbursement for RNs who fulfill this role.

DEFINITION OF RN FIRST ASSISTANT

The RNFA is a perioperative registered nurse who works in collaboration with the surgeon and health care team members to achieve optimal patient outcomes. The RNFA must have acquired the necessary knowledge, judgment, and skills specific to the expanded role of RNFA clinical practice. Intraoperatively, the RNFA practices at the direction of the surgeon and does not concurrently function as a scrub nurse.

SCOPE OF PRACTICE

All state boards of nursing recognize the role of the RNFA as being within the scope of nursing practice. Perioperative nursing is a specialized area of practice. Registered nurses practicing as first assistants in surgery are functioning in an expanded perioperative nursing role. Activities included in first assisting are further refinements of perioperative nursing practice and are executed within the context of the nursing process. First assisting behaviors are based on an extensive body of scientific knowledge. Certain of these behaviors include delegated medical functions that are unique to the perioperative RN qualified to practice as an RNFA. RN first assistant behaviors may vary depending on patient populations, practice environments, services provided, accessibility of human and fiscal resources, institutional policy, and state nurse practice acts.

Examples of RNFA behaviors in the perioperative arena include

♦ preoperative patient management in collaboration with other health care providers, including but not limited to,
  – performing preoperative evaluation/ focused nursing assessment,
  – communicating/collaborating with other health care providers regarding the patient plan of care, and
  – writing preoperative orders according to established protocols;
♦ intraoperative surgical first-assisting, including but not limited to,
  – using instruments/medical devices,
  – providing exposure,
  – handling and/or cutting tissue,
  – providing hemostasis, and
  – suturing; and
♦ postoperative patient management in collaboration with other health care providers in the immediate postoperative period and beyond, including but not limited to,
  – writing postoperative orders/operative notes according to established protocols,
  – participating in postoperative rounds, and
  – assisting with discharge planning and identifying appropriate community resources as needed.

PREPARATION OF THE RNFA

The complexity of knowledge and skill required to effectively care for recipients of perioperative nursing services compels nurses to be specialized and to continue their education beyond generic nursing programs. Perioperative nurses who wish to practice as RNFAs should develop a set of cognitive, psychomotor, and affective behaviors that demonstrate accountability and responsibility for identifying and meeting the needs of their perioperative patients.

374

Development of this set of behaviors begins with and builds upon the education program leading to licensure as an RN, which teaches basic knowledge, skills, and attitudes essential to the practice of perioperative nursing. Further preparation for the RNFA includes perioperative nursing practice with diversified experience culminating in the nurse achieving CNOR certification through the Competency and Credentialing Institute (CCI).

Additional preparation is then acquired through completion of an RNFA program that meets the "AORN standards for RN first assistant education programs" and is accepted by CCI. These programs should be equivalent to one academic year of formal, post-basic nursing study; consist of curricula that address all of the modules in the *Core Curriculum for the RN First Assistant*[1]; and award college credits or degrees and certificates of RNFA status upon satisfactory completion of all requirements. The RNFA programs should be associated with schools of nursing at universities or colleges that are accredited for higher education by an accrediting agency that is nationally recognized by the Secretary of the US Department of Education. The registered nursing program should be approved by a state licensing jurisdiction for nursing programs at the university, college, or community college level or by another national or regional agency that is nationally recognized by the Secretary of the US Department of Education as a specialized accrediting agency for nursing programs.

Each RNFA demonstrates behaviors that progress on a continuum from basic competency to excellence. When educational and experiential requirements have been met, the RNFA is encouraged to achieve and maintain certification status (CRNFA) through CCI, an independent entity.

QUALIFICATIONS FOR ENTRY INTO RNFA PRACTICE

AORN believes the minimum qualifications to practice as a RN first assistant are as follows:
- certification in perioperative nursing (CNOR);
- successful completion of an RNFA program that meets the "AORN standards for RN first assistant education programs" and is accepted by CCI; and

- compliance with statutes, regulations, and institutional policies relevant to RNFAs.

CLINICAL PRIVILEGING FOR THE RNFA

To determine if the RN qualifies for clinical privileges as a first assistant, an approval process should be established by the facility(ies) in which the individual will practice.

The process of granting clinical privileges should include mechanisms for
- assessing individual qualifications for practice,
- assessing continuing proficiency,
- evaluating annual performance,
- assessing compliance with relevant institutional and departmental policies,
- defining lines of accountability,
- retrieving documentation of participation as first assistant, and
- establishing systems for peer review that include a process for incorporating continuing education/contact hours relevant to RNFA practice.

Documentation of competency should be maintained within the facility.

The decision by an RN to practice as a first assistant must be made voluntarily and deliberately, with an understanding of the professional accountability that the role entails.

For additional sources of information, refer to the following AORN publications:
- *Standards, Recommended Practices, and Guidelines*
- *RN First Assistant Guide to Practice*
- *Core Curriculum for the RN First Assistant*

These publications are available from AORN's Perioperative Bookstore, (800) 755-2676 ext 1, or online at *http://www.aorn.org*.

For additional information regarding CRNFA certification, contact the Competency and Credentialing Institute (CCI), (888) 257-2667, or online at *http://www.http://www.cc-institute.org*.

NOTES

1. "American Colleges of Surgeons: Statement and qualifications for surgical privileges in approved hospitals," *Bulletin of the American College of Surgeons* 62 (April 1977) 12-13.

2. "Task force defines first assisting," *AORN Journal* (February 1984) 403-405.

Submitted in March 1984; adopted by the House of Delegates, Atlanta, March 5, 1984; proposed revision to Board of Directors in September 1992; adopted by the House of Delegates, Anaheim, Calif, March 4, 1993; proposed revision to Board of Directors in November 1997; adopted November 17, 1997; ratified by the House of Delegates, Orlando, April 2, 1998; proposed revision to Board of Directors in November 2003, ratified by House of Delegates, San Diego, March 25, 2004; sunset review: March 2009.

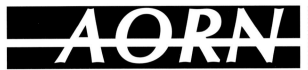

Association of periOperative Registered Nurses, Inc. • 2170 South Parker Road, Suite 300 • Denver, Colorado 80231-5711 • (303) 755-6300

STATEMENT ON THE ROLE OF THE SCRUB PERSON

PREAMBLE

Perioperative registered nurses provide care throughout a patient's surgical experience; the patient remains the focus of that care.[1,2] The scope of responsibility of perioperative registered nurses includes the scrub role as it relates to patient outcomes.[3]

Perioperative registered nurses have defined practice standards for the scrub person.[4-16] Perioperative registered nursing practice incorporates the cognitive, behavioral, and technical components of professional nursing.[2] When functioning in the scrub role, the perioperative registered nurse augments his or her ability to anticipate, plan for, and respond to the needs of the patient, surgeon, and other team members. The perioperative registered nurse is cognizant of patient responses to both planned and unplanned surgical events and contributes to the overall well-being of a patient by being vigilant in assessing the patient's condition as it is demonstrated within the surgical field and by visual monitoring devices. Perioperative registered nurses have performed the role of scrub person for more than 100 years.[1]

POSITION STATEMENT

AORN believes that to achieve optimal patient outcomes in the surgical environment, the perioperative registered nurse should maintain an active presence in performing the scrub role to ensure appropriate delegation and supervision of scrub duties and to maintain an integral link between scrub and circulating responsibilities.

AORN believes that with the continued technological advances in surgical care, a continued presence in the scrub role enhances the perioperative registered nurse's ability to assess and implement a plan of care (including the appropriate delegation of duties).

AORN believes individuals who are not licensed to practice professional nursing and who perform in the role of scrub person are performing a delegated technical function under the direct supervision of a perioperative registered nurse. In any state that has categories of unlicensed assistive individuals who are not under the jurisdiction of nursing, the role of the scrub person may be assigned to an unlicensed assistive individual. These technical functions are assigned by the perioperative registered nurse in charge, based on the level of training and competencies the unlicensed assistive individual may have.

AORN believes perioperative registered nurses performing in the role of the scrub person are practicing nursing.[1,2]

NOTES

1. "Perioperative patient focused model," in *Standards, Recommended Practices, and Guidelines* (Denver: AORN, Inc, 2004) 15-18.

2. L K Groah, *Operating Room Nursing: The Perioperative Role* (Reston, Va: Reston Publishing Co, 1983) 3-20.

3. "Perioperative patient outcomes," in *Standards, Recommended Practices, and Guidelines* (Denver: AORN, Inc, 2004) 197-206.

4. J Rothrock, "Concepts basic to perioperative nursing," in *Alexander's Care of the Patient in Surgery*, 12th ed, J C Rothrock, ed (St Louis: Mosby, 2003) 2-5.

5. "Recommended practices for surgical attire," in *Standards, Recommended Practices, and Guidelines* (Denver: AORN, Inc, 2004) 223-227.

6. "Recommended practices for sponge, sharp, and instrument counts," in *Standards, Recommended Practices, and Guidelines* (Denver: AORN, Inc, 2004) 229-234.

7. "Recommended practices for electrosurgery," in *Standards, Recommended Practices, and Guidelines* (Denver: AORN, Inc, 2004) 245-259.

8. "Recommended practices for endoscopic minimally invasive surgery," in *Standards, Recommended Practices, and Guidelines* (Denver: AORN, Inc, 2004) 267-271.

9. "Recommended practices for environmental responsibility," in *Standards, Recommended Practices, and Guidelines* (Denver: AORN, Inc, 2004) 281-284.

10."Recommended practices for surgical hand antisepsis/hand scrubs," in *Standards, Recommended Practices, and Guidelines* (Denver: AORN, Inc, 2004) 291-299.

11. "Recommended practices for safe care through identification of potential hazards in the surgical environment," in *Standards, Recommended Practices, and Guidelines* (Denver: AORN, Inc, 2004) 301-307.

12. "Recommended practices for laser safety in practice settings," in *Standards, Recommended Practices, and Guidelines* (Denver: AORN, Inc, 2004) 319-328.

13. "Recommended practices for standard and transmission-based precautions in the perioperative practice setting," in *Standards, Recommended Practices, and Guidelines* (Denver: AORN, Inc, 2004) 361-365.

14. "Recommended practices for maintaining a sterile field," in *Standards, Recommended Practices, and Guidelines* (Denver: AORN, Inc, 2004) 367-371.

15. "Recommended practices for sterilization in perioperative practice settings," in *Standards, Recommended Practices, and Guidelines* (Denver: AORN, Inc, 2004) 373-382.

16. "Recommended practices for surgical tissue banking," in *Standards, Recommended Practices, and Guidelines* (Denver: AORN, Inc, 2004) 385-395.

Original statement submitted: March 1988
Revised and adopted: March 1988, House of Delegates, Dallas. Reaffirmed: April 1995
Revised and ratified: April 2000.
Revised and ratified: April 2005, House of Delegates, New Orleans.
Sunset review: March 2009

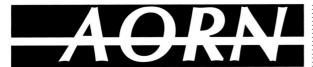
POSITION STATEMENT

Association of periOperative Registered Nurses, Inc. • 2170 South Parker Road, Suite 300 • Denver, Colorado 80231-5711 • (303) 755-6300

SAFE WORK/ON-CALL PRACTICES

PREAMBLE

Perioperative personnel are assigned designated times, in addition to their regular work hours, to be available on an "on-call" basis for unplanned, urgent, or emergent procedures or to provide care for patients whose procedures run past scheduled time periods. Call hours may vary from four hours to 72 hours or more. Actual hours worked during the call period are unpredictable and can range from 30 minutes to the entire length of the call period. Working sustained hours may affect safe patient care, strain existing human resources, create stress for perioperative staff members, and increase the potential for occupational injury due to prolonged work hours.

Traditionally, perioperative registered nurses have worked eight-hour shifts. Several new trends in perioperative staffing patterns include fewer but longer work days, in addition to on-call coverage.[1] Although on-call requirements may be assigned to perioperative nursing staff members on a rotating basis according to patient population, organizational needs, and demographic challenges, perioperative registered nurses may volunteer to take extra call to increase their income (eg, elective overtime). Perioperative registered nurses also may be directed to work beyond their scheduled work/call shift to augment staffing requirements, meet unexpected patient needs, or satisfy organizational expectations (eg, mandatory overtime). These new trends in staffing, other social and economic factors, and on-call hours have converged to create hazardous conditions that jeopardize patient and employee safety. Current research trending the number of hours worked per day by perioperative registered nurses is lacking. Anecdotal reports suggest perioperative staff nurses are working longer hours with fewer breaks and often inadequate time for rest between shifts.[2] Twenty-four hour call shifts are becoming more common.[3]

A large body of research exists about fatigue and sleep deprivation and their effect on performance. Research also describes the influence of circadian rhythms on alertness.[4] Sustained work hours and prolonged periods of wakefulness are among working conditions that may have a negative effect on human performance.[4-8] It has been reported that 17 hours without sleep can adversely affect performance to the equivalent of a blood alcohol concentration of 0.05%.[1] At 24 hours without sleep, performance degradation is equivalent to a blood alcohol concentration of 0.10%.[7] Definitions of intoxication are set by individual states and range from 0.08% to 0.10% blood alcohol concentration.[9] Current research identifies a relationship between preexisting fatigue, total number of hours worked, task intensity, and extended work periods, which exacerbate fatigue and increase the potential for error.[4]

Research also suggests that work periods of 12 hours or more are associated with a higher probability of making an error and an increase in risk-taking behaviors. For some cognitive tasks, peak performance is achieved at about five hours and then declines to its lowest levels after 12 to 16 hours.[4] Researchers have further established a link between working extended hours and medical error rates. According to studies, the medical error rate tripled after workers performed 12.5 hours of sustained activity.[3,6] Moreover, research has identified medication, procedural, documentation, and transcription errors as occurring more frequently as work hours increase.[3,10] Studies suggest a correlation between sleep deprivation and negative effects on memory, language/numeric skills, visual attention, and concentration.[11-13] In addition to creating a risk to patient safety, research reveals that sleep-deprived, fatigued people are at increased risk for personal injury on duty and when driving home after an extended work day.[6,14,15]

There is a consistent body of research demonstrating that most people require a minimum of eight hours of uninterrupted sleep per night to achieve normal levels of alertness during daytime hours. Although evidence indicates that reducing the sleep period by one hour may have little effect on alertness and performance if an individual is well-rested, reduced sleep when accompanied by an existing sleep debt diminishes performance and the ability of an individual to remain alert.[4] The literature indicates 10-hour, off-duty rest periods may not be sufficient to support an eight-hour sleep opportunity. To promote adequate sleep cycles of seven to eight hours, studies indicate optimal time between shift periods should be 16 hours.[4,16-18]

Self-assessment of fatigue often is inaccurate, with fatigue being underestimated. A noted discrepancy exists between subjective self-reports and psychophysiological measures. Impaired self-discernment of cognitive ability increases as sleep loss and fatigue increase. Higher-order cognitive brain functions and the ability to evaluate personal performance diminish as fatigue increases and sleep cycles shorten.[4] Environmental factors may contribute to masking perceptions of sleepiness and include, but are not limited to, noise, physical activity, nicotine, caffeine, thirst, hunger, excitement, and talking about something interesting. These behaviors, when used in an attempt to overcome sleepiness and/or exhaustion, also may contribute to escalations in fatigue.[19]

POSITION STATEMENT

AORN believes that on-call staffing plans should be based on strategies that minimize extended work hours, allow for adequate recuperation, and retain the perioperative registered nurse as circulator. AORN is committed to both patient and worker safety. AORN recognizes that research addressing sleep deprivation, fatigue, and patient outcomes related directly to perioperative nursing practice is limited. Human factors implications and evidence from existing research in other safety-sensitive industries (eg, medicine, the military, aviation) have significant implications in the development of perioperative work plans, including on-call schedules.

Recognizing the potential negative consequences of sleep deprivation and sustained work hours and further recognizing that adequate rest and recuperation periods are essential to patient and perioperative personnel safety, AORN suggests the following strategies.

♦ Perioperative registered nurses should not be required to work in direct patient care for more than 12 consecutive hours in a 24-hour period and not more than 60 hours in a seven-day period. Sufficient transition time is required for appropriate patient handoff and staff relief. Under extreme conditions exceptions to the 12-hour limit may be required (eg, disasters). Organization policy should outline exceptions to the 12-hour limitation. All worked hours (ie, regular hours and call hours worked) should be included in calculating total hours worked.[7,10,18]

♦ Off-duty periods should be inclusive of an uninterrupted eight-hour sleep cycle, a break from continuous professional responsibilities, and time to perform individual activities of daily living.[2,3,20]

♦ Arrangements should be made, in relation to the hours worked, to relieve a perioperative registered nurse who has worked on-call during his or her off shift and who is scheduled to work the following shift to accommodate an adequate off-duty recuperation period.

♦ The number of on-call shifts assigned in a seven-day period depends on the type of facility and should be coordinated with the number of sustained work hours and adequate recuperation periods mentioned above.

♦ An individual's ability to meet the anticipated work demand should be considered for on-call requirements. Limited research indicates older people are more likely than younger people to be adversely affected by sleep deprivation; however, there is no research specific to the effects of on-call assignment and a person's age.

♦ Orientation to on-call should be included in the orientation process and should be accomplished using the preceptor system (ie, having an experienced nurse serve as an immediate resource for the orientee). The time frame depends on the type of procedures and the scope of services.

♦ Perioperative registered nurses should uphold their ethical responsibility to patients and themselves to arrive at work adequately rested and prepared for duty.[10,21]

♦ Health care organizations should support perioperative RNs in changing cultural attitudes so that fatigue is recognized as an unacceptable risk to patient and worker safety rather than a sign of a worker's dedication to the job.[10]

This position statement articulates AORN's position regarding on-call practices for perioperative registered nurses based on available research at this time. It is the responsibility of each facility to determine its specific on-call policies and procedures based on patient need and available resources.

DEFINITIONS

On-call: A designated period of time, outside of designated hours of operation, during which perioperative RNs and other perioperative personnel are available to respond to patient care needs for unplanned circumstances or urgent or emergent procedures.

Call hours worked: This is the actual time the on-call perioperative registered nurse and other perioperative personnel are called in to the facility for a procedure.

Extended work period: Work schedules having a longer than normal workday; however, there is no clear consensus nor are there regulations about the length of the extended workday. Some sources regard time worked in excess of eight hours to be extended work periods, while others consider shifts longer than 12 hours to be extended shifts.[22,23]

Sustained work hours: Work periods of 12 or more hours with limited opportunity for rest and no opportunity for sleep.[8]

Off duty: A period of uninterrupted time during which an individual is free from work-related duties.[20]

Sleepiness: A physiological state. Deprivation or restriction of sleep increases sleepiness. Just as hunger and thirst are reversible by eating or drinking, respectively, sleep reverses sleepiness.[4]

Fatigue: A response to predefined conditions that has physiological and performance consequences. Fatigue is identified as deterioration in human performance arising as a consequence of changes in the physiological condition. Factors contributing to fatigue include, but may not be limited to, time on task, time and duty period duration, time since awake when beginning the duty period, acute and chronic sleep debt, circadian disruption, multiple time zones, and shift work.[4]

Circadian rhythms: Twenty-four-hour cycles of behavior and physiology generated by an internal biological clock located in the suprachiasmatic nuclei of the hypothalamus. It regulates the daily cyclical patterns of sleep and wakefulness. It compels the body to fall asleep and wake up and regulates hour-to-hour waking behavior reflected in fatigue, alertness, and cognitive performance.[24]

NOTES

1. Board on Health Care Services, Institute of Medicine, "Keeping patients safe: Transforming the work environment of nurses," National Academies Press, *http://www.nap.edu/openbook/0309090679/html/1.html* (accessed 10 Dec 2004).

2. A Page, "Appendix C: Work hour regulation in safety-sensitive industries," in *Keeping Patients Safe: Transforming the Work Environment of Nurses* (Washington, DC: National Academies Press, 2004) 384-435.

3. A E Rogers et al, "The working hours of hospital staff nurses and patient safety," *Health Affairs* 23 (July/August 2004) 202-212.

4. Battelle Memorial Institute, JIL Information Systems "An overview of the scientific literature concerning fatigue, sleep, and the circadian cycle" (January 1998), Federal Aviation Administration, *http://cf.alpa.org/internet/projects/ftdt/backgr/batelle.htm* (accessed 10 Dec 2004).

5. "The effect of health care working conditions on patient safety," *Evidence Report: Technology Assessment* 74 (March 2003) 1-3.

6. M R Rosekind et al, "Managing fatigue in operational settings 1: Physiological considerations and countermeasures," *Hospital Topics* 75 (Summer 1997) 23-30.

7. M Rosekind et al, "Managing fatigue in operational settings 2: An integrated approach," *Hospital Topics* 75 (Summer 1997) 31-35.

8. G P Kruger, "Sustained work, fatigue, sleep loss and performance: A review of the issues," *Work and Stress* 3 no 2 (1989) 129-141.

9. A Page, "Executive summary," in *Keeping Patients Safe: Transforming the Work Environment of Nurses* (Washington, DC: National Academies Press, 2004) 6.

10. D M Gaba, S K Howard, "Patient safety: Fatigue among clinicians and the safety of patients," *The New England Journal of Medicine* 347 (Oct 17, 2002) 1249-1255.

11. R P Hart et al, "Effect of sleep deprivation on first-year residents' response times, memory, and mood," *Journal of Medical Education* 62 (November 1987) 940-942.

12. R Rubin et al, "Neurobehavioral effects of the on-call experience in house staff physicians," *Journal of Occupational Medicine* 33 (January 1991) 13-18.

13. J Robbins, F Gottlieb, "Sleep deprivation and cognitive testing in internal medicine house staff," *Western Journal of Medicine* 152 (January 1990) 82-86.

14. A Gurjala et al "Petition to the Occupational Safety and Health Administration requesting that limits be placed on hours worked by medical residents (HRG publication #1570)," (April 30, 2001) Public Citizen, *http://www.citizen.org/publications/release.cfm?ID=6771* (accessed 10 Dec 2004).

15. R G Hughes, A E Rogers, "Are you tired?" *American Journal of Nursing* 104 (March 2004) 36-38.

16. N Kurumatani et al, "The effects of frequently rotating shiftwork on sleep and the family life of hospital nurses," *Ergonomics* 37 (June 1994) 995-1007.

17. G Kecklund, T Akerstedt, "Effects of timing of shifts on sleepiness and sleep duration," *Journal of Sleep Research* 4 no 2 (1995) 47-50.

18. A Page, "Work and workspace design to prevent and mitigate errors," in *Keeping Patients Safe: Transforming the Work Environment of Nurses* (Washington, DC: National Academies Press, 2004) 237.

19. S R Mohler, "Fatigue in aviation activities," *Aerospace Medicine* 37 (July 1966) 722-732.

20. D F Dinges et al, "Principles and guidelines for duty and rest scheduling in commercial aviation," Human Factors Research and Technology, *http://humanfactors.arc.nasa.gov/zteam/fcp/pubs/p.and.g.intro.html* (accessed 10 Dec 2004).

21. "AORN explications for perioperative nursing," in *Standards, Recommended Practices, and Guidelines* (Denver: AORN, Inc, 2004) 53-83.

22. "Extended/unusual work shifts," US Department of Labor, Occupational Safety and Health Administration, *http://www.osha.gov/SLTC/emergencypreparedness/guide/extended.html* (accessed 10 Dec 2004).

23. "OSH answers," Canadian Center for Occupational Health and Safety, *http://www.ccohs.ca/oshanswers/work_schedules/workday.html* (accessed 10 Dec 2004).

24. M H Kryger, T Roth, W C Dement, eds, *Principles and Practice of Sleep Medicine,* third ed (Philadelphia: W B Saunders Co, 2000) 319, 334.

Original statement adopted by the AORN Board of Directors in November 2004; ratified by the House of Delegates, New Orleans, in April 2005.
Sunset review: March 2009

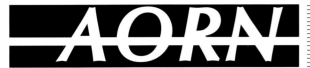
POSITION STATEMENT

Association of periOperative Registered Nurses, Inc. • 2170 South Parker Road, Suite 300 • Denver, Colorado 80231-5711 • (303) 755-6300

OPERATING ROOM STAFFING
SKILL MIX FOR DIRECT CAREGIVERS

PREAMBLE

A primary responsibility of perioperative nursing managers is to create an environment in which the safe care of the patient is the priority. Developing a staffing plan in which adequate numbers of competent perioperative registered nurses are available to care for patients and their family members is a critical component. Health care market forces (eg, lower reimbursement, a competitive health care environment) have compelled health care administrators to place pressure on perioperative nursing managers to reduce labor costs associated with staffing salaries. It is imperative that perioperative nursing managers understand factors influencing staffing patterns to maximize staffing resources. Perioperative nursing managers need to clearly articulate staffing ratio recommendations and provide justification to support them.

An important step in providing safe patient care is the development of a perioperative staffing ratio that provides the skill level necessary to promote optimum patient outcomes and efficient patient flow; is fiscally responsible; and satisfies federal, state, and local regulations. Some studies have demonstrated an association between lower RN staffing levels and adverse patient outcomes.[1-4]

The perioperative registered nurse is accountable for patient outcomes resulting from the nursing care provided during the perioperative experience. A perioperative registered nurse functioning in the circulating role must plan and direct the nursing care of every patient undergoing surgical and other invasive procedures, thus requiring a 1:1 perioperative RN:patient ratio.[5,6] The scrub role may be filled by an RN or a surgical technologist (ST)/licensed practical nurse (LPN). To this end, perioperative nursing managers must develop a staffing plan that integrates the perioperative registered

nurse into the circulating role and accommodates for skill diversity in the scrub role. Sufficient numbers of perioperative registered nurses are necessary to meet this objective.

Although there is no consensus among perioperative nursing managers related to OR skill mix ratios, a survey conducted by AORN indicates a 2:1 (67:33) RN:ST/LPN ratio. AORN's findings are consistent with current literature.[7-11]

POSITION STATEMENT

AORN believes that perioperative nursing managers in acute care and ambulatory facilities should maintain a minimum RN:ST/LPN ratio of 67:33 (two RNs to one ST/LPN) to provide two circulating nurses on nonanesthetist provider sedation procedures and procedures requiring a second circulating nurse and to provide additional RN resources when necessary.

AORN believes that OR staffing skill mix ratios must ensure that every patient undergoing a surgical or invasive procedure has a perioperative registered nurse in the role of circulator.[6]

AORN believes that OR staffing skill mix ratios must ensure that the core activities of perioperative nursing care (ie, assessment, diagnosis, outcome identification, planning implementation, evaluation) are completed by a perioperative registered nurse.[5]

AORN believes that OR staffing skill mix ratios should support the perioperative registered nurse functioning in both the scrub and circulating roles.

AORN believes that direct caregivers who are in orientation should not be included when calculating OR skill mix ratios.

DEFINITIONS

Direct staff caregivers: The direct caregivers in the OR are defined as those directly involved in providing care to patients undergoing surgical or other invasive procedures. For the purpose of this document, individuals providing direct patient care include perioperative registered nurses and STs/LPNs. Staffing policies for the OR should state the minimum number of personnel that will be provided for different types of surgical procedures. Procedure complexity and patient acuity may necessitate more than the minimum number of personnel identified.

Skill mix: Ratio of RNs to STs/LPNs providing direct patient care in the department.

NOTES

1. Agency for Healthcare Research and Quality, "Hospital nurse staffing and quality of care," in *Research in Action* (Rockville, Md: Agency for Healthcare Research and Quality, March 2004) 1-9.

2. Institute of Medicine, "Maximizing workforce capability," in *Keeping Patients Safe: Transforming the Work Environment of Nurses* (Washington, DC: National Academies Press, 2004) 171.

3. M A Blegen, C J Goode, L Reed, "Nurse staffing and patient outcomes," *Nursing Research* 47 (January/February 1998) 43-50.

4. A J Hartz et al, "Hospital characteristics and mortality rates," *The New England Journal of Medicine* 321 (Dec 21, 1989) 1720-1725.

5. "AORN official statement on unlicensed assistive personnel" in *Standards, Recommended Practices, and Guidelines* (Denver: AORN, Inc, 2004) 167.

6. "AORN statement on nurse-to-patient ratios," in *Standards, Recommended Practices, and Guidelines* (Denver: AORN, Inc, 2004) 157-158.

7. F Koch, "Staffing outcomes: Skill mix changes," *Seminars in Perioperative Nursing* 5 (January 1996) 32-35.

8. J Shamian, "Skill mix and clinical outcomes," *Canadian Operating Room Nursing Journal* 16 (June 1998) 36-41.

9. B Fernsebner, S Beyea, "Survey provides a snapshot of staffing challenges in the OR," *OR Manager* 17 (June 2001) 1, 10-13.

10. "Salary/career survey," *OR Manager* 19 (October 2003) 13.

11. "Salary/career survey," *OR Manager* 20 (October 2004) 15.

Original statement adopted by the AORN Board of Directors in November 2004; ratified by the House of Delegates, New Orleans, in April 2005.
Sunset review: March 2009

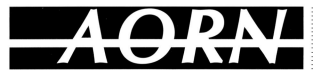

POSITION STATEMENT

Association of periOperative Registered Nurses, Inc. • 2170 South Parker Road, Suite 300 • Denver, Colorado 80231-5711 • (303) 755-6300

AORN POSITION STATEMENT ON WORKPLACE SAFETY

PREAMBLE

Perioperative nurses, along with others in the health care environment, are routinely faced with a wide array of occupational hazards that create a risk of personal injury in the workplace. A survey of registered nurses revealed that stress/overwork, disabling back injuries, and contracting a bloodborne disease were the top three health and safety concerns.[1,2] The National Institute for Occupational Safety and Health (NIOSH) reported that an estimated 600,000 to 800,000 percutaneous injuries occur annually to health care workers.[3] Reported information on needle sticks shows that nurses sustain the majority of these injuries.[3] Nurses practicing in the perioperative environment are at distinct risk for percutaneous injury due to prolonged exposure to open surgical sites, frequent handling of sharp instruments, and the presence of large quantities of blood and other potentially infectious body fluids.[4]

Back injuries pose a significant risk to perioperative nurses and are the most prevalent occupational injury in the health care industry.[5] Direct costs associated with occupational back injuries of health care providers average $37,000. Indirect costs associated with back injuries can range from $147,000 to $300,000.[5]

Key indicators to an organization's culture and commitment to ensure a safe workplace include maintaining safe equipment, providing adequate nurse staffing levels, and fostering safe work practices.[6] An unsafe workplace contributes to work-related injuries and diseases that often result in physical, emotional, and financial difficulties for perioperative nurses. Occupational injuries resulting from an unsafe workplace impact the health care organization by increased costs and a reduced ability to provide services. Occupational hazards in the workplace have been identified as a major contributor to nurses leaving the profession, contributing to the growing nursing shortage.[7]

BACKGROUND

The shortage of skilled registered nurses and other health care personnel has a major impact on the delivery of safe, quality patient care. The current shortage has become an area of grave concern for health care organizations and providers, the government, and consumers. Workplace safety is a primary concern of nurses and impacts their decision to continue working in the nursing profession. A safe workplace will have a positive impact on the retention and recruitment of qualified nurses to provide safe patient care.

The health care organization's commitment to workplace safety is an important factor influencing employee compliance with safe work practices. The workplace safety culture is of increasing importance as workloads increase, due to the effects of the nursing shortage, increased patient acuity, and emphasis on higher productivity.[8] One study demonstrated that strong support from senior management resulted in a reduced rate of occupational exposure to blood and body fluids.[8]

The multiple occupational hazards that create a risk of personal injury that perioperative nurses face in the workplace are both physical and psychosocial. Some of the workplace safety exposure issues identified in the perioperative setting include, but are not limited to, the following.[9]

1. Biological
   ♦ Exposure to bloodborne pathogens from percutaneous injuries, splashes, and other contact
   ♦ Exposure to infectious microorganisms
   ♦ Exposure to biological components of surgical smoke from use of lasers and electrosurgical units
   ♦ Exposure to the chemical and protein allergens in latex gloves
2. Ergonomic
   ♦ Static or awkward posture
   ♦ Standing for long periods of time in one position
   ♦ Back injuries

- Repetitive motion
- Moving patients or carrying heavy instruments and equipment
3. Chemicals
   - Anesthesia gases
   - Disinfecting/sterilizing agents
   - Cleaning agents
   - Specimen preservatives
4. Physical hazards
   - Fire
   - Electrical
   - Radiation
   - Lasers
   - Smoke plume
   - Compressed gases
5. Psychosocial
   - Long hours
   - Mandatory overtime
   - Demographic diversity
   - Nursing shortage
   - Call
   - Trauma
   - Burnout
   - Abuse—verbal and physical
   - Violence from staff, patients, patients' families, or nurses' families
6. Cultural
   - Tolerance of abuse from physicians
   - Lack of commitment by management to adhere to an optimal workplace safety program
   - Absence of respect from peers and other health care professionals
   - Absence of a code of conduct for all team members

WORKPLACE SAFETY STRATEGIES

AORN suggests the following strategies for developing and maintaining a safe workplace:

- The facility has the responsibility to establish and promote a safe work environment and strive to use best practice models (eg, magnet hospital status criteria, workplace of choice).
- Each facility should develop a comprehensive workplace safety program that includes a written plan for each topic covered in the program, a written plan to provide education on safety initiatives, and monitoring of compliance for employees and other health care providers.
- Every perioperative nurse is responsible for following safety policies and participating in the safety programs.

- The perioperative nurse has a responsibility to identify safety hazards, take appropriate action, and report them through the appropriate channels.

AORN'S POSITION

The Association is committed to the creation and maintenance of a safe perioperative work environment to protect all of those present in the workplace and provide safe patient care. AORN supports research that is directed toward creating and maintaining safe work environments. AORN further supports the Environmental Protection Agency (EPA), National Institute for Occupational Safety and Health (NIOSH), Occupational Safety and Health Association (OSHA), and state and local regulations that promote workplace safety in the perioperative environment.

NOTES

1. "Working conditions are major factor in retaining current nurse workforce," *Legislative Network for Nurses* 18 (Sept 10, 2001) 137.
2. "On-line health and safety survey, September 2001, Key finding," American Nurses Association/NursingWorld.org, *http://nursingworld.org/ surveys/keyfind.pdf* (accessed 8 Oct 2002).
3. "NIOSH alert: Preventing needlestick injuries in health care settings," US Department of Health and Human Services, National Institute for Occupational Safety and Health (November 1999) *http://www.cdc.gov/niosh/2000-108.html* (accessed 7 Oct 2002).
4. J Jagger, M Bentley, P Tereskerz, "Study of patterns and prevention of blood exposures in OR personnel," *AORN Journal* 67 (May 1998) 979-996.
5. D Blackmon, "Back injury prevention," *Surgical Services Management* 5 (July 1999) 43-46.
6. S Clarke et al, "Organizational climate, staffing, and safety equipment as predictors of needlestick injuries and near-misses in hospital nurses," *American Journal of Infection Control* 30 (June 2002) 207-216.
7. "Working conditions are major factor in retaining current nurse workforce," *Legislative Network for Nurses.*
8. R Gershon, et al, "Hospital safety climate and its relationship with safe work practices and workplace exposure incidents," *American Journal of Infection Control* 28 (July 2001) 211-221.
9. "Health care workers," US Department of Health and Human Services, National Institute for Occupational Safety and Health, *http://www.cdc.gov/niosh/healthpg. html#tb* (accessed 9 March 2003).

Original statement adopted by the AORN Board of Directors in February 2003.
Ratified by the House of Delegates, Chicago, in March 2003.
Sunset review: March 2008

STANDARDS OF
NURSING PRACTICE

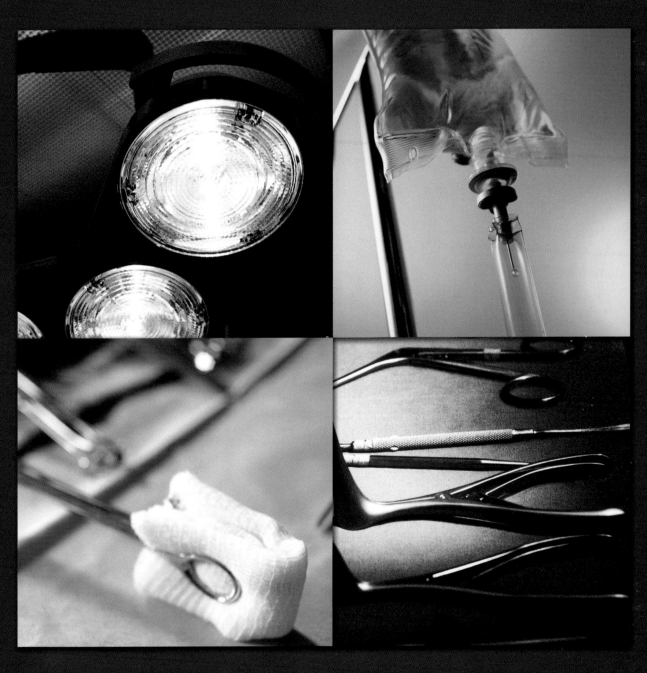

Section Two

Perioperative Patient Care Quality

Preamble

A fundamental precept of AORN is that it is the responsibility of professional registered nurses to ensure safe, high-quality nursing care to patients undergoing operative and other invasive procedures. The Association repeatedly has demonstrated its ongoing commitment to that premise through promulgation of standards of practice, support of perioperative nursing research, certification programs, competency statements, guidelines, guidance statements, recommended practices, and position statements.

The Association's first "Standards of nursing practice: OR" were developed with the American Nurses Association (ANA) Division of Medical Surgical Practice and printed in 1975. Subsequently, AORN provided its membership with a variety of programs and activities to assist nurses in the operating room in becoming aware of and using the standards to evaluate their professional practice. These standards were revised after data was collected from practicing nurses to determine the applicability and usefulness of the standards. The resulting revision, titled "Standards of perioperative nursing practice," was published in 1981. These standards were joined by "Standards of administrative nursing practice: OR" in 1982 and "Patient outcome standards for perioperative nursing" in 1985. In addition to standards of nursing practice, the Association began publishing recommended practices in the technical aspects of perioperative nursing in March 1975.

Perioperative nurses may validate and measure the quality of their practice by use of the "Competency statements in perioperative nursing," first published by AORN in 1986 and revised periodically, and the *Perioperative Nursing Data Set* (PNDS), published by AORN and first recognized by ANA in 1999.

The first perioperative nurse certification program was approved by the AORN House of Delegates in 1978 to "enhance quality patient care" and to "demonstrate accountability to the general public for nursing practice." Certification in perioperative nursing (CNOR) demonstrates the perioperative nurse's individual commitment to excellence in practice in the clinical setting as well as the Association's ongoing commitment to fostering excellence in the clinical setting. AORN encourages the achievement and maintenance of additional certifications applicable to various arenas of perioperative practice, such as first assisting (CRNFA), administration, nursing informatics, and other subspecialized arenas.

Further, resolutions and statements adopted by the House of Delegates consistently reiterate the primacy of the concern for quality and safety in patient care. The commitment to quality and safety has remained constant as each resolution or statement includes reference to the patient's entitlement to and nurses' obligation to provide safe, quality care.

Quality of care has three foci:

♦ quality of the service provided, which means the care given meets the expressed needs of the consumer;

♦ quality of process, meaning conformance to specifications or performance standards that demonstrate adherence to established standards; and perhaps the most important,

♦ quality as it relates to safe patient care.

Nurses have developed a scope and definition of practice that embraces those elements of health care that have been mandated by the consumer. The scope of practice includes independently assessing patient needs; making collaborative decisions relative to perioperative care; contributing to patient safety; and evaluating and monitoring care provided. Striving for excellence in practice, perioperative nurses actively participate in shaping the practice environment and identify clinical and organizational indicators for quality and performance improvement.

Operational definition of perioperative patient care quality

Perioperative patient care quality is based on nursing practice that encompasses accepted components of analysis and interpretation. These include the following:

Structure: Providing perioperative care within an environment that is conducive to its effective, safe, and efficient administration, as outlined in the AORN "Standards of perioperative administrative practice"[1] and the "Quality and performance improvement standards for perioperative nursing."[2]

Process: Meeting the needs of patients in a caring and safe manner and conforming to the standards of perioperative nursing practice. A goal-directed, interrelated series of actions, events, mechanisms, or steps.[3]

Outcome: Observable, measurable, physiological, and psychological responses to perioperative nursing interventions.[4] "The intended, or realistically expected, correction of the patient's problem by a certain point in time."[5]

NOTES

1. "Standards of perioperative administrative practice," in *Standards, Recommended Practices, and Guidelines* (Denver: AORN, Inc, 2003) 171-172.

2. "Quality and process improvement standards for perioperative nursing," in *Standards, Recommended Practices, and Guidelines* (Denver: AORN, Inc, 2004).

3. Joint Commission on Accreditation of Healthcare Organizations, "Glossary," in *Hospital Accreditation Standards* (Oakbrook Terrace, Ill: Joint Commission on Accreditation of Healthcare Organizations, 2002) 354.

4. S Beyea, ed, *Perioperative Nursing Data Set,* second ed (Denver: AORN, Inc, 2002) 21.

5. "Glossary," in *Standards, Recommended Practices, and Guidelines* (Denver: AORN, Inc 2003) 385.

Standards of Perioperative Nursing

The American Nurses Association (ANA) began developing standards in the late 1960s. The first, *Standards of Nursing Practice,* was published in 1973 and was a generic standard that focused on the nursing process. In 1974, ANA published *Standards of Medical-Surgical Nursing Practice* using the nursing process to describe nursing assessment, planning, implementation, and evaluation. A joint committee from the ANA Division on Medical-Surgical Nursing Practice and AORN determined that perioperative standards of practice would help ensure the quality of nursing care for surgical patients.[1]

The *Standards of Nursing Practice: Operating Room* were developed and published in 1975. The revised *Standards of Perioperative Nursing Practice,* published in 1981, were approved by the Executive committee of the ANA Division on Medical-Surgical Nursing Practice and the AORN Board of Directors. These standards reflect the definitions, purpose, and framework for standards of practice in the perioperative setting. These standards are used in conjunction with other documents that describe the practice of perioperative nursing. The ANA acknowledges the AORN "Standards of perioperative clinical practice" and "Standards of professional practice."

Standards Defined

Standards are authoritative statements that describe the responsibilities for which nursing practitioners are accountable. Standards reflect the values and priorities of the profession. They are a means to direct and evaluate professional nursing practice. When written in measurable terms, standards also define the nursing profession's accountability and responsibilities. Standards that relate to the practice of perioperative nursing focus on the individual experiencing surgical intervention. The dimensions of this practice range from perioperative assessment and planning to intraoperative intervention, to postoperative evaluation and documentation, which may occur in a variety of settings.

Organizing Principles

Standards describe a competent level of nursing practice and professional performance that is designed to achieve desired patient outcomes in the perioperative setting. The "Standards of perioperative nursing" are generic and apply to all registered nurses engaged in perioperative practice, regardless of clinical specialty, practice setting, or educational preparation.

Categories of Standards

The "Standards of perioperative nursing" may be categorized into structure, process, and outcome standards (Table 1).

Table 1 — Categories of Standards of Perioperative Nursing		
Structure	**Process**	**Outcome**
Administrative practice	Clinical practice Professional performance Quality improvement	Patient outcomes: Perioperative care

Structure standards

The "Standards of perioperative administrative practice" were developed to guide professionals in administrative roles and to provide a model for evaluating their practice. They are intended to assist agencies in establishing administrative practice in their settings.

Process standards

The "Standards of perioperative clinical practice" describe a competent level of perioperative nursing as demonstrated by assessment, diagnosis, outcome identification, planning, implementation, and evaluation. The nursing process encompasses all significant actions taken by the nurse in providing care to all patients and forms the foundation of clinical decision making.

Additional nursing responsibilities for all patients (eg, providing culturally and ethnically relevant care, maintaining a safe environment, educating patients about their illness, treatment, health promotion or self-care activities, planning for continuity of care) are subsumed within these standards.[2] The "Standards of perioperative professional performance" describe a competent level of behavior in the professional perioperative role, including activities related to providing quality of care, performance appraisal, pursuing education, practicing collegiality, ethical conduct, collaboration, efficient resource utilization, and participating in or conducting research. The scope of nurse's involvement in these standards may be dependent on his or her education, position, or practice environment.

While "Standards of perioperative professional performance" describe roles expected of all perioperative nurses, many other responsibilities comprise the hallmarks of a profession. The perioperative nurse should be self-directed and purposeful in seeking necessary knowledge and skills to advance career goals. Other activities, such as membership in a professional nursing organization and certification in specialty or advanced practice, are desirable methods to enhance the nurse's professionalism.

The "Quality improvement standards for perioperative nursing" assist members in developing a quality assessment/improvement program specific for their setting. The Joint Commission on Accreditation of Healthcare Organizations designed a model incorporating 10 steps for effective monitoring and evaluation.[3] The purpose of monitoring and evaluation activities is to examine the care provided, to identify problems or opportunities to improve quality and appropriateness of the care, and to improve the quality of care. *Quality assessment* measures care at a point in time but does not necessarily mean change or improvement. *Quality assurance* measures the level of care provided. *Quality improvement* includes aspects of assessment and assurance. AORN developed standards to assist with the monitoring and evaluation process.

Implementation of the quality assessment standards, with emphasis on continuous monitoring and evaluation, can provide the basis for selecting methods for quality improvement. The quality assessment/improvement process is best used when combined with all the resources perioperative nurses have available.

Outcome standards

The "Patient outcomes: Standards of perioperative care" describe a basic level of care the patient can expect to receive. Patient outcomes are a patient's observable and/or measurable physiological, psychosocial, and psychological responses.

Outcomes may be judged on the basis of patient achievement through collaborative planning and implementation of care. The achievement of patient outcomes from care provided by the health care team is a primary concern for the perioperative nurse in planning and implementing care during the perioperative period. Nursing activities contribute to outcome achievement but may not be the only factor involved.

The outcome standards focus on high-risk surgical patient problem areas. They reflect the perioperative nurse's scope of responsibility. The individual perioperative nurse can use the "Patient outcomes: Standards of perioperative care" to establish a data base to support current nursing practice, or as a rationale for change.

NOTES

1. "Standards of Perioperative Nursing Practice," in *AORN Standards and Recommended Practices for Perioperative Nursing* (Denver: Association of Operating Room Nurses, Inc, 1991) II:3-1.

2. American Nurses Association, *Standards of Clinical Nursing Practice*, manuscript submitted for publication, (Kansas City, Mo: American Nurses Association).

3. Joint Commission on Accreditation of Healthcare Organizations, *An Introduction to Joint Commission Nursing Care Standards* (Oakbrook, Ill: Joint Commission on Accreditation of Healthcare Organizations, 1991) 53-62.

Standards of Perioperative Administrative Practice

The following standards were revised by the Nursing Practices Committee and approved by the AORN Board of Directors in November 1996. They are a revision of the "Standards of Administrative Nursing Practice: OR" originally published in the June 1976 *AORN Journal* and the "Standards of Perioperative Administrative Practice" approved by the Board in November 1991.

The "Standards of Perioperative Administrative Practice" serve as the foundation upon which the perioperative setting is organized and managed. These structure standards are developed to guide professionals in administrative roles and to provide direction for evaluation of operational systems. These standards are broad in scope, definitive, relevant, and attainable, and they provide the framework for continuous quality improvement. The term *registered nurse administrator* is used to designate the individual responsible and accountable for the management of perioperative nursing services within a variety of settings.

Standard I

The administrative structure for perioperative services shall be developed and communicated.

A. A philosophy, purpose, and objectives are developed to guide perioperative services.
   1. The philosophy, purpose, and objectives are derived from the mission, vision, and values of the organization.
   2. Staff members participate in the ongoing development, implementation, and evaluation of the philosophy, purpose, and objectives for perioperative services.
   3. The philosophy, purpose, and objectives of perioperative services are applied universally throughout the organizational system.
B. An organizational plan for perioperative services is developed, communicated, implemented, and evaluated.
   1. The plan reflects the philosophy, purpose, and objectives of perioperative services.
   2. The plan defines the lines of formal authority, accountability, and communication for perioperative services.
   3. The plan describes the relationship of perioperative services to the whole of the organization.

C. A data management system is developed, maintained, and evaluated to support perioperative patient care and resource management.

Standard II

A registered nurse qualified by advanced education and management experience shall have administrative accountability for perioperative nursing services.

A. The registered nurse administrator demonstrates management and leadership skills.
B. The registered nurse administrator has experience and expertise in perioperative nursing.
C. The registered nurse administrator maintains competence in management through participation in continuing education or formal education.
D. The registered nurse administrator maintains awareness of local, state, and national legislative and regulatory activities affecting health care.
E. Only a registered nurse directs perioperative nursing care.

Standard III

The registered nurse administrator shall be accountable for planning perioperative nursing services.

A. The registered nurse administrator shares responsibility for the fiscal activities of perioperative nursing services as defined by the organization.
B. The registered nurse administrator allocates resources to meet the needs of the population served.
C. The registered nurse administrator collects data to facilitate planning decisions that address identified patient, family, and community needs and expectations.
D. The registered nurse administrator participates in strategic planning for the organization, integrating perioperative services into the organization as a whole.
E. The registered nurse administrator collaborates with risk management to plan and implement a program for perioperative services.
   1. Legal and regulatory requirements are met.
   2. Compliance with credentialing regulations is monitored.

Standard IV

The registered nurse administrator shall be accountable for the organization of perioperative nursing services.

A. The registered nurse administrator defines the lines of formal authority and communication.

B. The registered nurse administrator interprets and implements the scope of perioperative nursing practice.

   1. Processes that promote optimal patient outcomes are developed and implemented.

   2. Processes are consistent with nationally recognized professional standards and current nursing research and practice.

   3. Processes are in place to collect key data elements to demonstrate perioperative practice.

C. The registered nurse administrator promotes perioperative nursing research.

   1. Results of nursing research are used to develop perioperative care processes.

   2. Staff members are encouraged to initiate, promote, and support nursing research projects.

   3. Research findings and literature review are incorporated into policies and procedures guiding perioperative nursing care.

D. Through development of the performance evaluation tool, the registered nurse administrator implements an effective, ongoing program to monitor, assess, and improve the quality of care delivered to perioperative patients.

   1. Qualifications, competency, and necessary education to promote positive patient outcomes are defined for each staff function.

E. In collaboration with the governing body, management, and medical staff leaders, the registered nurse administrator participates in decision-making structures and processes for the organization.

Standard V

The registered nurse administrator shall be accountable for directing perioperative nursing services.

A. The registered nurse administrator interprets and implements the standards of nursing practice and nursing care.

B. Written policies and procedures guide perioperative services and are developed in collabora-

tion with appropriate departments, are consistent with the mission, and are appropriate to the scope and level of care.

C. The registered nurse administrator ensures that perioperative patient care is consistent with the level of care provided throughout the facility.

Standard VI

The registered nurse administrator shall be accountable for staffing perioperative nursing services.

A. The registered nurse administrator defines the qualifications, competencies, and staffing complement for perioperative nursing services.

   1. A master staffing plan is defined in writing and meets the needs of the population served and scope of services.

   2. Staff selection is based on facility needs and applicant qualifications.

   3. Staff assignments are based on patient needs, available resources, and staff competencies.

B. The registered nurse administrator defines the performance expectations for perioperative nursing staff members.

   1. Orientation programs are established and required for all staff members.

   2. A system for ongoing, periodic competency assessment is in place.

   3. Education programs are based on competency assessment, performance improvement initiative, and mandatory activities.

   4. Promotes ongoing development of staff members.

Standard VII

The registered nurse administrator shall be accountable for controlling perioperative nursing services.

A. The registered nurse administrator collaborates with community leaders and multidisciplinary groups in planning and designing a safe, functional, and effective therapeutic environment for patients, health care providers, and other individuals within the community.

B. Performance improvement activities are used to improve patient outcomes; defined in writing; consistent with the organizational mission, vision, and values; designed to meet the needs of key constituents; clinically validated and consistent with sound business practices; and designed to establish a baseline for measurement and assessment activities.

C. The registered nurse administrator ensures perioperative nursing service involvement in safety and infection surveillance programs.

Standard VIII

The registered nurse administrator shall be accountable for the identification and utilization of ethical processes to ensure positive patient outcomes.

A. Establishes an environment that promotes the delivery of patient care that is competent, ethical, and legal.

B. Promotes/ensures protection of human rights of all individuals in the perioperative setting.

1. Maintains privacy and confidentiality.
2. Fosters nondiscriminatory climate.
3. Maintains sensitivity to sociocultural diversity.

Standards of Perioperative Clinical Practice

The "Standards of perioperative clinical practice" and "Standards of perioperative professional performance" focus on the process of providing nursing care and performing professional role activities. These standards apply to all nurses in the perioperative setting and were developed by AORN using the ANA "Standards of clinical nursing practice."

It is the nurse's responsibility to meet these standards, assuming that adequate environmental working conditions and necessary resources are available to support and facilitate the nurse's attainment of these standards. Under certain conditions, nurses may not be able to fully meet the standards. It is important to recognize the link between working conditions and the nurse's ability to deliver care. It is the responsibility of employers or health care facilities to provide an appropriate environment for nursing practice.

Several related themes underlie the "Standards of perioperative clinical practice" and "Standards of perioperative professional performance." Nursing care must be individualized to meet a particular patient's unique needs and situation. This care should be provided in the context of disease or injury prevention, health promotion, health restoration, health maintenance, or palliative care. The cultural, racial, and ethnic diversity of the patient must always be taken into account in providing nursing services.

The nurse must respect the patient's goals and preferences in developing and implementing a plan of care. One of the nurse's primary responsibilities is patient education; therefore, nurses should provide patients with appropriate information to make informed decisions regarding their care and treatment. It is recognized, however, that some state regulations or institutional policies or procedures may prohibit full disclosure of information to patients.

The nurse's partnership with the patient and other health care providers is recognized in the standards. It is assumed that the nurse works with other health care providers in a coordinated manner throughout the process of caring for a surgical patient. The involvement of the patient, family, or significant others is paramount. The appropriate degree of participation expected of the patient, family, or other health care providers is determined by the clinical environment and the patient's unique situation.

Throughout the standards, terms such as *appropriate, pertinent,* and *realistic* are used. It is beyond the scope of documents such as these to account for all possible scenarios that the professional perioperative nurse may encounter in practice. The perioperative nurse will need to exercise judgment, based on education and experience, in determining what is appropriate, pertinent, or realistic. Further direction also may be available from documents such as recommended practices guidelines for care, agency standards, policies, procedures, protocols, and current research findings.

Summary

The "Standards of perioperative nursing" provide a mechanism to delineate the responsibilities of registered nurses engaged in practice in the perioperative setting. The standards of perioperative nursing and recommended practices serve as the basis for quality monitoring and evaluation systems; data bases; regulatory systems; the development and evaluation of nursing service delivery systems and organizational structures; certification activities; job descriptions and performance appraisals; agency policies, procedures and protocols; and educational offerings.

Standard I: Assessment

The perioperative nurse collects patient health data.

Interpretive statement:
Assessment is the systematic and ongoing collection of data, guided by the application of knowledge of physiological and psychological principles and experience, and is used to make judgments and predictions about a patient's response to illness or changes in life processes. Assessment is essential to establishing a nursing diagnosis and predicting outcomes. Assessment may occur in a variety of settings.

Criteria:
1. The priority of data collection is determined by the patient's immediate condition or needs, and the relationship to the proposed intervention. Pertinent data include, but are not limited to,

♦ current medical diagnoses and therapies;

♦ physical status and physiological responses;

♦ psychosocial status of the patient;

♦ cultural, spiritual, and lifestyle information;

♦ the individual's understanding, perceptions, and expectations of the procedure;

♦ previous responses to illness, hospitalizations, and surgical, therapeutic, or diagnostic procedures; and

♦ results of diagnostic studies.

2. Pertinent data are collected using appropriate assessment techniques.

3. Data collection involves the patient, significant others, and health care providers when appropriate. It may be accomplished through diverse means, such as interview, review of records, assessment, and/or consultation.

4. Data collection is systematic and ongoing.

5. Relevant data are documented in retrievable form.

Standard II: Diagnosis

The perioperative nurse analyzes the assessment data in determining diagnoses.

Interpretive statement:
The outcome of assessment is the potential for one or more nursing diagnoses. Nursing diagnoses are concise statements about actual, or high risk for, health problems/clinical conditions that are amenable to nursing intervention. Diagnoses result from analysis and interpretation of data about the patient's problems, needs, and health status.

Criteria:
1. Diagnoses are consistent with the assessment data.

2. Diagnoses are validated with the patient, significant others, and health care providers, when possible.

3. Diagnoses are documented in a manner that facilitates the determination of outcomes and plan of care.

Standard III: Outcome Identification

The perioperative nurse identifies expected outcomes unique to the patient.

Interpretive statement:
Patient outcomes are derived from nursing diagnoses and direct the interventions to correct, alter, or maintain the nursing diagnoses. Areas for the perioperative nurse to consider when formulating outcomes should include, but are not limited to,

♦ absence of infection;

♦ maintenance of skin integrity;

♦ absence of adverse effects through proper use of safety measures related to positioning, extraneous objects, and chemical, physical, and electrical hazards;

♦ maintenance of fluid and electrolyte balance;

♦ knowledge of the patient and significant others of the physiological and psychological responses to surgical intervention; and

♦ participation of the patient and significant others in the rehabilitation process.

Criteria:
1. Outcomes are derived from the diagnoses and are mutually formulated with the patient, significant others, and health care providers, when possible.

2. The patient's present and potential physical capabilities and behavioral patterns are congruent with the expected outcomes.

3. Outcomes are attainable with consideration to human and material resources available to the patient.

4. Outcome statements include measurable criteria for determining expected outcomes as a result of nursing interventions.

5. Outcomes include a time estimate for attainment.

6. Outcomes are prioritized.

7. Outcomes are communicated to appropriate people.

8. Outcomes are documented in a retrievable form.

9. Outcomes provide direction for continuity of care.

Standard IV: Planning

The perioperative nurse develops a plan of care that prescribes interventions to attain expected outcomes.

Interpretive statement:
The outcome statements become the guide for nursing interventions necessary to achieve the desired results. The individualized plan of care reflects the perioperative assessment and a logical sequence to attain outcomes. Priorities for the provision of nursing care are established by the perioperative nurse in collaboration with the patient, significant others, and health care providers. Examples of interventions performed include, but are not limited to,

- provision of information and supportive perioperative teaching specifically related to the surgical intervention and nursing care,
- identification of the patient,
- verification of the surgical site,
- verification of the operative consent and reports of essential diagnostic procedures,
- positioning according to physiological principles,
- adherence to principles of asepsis,
- provision of appropriate and properly functioning equipment and supplies for the patient,
- provision for comfort measures and supportive care to the patient,
- environmental monitoring and safety,
- evaluation of outcomes in relation to the identified interventions, and
- communication of intraoperative information to significant others and the health care team to provide for continuity of care.

Criteria:
1. The plan of care reflects current nursing practice.
2. The plan of care provides for continuity of care.
3. The plan of care specifies nursing diagnoses, interventions necessary to achieve the outcomes, and a logical sequence of interventions.
4. Human and materiel resources are available to implement the plan of care.

5. The plan of care is communicated to appropriate people.
6. Evidence of a plan of care is retrievable through documented intervention and evaluation of progress toward expected outcome.

Standard V: Implementation

The perioperative nurse implements the interventions identified in the plan of care.

Interpretive statement:
Interventions are consistent with the established plan of care and provide continuity of nursing care in the perioperative period. Interventions are based on expert opinion, scientific principles, and/or consensus. They reflect the rights and desires of the patient and significant others.

Criteria:
1. Interventions are consistent with the established plan of care.
2. Implementation of the plan of care is an ongoing process and is based on the patient's response.
3. Interventions reflect the rights and desires of the patient and significant others.
4. Interventions are implemented with safety, skill, and efficiency and are adjusted according to patient responses.
5. Interventions may be assigned or delegated as appropriate.
6. Interventions are documented and communicated verbally as appropriate to promote continuity of care.

Standard VI: Evaluation

The perioperative nurse evaluates the patient's progress toward attainment of outcomes.

Interpretive statement:
Evaluation is systematic and ongoing. It is based on observations and patient responses to nursing interventions; the effectiveness of interventions is evaluated in relation to the outcomes. Ongoing assessment data are used to revise diagnoses, the

plan of care, and/or outcomes as needed. The patient, significant others, and health care providers are involved in the evaluation process.

Criteria:

1. Evaluation of the effectiveness of interventions is systematic and ongoing.

2. The effectiveness of interventions is evaluated in relation to outcomes.

3. Documentation of the patient's progress toward achievable outcomes is retrievable.

4. Ongoing assessment data are used to revise diagnoses, outcomes, and the plan of care, as needed.

5. Revisions in diagnoses, outcomes, and the plan of care are documented.

6. The patient, significant others, and health care providers are involved in the evaluation process when appropriate.

Standards of Perioperative Professional Practice

Standard I: Quality of Practice

The perioperative nurse systematically evaluates the quality, safety, and appropriateness of nursing practice.

Interpretive statement:
The perioperative nurse engages in the evaluation of care delivery through a systematic quality and performance improvement process. This systematic approach uses specific steps to promote quality and safety in patient care.

Criteria:
1. The perioperative nurse participates in quality of care activities with a focus on nursing practice, safety, continuity of care, and outcomes. These activities are to be appropriate to the individual's position, education, and practice environment. Such activities may include
   - identifying and assigning responsibility for monitoring and evaluation activities,
   - delineating the scope of patient care activities or services,
   - identifying dimensions of performance,
   - developing quality indicators for each identified dimension of performance,
   - establishing thresholds for evaluation of the quality indicators,
   - collecting data related to the dimensions of performance and indicators,
   - evaluating care based on the cumulative data collected,
   - taking actions to improve care or services,
   - assessing the effectiveness of the action(s) taken and documenting the outcomes, and
   - communicating the data organization-wide.

2. Knowledge gained via the quality and performance improvement process is used to initiate change in nursing practice.

3. The perioperative nurse demonstrates that quality by applying that knowledge in a respectful, accountable, and ethical manner.

Standard II: Practice Evaluation

The perioperative nurse evaluates his or her practice in context with current professional practice standards, rules, and regulations.

Interpretive statement:
Practice evaluation is a process that includes defining and evaluating professional practice behaviors. This process demonstrates the accountability and responsibility for those practice behaviors The perioperative nurse is responsible for self-evaluation as well as receiving constructive feedback.

Criteria:
The perioperative nurse
- identifies the behaviors that support the level of performance desired within the perioperative setting, role, or situation;
- provides age-appropriate and culturally sensitive care;
- assesses perioperative practice behaviors on an ongoing basis, seeking constructive feedback;
- identifies areas for personal and professional development;
- develops and initiates an action plan to achieve professional development goals, which may include certification and advanced practice;
- periodically monitors and evaluates the progress of goal achievement; and
- participates in peer review.

Standard III: Education

The perioperative nurse acquires and maintains current knowledge in nursing practice.

Interpretive statement:
The purpose of professional development is to build on varied educational and experiential bases for the enhancement of perioperative nursing practice. The perioperative nurse has primary responsibility for his or her ongoing education and professional development.

Criteria:
The perioperative nurse
- completes an individualized orientation based on identified learning needs;
- acquires knowledge and skills appropriate to the specialty area, perioperative setting, role or situation;
- demonstrates accountability for maintaining competencies within the specific area of practice;

- participates in ongoing educational activities relevant to professional issues and trends in perioperative nursing; and
- participates in life-long learning.

Standard IV: Collegiality

The perioperative nurse interacts with and contributes to the professional growth of peers, colleagues, and others.

Interpretive statement:
The perioperative nurse has an obligation to support and advance the specialty and the profession by sharing his or her knowledge and expertise. The perioperative nurse interacts with colleagues to build and maintain the competencies necessary to provide safe, effective care to patients.

Criteria:
1. The perioperative nurse shares knowledge and skills. This is accomplished through a variety of methods, including, but not limited to,
   - providing inservice education, programs, seminars, and workshops;
   - precepting and mentoring;
   - role modeling;
   - publishing;
   - participating in professional organizations;
   - providing consultative services; and
   - participating in performance improvement activities.

2. The perioperative nurse provides peers with constructive feedback regarding their practice. This is facilitated through
   - the peer review process,
   - quality/performance improvement activities,
   - committee participation,
   - interdisciplinary teams, and
   - one-on-one discussions.

3. The perioperative nurse contributes to a supportive and healthy work environment using appropriate communication techniques.

4. The perioperative nurse is a role model for professional behavior.

Standard V: Collaboration

The perioperative nurse collaborates with the patient, family, health care team, and others in the conduct of professional nursing practice.

Interpretive statement:
Care of the perioperative patient requires cooperative efforts from many internal and external customers in order to achieve optimal outcomes. The perioperative nurse demonstrates accountability, flexibility, and communication skills when collaborating.

Criteria:
1. The perioperative nurse
   - communicates pertinent information relative to care,
   - consults with the health care team and others, and
   - makes referrals, including provisions for continuity of care, as needed.

2. The perioperative nurse has appropriate oversight and supervisory authority over unlicensed assistive personnel.

Standard VI: Ethics

The perioperative nurse's decisions and actions, on behalf of patients, are determined in an ethical manner.

Interpretive statement:
The basic human rights of individual patients are not forfeited when the patient enters the health care system. Care and services must be delivered without impeding these basic rights. The perioperative nurse is accountable to patients to safeguard these rights while providing appropriate nursing care or services in the perioperative setting. Nursing practice is guided by the *Code of Ethics for Nurses with Interpretive Statements* of the American Nurses Association.

Criteria:
1. The perioperative nurse acts as a patient advocate.

2. Patient confidentiality is maintained.

3. Care is delivered in a nonjudgmental and nondiscriminatory manner that is sensitive to cultural, racial, and ethnic diversity.

4. Care is delivered in a manner that preserves and protects patient autonomy, dignity, and rights.

5. The perioperative nurse uses available resources to help formulate ethical decisions.

Standard VII:
Evidence-Based Practice

The perioperative nurse uses research findings in evidence-based practice.

Interpretive statement:
Perioperative nursing practice is supported by research. The perioperative nurse uses evidence based on research to effect positive changes in patient outcomes. The perioperative nurse, regardless of position, education, or practice environment, participates in various aspects of research activities.

Criteria:
1. The perioperative nurse utilizes the best available evidence, preferably research data, to guide practice decisions.

2. Perioperative nurses participate in research by involvement in one or more of the following activities:
   - identifying clinical problems,
   - participating in data collection,
   - sharing research activities with others,
   - reading and critiquing research for application to practice,
   - participating on a research committee or in a study, and
   - using knowledge gained through research findings to initiate change.

Standard VIII: Resource Utilization

The perioperative nurse considers factors related to safety, effectiveness, efficiency, environmental concerns, and cost in planning and delivering patient care.

Interpretive statement:
The perioperative nurse identifies and promotes the most cost-effective and environmentally conscientious method of providing safe and effective patient care in accordance with established standards.

Criteria:
1. The perioperative nurse
   - evaluates factors related to safety, effectiveness, availability, cost, and impact on practice;

   - assigns tasks or delegates care based on the needs of the patient, potential for harm, and the knowledge and skills of the provider selected; and
   - assists the patient and family to become informed economic consumers in identifying appropriate services available to address perioperative patient needs.

2. The perioperative nurse utilizes technical advances in clinical care and information systems.

Standard IX: Leadership

The perioperative nurse provides leadership in the profession and professional practice setting.

Interpretive statement:
The perioperative nurse leader has the responsibility to display professionalism at all times. The perioperative nurse provides leadership in the profession and in the professional practice setting. The perioperative nurse has the responsibility to preserve the integrity and safety of perioperative patient care, and, to maintain competencies by continuing personal and professional growth through leadership development.

Criteria:
1. The perioperative nurse displays leadership by
   - supervising the assigned licensed and unlicensed caregivers,
   - holding self and team accountable for actions taken, and
   - being reliable to the team, the patient, and the organization.

2. The perioperative nurse leader works to create and maintain a healthy environment in local, regional, national, or international communities by
   - embracing life-long learning;
   - being a "systems thinker" and possessing the skills to develop processes;
   - strategizing;
   - planning, both in the short and long term;
   - using analytical skills to make changes; and
   - participating in perioperative research.

3. The perioperative nurse leader directs the coordination of perioperative care across settings and among caregivers.

4. The perioperative nurse leader promotes advancement of perioperative nursing through involvement with professional organizations by
   ♦ taking an active role in the organization,
   ♦ encouraging all team members to be active, and
   ♦ sharing information received through the organizations with team members.

5. The perioperative nurse leader works toward influencing policy-making to improve patient care organization-wide by
   ♦ being prepared to discuss issues that affect the patients in the perioperative setting at all levels of the organization, and
   ♦ participating in various performance improvement activities in the organization.

RESOURCES

AACN White Paper, "Hallmarks of the professional nursing practice environment." Washington, DC: American Association of Colleges of Nursing, January 2002.

"AORN explications for perioperative nursing," in *Standards, Recommended Practices, and Guidelines*. Denver: AORN, Inc, 2004, 53-84.

Bailes, B. "Evidence-based practice guidelines—One way to enhance clinical practice." *AORN Journal* 75 no 6 (June 2002) 1166-1167.

Seifert, P. "Ethics in perioperative practice—Duty to self," *AORN Journal* 76 no 2 (August 2002) 306-313.

Originally published as "Standards of perioperative professional performance" in the 1992 Standards and Recommended Practices for Perioperative Nursing.
Revised; approved by the AORN Board of Directors in October 2003.

Quality and Performance Improvement Standards for Perioperative Nursing

The 2002 AORN Nursing Practices Committee (NPC) was charged with the review and revision of the "Quality improvement standards for perioperative nursing" developed by the 1990 NPC.

Over time, health care has used many different terms to denote the processes used to improve patient care, such as quality assurance (QA), continuous improvement (CI), and continuous quality improvement (CQI). Quality cannot be assured, but it can be measured, assessed, and improved. Perioperative nurses should strive continuously to improve the care provided to patients in the perioperative setting.

Quality improvement (QI) and performance improvement (PI) are the newest terms used in the quest for excellence. They are two different methodologies that are linked together and continuously developing. "QI examines processes in order to improve them. PI addresses human performance within organizations at the individual, process, and organizational levels."[1] The origin of QI is based in industry and has more of a management and process focus; PI focuses more on the people, their motivation, and the tools (eg, work design, technical support, supervision, safety) they use to achieve the goals of the organization.

Government-funded peer review organizations (PROs), Medicare/Medicaid reimbursement regulations, laws generated at the federal and state levels, and private health insurers' standards have refocused the efforts required to assess patient care systematically. The recent focus of regulatory bodies and the Joint Commission on Accreditation of Healthcare Organizations (JCAHO) has placed greater emphasis on patient safety and reducing the errors that have resulted, at times, in patient deaths. The Institute of Medicine's 1999 report, *To Err Is Human: Building a Safer Health System*," states, "Although there are many kinds of standards in health care, especially those promulgated by licensing agencies and accrediting organizations, few standards focus explicitly on issues of patient safety."[2]

The Joint Commission states, "The goal of the improving organization performance function is to ensure that the organization designs processes well and systematically monitors, analyzes, and improves its performance to improve patient outcomes. Value in health care is the appropriate balance between good outcomes, excellent care and services, and costs. To add value to the care and services provided, organizations need to understand the relationship between perception of care, outcomes, and costs, and how the three issues are affected by processes carried out by the organization. An organization's performance of important functions significantly affects the quality and value of its services."[3] JCAHO bases its evaluation of an institution's QI/PI activities on

♦ designing processes,
♦ monitoring performance through data collection,
♦ analyzing current performance, and
♦ improving and sustaining improved performance.

An effective quality/performance improvement plan should be consistent with the philosophy, mission, and strategic goals of the organization. Departmental initiatives should be systematic, written, and communicated to leaders, practitioners, and staff. The plan should provide reliable data that is integrated into an organization-wide plan. Implementation of QI/PI standards may provide the basis for selecting mechanisms that measure outcomes and maintain systems to analyze and trend data and corrective actions that result in improved, safer patient care.

Staff participation and a multidisciplinary approach to the program enhance the awareness of personnel providing direct and indirect care and enable challenges to be funneled into opportunities for improvement. Documentation should show that all aspects of care in the department conform to contemporary standards of clinical practice and that data are used to study and improve the quality of care.

AORN's *Standards, Recommended Practices, and Guidelines* should be used as a resource when establishing a QI/PI program. Organizations, depending on their size, resources, and commitment to QI/PI, may have a central department, task force, or steering committee to oversee, expedite, and guide departments in achieving the goals of their QI/PI plan.

Standard I

Assign responsibility for monitoring and evaluation activities.

Interpretive statement 1:
The director and/or the designee (eg, manager or other individual[s] responsible for the department) assume overall responsibility for the monitoring and evaluation processes within the department and in the department's participation in the organization-wide performance improvement plan.

Criteria:
1. The director actively participates in and supports the program.

2. The director may select an individual (ie, designee) to be responsible for the department's overall participation in the QI/PI plan.

3. The director/designee selects the individual/ team responsible for each QI/PI project. The team may include, but is not limited to,
   ♦ staff nurses,
   ♦ ancillary staff members,
   ♦ educators,
   ♦ medical director/chief of services,
   ♦ members of the medical staff
   ♦ OR director/supervisor,
   ♦ QI/PI coordinator, and
   ♦ representatives from any departments involved in the process.

4. The director collaborates with other disciplines and departments that share responsibility for QI/PI activities.

Interpretive statement 2:

The director/designee or other responsible individual(s) develops a mechanism for ensuring that departmental initiatives are congruent with the organization-wide QI/PI plan. The departmental initiatives are integrated and communicated throughout the organization.

Criteria:

1. The plan reflects a departmental and organization-wide commitment to patient care excellence.

2. The plan is communicated through organization-wide and unit-based staff development programs.

3. The plan is evaluated and revised at least annually to determine program appropriateness and effectiveness.

4. The plan describes the roles and responsibilities of those involved in quality improvement/performance improvement. This plan may be in the form of a narrative statement, outline, flow chart, or team charter.

5. The plan describes the monitoring and evaluation activities. These may include, but are not limited to,
   ♦ delineating scope of care,
   ♦ identifying important functions and processes,
   ♦ prioritizing areas for improvement,
   ♦ collecting and analyzing data,
   ♦ evaluating patient care,
   ♦ resolving problem areas and/or improving processes that affect patient care,
   ♦ documenting results,
   ♦ communicating findings, and
   ♦ maintaining improvements.

6. The plan identifies collaborating disciplines/ departments that share responsibilities and are interdependent in QI/PI. These activities may include, but are not limited to,
   ♦ contracted services,
   ♦ engineering,
   ♦ environmental services,
   ♦ infection control,
   ♦ laboratory,
   ♦ materials management,
   ♦ medical staff,
   ♦ nursing units,
   ♦ pharmacy,
   ♦ radiology,
   ♦ risk management/safety, and
   ♦ special care units.

7. The plan describes the schedule of the quality QI/PI plan. This may include, but is not limited to, schedule of meetings, schedule of times, and locations of monitoring and evaluation activities.

8. The plan reflects the uniqueness of nursing activities performed in the perioperative setting and the outcomes of perioperative patient care.

Standard II

Delineate the scope of patient care activities or services.

Interpretive statement:

The scope of patient care activities or services describes who is served, what services are provided, who provides the services, physical sites, and times that services are provided.

Criteria:

1. The patient population assessment/description may include, but is not limited to,
   ♦ patient acuity,
   ♦ patient socioeconomic status,
   ♦ demographics,
   ♦ support systems, and
   ♦ clinical conditions/diagnoses.

2. Customers are identified, and they are relevant to the type of service provided. Customers may include, but are not limited to,
   ♦ employees,
   ♦ patients,
   ♦ families,
   ♦ practitioners,
   ♦ purchasers, and
   ♦ suppliers.

3. Clinical care activities and nursing services are determined. These may include, but are not limited to,
   ♦ circulating;
   ♦ scrubbing;
   ♦ first assisting;
   ♦ patient education;
   ♦ resource nurses/advanced practitioners (eg, clinical nurse specialists, nurse practitioners); and
   ♦ others identified in AORN's *Standards, Recommended Practices, and Guidelines.*

4. Services provided in the department are inventoried. Services may include, but are not limited to,
   ♦ cardiovascular/thoracic,
   ♦ endoscopy,
   ♦ general surgery,
   ♦ ophthalmology,
   ♦ orthopedics,
   ♦ otolaryngology,
   ♦ obstetrics and gynecology,
   ♦ neurosurgery,
   ♦ pediatrics, and
   ♦ pain management.

5. Departmental practitioners are listed by job title and level of expertise. Individuals who contribute to departmental care and activities may include, but are not limited to,
   ♦ advanced practice nurses,
   ♦ registered nurses,
   ♦ licensed practical/vocational nurses, and
   ♦ unlicensed assistive personnel.

6. Other practitioners/personnel who share patient care responsibilities are listed. These may include, but are not limited to,
   ♦ ancillary departments,
   ♦ contracting agencies,
   ♦ employed caregivers, and
   ♦ physicians.

7. The physical site is described. The description may include, but is not limited to,
   ♦ number and type of suites/rooms,
   ♦ their proximity to each other, and
   ♦ support areas.

8. Dates, days, and hours of operation are described.

9. Suites/rooms are identified by type of service provided.

10. Staffing plans/patterns that support services are identified.[4] A rationale is given for the chosen staffing, and a mechanism is in place to evaluate the effectiveness.

Standard III

Identify processes impacting the quality and safety of patient care.

Interpretive statement:
High-volume, high-risk, and/or problem-prone processes are identified.

Criteria:
1. High-volume types of patient care activities are those performed on a frequent or daily basis to a large volume of patients. High-volume types include, but are not limited to,
   ♦ procedures that occur frequently (eg, cholecystectomy, laparoscopy, cataract extraction);
   ♦ nursing activities frequently performed for patients (eg, placement of electrosurgical dispersive pad, administration of medication, aseptic technique); and
   ♦ nursing care that affects a large number of patients (eg, patient assessments, patient education, discharge planning, intravenous therapy, pain management).

2. High-risk processes are those that carry a greater potential for liability and/or patient injury. High-risk areas may include, but are not limited to,
   ♦ patients at risk of serious consequences (eg, patients with a history of difficult airway management or a high risk assessment for DVT/PE, physiologically compromised patients, elderly patients, children, neonatal patients);
   ♦ complex or high-risk procedures that are performed infrequently;
   ♦ care delivered that was inconsistent with nursing standards or guidelines (eg, incorrect counts, wrong site/side surgery or failure to verify procedure[s] or patient identity, medication errors, improper positioning, breaks in aseptic technique, lack of appropriate patient education);
   ♦ acts of omission/commission;
   ♦ patients receiving moderate or deep sedation (refer to JCAHO Standards [TX2]); and
   ♦ patients undergoing multiple procedures or recurrent surgeries.

3. Problem-prone processes identify departmental problem areas. Problem-prone areas may include, but are not limited to,
   ♦ procedures and/or care that cause patient and/or staff anxiety;

♦ activities known to generate a number of incident reports;

♦ activities needing increased efficiency (eg, surgery schedule management, instrument processing);

♦ equipment known to have a high risk or incidence of user error (eg, new equipment, infrequently used equipment, equipment that has been modified).

Standard IV

Systematic performance measures (ie, indicators) and/or priority areas are identified as opportunities for improvement based on the functions and processes of the perioperative episode.

Interpretive statement:
Performance measures (ie, indicators) should relate to the structure, process, or outcome of care and/or service.

Criteria:
1. Structure measures based on the AORN "Standards of perioperative administrative practice" relate to physical, fiscal, and organizational elements that require
   ♦ establishing, controlling, and monitoring a safe perioperative environment (eg, technical and aseptic practice, electrical safety, physical facilities, occupational safety);
   ♦ assessing, managing, and monitoring fiscal resources (eg, equipment, supplies, personnel, time); and
   ♦ communicating and implementing organizational elements (eg, standards of nursing practice, such as care and professional performance, policies and procedures, staffing patterns, orientation, staff development activities, quality assessment plans).
2. Process measures based on the AORN "Standards of perioperative clinical practice" and "Standards of perioperative professional practice" focus on activities of the nurse or process of nursing that require
   ♦ implementation of the nursing process;
   ♦ management of complications; and
   ♦ adherence to policies and procedures (eg, correct site/side and identity verification, safe medication administration, specimen labeling, counting, positioning).

3. Outcome measures based on the AORN "Perioperative patient outcomes" relate to patient status following delivery of care that requires
   ♦ emphasis on adverse events and complications; and
   ♦ evaluation of measurable changes in patient health status (eg, free from injury, infection, nerve damage, altered skin integrity).
4. When selecting performance measures (ie, indicators), consideration should be given to the following issues:
   ♦ departmental and organizational quality and safety goals;
   ♦ accreditation standards and regulatory requirements;
   ♦ perioperative clinical and service topics of national or local interest;
   ♦ topics of greatest concern to patients and the community; and
   ♦ trends of near misses for the purposes of improving processes.

Standard V

Establish performance expectations.

Interpretive statement 1:
The baselines for each of the measures are determined based on the measurement of the current process.

Criteria:
1. Baseline data should be gathered to establish the current level of performance.
2. Baseline data is used as a starting point for measurement.

Interpretive statement 2:
The baseline is evaluated and a determination is made whether there is an opportunity for improvement.

Criteria:
1. Evaluation of the baseline may be accomplished through analysis of collected data, peer review, literature review, etc.
2. A plan for improvement is thoughtfully designed. Tools such as flowcharts and process diagrams may be used to assist in identifying areas of the process with potential for failure.

Standard VI

Collect and organize data for evaluation.

Interpretive statement 1:
Data sources and methods of data collection/organization for each indicator are identified to establish a baseline of performance.

Criteria:
1. Existing sources of data are used. These may include, but are not limited to,
   ♦ surgery schedule log,
   ♦ staffing schedule,
   ♦ incident reports,
   ♦ perioperative documentation,
   ♦ occurrence screens,
   ♦ patient questionnaires,
   ♦ patient records,
   ♦ personnel credentialing/inservice records, and
   ♦ postoperative visit/call log.
2. Other sources for data collection are used. These may include, but are not limited to,
   ♦ direct observation of and inquiries regarding staff and patient care activities, and
   ♦ physical site inspections.
3. Individuals collecting data have appropriate skill levels for the task being monitored and have the information system—or access to an individual who does—for inputting data and formulating meaningful reports.
4. Methods of data collection are concurrent and retrospective. These methods may include, but are not limited to,
   ♦ chart review,
   ♦ departmental reporting forms,
   ♦ focused review,
   ♦ occurrence screening,
   ♦ peer review,
   ♦ interviews, and
   ♦ questionnaires/surveys.
5. Personnel are provided adequate time to participate in data collection and entry.
6. Personnel are encouraged to report incidents, adverse events, and hazardous conditions without fear of punitive action or retribution.

Interpretive statement 2:
The frequency of data collection and the sample size are sufficient to accumulate the necessary data.

Criteria:
1. The frequency of data collection is determined by the type of care or activity being monitored. This may include, but is not limited to,
   ♦ the number of patients affected,
   ♦ the degree of risk involved,
   ♦ the frequency of the event,
   ♦ the significance of the event or activity being monitored, and
   ♦ the extent to which the important aspect of care has been demonstrated to be problem free.
2. Data collection includes all sentinel events (eg, deaths, serious perioperative complications, near misses).
3. Data collection for performance measures is ongoing. A calendar of events is established to determine frequency of data collection for each indicator.
4. Sampling can be used to gather measurement data. Criteria such as volume, risk, and new procedure or provider can be used to determine an adequate sample size.[5]

Interpretive statement 3:
Data are organized, synthesized, and reported to allow for an accurate analysis of performance.

Criteria:
1. The quality of the data is evaluated to determine accuracy. This may be evaluated by answering questions such as the following.
   ♦ Have all cases that were to be included in the study population been identified and reviewed?
   ♦ Have all required data fields on the data collection instrument been completed?
   ♦ Did the data gatherer(s) follow their explicit data collection instructions?
   ♦ If the data were entered into a computerized database, did the edit/validation checks confirm the accuracy of the data?
   ♦ If the data were obtained through electronic data transfer, did the edit/validation checks confirm the accuracy of the data?
2. Data collected over a period of time for each measure are aggregated for analysis purposes.
3. Aggregated measurement data are used to identify trends or patterns of performance that might not otherwise be evident in case-by-case review.
4. Statistical analysis techniques and comparative measurement data from outside sources are used to evaluate aggregated measurement data to identify significant undesirable variation from expected performance.

Standard VII

Evaluate care based on data collected.

Interpretive statement 1:
Analysis and evaluation of ongoing, collected data determines the need for action to improve the process(es).

Criteria:
1. Action is taken on adverse trends and patterns. The goal is for the care given to be congruent with perioperative nursing standards.
2. Analysis and evaluation of data collection is timely and provides efficacious opportunities for modifying actions/processes.

Interpretive statement 2:
Measurement data are compared with performance expectations.

Criteria:
1. Performance expectations are compared with actual performance to evaluate compliance with perioperative nursing standards of care and other important aspects of patient care and service.
2. Analysis of measurement data determines the need for more in-depth evaluation and/or initiation of an improvement project.
3. When performance consistently meets or exceeds expectations, the need for continued monitoring of that aspect of care/service is evaluated.
4. Evaluation of performance measurement data is timely.

Interpretive statement 3:
Initiate evaluation of important single events.

Criteria:
1. When an important single event occurs, a root cause analysis will be initiated in accordance with the organization's patient safety policies.
2. People knowledgeable about the systems and processes that affected the occurrence of the event are involved in the evaluation.
3. Evaluation of important single events are coordinated with other involved disciplines or departments.

Standard VIII

Take actions to improve care and services.

Interpretive statement 1:
Action plans/solutions are developed, supported, and approved at the appropriate levels and enacted to solve problems or improve care.

Criteria:
1. Identify the cause(s) of undesirable performance.
2. Corrective action plans are developed based on a thorough understanding of the process problems that are contributing to undesirable performance.
3. Actions are taken to correct defects in systems and/or processes. Actions may include revision of policies and procedures, staffing modifications, judicious use of equipment and supplies, and/or correction of communication or teamwork problems.
4. Relevant knowledge-based information is considered when developing action plans.
5. The plan of corrective action includes who or what is expected to change, individual(s) responsible for implementing the change, what action is needed to bring about the change, and when the change is expected to occur.
6. The action plan/solutions are forwarded to the body that has the authority to act, if the needed action exceeds the authority of the department. This may include, but is not limited to, the
   ♦ administration,
   ♦ board of trustees,
   ♦ chief of service,
   ♦ nursing/medical staff peer review committees,
   ♦ ethics committee, and
   ♦ OR committee.

Interpretive statement 2:
Actions for improvement are appropriate to the cause, scope, and severity of the problem.

Criteria:
1. Active reporting of errors and breaches in patient safety should be embraced without punitive action.
2. Whenever possible, corrective actions should be of a non-punitive nature. They should be viewed as an opportunity for education and process improvement of the individual(s) involved, the department, and even the institution.
3. Punitive measures can be counterproductive to the goals of QI/PI and should only be used when appropriate (eg, blatant failure to follow policy resulting in injury and/or liability).

4. Actions are taken to correct knowledge deficits. Actions related to insufficient knowledge may require staff development, referral to other resources, and/or recommendations for continuing education.
5. Actions are taken to correct defects in the system. Actions related to systems may require revision of policies and procedures, staffing modifications, judicious use of equipment and supplies, a change in process, and/or correction of communication problems.
6. Actions are taken to correct deficient behavioral performances. Actions related to behavior or performance may require, but are not limited to,
   ◆ education and training;
   ◆ mentoring;
   ◆ counseling;
   ◆ increased supervision;
   ◆ peer review; and
   ◆ transfer, suspension, termination, or other disciplinary action.

Standard IX

Assess the effectiveness of action(s) and document outcomes.

Interpretive statement 1:
Actions are evaluated based on outcomes.

Criteria:
1. Actions delegated to individuals or disciplines for problem solving are monitored.
2. Effectiveness of actions is assessed through continuous monitoring of care. If an opportunity to improve care is identified and improvement does not occur, the action needs to be reevaluated.
3. A time line is established for reevaluation.
4. Further investigation of the cause of the problem and evaluation to identify the less obvious elements that contributed to the failure of the action plan must take place.

Interpretive statement 2:
Document the action plan and the method of communication.

Criteria:
1. A system is established to document the problem-solving process and the effectiveness in improving care or resolving the problem.

2. A system is established to document the results of the action plan, including trends and patterns that affect action.

Standard X

Communicate relevant information to the appropriate individuals, organization-wide, while maintaining confidentiality.

Interpretive statement 1:
The written organization-wide QI/PI plan identifies appropriate channels of communication.

Criteria:
1. Intradepartmental communication channels include, but are not limited to,
   ◆ minutes of departmental meetings,
   ◆ staff meetings, and
   ◆ summary reports.
2 Conclusions, recommendations, actions, and findings are communicated to
   ◆ departmental staff,
   ◆ appropriate medical staff committees,
   ◆ administration,
   ◆ interdisciplinary committees,
   ◆ organization-wide QI/PI committee,
   ◆ governing body, and
   ◆ accreditation and/or regulatory agencies as appropriate.
3. Confidentiality of QI/PI data is maintained. Maintenance of QI/PI data and all related communications shall comply with
   ◆ federal Health Insurance Portability and Accountability Act (HIPAA) privacy and confidentiality regulations,
   ◆ pertinent state regulations governing privacy and confidentiality of peer review and quality/performance data, and
   ◆ organizational privacy and confidentiality policies and procedures.

Interpretive statement 2:
Personnel are informed of the conclusions, recommendations, actions, and findings.

Criteria:
1. Regularly scheduled staff and/or departmental meetings include quality improvement/performance improvement reports and activities.
2. Identified opportunities to improve care are addressed through staff development offerings, deploying changes in process and practice to staff.

Interpretive statement 3:

Results of the organization-wide quality improvement/performance improvement monitoring activities provide the opportunity to improve care and may have applicability in other areas in the organization.

Criteria:

1. Medical staff, administration, and the governing body use outcomes to determine clinical privileges and credentialing decisions.
2. Departmental managers use outcomes to objectively monitor staff performance, develop short- and long-range plans, measure performance, and contain costs
3. Clinical practitioners use the outcomes of the QI/PI activities for self-assessment and peer review activities.

Models and Improvement Processes

The models and processes for performing QI/PI are numerous. More than one model can be used in an effective QI/PI program. No matter which method or model is used, the goal is to "Do the right thing, and do the right thing well."[3] AORN and the NPC are not endorsing any one model or any accrediting body. **Note:** More information is available in the *Notes* and *Resources* listed, or by using the Internet and searching under the terms *quality improvement* and *performance improvement*.

Glossary

Assessment: For purposes of performance improvement, the systematic collection and review of patient-specific data.

"For purposes of patient assessment, the process established by an organization for obtaining appropriate and necessary information about each individual seeking entry into a health care setting or service. The information is used to match an individual's need with the appropriate setting, care level, and intervention."[6]

Baseline: "A set of critical observations or data used for comparison or a control."[7]

Clinical practice guidelines: Systematically developed statements to assist practitioner and patient decisions about appropriate health care for specific clinical circumstances.

Concurrent: An activity that takes place in real time; care in progress.

Failure Mode and Effects Analysis (FMEA): A proactive approach to prevent or lessen the chances of a sentinel event from occurring, or reducing the risk/liability when an event occurs. This differs from root cause analysis, which is done after a sentinel event occurs and is a retrospective review of a process or processes. As with other QI/PI models, FMEA is an analysis technique drawn from non-medical industry. FMEA is an exercise that allows identification of the probabilities for "failure" at any point in the implementation of a process. In utilizing this technique, three questions must be answered:

♦ What are the steps of the process?
♦ Where is the process most likely to fail?
♦ How can we minimize the effects of these failures?

FMEA incorporates many of the same tools that are used in other QI/PI models. In determining the possible effects of potential failures, it is possible to quantify the likelihood, severity, and probability of detecting and preventing each failure. This allows providers to determine how critical each failure will be and give it a priority ranking. It allows one to avoid errors or failures before putting new processes in place.

JCAHO, in its leadership standards, addresses the requirements for the use of FMEA and root cause analysis by organizations seeking accreditation. These requirements are specific to the level of care provided by the organization.

Focused review: A formal review of one particular indicator, procedure, or practitioner over a specified time frame. It can be retrospective or concurrent.

Goal: The result that a department, service, or organization aims to accomplish. Also, a statement of attainment/achievement that is proposed to be accomplished or attained.[8]

Hazard analysis: The process of collecting and evaluating information on the circumstances leading to a higher risk for adverse outcomes. These circumstances or conditions are not related to the disease process or the condition for which the patient is being treated.

High risk: Patients at risk if the aspect of care is not provided correctly and in a timely manner. It may be that the patient themselves are at risk due to physical status, or it may be that the complexity and/or risk of complications related to the procedure puts the patient at risk.

High volume: The procedures or treatments that occur frequently, on a regular basis, or affect a large patient population.

Important aspects of care: Clinical or service-related activities that involve a high volume of patients, entail a high degree of risk for patients, or tend to produce problems for staff or patients. Such activities are deemed most important for purposes of monitoring and evaluation.[8]

Indicator: Well-defined, measurable, objective statement related to the structure, process, or outcomes of care; direct attention to problems or opportunities to improve care.[8]

Methodology: The strategies, models, or steps for gathering and analyzing the data in the quality improvement/performance improvement process.

Near miss: "Any process variation that did not affect the outcome, but for which a recurrence carries a significant chance of a serious adverse outcome. Such a near miss falls within the scope of the definition of a sentinel event, but outside the scope of those sentinel events that are subject to review by the Joint Commission under its Sentinel Event Policy."[6]

Nursing process: A systematic approach to nursing practice utilizing problem-solving techniques, including the components of assessment, planning, implementation, and evaluation.

Occurrence screens: Data that are used to identify individual variations in care, which are reviewed and confirmed by peer review and entered into a database to identify trends and/or patterns.[8]

Outcome identification: The intended, or realistically expected, correction of the patient's problem by a certain point in time.

Peer review: The examination and evaluation by associates of a practitioner's clinical practice. Individuals are evaluated by recognized, established standards. Physicians review physicians, registered nurses review registered nurse, etc.

Performance expectation: The desired condition or target level for each performance measure.

Performance measure: A quantitative tool (eg, rate, ratio, index, percentage) that provides an indication of an organization's performance in relation to a specified process or outcome. (See also *process measure* and *outcome measure*.)[6]

Population: The entire set of individuals sharing some common characteristics (eg, all patients with a particular disease, undergoing the same procedure, or of the same demographics).

Problem-prone: Those processes or steps that commonly generate incidents or barriers for patients and/or staff.

Process: A goal-directed, interrelated series of actions, events, mechanisms, or steps. An interrelated series of events, activities, actions, mechanisms, or steps that transform inputs into outputs.[6]

Retrospective: A review that begins with a current manifestation and links this effect to some occurrence in the past; post-discharge or post-procedure; not concurrent.

Root cause analysis: "A process for identifying the basic or causal factors that underlie variation in performance, including the occurrence or possible occurrence of a sentinel event. A root cause analysis focuses primarily on systems and processes, not individual performance. It progresses from special causes in clinical processes to common causes in organizational processes and identifies potential improvements in processes or systems that would tend to decrease the likelihood of such events in the future, or determines, after analysis that no such improvement opportunities exist."[9]

Sentinel event: "An unexpected occurrence involving death or serious physical or psychological injury, or the risk thereof. Serious injury specifically includes loss of limb or function. The phrase 'or the risk thereof' includes any process variation for which a recurrence would carry a significant chance of a serious adverse outcome. Such events are called 'sentinel' because they signal the need for immediate investigation and response."[9]

Standard: "A statement that defines the performance expectations, structures, or processes that must be substantially in place in an organization to enhance the quality of care."[6]

Structure: Organizational characteristics, fiscal resources, and management qualifications of health professionals; physical facilities and equipment; environment where care takes place.[10]

NOTES

1. T Bornstein, "Quality improvement and performance improvement: Different means to the same end?" *QA Brief* 9 (Spring 2001) http://www.qaproject.org/pdf/engv9n1.pdf (accessed 5 March 2003).

2. Institute of Medicine, *To Err is Human: Building a Safer Health System* (Washington, DC: National Academy Press, 2000) 114.

3. Joint Commission on Accreditation of Healthcare Organizations, "Improving organization performance," in *Hospital Accreditation Standards* (Oakbrook Terrace, Ill: Joint Commission on Accreditation of Healthcare Organizations, 2002) 161, 163.

4. Joint Commission on Accreditation of Healthcare Organizations, "Management of human resources," in

Hospital Accreditation Standards (Oakbrook Terrace, Ill: Joint Commission on Accreditation of Healthcare Organizations, 2002) 234.

5. Joint Commission on Accreditation of Healthcare Organizations, "Management of information," in *Hospital Accreditation Standards* (Oakbrook Terrace, Ill: Joint Commission on Accreditation of Healthcare Organizations, 2002) 254.

6. Joint Commission on Accreditation of Healthcare Organizations, "Glossary," in *Hospital Accreditation Standards* (Oakbrook Terrace, Ill: Joint Commission on Accreditation of Healthcare Organizations, 2002) 331, 346, 351, 354, 360.

7. *Merriam-Webster's Collegiate Dictionary,* 10th ed (Springfield, Mass: Merriam-Webster, Inc., 1993) 95.

8. L A Kepler, E A Stuart, J Kiefel, "Ten-step template," *QRC Advisor* 6 (April 1990) 1-3.

9. Joint Commission on Accreditation of Healthcare Organizations, "Sentinel events," in *Hospital Accreditation Standards* (Oakbrook Terrace, Ill: Joint Commission on Accreditation of Healthcare Organizations, 2002) 51, 52.

10. Joint Commission on Accreditation of Healthcare Organizations, "Official accreditation policies and procedures," in *Hospital Accreditation Standards* (Oakbrook Terrace, Ill: Joint Commission on Accreditation of Healthcare Organizations, 2002) 48-49.

Resources

AORN, Inc. *Standards, Recommended Practices, and Guidelines.* Denver: AORN, Inc. Annual edition.

Joint Commission Resources. *Failure Mode and Effects Analysis in Health Care: Proactive Risk Reduction.* Oakbrook Terrace, Ill: Joint Commission on Accreditation of Healthcare Organizations, 2002.

Joint Commission Resources. *A Guide to Performance Measurement for Hospitals.* Oakbrook Terrace, Ill: Joint Commission on Accreditation of Healthcare Organization, 2000.

Joint Commission Resources. *A Pocket Guide to Using Performance Improvement Tools.* Oakbrook Terrace, Ill: Joint Commission on Accreditation of Healthcare Organization, 1996.

Joint Commission Resources. *Tools for Performance Measurement in Health Care: A Quick Reference Guide.* Oakbrook Terrace, Ill: Joint Commission on Accreditation of Healthcare Organization, 2002.

Organizational Dynamics. *Quality Action Teams: Team Members' Workbook.* Burlington, Mass: Organizational Dynamics, 1987.

Schroeder, P, ed. *Journal of Nursing Care Quality* Published quarterly by Lippincott Williams & Wilkins, Philadelphia.

Shewhart, W A; Deming, W E. *Statistical Method from the Viewpoint of Quality Control.* New York: Dover Publications, 1986.

Spath, P L. *Fundamentals of Health Care Quality Management.* Forest Grove, Ore: Brown-Spath & Associates, 2000.

Originally published as "Quality improvement standards for perioperative nursing" in the 1992 Standards and Recommended Practices for Perioperative Nursing.

Revised; approved by the AORN Board of Directors in June 2003.

Perioperative Patient Outcomes

The "Patient outcome standards for perioperative care" were developed by the AORN Nursing Practices Committee and approved by the AORN Board of Directors in November 1983. In November 1991, these standards were renamed "Patient outcomes: Standards of perioperative care." This change was intended to reflect that standards of care describe the desired results that patients can expect to receive during surgical and other diagnostic or therapeutic interventions. In 1995, the Data Elements Coordinating Committee (DECC) charged the DECC outcomes subcommittee with revising the standards. This revision was integral to the committee's work of developing perioperative nursing data elements. The most recent revision of these patient outcomes occurred in 2001 as part of a revision of the first edition of the *Perioperative Nursing Data Set*. Each of these outcome statements can be used in research, teaching, practice, policy development, and information systems.

Patient outcomes are observable, measurable physiologic and psychosocial responses to perioperative nursing interventions. These outcomes, interpretive statements, and accompanying outcome indicators provide a framework for measuring patient responses. Patient outcomes reflect collaborative, interdisciplinary efforts and independent nursing activities. The achievement of patient outcomes is of primary concern for perioperative nurses in assessing, planning, implementing, and evaluating care. Documentation is a means to record and communicate patients' experiences and responses to perioperative plans of care.

The outcome standards focus on high-risk areas for patients undergoing operative or other invasive procedures. They reflect the nurse's scope of responsibility in all phases of the perioperative period. The individual perioperative nurse may use the standards to establish a database to support current nursing practice or as a rationale for practice changes.

As recipients of care, patients are entitled to the assurance of privacy, confidentiality, personal dignity, and quality health services. The delivery of patient-focused care is guided by ethical, legal, and moral principles. These principles are inherent and serve as a foundation for perioperative nursing practice, and are paramount in achieving optimal patient outcomes.

Physiologic responses, behavior responses, and patient safety, each a domain of the "Perioperative patient focused model" described elsewhere in this publication, provide the organizational framework for the outcome statements. Each domain represents specific phenomena of concern to perioperative nurses and the needs of surgical patients and their families. Within the "Perioperative patient focused model," each domain is in continuous interaction with the health system encircling the focus of perioperative nursing practice: the patient. The fourth domain, the health system, is comprised of the structural data elements and focuses on clinical processes and outcomes. The perioperative nurse intervenes to assist the surgical patient to achieve the highest attainable health (ie, physiological, behavioral, and safety) outcomes throughout the perioperative experience.

Editor's note: Each outcome statement is accompanied by a unique identifier for that outcome statement. Please refer to the *Perioperative Nursing Data Set*, second ed, S Beyea, ed (Denver: AORN, 2002), for complete information.

Assumptions

- Successful achievement of outcomes may be dependent on the patient's preoperative status.
- The perioperative RN is to be actively involved in identifying potential hazards in the practice setting and in implementing appropriate interventions.
- The patient has the right to know the risks of operative or other invasive procedures and the right to qualified, competent personnel.
- The perioperative nurse uses all phases of the nursing process.
- Outcomes are not mutually exclusive of each other and may overlap.
- The patient expects to have an operative or other invasive procedure for an intended therapeutic effect without injury.
- In this document, the term *signs* refers to objective, observable phenomena, and the term *symptoms* refers to subjective, patient-reported phenomena.
- The patient is the primary partner in care. The responsible caregiver, significant other, or family member may perform this role if the patient is unable to do so.

DOMAIN: Perioperative Safety

The patient is free from signs and symptoms of injury caused by extraneous objects. (O2)

Interpretive statement:
Performance of an operative or other invasive procedure requires the use of a variety of equipment (eg, IVs, tracheostomy tubes, pneumatic tourniquet, thermal blanket, and sequential compression devices). Prevention of injury requires application of knowledge regarding each item used during the operative or invasive procedure. Care must be taken to ensure the proper use and coordination of these items so they may serve their intended therapeutic purposes. Factors independent of nursing care can contribute to injury. These include, but are not limited to,
- duration of use of object or contact with object,
- length of procedure, and
- faulty equipment.

Outcome indicators:
- *Skin condition (general):* smooth, intact, and free of ecchymosis, cuts, abrasions, shear injury, rash, or blistering.
- *Skin condition (IV site):* free of discoloration, swelling, or induration.
- *Neuromuscular status:* flexes and extends extremities without assistance; denies numbness or tingling of extremities.
- *Cardiovascular status:* heart rate and blood pressure within expected ranges; peripheral pulses present and equal bilaterally; skin warm to touch.

The patient is free from signs and symptoms of chemical injury. (O3)

Interpretive statement:
Hazards arise from the use of a variety of chemicals in the perioperative environment. Prevention of chemical injury requires application of knowledge of the proper use of each chemical compound. Preexisting patient conditions (eg, open wounds, skin condition, immune status, previous chemical exposure) can influence patient susceptibility to chemical injury. Length of exposure to a chemical may increase the likelihood of injury. These chemicals include, but are not limited to,

- cleaning solutions,
- skin prep solutions,
- pharmaceuticals (eg, irrigation solutions),
- methylmethacrylate, and
- tissue preservatives (eg, formalin).

Outcome indicators:
- *Skin condition (wound):* Skin prepared for surgical incision is free of redness, rash, abrasion, or blistering.
- *Skin condition (general):* smooth, intact, and free of ecchymosis, redness, cuts, abrasions, shear injury, hives, rash, or blistering.
- *Respiratory status:* respirations free of dyspnea, wheezing, or stridor; oxygen saturation (SaO_2) within expected range.
- *Cardiovascular status:* heart rate and blood pressure within expected ranges; peripheral pulses present and equal bilaterally; skin warm to touch.
- *Gastrointestinal status:* free of nausea, vomiting, or diarrhea following exposure to chemical agents.

The patient is free from signs and symptoms of electrical injury. (O4)

Interpretive statement:
Prevention of electrical injury requires application of principles of electrosurgical safety, routine maintenance, and knowledge of potential hazards. Performance of the operative or other invasive procedure relies on many electrical devices, notably the electrosurgical unit (ESU). Electrical equipment must be used according to manufacturers' documented instructions.

Outcome indicators:
- *Skin condition (dispersive electrode and potential alternative ground injury):* smooth, intact, and free of ecchymosis, blisters, or redness.
- *Neuromuscular status:* flexes and extends extremities without assistance; denies numbness or tingling of extremities.
- *Cardiovascular status:* heart rate and blood pressure within expected ranges; peripheral pulses present and equal bilaterally; skin warm to touch.
- *Pain perception:* denies acute pain or discomfort at dispersive electrode ground site.

The patient is free of signs and symptoms of injury related to positioning. (O5)

Interpretive statement:
Prevention of positioning injury requires application of the principles of body mechanics, ongoing assessment throughout the perioperative period, and coordination with the entire health care team. Preexisting conditions (eg, poor nutritional status, extremes of age, vascular insufficiency, diabetes, impaired nerve function) may increase the patient's risk of injury. Other factors, independent of nursing care (eg, type and length of procedure, type of anesthesia), can contribute to the risk of positioning injury.

Outcome indicators:
- *Skin condition (general):* smooth, intact, and free of ecchymosis, cuts, abrasions, shear injury, or blistering.
- *Cardiovascular status:* heart rate and blood pressure within expected ranges; peripheral pulses present and equal bilaterally; skin warm to touch
- *Neuromuscular status:* flexes and extends extremities without assistance; denies numbness or tingling of extremities.

The patient is free from signs and symptoms of laser injury. (O6)

Interpretive statement:
Prevention of laser injury requires application of laser safety principles, coordination with the entire health care team, and knowledge of hazards. Policies that address credentialing of personnel, laser safety, and maintenance must be in accordance with national regulatory standards and manufacturers' documented instructions.

Outcome indicators:
- *Skin condition (general):* smooth, intact, and free of unexplained edema, redness, or tenderness in nontargeted area.
- *Vision:* vision equal to preoperative status (nonopthalmologic patient); vision in non-operative eye unaffected (opthalmologic patient).
- *Pain perception:* denies corneal pain or discomfort in nontargeted areas.

The patient is free from signs and symptoms of radiation injury. (O7)

Interpretive statement:
Prevention of radiation injury requires the application of principles of physics and radiologic safety standards. Policies addressing education, credentialing, and radiologic safety and maintenance must be in accordance with national regulatory standards and manufacturers' documented instructions. Preexisting patient conditions (eg, length of and/or previous exposure) can influence the patient's susceptibility to radiologic injury.

Outcome indicators:
- *Skin condition (general):* smooth, intact, and free of unexplained edema, redness, blistering, or tenderness in nontargeted areas.
- *Cognition:* responds appropriately to questioning; memory intact.

The patient is free from signs and symptoms of injury related to transfer/transport. (O8)

Interpretive statement:
Prevention of patient injury during transfer/transport requires application of principles of body mechanics, knowledge of transfer/transport techniques and equipment, and coordination of the entire health care team. Appropriate restraints or safety devices are used in accordance with regulatory standards and manufacturers' documented instructions. The condition of the patient will determine the type of health care providers necessary during transfer/transport to ensure safety. Adequate numbers of trained personnel shall attend the patient during transfer/transport activities. The patient may be able to assist in these activities to ensure safety.

Outcome indicators:
- *Skin condition (general):* smooth, intact, and free of ecchymosis, cuts, abrasions, shear injury, or blistering.
- *Musculoskeletal status:* flexes and extends extremities with ease.
- *Pain perception:* reports comfort during and after transfer/transport.

The patient receives appropriate medication(s), safely administered during the perioperative period. (O9)

Interpretive statement:
Medications administered must be within the defined scope of nursing practice. Safe administration of medications during the perioperative period requires knowledge of the intended purpose and side effects of each medication and the patient's condition and current medication usage. Documentation should reflect name, dose, route, time, and effects of all medications administered.

Outcome indicators:
- *Clinical documentation:* name, dose, route, time, and effects of medications administered as ordered and recorded in a manner consistent with the facility's policy.
- *Cognition:* states understanding of purpose, effects, and side effects of medications administered.

DOMAIN: Physiologic Responses

The patient is free from signs and symptoms of infection. (O10)

Interpretive statement:
Prevention of infection requires the application of the principles of microbiology and aseptic practice. Measurement of this outcome is based on the stages of wound healing and the Centers for Disease Control and Prevention (CDC) guidelines defining surgical site infections as occurring 30 days postoperative and up to 1 year for transplant surgery. Preexisting patient conditions and other factors independent of nursing care can contribute to the development of infections. These factors include, but are not limited to:
- procedure type;
- organ systems involved;
- tissue trauma;
- wound class (ie, clean, clean contaminated, contaminated, dirty);
- presence of devices (eg, urinary catheters, IVs, invasive monitoring devices, endotracheal tubes);
- procedure length;
- implants;
- administration of prophylactic antibiotics;
- surgical technique; and
- practice setting.

Outcome indicators:
- *Immune status:* afebrile; leukocyte count three to 30 days postoperative within expected range.
- *Skin condition (surgical wound):* incision approximated and free of heat, redness, induration, swelling, or foul odor; drains covered with sterile dressing and/or connected to continuous drainage; wound class identified.
- *Medication regimen:* preoperative antibiotics given according to recommended guidelines; no antibiotic use three to 30 days postoperative.
- *Clinical documentation:* wound class and infection control interventions and measures documented according to facility policy.

The patient has wound/tissue perfusion consistent with or improved from baseline levels established preoperatively. (O11)

Interpretive statement:
Adequate wound/tissue perfusion is necessary to promote optimal healing and maintain cellular function. Preexisting conditions (eg, diabetes, vascular disease) and patient behaviors (eg, smoking) can interfere with the adequate perfusion of both oxygen and nutrients.

Outcome indicators:
- *Skin condition (general):* conjunctiva and/or mucous membranes pink; free of cyanosis or pallor.
- *Skin condition (surgical wound):* incision edges approximated; free of ischemia (pallor, cyanosis, erythema).
- *Vital signs:* temperature, pulse, and respirations within expected ranges.
- *Cardiovascular status:* heart rate and blood pressure within expected ranges; peripheral pulses present and equal bilaterally; skin warm to touch; capillary refill less than 3 sec.

The patient is at or returning to normothermia at the conclusion of the immediate postoperative period. (O12)

Interpretive statement:
The patient must be at or near normal temperature for basal metabolic processes to occur. A core

temperature is preferred to assess thermoregulation. Alterations in temperature, either above or below normothermia, interfere with optimal recovery from anesthesia, thereby increasing the probability of negative postoperative sequelae. Surgical intervention may include intentional alternations in body temperature.

Outcome indicators:
- *Vital signs:* temperature, pulse, and respirations within expected ranges.
- *Cardiovascular status:* heart rate and blood pressure within expected ranges; peripheral pulses present and equal bilaterally; skin warm to touch; capillary refill less than 3 sec.
- *Skin condition (general):* free of shivering (rigor); free of cyanosis or pallor.

The patient's fluid, electrolyte, and acid-base balances are consistent with or improved from baseline levels established preoperatively. (O13)

Interpretive statement:
Continuous monitoring of fluid loss, replacement, and acid-base balance occurs during the perioperative period. Fluid electrolyte and acid-base balances are critical for optimal recovery from anesthesia and surgery.

Outcome indicators:
- *Skin condition (general):* free of new or increasing edema in dependent areas; conjunctiva and/or mucous membranes pink; free of cyanosis or pallor.
- *Vital signs:* temperature, pulse, and respirations within expected ranges.
- *Cardiovascular status:* heart rate and blood pressure within expected ranges; peripheral pulses present and equal bilaterally; skin warm to touch; capillary refill less than 3 sec.
- *Renal status:* output greater than 30 mL/hr; specific gravity 1.010 to 1.030.
- *Laboratory values:* arterial blood gases, serum electrolytes, and hemodynamic monitoring values (if ordered/available) within expected ranges.

The patient's respiratory function is consistent with or improved from baseline levels established preoperatively. (O14)

Interpretive statement:
Adequate pulmonary function is essential to maintain oxygenation and elimination of carbon dioxide. Adequate pulmonary function is critical for optimal recovery and the prevention of hypoventilation, which can lead to cardiac arrest, permanent brain injury, and death.

Outcome indicators:
- *Cognition:* answers questions appropriately; memory intact.
- *Affective response:* awake; cooperative with plan of care.
- *Vital signs:* blood pressure, temperature, and pulse within expected ranges.
- *Respiratory status:* oxygen saturation (SaO_2) within expected range; rate, depth, and symmetry of respirations unchanged or improved from preoperative assessment; breath sounds free of adventitious sounds.
- *Skin condition (general):* conjunctiva and/or mucous membranes pink; free of cyanosis or pallor.

The patient's cardiovascular function is consistent with or improved from baseline levels established preoperatively. (O15)

Interpretive statement:
Adequate cardiac output is essential to maintain perfusion of tissues. Cardiovascular function contributes to tissue perfusion of oxygen and nutrients, removal of cellular waste, and temperature regulation. Cardiac monitoring can be invasive or noninvasive depending on the type of procedure.

Outcome indicators:
- *Cardiovascular status:* heart rate and blood pressure within expected ranges; peripheral pulses present and equal bilaterally; skin warm to touch; capillary refill less than 3 sec.
- *Respiratory status:* oxygen saturation (SaO_2) within expected range; rate, depth, and symmetry of respirations unchanged or improved from preoperative assessment; free of adventitious breath sounds.

- *Skin condition (general):* conjunctiva and/or mucous membranes pink; free of cyanosis or pallor.
- *Renal status:* output greater than 30 mL/hr; specific gravity 1.010 to 1.030.

The patient demonstrates and/or reports adequate pain control throughout the perioperative period. (O29)

Interpretive statement:
Patient comfort and pain relief is critical to recovery from anesthesia and surgery. Methods to alleviate or reduce pain and/or discomfort may include pharmacologic and/or nonpharmacologic means.

Outcome indicators:
- *Pain perception:* patient reports pain controlled based on a recognized pain scale (eg, less than 4 on a 1–10 scale); facial expression relaxed; rests comfortably; denies discomfort in nontargeted areas.
- *Cognition:* uses pain scale appropriately to describe level of discomfort.
- *Affective response:* cooperative with plan of care; relaxed body position; verbalizes ability to cope.
- *Vital signs:* blood pressure, pulse, and respiration within expected ranges.
- *Patient satisfaction:* reports satisfaction with level of pain control.

The patient's neurological function is consistent with or improved from baseline levels established preoperatively. (O30)

Interpretive statement:
Adequate neurologic output is essential to maintain affective, cognitive, and neuromuscular function. Neurologic procedures are classified as cranial (brain and accessory structures), spinal (cord and nerves), and peripheral (all other neural tissue). Neurologic status can be measured by noninvasive or invasive methods depending on the type of procedure.

Outcome indicators:
- *Cognition:* responds appropriately to questioning; memory intact.
- *Affective response:* awake; cooperative with plan of care.

- *Psychomotor response:* verbal and motor responses equal to or improved from baseline levels; free of abnormal posturing; follows commands appropriately.
- *Neuromuscular status:* flexes and extends extremities; denies numbness or tingling of extremities; pupils equal and reactive to light; swallows without difficulty; reports vision unchanged; tremors decreased from baseline.
- *Cardiovascular status:* heart rate and blood pressure within expected ranges; peripheral/intracranial pulses present and equal by Doppler; skin warm to touch; capillary refill less than 3 sec.
- *Skin condition (general):* smooth, intact, and free of ecchymosis, cuts, abrasions, shear injury, rash, or blistering.

DOMAIN: Behavioral Responses— Patient and Family

The patient demonstrates knowledge of expected responses to the operative or invasive procedure. (O31)

Interpretive statement:
The patient needs information regarding the expected outcomes, benefits, risks, surgical experience, and recovery process related to the planned operative or other invasive procedure. The information is shared with the patient's family or significant others according to the patient's preference.

Outcome indicators:
- *Cognition:* describes sequence of planned procedure; repeats instructions correctly; asks questions based on information provided; participates in plan of care.
- *Affective response:* calm; cooperates with plan of care; relaxed facial expression; verbalizes ability to cope.
- *Psychomotor skills:* correctly demonstrates deep breathing, coughing, leg exercises, wound care.
- *Supportive resources:* family demonstrates willingness to be actively involved in rehabilitation.
- *Patient satisfaction:* verbalizes satisfaction with content and process of teaching.

The patient demonstrates knowledge of nutritional requirements related to the operative or other invasive procedure. (O18)

Interpretive statement:
The patient needs information regarding nutritional requirements related to the operative or other invasive procedure. The information is shared with the patient's family or significant others according to the patient's preference.

Outcome indicators:
- *Cognition:* repeats instructions correctly; asks questions based on information provided; verbalizes ability to manage dietary requirements; describes preferred foods/fluids consistent with dietary requirements.
- *Affective response:* verbalizes understanding of the importance of balanced diet to facilitate healing.
- *Supportive resources:* family demonstrates willingness to obtain appropriate food and assist with meal preparation.
- *Patient satisfaction:* verbalizes satisfaction with content and process of teaching.

The patient demonstrates knowledge of medication management. (O19)

Interpretive statement:
The patient needs information regarding administration and management of medication. The information is shared with the patient's family or significant others according to the patient's preference.

Outcome indicators:
- *Cognition:* repeats instructions correctly; asks questions based on information provided; states dose, purpose, frequency, route, side effects, and symptoms to report for each medication.
- *Affective response:* verbalizes acceptance of medication administration responsibility.
- *Psychomotor skills:* demonstrates how to care for surgical wound; prepares and self-administers injectable medication appropriately; demonstrates procedure required prior to medication administration (eg, pulse check).
- *Supportive resources:* family demonstrates willingness to be actively involved in medica-

tion management, including medication acquisition.
- *Patient satisfaction:* verbalizes satisfaction with medication teaching and information provided.

The patient demonstrates knowledge of pain management. (O20)

Interpretive statement:
The patient needs information regarding pain assessment and management plan, realistic outcomes, and pharmacologic and nonpharmacologic methods of pain management. The pain management plan reflects the patient's age, cultural background, and previous experiences with pain and surgery.

Outcome indicators:
- *Cognition:* repeats instructions correctly; asks questions based on information provided; states dose, purpose, frequency, route, and which side effects from pain medication(s) to report; evaluates effect of pain medication using a recognized pain scale; recognizes the importance of timing of administration.
- *Affective response:* verbalizes willingness to accept responsibility for medication administration; agrees to notify health care provider with worsening or uncontrolled pain.
- *Psychomotor skills:* prepares and self-administers injectable medication appropriately; demonstrates ability to use patient controlled analgesic device.
- *Supportive resources:* family demonstrates willingness to be actively involved in pain management plan, including medication acquisition.
- *Patient satisfaction:* verbalizes satisfaction with pain management teaching and information provided.

The patient participates in the rehabilitation process. (O21)

Interpretive statement:
The patient can expect continuity of care. The rehabilitation process begins with the initial patient contact. Appropriate resources are identified and referrals are initiated to support continuity of care throughout the perioperative experience.

Outcome indicators:

♦ *Cognition:* repeats instructions correctly; asks questions based on information provided; verbalizes expected sequence of events for rehabilitation plan; states activities to avoid/limit during recovery process.

♦ *Affective response:* cooperates with plan of care; verbalizes willingness to participate in rehabilitation plan and ability to cope.

♦ *Psychomotor skills:* correctly demonstrates techniques required for postoperative recovery (eg, deep breathing, coughing, leg exercises, wound care).

♦ *Supportive resources:* family demonstrates willingness to be actively involved in rehabilitation; transportation is available for follow-up visits; states date and time for follow-up appointments.

♦ *Patient satisfaction:* verbalizes satisfaction with content and process of teaching.

The patient demonstrates knowledge of wound healing. (O22)

Interpretive statement:
The patient needs information regarding wound healing and management. Wound healing is a complex and highly organized physiological response caused by intentional or accidental injury to tissue. The information is shared with the patient's family or significant others according to the patient's preference.

Outcome indicators:

♦ *Cognition:* repeats instructions correctly; asks questions based on information provided; verbalizes expected sequence for wound healing; describes plan for wound care correctly.

♦ *Affective response:* cooperates with plan of care; verbalizes ability to manage and cope with wound care.

♦ *Psychomotor skills:* correctly demonstrates postoperative wound care.

♦ *Supportive resources:* family demonstrates willingness to be actively involved in wound care.

♦ *Patient satisfaction:* verbalizes satisfaction with content and process of teaching.

The patient participates in decisions affecting his or her perioperative plan of care. (O23)

Interpretive statement:
Clinical processes support the patient's informed decision-making process in accordance with facility and regulatory standards. The patient receives timely and accurate information regarding diagnosis, surgery, and treatment options, and has his or her questions answered. Care is individualized, and the perioperative plan of care addresses the unique needs of each patient related to

♦ informed surgical consent,

♦ informed consent for research/clinical trials, and

♦ decisions related to self-determination, including resuscitative measures, life-sustaining treatment, and end-of-life decisions.

Outcome indicators:

♦ *Cognition:* verbalizes understanding of treatment options; describes sequence of planned procedure; repeats provided information correctly; asks questions based on information provided; participates in plan of care.

♦ *Affective response:* verbalizes concerns about decisions.

♦ *Clinical documentation:* surgical consent for procedure is signed; Self-Determination Act is implemented according to patient wishes.

♦ *Supportive resources:* family participates in perioperative plan of care according to patient's preference.

♦ *Patient satisfaction:* expresses satisfaction with level of involvement in plan of care and decision-making process.

The patient's care is consistent with the perioperative plan of care. (O24)

Interpretive statement:
The patient receives quality health services and continuity of care consistent with the planned intervention. The continuity of care is evident in the plan of care from the preoperative period through rehabilitation.

Outcome indicators:
- *Cognition:* describes sequence of planned procedure; repeats instructions correctly; asks questions based on information provided; participates in plan of care.
- *Clinical documentation:* plan of care is documented and reflects individual preferences.
- *Supportive resources:* family demonstrates willingness to participant in plan of care.
- *Patient satisfaction:* expresses satisfaction with delivered care.

The patient's right to privacy is maintained. (O25)

Interpretive statement:
Confidentiality of patient information is an integral component of patient privacy. Caregivers protect patients from undue physical exposure or unwarranted invasions of privacy.

Outcome indicators:
- *Affective response:* verbalizes feelings of safety and privacy.
- *Skin condition (general):* skin exposure is limited to that required for the operative/invasive procedure.
- *Clinical documentation:* personnel are identified and limited to authorized staff only; personal belongings are identified and secured; only authorized personnel have access to patient records.
- *Patient satisfaction:* patient and family verbalize satisfaction with privacy measures.

The patient is the recipient of competent and ethical care within legal standards of practice. (O26)

Interpretive statement:
The perioperative patient is entitled to qualified and skilled care providers. Health care professionals are responsible for maintaining requirements and qualifications for competent practice.

Outcome indicators:
- *Administrative policy:* clinicians practice in a manner consistent with credentialing policies; records are maintained and document

professional nursing staff competence licensure and continuing education; perioperative care plans are based on ethical concepts and principles; variances in care are documented and corrective action taken.
- *Patient satisfaction:* patients report that care is competent, ethical, and within legal standards.

The patient receives consistent and comparable care regardless of the setting. (O27)

Interpretive statement:
The perioperative patient receives care that fosters a positive self-image and preserves personal dignity. Caregivers respect patients and provide nondiscriminatory and nonprejudicial care.

Outcome indicators:
- *Administrative policy:* care is consistent with professional and regulatory standards of care and the facility's human rights policy.
- *Performance improvement:* quality improvement indicators demonstrate consistent quality of care across patient populations.
- *Patient satisfaction:* patients report high levels of satisfaction with the delivery of care.

The patient's value system, lifestyle, ethnicity, and culture are considered, respected, and incorporated in the perioperative plan of care. (O28)

Interpretive statement:
The implementation of the perioperative plan of care incorporates, but is not limited to, the patient's
- cultural and/or ethnic practices,
- spiritual or religious beliefs,
- psychosocial barriers and/or support systems,
- physical and/or cognitive limitations,
- language barriers, and
- age or developmental stage.

Outcome indicators:
- *Cognition:* communicates personal needs related to lifestyle, religion, ethnicity, and culture.

- *Affective response:* verbalizes individual needs and indicates whether they are met.
- *Clinical documentation:* plan of care addresses patient's preferences and needs; cultural/religious practices that influence care are recorded; required interpreter services are facilitated; clinical documents reflect age-specific, functional, physical, or cognitive needs.
- *Patient satisfaction:* states that care is individualized and provided in a nondiscriminatory, nonjudgmental manner.

AORN Standards for RN First Assistant Education Programs

Registered nurse first assistant (RNFA) education programs are designed to provide RNs with the educational preparation necessary to assume the role of the first assistant in operative and other invasive procedures. These programs should be equivalent to one academic year of formal, post-basic nursing study; consist of curricula that address all of the modules in the *Core Curriculum for the RN First Assistant*[1]; and award college credits and degrees or certificates of RNFA status upon satisfactory completion of all requirements. The RNFA programs should be associated with schools of nursing at universities or colleges that are accredited for higher education by an accrediting agency that is nationally recognized by the Secretary of the US Department of Education. The registered nursing program should be approved by a state licensing jurisdiction for nursing programs at the university, college, or community college level or by another national or regional agency that is nationally recognized by the Secretary of the US Department of Education as a specialized accrediting agency for nursing programs.

The "Standards for RN first assistant education programs" serve as the foundation upon which RNFA programs are developed and implemented. These standards are intended to guide program administrators and faculty in designing and evaluating curricula. These standards are broad in scope, definitive, relevant, and attainable, and they provide the framework for RNFA education. AORN's "Official statement on RN first assistants"[2] should be recognized by all institutions offering RNFA programs.

Standard I

Preadmission requirements for RNFA education programs shall include the following.

A. General admission requirements as determined by each educational institution.

B. Proof of licensure to practice as an RN in the state in which the clinical internship will be undertaken.

C. Verification of certification as one of the following:
   1. CNOR or CNOR eligible, or
   2. board certified or board eligible as an advanced practice nurse (APN).

Important Note

When choosing an RNFA program, prospective students are advised to use these education standards to evaluate each program under consideration. AORN holds all prospective students accountable for reviewing the list of programs that the Competency and Credentialing Institute (CCI, formerly Certification Board Perioperative Nursing [CBPN]) deems acceptable for those applicants wishing to sit for RNFA certification examination. For more information, contact CCI at (888) 257-2667 or *http://www.cc-institute.org.*

APNs without competence in intraoperative patient care must undergo an assessment regarding clinical skills and knowledge. If it is determined that skills and knowledge are deficient, faculty in the educational institution shall develop a plan to remediate identified deficiencies.
   3. Certification must be submitted before program completion.

D. Cardiopulmonary resuscitation (CPR) or basic cardiac life support certification (BCLS) is required; advanced cardiac life support (ACLS) is preferred.

E. Letters of recommendation attesting to the years of experience as an RN and knowledge, judgment, and skills specific to surgical patient care.

Standard II

The didactic component of the curriculum for RNFA education programs shall be designed and evaluated based on a course description that identifies course content, faculty, length of the course, instructional and evaluation methodologies, and instructional resources.

A. Course content shall emphasize the expanded functions unique to the RNFA during operative and other invasive procedures, including, but not limited to,
   1. preoperative patient management in collaboration with other health care providers, including, but not limited to,
      – performing a preoperative evaluation/ focused nursing assessment,

---

– communicating or collaborating with other health care providers regarding the patient's plan of care, and

– writing preoperative orders according to established protocols;

2. intraoperative surgical first-assisting, including, but not limited to,

– using instruments and medical devices,
– providing exposure,
– handling and cutting tissue,
– providing hemostasis, and
– suturing;

3. postoperative patient management in collaboration with other health care providers in the immediate postoperative period and beyond, including, but not limited to,

– writing postoperative orders and operative notes according to established protocols,
– participating in postoperative rounds, and
– assisting with discharge planning and identifying appropriate community resources as needed.[2]

B. A multidisciplinary faculty should include

1. a perioperative nurse with a master of science in nursing degree,
2. a CNOR/RNFA or certified RNFA (CRNFA), and
3. a board-certified surgeon.

C. The course shall be a minimum of one academic semester of study, including student assignments, classroom instruction, and laboratory practicums.

D. Instructional methodologies shall include, but not be limited to, lecture, interactive discussion, independent study, instructional media, demonstration/return demonstration, and laboratory practicums.

E. Evaluation methodologies shall include, but not be limited to, written examinations, laboratory practicums, and independent critical thinking assignments.

F. Instructional resources shall include

1. *Core Curriculum for the RN First Assistant*[1] and
2. texts or other instructional media that include anatomy and physiology, operative and other invasive procedures, and preoperative and postoperative patient assessment and management.

Standard III

Specific requirements for the clinical component shall include:

A. Successful completion of all requirements of the didactic component, and

B. Evidence of current personal professional liability insurance for RNFA practice.

Standard IV

The clinical component of the curriculum for RNFA education programs shall be designed and evaluated based on a course description that identifies course content, faculty, length of the course, instructional and evaluation methodologies, and instructional resources.

A. Course content emphasizes the expanded functions unique to the RNFA intern during operative and other invasive procedures, including, but not limited to,

1. preoperative patient management in collaboration with other health care providers, including, but not limited to,

– performing and documenting preoperative evaluation/focused nursing assessment,
– communicating and collaborating with other health care providers regarding the patient plan of care, and
– writing preoperative orders according to established protocols;

2. validated documentation of intraoperative surgical first-assisting clinical experience, including, but not limited to,

– using instruments and medical devices,
– providing exposure,
– handling and cutting tissue,
– providing hemostasis, and
– suturing;

3. postoperative patient management in collaboration with other health care providers in the immediate postoperative period and beyond, including, but not limited to,

– writing postoperative orders and operative notes according to established protocols,
– participating in postoperative rounds, and
– assisting with discharge planning and identifying appropriate community resources as needed.[2]

B. A multidisciplinary faculty should include
1. a board-certified surgeon in the RNFA intern's primary area of practice,
2. an RNFA program faculty member, and
3. an RNFA/CRNFA mentor if available and/or desired by the student.
C. The clinical course shall be a minimum of one academic semester and shall include, but not be limited to, intern assignments as assistant at surgery and patient care management.
D. Instructional methodologies shall include, but not be limited to, physician-supervised clinical activities, assigned independent learning activities, a self-evaluative learning diary, a clinical case study project, and a surgical intervention participation log.
E. Evaluation methodologies shall include, but not be limited to, completion of assigned independent learning activities, a self-evaluative learning diary, a clinical case study project, preceptor evaluations, a surgical intervention participation log, and mentor evaluations when applicable. Students must satisfactorily complete all requirements. The RNFA program faculty reviews all documentation. The surgeon preceptor provides a summative evaluation of achievement of competence and a letter of recommendation based on all required learning activities, as does the RNFA/CRNFA mentor when applicable.
F. Instructional resources shall include
1. *Core Curriculum for the RN First Assistant,*[1]
2. texts or other instructional media, and
3. consultation and collaboration with other health care providers.

Glossary

Faculty: A person who is appointed by the educational institution to design, teach, or evaluate a course of instruction.

Advanced practice nurse (APN): Advanced practice nurse is a term used to refer to an RN prepared at the graduate level who has met advanced educational and clinical practice requirements for a particular and unique clinical practice focus. There are four principle types of APNs, including nurse practitioner (NP), clinical nurse specialist (CNS), certified nurse midwife (CNM), and certified RN anesthetist (CRNA).[3,4]

CNOR: "The documented validation of the professional achievement of identified standards of practice by an individual registered nurse providing care for patients before, during, and after surgery."[5]

CRNFA: "The documented validation of the professional achievement of identified standards of practice by an individual registered nurse first assistant providing care for patients before, during, and after surgery."[6]

Preceptor: One who teaches, counsels, inspires, serves as a role model, and supports the growth and development of the novice for a fixed and limited period.

Mentor: One who provides encouragement and acts as a guide and facilitator while modeling professional nursing behaviors.[7]

NOTES
1. R E Vaiden, J C Rothrock, V J Fox, eds, *Core Curriculum for the RN First Assistant* (Denver: AORN, Inc, 2000).
2. "Official statement on RN first assistants," in *Standards, Recommended Practices, and Guidelines* (Denver: AORN, Inc, 2005) 237-238.
3. "Certification and regulation of advanced practice nurses," American Association of Colleges of Nursing, *http://www.aacn.nche.edu/Publications/ positions/cerreg.htm* (accessed 10 Jan 2005).
4. "Advanced practice nursing: A new age in health care," American Nurses Association, *http://www.nursingworld.org/readroom/fsadvprc.htm* (accessed 10 Jan 2005).
5. "2005 CNOR certification," Certification Board Perioperative Nursing, *http://www.certboard.org/cnor/cert/ gen_info.htm* (accessed 10 Jan 2005).
6. "2005 CRNFA certification," Certification Board Perioperative Nursing, *http://www.certboard.org/crnfa/cert/ gen_info.htm* (accessed 10 Jan 2005).
7. "AORN resolution on responsibility for mentoring," in *Standards, Recommended Practices, and Guidelines* (Denver: AORN, Inc, 2004) 156.

Originally published March 1995, AORN Journal, as "AORN recommended education standards for RN first assistant programs." Revised December 2004; approved by the AORN Board of Directors in February 2005.

> **Editor's note:** *These recommended education standards were developed by the RN First Assistant Specialty Assembly in July 1994 and were approved by the AORN Board of Directors in November 1994. Revisions took place in November 1995; October 1996; October 1998; and most recently, as noted on the previous page, in December 2004.*

RECOMMENDED PRACTICES FOR PERIOPERATIVE NURSING

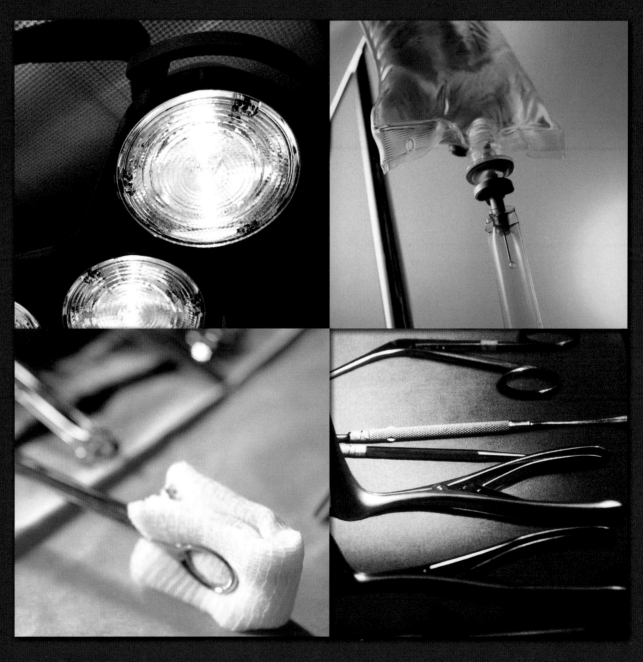

Section Three

Introduction

This section contains recommended practices concerning aseptic and technical aspects of perioperative nursing practice. They are based on principles of microbiology, research, review of the scientific literature, and the opinions of experts knowledgeable in the subject. The AORN recommended practices are written by selected members of the Association and liaisons from the Centers for Disease Control and Prevention, the Association for Professionals in Infection Control and Epidemiology, the American Society of Healthcare Central Service Professionals, the International Association of Healthcare Central Service Materiel Management, the American College of Surgeons, and the American Society of Anesthesiologists.

These recommended practices represent the Association's official position on questions of aseptic and technical practices performed by perioperative nurses. The recommended practices appearing in this edition have been approved by the AORN Recommended Practices Committee and the AORN Board of Directors. In general, recommended practices are written in broad terms and are based on principals of aseptic practice and infection control. They are intended to serve as the basis for policy and procedure development in perioperative practice settings. The recommended practices address both human behaviors and the use, care, and processing of medical devices in the perioperative practice setting. The recommended practices are intended to define correct nursing practices and to promote patient safety.

AORN's recommended practices are intended as achievable and represent what is believed to be an optimal level of aseptic and technical practice. No attempt has been made to gain consensus among users, manufacturers, and consumers of any material or product. **Compliance with the AORN recommended practices is voluntary.**

Within the context of the recommended practices, "may" is used to indicate that a course of action is permissible within the limits of the recommended practice; and "can" is used as a statement of possibility and capability. The use of "should" indicates that a certain course of action is recommended. "Must" is used only to describe unavoidable situations, including those mandated by government regulation and accreditation organization standards.

Application in Practice

Application of the recommended practices in individual work settings requires close examination of existing policies and procedures. This review may indicate that revised or new policies and/or procedures are necessary. Individual commitment, professional conscience, and the setting in which perioperative nursing is practiced must guide the nurse in implementing these recommended practices. Variations in practice settings and clinical situations may determine the degree to which the recommended practice can be fulfilled.

Recommended Practices and the PNDS

The Perioperative Nursing Data Set (PNDS) was recognized by the American Nurses Association in 1999 and published by AORN in the first edition of *Perioperative Nursing Data Set: The Perioperative Nursing Vocabulary*. The PNDS should be used when documenting perioperative nursing care. Use of standardized nomenclature will facilitate data capture and analysis for safe, quality patient care. As the recommended practices are reviewed and updated, information regarding the application of the PNDS will be included as appropriate.

This standardized language consists of a collection of data elements (ie, the PNDS) and includes perioperative nursing diagnoses, interventions, and outcomes. The perioperative patient focused model provides the conceptual framework for the PNDS and the model for perioperative nursing practice. The patient and his or her family members are at the core of the model, which depicts perioperative nursing in four domains and illustrates the relationship between the patient, his or her family members, and care provided by the perioperative professional registered nurse. The patient-centered domains are

D1 Safety,

D2 Physiological responses to surgery,

D3 Patient and family member behavioral responses to surgery, and

D4 Health system in which perioperative care is provided.

Each data element in the PNDS is represented by a unique identifier. The domains are represented by the letter "D" followed by numbers one to four to indicate the particular domain being addressed. Nursing diagnoses are represented by the letter "X" and a number unique to the diagnosis; interventions are represented by the letter "I" and a unique number; and outcomes are represented by the letter "O" and a unique number. These designations are used in the recommended practices as appropriate.

Introduction

Revision Process

Each recommended practice is reviewed and revised as appropriate at regular periodic intervals. Although only a portion of the recommended practices may be updated for publication in any given year, all 29 recommended practices are under continuous scrutiny by the AORN Recommended Practices Committee, which is charged with keeping them up to date. A newly developed recommended practice, "Specimen care and handling," makes its first appearance in this edition. In addition, five recommended practices have been revised for 2006:

- Sponge, Sharps, and Instruments Counts
- Maintaining a Sterile Field
- Sterilization
- Tissue Banking
- Traffic Patterns

The important task of overseeing AORN's recommended practices is ongoing; that is, the work of the Recommended Practices Committee overlaps from one term of office to the next. Thus, one committee is always building on the efforts of previous committees by revising and updating their work to keep pace with changes in nursing practice, nursing and medical research, and surgical technology.

AORN began publishing recommended practices in March 1975. A compilation was printed in March 1978 in *AORN Standards of Practice*. The book at hand contains revisions of those previously published recommended practices as well as new ones developed since 1978.

AORN gratefully acknowledges the work of the 2005–2006 Recommended Practices Committee

COMMITTEE CHAIR
Victoria M. Steelman, RN, PhD, CNOR
Advanced Practice Nurse, Perioperative Nursing
University of Iowa Hospitals & Clinics
Coralville, Iowa

COMMITTEE MEMBERS
Nancy Chobin, RN, AAS, CSPDM, ACSP
St Barnabas Health Care System
West Orange, New Jersey

Alice S. Comish, RN, BSN, CNOR
Director, Surgical Technology Program
Our Lady of the Lake College
Baton Rouge, Louisiana

Deborah A. Gering, RN, BSN, CNOR
Clinical Manager, OR Services
Sinai-Grace Hospital
Detroit, Michigan

Judith L. Goldberg, RN, BSN, CNOR
Clinical Educator
William W Backus Hospital
Norwich, Connecticut

Brenda Jeffers, RN, MS, CNOR
Ottumwa Regional Health Center
Ottumwa, Iowa

Diana S. Mc Dowell, RN, MSN, CNOR
Chief Quality Coordinator
Clarian Health Partners Inc
Indianapolis, Indiana

Andrea Spalter, RN, MSN, CNOR
University of Kansas Hospital
Kansas City, Missouri

COMMITTEE LIAISONS
American College of Surgeons
H. David Reines, MD

**American Society for Healthcare
Central Service Professionals**
Paul Hess, RN, BSN, CRCST, ACSP

American Society of Anesthesiologists
Joseph P. Annis, MD

**Association for Professionals in
Infection Control and Epidemiology**
Ardene L. Nichols, BSN, RN, MSN, CNS, CNOR, PAHM

Centers for Disease Control and Prevention
Elizabeth Bolyard

AORN BOARD LIAISON
Susan Banschbach, RN, BSN, CNOR, MSN
St Francis Hospital
Tulsa, Oklahoma

AORN STAFF LIAISONS
Ramona L. Conner, RN, MSN, CNOR
Perioperative Nursing Specialist
AORN Center for Nursing Practice

Margi Stewart
Research Librarian
AORN Center for Nursing Practice

Bonnie Kibbe
Administrative Assistant
AORN Center for Nursing Practice

Recommended Practices for Managing the Patient Receiving Moderate Sedation/Analgesia

The following recommended practices were developed by the AORN Recommended Practices Committee and have been approved by the AORN Board of Directors. They were presented as proposed recommended practices for comments by members and others. They are effective January 1, 2002.

These recommended practices are intended as achievable recommendations representing what is believed to be an optimal level of practice. Policies and procedures will reflect variations in practice settings and/or clinical situations that determine the degree to which the recommended practices can be implemented.

AORN recognizes the numerous types of settings in which perioperative nurses practice. These recommended practices are intended as guidelines adaptable to various practice settings. These practice settings include traditional ORs, ambulatory surgery units, physicians' offices, cardiac catheterization suites, endoscopy suites, radiology departments, and all other areas where operative and other invasive procedures may be performed.

Purpose

The use of moderate sedation/analgesia allows patients to tolerate unpleasant procedures while maintaining adequate cardiorespiratory function, protective reflexes, and the ability to respond purposefully to verbal and/or tactile stimulation.[1]

Moderate sedation/analgesia is a specific level or depth of sedation in the continuum of sedation (Table 1). It is not always possible to gauge how a patient may respond to sedation; therefore, the health care professional intending to produce moderate sedation/analgesia should be able to rescue patients whose level of consciousness progresses to deep sedation. The possibility that the patient may enter a deeper state, such as general anesthesia, must be considered, and rescue measures by credentialed anesthesia care providers must be available.[2]

These recommended practices provide guidelines for RNs who manage the care of patients receiving moderate sedation/analgesia. Patient selection for moderate sedation/analgesia should be based on established criteria developed through interdisciplinary collaboration by health care professionals. The type of monitoring used with patients who receive moderate sedation/analgesia, the medications selected, and the interventions taken must be within the legally defined scope of practice for perioperative RNs.[3]

Certain patients are not candidates for moderate sedation/analgesia monitored by RNs. Such patients may require more extensive sedation and should be identified, monitored, and managed by credentialed anesthesia care providers, surgeons, or other physicians.[4]

Recommended Practice I

Registered nurses should understand the goals and objectives of moderate sedation/analgesia.

1. The primary goal of moderate sedation/analgesia is to reduce the patient's anxiety and discomfort. Moderate sedation/analgesia also can facilitate cooperation between the patient and caregivers.[5] Moderate sedation/analgesia produces a condition in which the patient exhibits a depressed level of consciousness and an altered perception of pain but retains the ability to respond appropriately to verbal and/or tactile stimulation and maintains protective reflexes.

2. The RN should be knowledgeable about the following desired outcomes when moderate sedation/analgesia medications are administered:
   ♦ alteration of mood;
   ♦ enhanced cooperation;
   ♦ alteration in perception of pain;
   ♦ maintenance of consciousness;
   ♦ maintenance of intact protective reflexes;
   ♦ minimal variation of vital signs;
   ♦ some degree of amnesia; and
   ♦ a rapid, safe return to activities of daily living.[6]

3. The RN may be responsible for administering ordered medications based on the patient's response and according to established protocols and defined scope of practice. Adequate preoperative patient preparation and verbal reassurances from the RN facilitate the desired effects of moderate sedation/analgesia and may allow for a decrease in the dosages of opioids and sedatives.[7]

Recommended Practice II

The RN managing the nursing care of the patient receiving moderate sedation/analgesia should have no other responsibilities that would require leaving the patient unattended or compromising continuous patient monitoring during the procedure.

Table 1

CONTINUUM OF DEPTH OF SEDATION				
	Minimal sedation	**Moderate sedation/ analgesia**	**Deep sedation/ analgesia**	**General anesthesia**
Responsiveness	Normal response to verbal stimulation	Purposeful response to verbal or tactile stimulation*	Purposeful response following repeated or painful stimulation*	Unarousable even with painful stimulus
Airway	Unaffected	No intervention required	Intervention may be required	Intervention often required
Spontaneous ventilation	Unaffected	Adequate	Intervention may be inadequate	Frequently inadequate
Cardiovascular function	Unaffected	Usually maintained	Usually maintained	May be impaired

* Reflex withdrawal from a painful stimulus in not considered a purposeful response.

Continuum of Depth of Sedation *is reprinted with permission of the American Society of Anesthesiologists, 520 N Northwest Highway, Park Ridge, Ill 60068-2573.*

1. There should be an additional RN serving as the circulating nurse during any procedure in which a patient receives moderate sedation/ analgesia. Continuous monitoring of the patient's physiological and psychological status by a competent RN leads to early detection of potential complications and increases the likelihood of positive outcomes.[8]

Recommended Practice III

The RN should be clinically competent, possessing the skills necessary to manage the nursing care of the patient receiving moderate sedation/analgesia.

1. Health care facilities should provide or make available competency-based education programs for all RNs who manage the care of patients receiving moderate sedation/analgesia. These programs should include a competency-validation process for evaluating and documenting RNs' demonstration of relevant knowledge, skills, and abilities. Standardized competency-based programs establish baseline educational requirements and ensure comparable training throughout a facility. Evaluation and documentation of competence should occur on a periodic basis according to the health care facility's policies and procedures and according to regulatory requirements.[9]

2. At a minimum, any RN monitoring the patient receiving moderate sedation/analgesia should be competent in basic life support. Additional skills for the RN should be defined by the health care facility's policies and procedures and may include advanced cardiac life support (ACLS) certification. Health care professionals with ACLS skills should be readily available during all procedures involving moderate sedation/analgesia. The RN monitoring the patient should demonstrate the following skills and knowledge of

   ◆ proper patient selection and screening;
   ◆ anatomy and physiology;
   ◆ total patient care parameters, including, but not limited to, respiratory rate, oxygen saturation, blood pressure, cardiac rate, and level of consciousness;
   ◆ pharmacology of medications used to induce and reverse sedation/analgesia;
   ◆ respiratory physiology, airway management, and the use of oxygen delivery devices;
   ◆ the function and use of monitoring equipment;
   ◆ cardiac dysrhythmia interpretation;
   ◆ possible complications and contraindications related to the use of moderate sedation/analgesia medications; and
   ◆ age-appropriate needs and responses of patients.[10]

3. For patient safety, it is essential that the RN monitoring the patient receiving moderate sedation/analgesia understands how to operate monitoring equipment.

Recommended Practice IV

Each patient receiving moderate sedation/analgesia should be assessed physiologically and psychologically before the procedure. The assessment should be documented in the patient's record.

1. A preoperative assessment helps determine a patient's suitability for RN-monitored moderate sedation/analgesia by identifying potential risk factors for undesirable outcomes. The monitoring RN should conduct the assessment and include data from numerous sources, such as chart review, patient physical assessment and interview, and consultation with other health care providers as appropriate.[11] The preoperative patient assessment should include, but not be limited to,
   - chief complaint;
   - level of consciousness;
   - potential airway problems;
   - orientation and cognitive state;
   - emotional state;
   - communication ability;
   - patient's perception and understanding of the procedure and moderate sedation/analgesia;
   - history and physical examination;
   - current laboratory values;
   - current medications, including alternative and/or complementary preparations;
   - medication allergies/sensitivities;
   - current medical problems;
   - surgical history;
   - tobacco use and substance abuse history; and
   - baseline information, including vital signs, height, weight, and age.

2. Indication of the patient's appropriateness for the procedure also should include the American Society of Anesthesiologists (ASA) physical status classification. Patients classified as P1 or P2 are considered appropriate for RN-monitored moderate sedation/analgesia. Patients with a classification of P3 may be appropriate and should be evaluated on an individual basis. Any ASA physical status classification higher than P3 is consid-

ered inappropriate for RN monitoring during moderate sedation/analgesia.[12] The ASA physical status classification is described in Table 2.

3. After analysis of assessment data and verification of written consent for the procedure and planned sedation/analgesia, the monitoring RN should develop an individualized care plan for the patient. The assessment findings and care plan should be documented in the patient's record.

Recommended Practice V

The RN managing the nursing care of the patient receiving moderate sedation/analgesia should be proficient in equipment selection and use and should ensure that the necessary equipment is available and working properly.

1. Monitoring equipment provides the RN with patient data to identify risks and/or complications during a procedure. Airway management devices provide the needed safety equipment to decrease the risk of adverse outcomes that potentially can occur during moderate sedation/analgesia. The following equipment should be present and ready for use in the room in which moderate sedation/analgesia is administered:
   - oxygen and delivery devices,
   - suction apparatus,
   - noninvasive blood pressure device,
   - electrocardiograph,
   - pulse oximeter, and
   - narcotic and sedative reversal agents.[13]

2. Before moderate sedation/analgesia medications are administered, an oxygen delivery device should be in place or immediately available, an IV access line should be established, and appropriate hemodynamic monitoring devices should be in place.[14] The type of IV access chosen will vary depending on health care facilities' policies and procedures and physicians' preferences. Continuous IV access provides a means for administering medications used for moderate sedation/analgesia and for implementing emergency medications and fluids to counteract adverse medication effects.[15]

3. An emergency cart with resuscitative medications, including narcotic and sedative reversal medications; resuscitative equipment, such as a

Table 2

PHYSICAL STATUS CLASSIFICATION	
Definition of patient status[1]	**Example**
P1—Normal healthy patient	No physical or psychological disturbances
P2—Patient with a mild systemic disease	Asthma, obesity, diabetes mellitus
P3—Patient with a severe systemic disease	Cardiovascular disease that limits activity; severe diabetes with systemic complications
P4—Patient with a severe systemic disease that is a constant threat to life	Severe cardiac, pulmonary, renal, hepatic, or endocrine dysfunction
P5—Moribund patient who is not expected to survive without surgical intervention	Surgery is a resuscitative effort, major multisystem trauma
P6—Declared brain dead patient whose organs are being removed for donor purposes	Organ donor being maintained by life support equipment

NOTE

1. "The ASA physical status classification system," American Society of Anesthesiologists, http://www.asahq.org/ ProfInfo/ PhysicalStatus.html (accessed 27 Sept 2001).

defibrillator, suction, and airways; and a positive pressure breathing device should be immediately accessible in every location in which moderate sedation/ analgesia is being administered.[16] Medication overdoses or adverse reactions may cause respiratory depression, hypotension, or impaired cardiovascular function requiring immediate intervention and/or cardiopulmonary resuscitation.

Recommended Practice VI

Each patient who receives moderate sedation/ analgesia should be monitored for adverse reactions to medications and for physiological and psychological changes.

1. Observing the patient for desired therapeutic medication effects, preventing avoidable medication reactions, detecting and managing unexplained adverse reactions early, and accurately documenting the patient's response are integral components of the monitoring process. The RN monitoring the patient should monitor the following parameters:

   ♦ respiratory rate and effort,
   ♦ oxygen saturation,
   ♦ blood pressure,
   ♦ cardiac rate and rhythm,
   ♦ level of consciousness,
   ♦ comfort level/tolerance to procedure, and
   ♦ skin condition.[17]

2. The RN should understand the pharmacology of moderate sedation/analgesia medications and reversal agents, including the following factors:

   ♦ indications and dosages,
   ♦ contraindications,
   ♦ adverse reactions and emergency management techniques,
   ♦ interactions with other medications,
   ♦ onset and duration of action, and
   ♦ desired effects.[18]

3. Patient anxiety and medications used for moderate sedation/analgesia may cause rapid, adverse physiological responses in the patient. Early detection of such responses allows for rapid intervention and treatment. Desirable effects of moderate sedation/analgesia include, but are not limited to,

   ♦ intact protective reflexes,
   ♦ relaxation,
   ♦ comfort,
   ♦ cooperation,
   ♦ appropriate level of verbal communication,
   ♦ patent airway with adequate ventilatory exchange, and
   ♦ easy arousal from sleep.[19]

4. Sedatives may cause somnolence, confusion, diminished reflexes, depressed respiratory and cardiovascular functions, and coma. Opioids may cause respiratory depression, hypotension, nausea, and vomiting. Oversedation and adverse reactions may occur any time during the procedure and may be reversible. Any undesirable changes in patient condition should be reported immediately to the physician. Undesirable effects of moderate sedation/analgesia include, but are not limited to,

   ♦ aspiration,
   ♦ severely slurred speech,
   ♦ unarousable sleep,
   ♦ hypotension or hypertension,
   ♦ agitation,
   ♦ combativeness,

♦ respiratory depression,

♦ airway obstruction, and

♦ apnea.[20]

Recommended Practice VII

Documentation of the patient's care during moderate sedation/analgesia should be consistent with AORN's "Recommended practices for documentation of perioperative nursing care."[21]

1. Documentation should include a patient assessment, prioritized nursing diagnoses, identification of desired outcomes, planned interventions, and patient responses. Perioperative RNs use the nursing process to manage the care of the patient receiving moderate sedation/analgesia.

2. Documentation of nursing interventions promotes continuity of patient care and improves communication among health care team members. It provides a mechanism for comparing actual versus expected patient outcomes.[22] Perioperative documentation should include

   ♦ preoperative assessment;

   ♦ actual and potential nursing diagnoses, such as

   – anxiety related to the unfamiliar environment and procedure,

   – ineffective breathing patterns or impaired gas exchange related to altered level of consciousness or airway obstruction,

   – knowledge deficit related to poor recall secondary to medication effects,

   – increased or decreased cardiac output related to medication effects on the myocardium,

   – injury related to altered level of consciousness; and

   ♦ nursing interventions and the patient's responses, including

   – dosage, route, time, and effects of all medications and fluids used;

   – IV site location, type and amount of fluids administered, including blood and blood products, monitoring devices, and equipment used;

   – physiological data from continuous monitoring at five- to 15-minute intervals and upon significant events;

   – level of consciousness;

   – untoward significant patient reactions and their resolution; and

   – postoperative evaluation based on preoperative assessment data.

3. The Perioperative Nursing Data Set (PNDS) should be used to document the patient's care during moderate sedation/analgesia. This standardized nursing vocabulary developed by AORN can be used to improve clinical documentation and communication between clinicians and practice settings. The PNDS includes nursing diagnoses, nursing interventions, and nurse-sensitive patient outcomes. This data set has received official recognition by the American Nurses Association.[23]

Recommended Practice VIII

Patients who receive moderate sedation/analgesia should be monitored postoperatively, receive verbal and written discharge instructions, and meet specified criteria before discharge.

1. Postoperative patient care, monitoring, and discharge criteria should be consistent for all patients. Recovery time will depend on the type and amount of sedation/analgesia given, procedure performed, and facility policy. Postoperative monitoring should include respiratory rate, cardiac rate and rhythm, level of consciousness, oxygen saturation, and blood pressure. The wound/dressing condition, patency of any lines or drainage tubes, and the pain level of the patient also should be monitored postoperatively.[24]

2. Discharge criteria should be developed by representatives from nursing, medicine/surgery, and anesthesia services. These are specifically for assessing and determining the patient's readiness for discharge and home care. They should reflect indications that the patient has returned to a safe physiological level. These discharge criteria should include, but are not limited to,

   ♦ adequate respiratory function,

   ♦ stability of vital signs,

   ♦ preoperative level of consciousness,

   ♦ intact protective reflexes,

   ♦ return of motor/sensory control,

   ♦ absence of protracted nausea,

   ♦ adequate state of hydration,

♦ skin color and condition,

♦ wound/dressing condition, and

♦ reasonable pain management.[25]

3. Patients and/or significant others should receive verbal and written discharge instructions and be able to verbalize an understanding of the instructions to the RN. Written preoperative and postoperative instructions, as well as verbalization of understanding, is encouraged because medications used for moderate sedation/analgesia may cause significant amnesia that directly affects recall ability. A copy of the instructions should be given to the patient and a copy should be placed in the patient's medical record.[26]

Recommended Practice IX

Policies and procedures for managing patients who receive moderate sedation/analgesia should be written, reviewed periodically, and readily available within the practice setting.

1. Policies and procedures are operational guidelines that are used to minimize patient risk factors, standardize practice, direct staff members, and establish guidelines for continuous performance improvement activities. Policies and procedures should establish authority, responsibility, and accountability.[27] Policies and procedures for managing patients receiving moderate sedation/analgesia should include, but are not limited to,

♦ patient selection criteria,

♦ extent of and responsibility for monitoring,

♦ necessary monitoring equipment,

♦ medications that may be administered by the RN,

♦ documentation of patient care, and

♦ discharge criteria.

Glossary

American Society of Anesthesiologists physical status classification: An anesthesia risk evaluation using predetermined criteria defined by the American Society of Anesthesiologists. This system ranks patient physical status on a scale of one to six to determine appropriate patient selection for anesthesia.

Deep sedation/analgesia: A medication-induced depression of consciousness that allows patients to respond purposefully after repeated or painful stimulation. The patient cannot be aroused easily, and the ability to independently maintain a patent airway may be impaired with spontaneous ventilation possibly inadequate. Cardiovascular function usually is adequate and maintained.

General anesthesia: Patients cannot be aroused, even by painful stimulation, during this medication-induced loss of consciousness. Patients usually require assistance in airway maintenance and often require positive pressure ventilation due to depressed spontaneous ventilation or depression of neuromuscular function. Cardiovascular function also may be impaired.

Minimal sedation: A medication-induced state that allows patients to respond normally to verbal commands. Cognitive function and coordination may be impaired, but ventilatory and cardiovascular functions remain unaffected.

Moderate sedation/analgesia: A minimally depressed level of consciousness that allows a surgical patient to retain the ability to independently and continuously maintain a patent airway and respond appropriately to verbal commands and physical stimulation.

Monitoring: Clinical observation that is individualized to patient needs based on data obtained from preoperative patient assessments. The objective of monitoring patients who receive moderate sedation/analgesia is to improve patient outcomes. Monitoring includes the use of mechanical devices and direct observation.

Opioid: Pharmacological agent that produces varying degrees of analgesia and sedation and relieves pain. Fentanyl, morphine, and hydromorphone are opioid analgesic medications that may be used for moderate sedation/analgesia.

Sedative: Pharmacological agent that reduces anxiety and may induce some degree of short-term amnesia. Diazepam and midazolam are two benzodiazepines commonly used for sedation.

NOTES

1. American Society of Anesthesiologists, Inc, "Practice guidelines for sedation and analgesia by non-anesthesiologists," *Anesthesiology* 84 (February 1996) 459-471; Joint Commission on Accreditation of Healthcare Organizations, "Standards, intent statements, and examples for sedation and anesthesia care," in *Comprehensive Accreditation Manual for Hospitals, Update 3, August 2000* (Oakbrook Terrace, Ill: Joint Commission on Accreditation of Healthcare Organizations, 1999) TX15-TX19.

2. L L Yaney, "Intravenous conscious sedation: Physiologic, pharmacologic, and legal implications for nurses," *Journal of Intravenous Nursing* 21 (January/February 1998) 9-19; Joint Commission on Accreditation of Healthcare Organizations, "Standards, intent statements, and examples for sedation and anesthesia care," TX15-TX19.

3. "Endorsement of position statement on the role of the registered nurse (RN) in the management of patients receiving IV conscious sedation for short-term therapeutic, diagnostic, or surgical procedures," American Nurses Association, http://www.ana.org/readroom/position/joint/jtsedate.htm (accessed 27 Sept 2001); J Odom, "Conscious sedation in the ambulatory setting," *Critical Care Nursing Clinics of North America* 9 (September 1997) 361-370.

4. Odom, "Conscious sedation in the ambulatory setting," 361-370; D Dlugose, "Risk management considerations in conscious sedation," *Critical Care Nursing Clinics of North America* 9 (September 1997) 429-440; L Landrum, "A nursing guide to conscious sedation: Clarification of current practice issues," *Critical Care Nursing Clinics of North America* 9 (September 1997) 411-418; D S Watson, *Conscious Sedation/Analgesia* (St Louis: Mosby Year Book, Inc, 1998) 15-16.

5. American Society of Anesthesiologists, Inc, "Practice guidelines for sedation and analgesia by non-anesthesiologists," 459-471; J D Waegerle, "Practical considerations of intravenous sedation for the perioperative nurse," *Seminars in Perioperative Nursing* 7 (January 1998) 21-28.

6. Watson, *Conscious Sedation/Analgesia,* 15-16; Landrum, "A nursing guide to conscious sedation: Clarification of current practice issues," 411-418.

7. Yaney, "Intravenous conscious sedation: Physiologic, pharmacologic, and legal implications for nurses," 9-19; Watson, *Conscious Sedation/Analgesia,* 15-16; Dlugose, "Risk management considerations in conscious sedation," 429-440.

8. "Endorsement of position statement on the role of the registered nurse (RN) in the management of patients receiving IV conscious sedation for short-term therapeutic, diagnostic, or surgical procedures"; Joint Commission on Accreditation of Healthcare Organizations, "Standards, intent statements, and examples for sedation and anesthesia care," TX16-TX19; Waegerle, "Practical considerations of intravenous sedation for the perioperative nurse," 21-28; D L Janikowski, C A Rockefeller, "Awake and talking: Ambulatory surgery and conscious sedation," *Nursing Economics* 16 (January/February 1998) 37-43; M Kost, "Conscious sedation: Guarding your patient against complications," *Nursing 99* (April 1999) 34-39; Dlugose, "Risk management considerations in conscious sedation," 429-440; Odom, "Conscious sedation in the ambulatory setting," 361-370; Watson, *Conscious Sedation/Analgesia,* 28, 74; American Society of Anesthesiologists, Inc, "Practice guidelines for sedation and analgesia by non-anesthesiologists," 459-471.

9. Joint Commission on Accreditation of Healthcare Organizations, "Standards, intent statements, and examples for sedation and anesthesia care," TX15-TX19; Waegerle, "Practical considerations of intravenous sedation for the perioperative nurse," 21-28; Janikowski, Rockefeller, "Awake and talking: Ambulatory surgery and conscious sedation," 37-43.

10. "Endorsement of position statement on the role of the registered nurse (RN) in the management of patients receiving IV conscious sedation for short-term therapeutic, diagnostic, or surgical procedures"; American Society of Anesthesiologists, Inc, "Practice guidelines for sedation and analgesia by non-anesthesiologists," 459-471; Landrum, "A nursing guide to conscious sedation: Clarification of current practice issues," 411-418; Watson, *Conscious Sedation/Analgesia,* 72-74; Waegerle, "Practical considerations of intravenous sedation for the perioperative nurse," 21-28.

11. American Society of Anesthesiologists, Inc, "Practice guidelines for sedation and analgesia by non-anesthesiologists," 459-471; Joint Commission on Accreditation of Healthcare Organizations, "Standards, intent statements, and examples for sedation and anesthesia care," TX15-TX19; Dlugose, "Risk management considerations in conscious sedation," 429-440; Kost, "Conscious sedation: Guarding your patient against complications," 34-39; R Bryan, "Administering conscious sedation: Operational guidelines," *Critical Care Nursing Clinics of North America* 9 (September 1997) 289-300.

12. Watson, *Conscious Sedation/Analgesia,* 20; Odom, "Conscious sedation in the ambulatory setting," 361-370; Dlugose, "Risk management considerations in conscious sedation," 429-440.

13. Dlugose, "Risk management considerations in conscious sedation," 429-440; American Society of Anesthesiologists, Inc, "Practice guidelines for sedation and analgesia by non-anesthesiologists," 459-471; Joint Commission on Accreditation of Healthcare Organizations, "Standards, intent statements, and examples for sedation and anesthesia care," TX15-TX19; "Endorsement of position statement on the role of the registered nurse (RN) in the management of patients receiving IV conscious sedation for short-term therapeutic, diagnostic, or surgical procedures"; Watson, *Conscious Sedation/Analgesia,* 27-38.

14. "Endorsement of position statement on the role of the registered nurse (RN) in the management of patients receiving IV conscious sedation for short-term therapeutic, diagnostic, or surgical procedures"; Kost, "Conscious sedation: Guarding your patient against complications," 34-39; Dlugose, "Risk management considerations in conscious sedation," 429-440; American Society of Anesthesiologists, Inc, "Practice guidelines for sedation and analgesia by non-anesthesiologists," 459-471.

15. "Endorsement of position statement on the role of the registered nurse (RN) in the management of patients receiving IV conscious sedation for short-term therapeutic, diagnostic, or surgical procedures"; American Society of Anesthesiologists, Inc, "Practice guidelines for sedation and analgesia by non-anesthesiologists," 459-471; Odom, "Conscious sedation in the ambulatory setting," 361-370.

16. "Endorsement of position statement on the role of the registered nurse (RN) in the management of patients receiving IV conscious sedation for short-term therapeutic, diagnostic, or surgical procedures"; Odom, "Conscious sedation in the ambulatory setting," 361-370; Landrum, "A nursing guide to conscious sedation: Clarification of current practice issues," 411-418; Yaney, "Intravenous conscious sedation: Physiologic, pharmacologic, and legal

implications for nurses," 9-19; American Society of Anesthesiologists, Inc, "Practice guidelines for sedation and analgesia by non-anesthesiologists," 459-471.

17. "Endorsement of position statement on the role of the registered nurse (RN) in the management of patients receiving IV conscious sedation for short-term therapeutic, diagnostic, or surgical procedures"; Odom, "Conscious sedation in the ambulatory setting," 361-370; Yaney, "Intravenous conscious sedation: Physiologic, pharmacologic, and legal implications for nurses," 9-19; American Society of Anesthesiologists, Inc, "Practice guidelines for sedation and analgesia by non-anesthesiologists," 459-471; Watson, *Conscious Sedation/Analgesia,* 27-38.

18. Odom, "Conscious sedation in the ambulatory setting," 361-370; Yaney, "Intravenous conscious sedation: Physiologic, pharmacologic, and legal implications for nurses," 9-19; Waegerle, "Practical considerations of intravenous sedation for the perioperative nurse," 21-28; Dlugose, "Risk management considerations in conscious sedation," 429-440.

19. Landrum, "A nursing guide to conscious sedation: Clarification of current practice issues," 411-418; American Society of Anesthesiologists, Inc, "Practice guidelines for sedation and analgesia by non-anesthesiologists," 459-471; Kost, "Conscious sedation: Guarding your patient against complications," 34-39; Watson, *Conscious Sedation/Analgesia,* 14.

20. Kost, "Conscious sedation: Guarding your patient against complications," 34-39; Bryan, "Administering conscious sedation: Operational guidelines," 289-300; Watson, *Conscious Sedation/Analgesia,* 14; Yaney, "Intravenous conscious sedation: Physiologic, pharmacologic, and legal implications for nurses," 9-19.

21. "Recommended practices for documentation of perioperative nursing care," in *Standards, Recommended Practices, and Guidelines* (Denver: AORN, Inc, 2001) 199-201.

22. J C Rothrock, "Generic care planning: AORN patient outcome standards," in *Perioperative Nursing Care Planning,* second ed, J C Rothrock, ed (St Louis: Mosby-Year Book, Inc, 1996) 91.

23. S Beyea, ed, *Perioperative Nursing Data Set,* second ed (Denver: AORN, Inc, 2002) 4, 13.

24. American Society of Anesthesiologists, Inc, "Practice guidelines for sedation and analgesia by non-anesthesiologists," 459-471; Bryan, "Administering conscious sedation: Operational guidelines," 289-300; Watson, *Conscious Sedation/Analgesia,* 98-100.

25. American Society of Anesthesiologists, Inc, "Practice guidelines for sedation and analgesia by non-anesthesiologists," 459-471; Bryan, "Administering conscious sedation: Operational guidelines," 289-300; Watson, *Conscious*

Sedation/Analgesia, 101-103; Odom, "Conscious sedation in the ambulatory setting," 361-370; Joint Commission on Accreditation of Healthcare Organizations, "Standards, intent statements, and examples for sedation and anesthesia care," TX15-TX19.

26. Odom, "Conscious sedation in the ambulatory setting," 361-370; Watson, *Conscious Sedation/Analgesia,* 103.

27. Joint Commission on Accreditation of Healthcare Organizations, "Standards, intent statements, and examples for sedation and anesthesia care," TX15-TX19.

RESOURCES

"Endorsement of position statement on the role of the registered nurse (RN) in the management of patients receiving IV conscious sedation for short-term therapeutic, diagnostic, or surgical procedures," American Nurses Association, http://www.ana.org/readroom/position/joint/jtsedate.htm (accessed 26 Sept 2001).

Foster, F. "Conscious sedation: Coming to a unit near you," *Nursing Management* (April 2000) 45-51.

Hayes, J S, et al. "Oral meperidine, atropine, and pentobarbital for pediatric conscious sedation," *Pediatric Nursing* 26 (September/October 2000) 500-504.

Poe, S, et al. "Ensuring safety of patients receiving sedation for procedures: Evaluation of clinical practice guidelines," *Journal on Quality Improvement* 27 (January 2001) 28-41.

"Policy statement: Guidelines for monitoring and management of pediatric patients during and after sedation for diagnostic and therapeutic procedures (RE9252)," American Academy of Pediatrics, http://www.aap.org/policy/04789.html (accessed 27 Sept 2001).

"Revisions to anesthesia care standards," Joint Commission on Accreditation of Healthcare Organizations, http://www.jcaho.org/standard/aneshap.html (accessed 26 Sept 2001).

Shields, R E. "A comprehensive review of sedative and analgesic agents," *Critical Care Nursing Clinics of North America* 9 (September 1997) 281-288.

Originally published April 1993, *AORN Journal,* as "Recommended practices for monitoring the patient receiving intravenous conscious sedation."

Revised; published January 1997, *AORN Journal,* as "Recommended practices for managing the patient receiving conscious sedation/analgesia."

Reformatted July 2000.

Revised November 2001; published March 2002, *AORN Journal.*

Recommended Practices for Cleaning, Handling, and Processing Anesthesia Equipment

The following recommended practices were developed by the AORN Recommended Practices Committee and have been approved by the AORN Board of Directors. They were presented as proposed recommended practices for comment to members and others. These recommended practices are effective January 1, 2005.

These recommended practices are intended as achievable recommendations representing what is believed to be an optimal level of practice. Policies and procedures will reflect variations in practice settings or clinical situations that determine the degree to which the recommended practices can be implemented.

AORN recognizes the numerous types of settings in which perioperative nurses practice. These recommended practices are intended to provide guidance for various practice settings, including traditional ORs, ambulatory surgery units, physicians' offices, cardiac catheterization suites, endoscopy suites, radiology departments, and all other areas where operative and other invasive procedures may be performed.

Purpose

Anesthesia equipment is a potential vector in the transmission of microorganisms. Proper handling and processing of medications, supplies, and equipment can reduce the risk of infection to the patient. These recommended practices provide guidelines for the handling, cleaning, disposal, and reprocessing of anesthesia equipment and instrumentation.

Recommended Practice I

Anesthesia equipment that comes in contact with the vascular system or sterile body tissue should be sterile at the time of use.

1. Items such as IV catheters, tubing, and stopcocks; syringes and needles; and medication vials and ampules are considered critical items. The Centers for Disease Control and Prevention (CDC) uses Spaulding's criteria to determine the potential for transmission of infectious agents. In this classification, items contacting the vascular system or sterile tissues pose the greatest risk of infection and are classified as critical.[1] Using sterile items when contacting the vascular system or sterile tissues minimizes the risk of infection.

2. Aseptic technique should be used when preparing medications. Breaks in aseptic technique have contaminated IV anesthetic agents and medications, resulting in clusters of infections.[2-9] Good practices include
   - performing hand hygiene before preparing medications,
   - cleaning vial stoppers before puncturing them,
   - using multiple needles to withdraw medication into multiple syringes,
   - not transferring syringes of unused medication between patients, and
   - not storing syringes of propofol at room temperature for the day.

   Medications should be stored in a clean area. Personnel should perform basic hand hygiene according to the CDC's "Guideline for hand hygiene in health-care settings,"[10] before preparing medication. Vial stoppers should be cleaned with alcohol before they are punctured. Single-dose vials should be used for only one patient. Syringes of unused medication should be discarded at the end of the procedure. Propofol should be withdrawn immediately before administration.

3. Aseptic technique should be used when administering medications. Bacteria from hands can contaminate syringes and their contents.[11-16] Multidose vials have been found to be contaminated.[17] Syringe contents have been found to contain blood or bloodborne pathogens after one injection or entry into IV tubing.[13,18-23] Using a common syringe in the IV tubing ports of more than one patient has transmitted infectious diseases.[9,24] Syringes and needles should be used for only one application (eg, one syringe and one needle per entry into a multidose vial). Intravenous tubing ports should be cleaned with alcohol before they are punctured with a needle.

Recommended Practice II

Anesthesia equipment that comes in contact with mucous membranes should be sterilized or undergo high-level disinfection before use.

1. Reusable items (eg, airways, breathing circuits, connectors, fiberoptic endoscopes, forceps, laryngoscope blades, masks, self-inflating bags,

some laryngeal mask airways [LMAs], transducer tubing, transesophageal probes) are considered semicritical. The CDC has determined that their potential for transmitting infectious agents is significant and has classified these items as semicritical.[1]

2. Reusable semicritical items should be cleaned as the first step in reprocessing. Removal of organic material provides optimal conditions for proper exposure of equipment to disinfectants and sterilants.[1,25,26] Rigid laryngoscopes should be disassembled and all components cleaned, including handles. Some automated pasteurization equipment has a cleaning step within the pasteurizing cycle.

3. Clean, semicritical reusable items should be processed by high-level disinfection, pasteurization, or sterilization with a US Food and Drug Administration (FDA)-approved agent, according to AORN's "Recommended practices for high-level disinfection" or "Recommended practices for sterilization in the practice setting."[27,28] Written instructions from the manufacturers of reprocessing equipment, chemicals, and instruments should be followed. High-level disinfection kills vegetative bacteria, tubercle bacilli, some spores, fungi, and viruses.[1] The CDC recommends that reusable semicritical items be high-level disinfected, pasteurized, or sterilized to minimize the risk of transmission of infectious agents.[1] This recommendation is supported by professional organizations, including the Association for Professionals in Infection Control and Epidemiology, Inc (APIC), the American Society of Anesthesiologists (ASA), and the American Association of Nurse Anesthetists (AANA).[1,29,30] Inadequately disinfected laryngoscope blades have been implicated in clusters of infections.[31-33] Laryngoscopes should be disassembled and all parts thoroughly cleaned and the blades high-level disinfected before they are reassembled. Some LMAs are designed for limited reuse. Manufacturers' instructions should be followed.

4. Flexible endoscopes should be processed according to AORN's "Recommended practices for cleaning and processing endoscopes and endoscope accessories,"[34] and the manufac-

turer's written instructions. Infections have been transmitted when flexible endoscopes have been reprocessed in an automated endoscope reprocessor with the biopsy port caps off or adapters that were incompatible with the equipment.[35,36] Users of this equipment should verify compatibility of the reprocessor with the endoscope and that adapters are approved by the manufacturer of the reprocessing equipment for use with the particular endoscope being processed. Manufacturers' written instructions should be followed.

5. Residual chemicals should be removed and the reprocessed item thoroughly dried before storage or use on a patient. Residual chemicals on items have led to allergic reactions and tissue burns.[37] Chemical stains have occurred when orthophthalaldehyde was not rinsed off adequately before use.[38] Users of chemical disinfectants should verify the appropriateness of the chemical's use on items being disinfected and thoroughly rinse the items according to the manufacturer's written instructions. These recommendations may include a triple rinse. Disinfected items should be dried thoroughly and stored in manner that prevents recontamination or damage. Use of contaminated tap water to rinse semicritical items has resulted in transmission of *Pseudomonas aeruginosa*.[39-43] This agent proliferates in the channels of endoscopes.[39,40,43] Items should be rinsed with sterile water after the chemical disinfection process. If sterile water is not used, the item should be rinsed first with water and then with 70% alcohol, and it should be thoroughly dried, along with its lumens and channels.[43]

6. Disinfected semicritical items should be stored in a clean location in a manner that prevents recontamination or damage. Storing semicritical items in a clean location minimizes the risk of contamination with pathogens before use. Endoscopes should be stored vertically with control valves, caps, and hoods removed.[43]

7. Personnel should be trained in the reprocessing procedures and equipment. Training personnel regarding the complexities of the equipment, chemicals, and processes used minimizes the risk of human error.

8. Quality control of reprocessing procedures should be performed and documentation maintained in accordance with
   ♦ AORN's "Recommended practices for high-level disinfection,"[27]
   ♦ AORN's "Recommended practices for sterilization in the practice setting,"[28] and
   ♦ manufacturers' written instructions.

Quality control measures provide assurance that mechanical and chemical conditions are optimal for high-level disinfection. Documentation provides a mechanism for process improvement and investigation of adverse events.

Recommended Practice III

Anesthesia equipment contacting intact skin should be clean at the time of use.

1. Items such as blood pressure cuffs, electrocardiogram (ECG) leads, and oximeter probes that contact only intact skin are considered noncritical. The CDC
   ♦ has determined that the potential for transmission of infectious agents is lower when items contact only intact skin,
   ♦ has classified these items as noncritical, and
   ♦ recommends low-level disinfection.[1]

2. Reusable items and surfaces contacting intact skin (eg, blood pressure cuffs, ECG leads, skin temperature probes) should be cleaned between use on patients. Cleaning removes organic and inorganic material, which allows the disinfectant to contact all surfaces.[1,25,26]

3. Reusable laryngoscope handles should be cleaned and low-level disinfected between patients. Laryngoscope handles become contaminated during airway management. In studies, 40% to 50% of handles tested positive for blood.[44,45] Cleaning and disinfecting these handles minimizes the risk of transmission of bloodborne pathogens. The disinfectant selected should be registered with the Environmental Protection Agency (EPA) for use as a hospital disinfectant and used according to the manufacturer's written instructions.[46]

4. Reusable noncritical items should be low-level disinfected between patients. Low-level disinfection with an EPA-registered hospital disinfection with an EPA-registered hospital disinfection with an EPA-registered hospital disinfectant kills most bacteria and some viruses and fungi but may not kill tubercle bacilli or bacterial spores.[1] After subjection to low-level disinfection, the device is considered safe to come in contact with intact skin.

5. Surfaces of anesthesia equipment that are touched by personnel while they are providing patient care or handling contaminated items should be cleaned and low-level disinfected between use on patients, according to manufacturers' written instructions. Surfaces of anesthesia equipment become contaminated with oral secretions and blood during surgical procedures.[47-50] Researchers have found occult or visible blood on 29.5% to 35.5% of anesthesia machines, carts, and monitors.[47,48] Blood also has been found on ventilator controls, flow meter knobs, vapor controls, ECG leads, oximeter probes, and blood pressure cuffs (ie, 25% to 64.3%).[48] Surfaces of anesthesia carts, drawer handles, touch screens, flow meter knobs, ventilator controls, ECG leads, oximeter probes, and blood pressure cuffs should be cleaned and disinfected between use on patients. Other surfaces known to have been touched during patient care also should be cleaned and disinfected between patients.

6. Exterior surfaces of anesthesia equipment (eg, anesthesia cart, machine, monitors) that are not knowingly contaminated during patient care should be terminally low-level disinfected at the end of the day according to manufacturers' written instructions. Contact with blood and body fluids is routinely associated with tasks performed by anesthesia care providers.[50] These surfaces may become contaminated during use, without the knowledge of the provider.[51] Low-level disinfection with an EPA-registered hospital disinfectant renders the surfaces safe to contact intact skin.[1] Manufacturers recommend specific agents to clean complex electronic equipment. These instructions should be followed.

Recommended Practice IV

Single-use items (eg, breathing circuits, endotracheal tubes, filters, needles, some LMAs, stylets, suction catheters, syringes) should be used once and discarded in accordance with local, state, and federal regulations.

1. Single-use items should be used for a single patient and not reused on subsequent patients. Patient care equipment and supplies are potential vectors of microorganisms and can transmit infectious agents. Safe cleaning and reuse of single-use items has not been established. These items should be discarded after use on a single patient.

2. Single-use items should not be reprocessed unless requirements for validation testing can be met. Reuse of items designed for single use creates the potential for injury related to mechanical failure, residual bioburden, and chemical residue from the reprocessing agent. For these reasons, reprocessing of items designed for single use is regulated by the FDA. Under the Federal Food, Drug, and Cosmetic Act, facilities reprocessing single-use devices must meet all regulatory requirements of a device manufacturer, including
   ♦ facility registration and device listing,
   ♦ premarket clearance or approval,
   ♦ labeling,
   ♦ corrections and removals,
   ♦ medical device tracking,
   ♦ medical device reporting, and
   ♦ quality system regulation.[52]

   These requirements exceed the capabilities of most perioperative settings.

Recommended Practice V

Anesthesia equipment should meet performance and safety criteria established by the practice setting and that is consistent with the manufacturer's written instructions.

1. Written information regarding safety and testing methods, warranties, and a manual for maintenance and inspections should be obtained from the manufacturer for all anesthesia equipment. These manuals help in developing operational, safety, and maintenance guidelines. Recommendations vary by manufacturer and equipment model. Manuals should be maintained for each.

2. Anesthesia equipment should be assigned an identification number. Identification numbers allow for documentation of inspections, safety checks, preventive maintenance, repairs, and tracking in the event of a patient or equipment problem.

3. Before placing anesthesia equipment into service, the safety features of the equipment should be tested by qualified, trained personnel, according to manufacturers' written instructions. These tests should be specific to the type and model of equipment involved and include, but not be limited to, calibrations and alarms. Testing the equipment before initial use minimizes the risk of patient injury resulting from faulty equipment.

4. Before use, anesthesia equipment should be tested according to manufacturers' written instructions and the safety standards of the facility. This check provides assurance that basic safety features of the equipment are operational. The FDA's "Anesthesia apparatus checkout recommendations" can be adapted for this purpose.[53]

5. Routine maintenance of anesthesia machines should be conducted on a regular schedule by qualified, trained personnel, according to manufacturers' written instructions. Regular preventive maintenance minimizes the risk of mechanical failure of anesthesia equipment.

6. Any equipment not meeting safety standards should be removed from service. Equipment failing safety checks poses a risk to patients and/or personnel. Removal of the equipment minimizes these risks. The ASA has published guidelines for determining when anesthesia machines should be considered obsolete.[54] Obsolete machines and equipment should be replaced.

7. Before use on a patient susceptible to malignant hyperthermia (MH), the anesthesia machine should be prepared in a manner that minimizes trace anesthetic agents. Halogenated anesthetic agents may trigger MH in susceptible patients.[55] Removing traces of these agents minimizes this risk. The Malignant Hyperthermia Association of the United States recommends changing the soda lime and breathing circuit, draining and inactivating vaporizers, and flushing the machine with 10 L of air or oxygen for 10 minutes before using the machine for an MH-susceptible patient.[56]

8. Equipment containing mercury should be replaced with alternatives that are mercury-free. Mercury poses a risk to patients and personnel as well as the environment. Removing mercury from the health care environment minimizes these risks.[57]

Recommended Practice VI

Internal components of the anesthesia machine breathing circuit should be cleaned regularly.

1. Reusable absorbers and valves should be cleaned on a regular basis according to manufacturers' written instructions. Particular attention should be given to the valves. An appropriate and cost-effective schedule for reprocessing has not been established.[58] Single-use absorbers are available and should be used for only one patient. Routine sterilization or high-level disinfection of the internal components of anesthesia machines is unnecessary.[29,30,58]

2. Anesthesia ventilator bellows should be cleaned regularly according to manufacturers' written instructions.

3. Soda lime should be changed according to the manufacturer's written instructions. Soda lime canisters do not filter bacteria adequately.[59-61] In one study, 40% of bacteria passed through the soda lime.[61] The bactericidal activity of soda lime also is unreliable.[61,62] *Mycobacterium tuberculosis* has been found to survive three hours in soda lime.[61] Soda lime, therefore, should not be used as the only method of filtration. Canisters and contents should be replaced according to the manufacturer's written instructions.

4. Routine use of single-use breathing circuits with bacterial filters should be considered. Bacteria circulate through the anesthesia circuit and proliferate inside the absorber and accessories.[63-65] Filters prevent microorganisms from contaminating the ventilator and escaping into the OR through the positive pressure relief valve of the waste gas scavenging system.[62,66-73] Research findings indicate that the absence of bacterial filters does not lead to an increased rate of nosocomial pneumonias.[58,74] In one investigation, however, contamination of the anesthetic circuit was identified as the likely cause of transmission of hepatitis C virus.[75] Currently, there is no consensus about the routine use of bacterial filters.[29,30,58,76,77] For patients with known or suspected tuberculosis, the CDC, ASA, and AANA recommend using a bacterial filter between the patient and breathing circuit.[29,30,58] The Canadian Society of Anesthesiologists also recommends use of bacterial filters for patients with severe acute respiratory syndrome (SARS).[78] With the increased prevalence of tuberculosis, increased numbers of immunocompromised patients, and the advent of SARS, it is prudent to consider the routine use of bacterial filters on the inspiratory and expiratory limbs of the anesthesia circuit. Some single-use circuits have a heat and moisture exchanger equipped with these filters. Reusable circuits should be cleaned and undergo high-level disinfection, pasteurization, or sterilization between use on patients.

5. Humidifiers should be used and cleaned according to manufacturers' written instructions. The water in humidifiers is heated to temperatures that reduce or eliminate microbial growth.[79] Tap water may contain stationary-phase forms of *Legionella pneumophila,* which are heat resistant.[66] Sterile water should be used in humidifiers.[58,79-81] Reusable humidifying chambers should undergo sterilization or high-level disinfection between patient uses.[58,79] Single-use chambers should be discarded after use on one patient.

Recommended Practice VII

Waste must be disposed of in a manner consistent with local, state, and federal regulations.

1. Biohazardous waste should be placed in a biohazardous waste bag. Some anesthetic waste poses a risk of transmission of bloodborne pathogens. Placing it in designated biohazardous containers alerts handlers to this risk. Management of biohazardous waste within the health care facility is regulated by the Occupational Safety and Health Administration (OSHA).[82] State and local laws also apply. Perioperative professionals should be aware of and act in accordance with these laws.

2. Sharps should be handled in a manner that minimizes the risk of percutaneous injury. To minimize the risk of injury from contaminated sharps, OSHA requires that puncture-resistant sharps containers be located at the point of use.[82] Placing the container next to or on the anesthesia equipment meets this expectation. Sharps should be placed directly into the container.

3. Waste that is hazardous upon disposal must be managed in a way that minimizes environmental impact. Some waste poses a risk to the environment (eg, alcohol, bezoin, epinephrine, mercury). This waste is classified by the EPA as hazardous upon disposal and is regulated under the Resource Conservation and Recovery Act.[83] The EPA requires that this waste be placed in hazardous waste containers at the point of use to alert handlers to the need to take precautions upon its disposal.[84] State and local laws also may apply.

Recommended Practice VIII

Potential hazards to perioperative personnel that are associated with handling and processing clean and contaminated anesthesia equipment (eg, exposure to infectious organisms, chemicals) should be identified, and practices should be established to reduce the risk of injury.

1. Contaminated sharps must be discarded in a puncture-resistant container at the point of use. Immediate disposal of sharps prevents injuries to people unaware of the location of the sharp and is required by OSHA.[82]

2. All personnel involved with cleaning and processing anesthesia equipment should practice according to AORN's "Recommended practices for standard and transmission-based precautions."[85] These precautions define general measures for infection control.

3. Anesthesia equipment should be processed using methods that reduce the risk of exposure to pathogens and injury. Manual cleaning methods that minimize splashing, spraying, spattering, and generation of droplets protect personnel from exposure to blood, body fluids, and cleaning agents.

4. Personnel must be apprised of the hazards in the workplace, including chemicals used for reprocessing anesthesia equipment. Knowledge of the hazards in the workplace, preventive measures, and exposure management minimize the risk of injury to employees and are required by OSHA.[86]

5. Personal protective equipment (PPE) must be provided to minimize the risk of exposure to bloodborne pathogens and chemicals used in the workplace. Use of barrier protection minimizes the risk of exposure to bloodborne pathogens by personnel performing tasks likely to generate contact with blood. According to OSHA regulations, employers are required to provide PPE (eg, gloves, gown, mask, protective eyewear, face shield) for their employees.[82]

6. Personnel should actively participate in the evaluation of engineering devices and work practice controls to minimize the risk of exposure to bloodborne pathogens. Active participation in the selection of PPE and practices provides the best opportunity for designing a safer workplace. According to OSHA regulations, employers are required to solicit nonmanagerial employee input during evaluation of engineering devices and work practice controls to minimize exposures to bloodborne pathogens.[87]

Recommended Practice IX

Anesthesia equipment should be handled, cleaned, processed, or discarded in the same manner in all areas of the practice setting.

1. Guidelines should be developed and approved by appropriate mechanisms and governing bodies in the practice setting. Equipment may be located in satellite areas (eg, labor and delivery). Guidelines should be consistent throughout the practice setting because all patients are entitled to the same standard of care.[88]

Recommended Practice X

Policies and procedures on cleaning and processing anesthesia equipment should be developed, reviewed periodically, and readily available in the practice setting.

1. These recommended practices should be used as guidelines for developing policies and procedures in the practice setting. Policies and procedures establish authority, responsibility, and accountability for cleaning, handling, and processing anesthesia equipment and serve as operational guidelines. Policies and procedures also help in developing performance improvement activities.

2. Policies and procedures for cleaning and processing anesthesia equipment should include, but not be limited to,
   - disposal of single-use items,
   - equipment maintenance programs,
   - equipment quality checks,
   - personal protection,
   - personnel education,
   - processing reusable equipment, and
   - waste disposal.

Glossary

Anesthesia equipment: Equipment used to provide anesthesia and/or monitor the patient under sedation or anesthesia.

Cleaning: A process using friction, detergent, and water to remove organic debris.

Critical item: An item that contacts the vascular system or enters sterile tissue, posing the highest risk of transmission of infection.

High-level disinfection: A process that uses a government-registered agent that kills vegetative bacteria, tubercle bacilli, some spores, fungi, and lipid and nonlipid viruses, given appropriate concentration, submersion, and contact time.

Low-level disinfection: A process by which most bacteria, some viruses, and some fungi are killed. This process may not kill resistant organisms, such as mycobacterium tubercle or bacterial spores.

Noncritical item: An item that comes in contact with intact skin but not with mucous membranes, sterile tissue, or the vascular system.

Pasteurization: A process that employs time and hot water (ie, 160° to 170° F [21.7° C to 25° C] for 30 minutes) for high-level disinfection. The intensity of heat and duration of exposure must be determined by the manufacturer of the pasteurization unit and the manufacturer of the product or device to be cleaned.

Semicritical item: An item that comes in contact with mucous membranes or with skin that is not intact.

NOTES

1. W A Rutala, APIC Guidelines Committee, "APIC guideline for selection and use of disinfectants," *American Journal of Infection Control* 24 (August 1996) 313-342.

2. Centers for Disease Control and Prevention, "Postsurgical infections associated with an extrinsically contaminated intravenous anesthetic agent—California, Illinois, Maine, and Michigan, 1990," *Morbidity and Mortality Weekly Report* 39 (June 29, 1990) 426-427, 433.

3. M J Daily, J B Dickey, K H Packo, "Endogenous Candida endophthalmitis after intravenous anesthesia with propofol," *Archives of Ophthalmology* 109 (August 1991) 1081-1084.

4. M E Villarino et al, "Postsurgical infectious associated with an extrinsically contaminated intravenous anesthetic agent," program and abstracts of the 31st Interscience Conference on Antimicrobial Agents and Chemotherapy, Chicago, 29 Sept-2 Oct 1991.

5. B Veber et al, "Severe sepsis after intravenous injection of contaminated Propofol," *Anesthesiology* 80 (March 1994) 712-713.

6. K Kidd-Ljunggren et al, "Nosocomial transmission of hepatitis B virus infection through multiple-dose vials," *Journal of Hospital Infection* 43 (September 1999) 57-62.

7. M J Kuehnert et al, "Staphylococcus aureus bloodstream infections among patients undergoing electroconvulsive therapy traced to breaks in infection control and possible extrinsic contamination by Propofol," *Anesthesia and Analgesia* 85 (August 1997) 420-425.

8. M Massari et al, "Transmission of hepatitis C virus in a gynecological surgery setting," *Journal of Clinical Microbiology* 39 (August 2001) 2860-2863.

9. Centers for Disease Control and Prevention, "Transmission of hepatitis B and C viruses in outpatient settings—New York, Oklahoma, and Nebraska, 2000-2002," *Morbidity and Mortality Weekly Report* 52 (Sept 26, 2003) 901-906.

10. J M Boyce, D Pittet, "Guideline for hand hygiene in health-care settings: Recommendations of the Healthcare Infection Control Practices Advisory Committee and the HICPAC/SHEA/APIC/ISAD Hand Hygiene Taskforce," *Morbidity and Mortality Weekly Report* 51 (Oct 25, 2002) (RR16) 1-44.

11. C E Blogg, M A Ramsey, J D Jarvis, "Infection hazard from syringes," *British Journal of Anaesthesia* 46 (April 1974) 260-262.

12. M R Lessard et al, "A microbiological study of the contamination of the syringes used in anaesthesia practice," *Canadian Journal of Anaesthesia* 35 (November 1988) 567-569.

13. C T Lutz et al, "Allergy testing of multiple patients should no longer be performed with a common syringe," *The New England Journal of Medicine* 310 (May 17, 1984) 1335-1337.

14. J W Koepke, J C Selner, "Allergy testing of multiple patients with a common syringe," *The New England Journal Medicine* 311 (Nov 1, 1984) 1188-1189.

15. D J Shulan et al, "Contamination of intradermal skin test syringes," *Journal of Allergy and Clinical Immunology* 76 (August 1985) 226-227.

16. J W Koepke et al, "Viral contamination of intradermal skin test syringes," *Annals of Allergy* 55 (December 1985) 776-778.

17. A Carbonne et al, "Patient to patient transmission of hepatitis C in surgery clinic through multi-dose vials," abstract presented at the 13th annual meeting of the Society for Healthcare Epidemiology of America, Arlington Va, 5-8 April 2003.

18. A Fleming, A C Ogilvie, "Syringe needles and mass inoculation technique," *British Medical Journal* 1 (March 17, 1951) 543-546.

19. R R Hughes, "Post-penicillin jaundice," *British Medical Journal* 2 (Nov 9, 1946) 685-688.

20. R Uren, C Commens, R Howman-Giles, "Intradermal injections: A potential health hazard?" *Medical Journal of Australia* 161 (August 994) 226.

21. H A Hein et al, "Recapping needles in anesthesia—Is it safe?" *Anesthesiology* 67 (September 1987) A161.

22. C A Trepanier et al, "Risk of cross-infection related to the multiple use of disposable syringes," *Canadian Journal of Anaesthesia* 37 (March 1990) 156-159.

23. J L Parlow, "Blood contamination of drug syringes used in anaesthesia," *Canadian Journal of Anaesthesia* 36 suppl (1989) S61-S62.

24. B Meier, "Reuse of needle at hospital infects 50 with hepatitis C," *New York Times,* Oct 10, 2002.

25. Association for the Advancement of Medical Instrumentation, "Safe handling and biological decontamination of reusable medical devices in health care facilities and in nonclinical settings; ANSI/AAMI ST35" (Arlington, Va: Association of the Advancement of Medical Instrumentation, 2003) 16.

26. "Sterilization or disinfection of medical devices: General principles," Centers for Disease Control and Prevention, *http://www.cdc.gov/ncidod/hip/sterile/sterilgp.htm* (accessed 24 Sept 2004).

27. "Recommended practices for high-level disinfection," in *Standards, Recommended Practices, and Guidelines* (Denver: AORN, Inc, 2004) 235-240.

28. "Recommended practices for sterilization in the practice setting," in *Standards, Recommended Practices, and Guidelines* (Denver: AORN, Inc, 2004) 373-384.

29. American Society of Anesthesiologists Committee on Occupational Health of Operating Room Personnel, *Recommendations for Infection Control for the Practice of Anesthesiology,* second ed (American Society of Anesthesiologists: Park Ridge, Ill, 1998). Also available at *http://www.asahq.org/publicationsAndServices/infectioncontrol.pdf* (accessed 24 May 2004).

30. American Association of Nurse Anesthetists, *Infection Control Guide* (Park Ridge, Ill: American Association of Nurse Anesthetists, 1997) 13-23.

31. J E Foweraker, "The laryngoscope as a potential source of cross-infection," *Journal of Hospital Infections* 29 (April 1995) 315-316.

32. T J Neal et al, "The neonatal laryngoscope as a potential source of cross-infection," *Journal of Hospital Infections* 30 (August 1995) 315-317.

33. K E Nelson et al, "Transmission of neonatal listerosis in a delivery room," *American Journal of Diseases of Children* 139 (September 1985) 903-905.

34. "Recommended practices for cleaning and processing endoscopes and endoscope accessories," in *Standards, Recommended Practices, and Guidelines* (Denver: AORN, Inc, 2004) 261-266.

35. Centers for Disease Control and Prevention, "Bronchoscopy-related infections and pseudoinfections—New York, 1996 and 1998," *Morbidity and Mortality Weekly Report* 48 (July 9, 1999) 557-560.

36. US Department of Health and Human Services, "Infections from inadequately processed endoscopes," *User Facility Reporting* 28 (Fall 1999) 1-5.

37. "Manufacturer and User Facility Device Experience Database. Report Numbers 2084725-2002-00033; 2084725-2003-00084; 2084725-2004-00010; 2084725-2004-00003; 2084725-2004-00011; 2084725-2004-00012; 3003723454-2004-0001," US Food and Drug Administration, *http://www.accessdata.fda.gov/scripts/cdrh/cfdocs/cfMAUDE/Search.cfm* (accessed 30 Sept 2004).

38. "Manufacturer and User Facility Device Experience Database. Report Numbers 2084725-2003-00008; 3003723454-2004-0001," US Food and Drug Administration, *http://www.accessdata.fda.gov/scripts/cdrh/cfdocs/cfMAUDE/Search.cfm* (accessed 30 Sept 2004).

39. H J O'Conner, J R Babb, G A Ayliffe, "*Pseudomonas aeruginosa* infection in endoscopy," *Gastroenterology* 93 (December 1987) 1451.

40. J I Allen et al, "*Pseudomonas* infection of the biliary system resulting from use of contaminated endoscope," *Gastroenterology* 92 (March 1987) 759-763.

41. D E Low et al, "Infectious complications of endoscopic retrograde cholangio-pancreatography. A prospective assessment," *Archives of Internal Medicine* 140 (August 1980) 1076-1077.

42. M J Arfa, D L Sitter, "In-hospital evaluation of contamination of duodenoscopes: A quantitative assessment of the effect of drying," *Journal of Hospital Infections* 19 (October 1991) 89-98.

43. C J Alvarado, M Reichelderfer, "APIC guideline for infection prevention and control in flexible endoscopy," *American Journal of Infection Control* 18 (April 2000) 138-155.

44. R C Morell et al, "A survey of laryngoscope contamination at a university and a community hospital," *Anesthesiology* 80 (April 1994) 960.

45. R A Phillips, W P Monaghan, "Incidence of visible and occult blood on laryngoscope blades and handles," *AANA Journal* 65 (June 1997) 241-246.

46. Centers for Disease Control and Prevention, "Guidelines for environmental infection control in health-care facilities: Recommendations of CDC and the Healthcare Infection Control Practices Advisory Committee (HICPAC)," *Morbidity and Mortality Weekly Report* 52 (June 6, 2003) No RR-10 22.

47. J R Hall, "Blood contamination of anesthesia equipment and monitoring equipment," *Anesthesia and Analgesia* 78 (June 1994) 1136-1139.

48. S M Perry, W P Monghan, "The prevalence of visible and/or occult blood on anesthesia and monitoring equipment," *Journal of the American Association of Nurse Anesthetists* 69 (February 2001) 44-48.

49. H Arkoff, R A Ortega, "Touchscreen technology: Potential source of cross-infections," *Anesthesia and Analgesia* 75 (December 1992) 1073.

50. M S Kristensen, E Sloth, T K Jensen, "Relationship between anesthetic procedure and contact of anesthesia personnel with patient body fluids," *Anesthesiology* 73 (October 1990) 619-624.

51. L A Herwaldt, J M Pottinger, S A Coffin, "Nosocomial infections associated with anesthesia," in *Hospital Epidemiology and Infection Control,* third ed, C G Mayhall ed (Philadelphia: Lippincott Williams & Wilkins, 2004).

52. US Food and Drug Administration, "Important enforcement date for reprocessing single-use devices," *User Facility Reporting* 39 (Summer 2002). Also available at *http://www.fda.gov/cdrh/fusenews/ufb39.html#1* (accessed 24 Sept 2004).

53. "Anesthesia apparatus checkout recommendations, 1993," US Food and Drug Administration, *http://www.fda.gov/cdrh/humfac/anesckot.html* (accessed 24 Sept 2004).

54. "Guidelines for determining anesthesia machine obsolescence," American Society of Anesthesiologists, *http://www.asahq.org/PublicationsAndServices/machine obsolescense.pdf* (accessed 24 Sept 2004).

55. B Abraham et al, "Malignant hyperthermia susceptibility: Anaesthetic implications and risk stratification," *Quarterly Journal of Medicine* 90 (January 997) 13-18.

56. "Medical FAQs," Malignant Hyperthermia Association of the United States, *http://www.mhaus.org/index.cfm/fuseaction/Content.Display/PagePK/MedicalFAQs.cfm* (accessed 24 Sept 2004).

57. "Reducing mercury use in healthcare: Promoting a healthier environment: A how-to manual," US Environmental Protection Agency, *http://www.epa.gov/glnpo/bnsdocs/merchealth* (accessed 24 Sept 2004).

58. Centers for Disease Control and Prevention, "Guidelines for prevention of nosocomial pneumonia, 2003," *Morbidity and Mortality Weekly Report* 53 (March 26, 2004) (RR03) 1-36.

59. G E Dryden, "Risk of contamination from the anesthesia circle absorber: An evaluation," *Anesthesia and Analgesia* 48 (November/December 1969) 939-943.

60. J R Jenkins, W M Edgar, "Sterilization of anaesthetic equipment," *Anaesthesia* 19 (April 1964) 177-190.

61. P M Murphy, R B Fitzgeorge, F Barrett, "Viability and distribution of bacteria after passage through a circle anaesthetic system," *British Journal of Anaesthesia* 66 (March 1991) 300-304.

62. D T Leijten, V S Rejger, R P Mouton, "Bacterial contamination and the effect of filters in anaesthetic circuits in a simulated patient model," *Journal of Hospital Infections* 21 (May 1992) 51-60.

63. G E Dryden, "Uncleaned anesthesia equipment," *JAMA* 233 (September 1975) 1297-1298.

64. B C Stratford, R R Clark, S Dixson, "The disinfection of anaesthetic apparatus," *British Journal of Anaesthesia* 36 (August 1964) 471-476.

65. "Bacterial contamination of anesthesia machines revealed," *Excerpta Medica* (Lawrenceville, NJ: Convention Reporter, 1991) 12-14.

66. H Aranha-Creado et al, "Removal of *Mycobacterium* species by breathing circuit filters," *Infection Control and Hospital Epidemiology* 18 (April 1997) 252-254.

67. A J Berry, F S Nolte, "An alternative strategy for infection control of anesthesia breathing circuits: A laboratory assessment of the Pall HME filter," *Anesthesia and Analgesia* 72 (May 1991) 651-655.

68. I Hogbarth, "Anaesthetic machine and breathing system contamination and the efficacy of bacterial/viral filters," *Anaesthesia and Intensive Care* 25 (April 1996) 154-163.

69. G Lloyd et al, "Barriers to hepatitis C transmission within breathing systems: Efficacy of a pleated hydrophobic filter," *Anaesthesia and Intensive Care* 25 (June 1997) 235-238.

70. H H Luttropp, L Berntman, "Bacterial filters protect anaesthetic equipment in a low-flow system," *Anaesthesia* 48 (June 1993) 520-523.

71. J Rathgeber et al, "Prevention of patient bacterial contamination of anaesthesia-circle-systems: A clinical study of the contamination risk and performance of different heat and moisture exchanges with electret filter (HMEF)," *European Journal of Anaesthesia* 14 (July 1997) 368-373.

72. G M Shiotani et al, "Prevention of contamination of the circle system and ventilators with a new disposable filter," *Anesthesia and Analgesia* 50 (September/October 1971) 844-845.

73. C Smith et al, "An evaluation of one and two airflow filters preventing the movement of bacterial through the anesthesia circle system," *Journal of the American Association of Nurse Anesthetists* 64 (April 1996) 153-156.

74. S Van Hassel et al, "Bacterial filters in anesthesia: Results of nine years of surveillance," *Infection Control and Hospital Epidemiology* 20 (January 1999) 58-60.

75. K Chant et al, "Investigation of possible patient-to-patient transmission of hepatitis C in a hospital," *New South Wales Public Health Bulletin* 5 (May 1994) 47-51.

76. Association of Anaesthetists of Great Britain and Ireland, *Infection Control in Anaesthesia* (London: The Association of Anaesthetists of Great Britain and Ireland, 2002) 4.

77. "Policy on infection control in anaesthesia, 1995," Australian and New Zealand College of Anaesthetists, *http://www.medeserv.com.au/anzca/pdfdocs/P28_1995.PDF* (accessed 25 Sept 2004).

78. "Anesthetic management of a SARS-Infected patient," Canadian Society of Anesthesiologists, *http://www.asahq.org/clinical/pracadvsars.htm* (accessed 25 Sept 2004).

79. Centers for Disease Control and Prevention, "Guidelines for prevention of nosocomial pneumonia," *Morbidity and Mortality Weekly Report* 46 (Jan 3, 1997) (RR-1) 1-77.

80. P M Anrow et al, "Nosocomial Legionnaire's disease caused by aerosolized tap water from respiratory devices," *Journal of Infectious Diseases* 146 (October 1982) 460-467.

81. D E Craven, T A Goularte, B J Make, "Contaminated condensate in mechanical ventilator circuits: A risk factor for nosocomial pneumonia?" *American Review of Respiratory Disease* 129 (April 1984) 625-628.

82. "Bloodborne pathogens—1910.1030," US Department of Labor Occupational Safety and Health Administration, *http://www.oshaslc.gov/pls/oshaweb/owadisp.show_document?p_table=STANDARDS&p_id=10051* (accessed 25 Sept 2004).

83. "RCA online," US Environmental Protection Agency, *http://www.epa.gov/rcraonline* (accessed 25 Sept 2004).

84. "Identification and listing of hazardous waste," in *Electronic Code of Federal Regulations (e-CFR)* 40: Protection of Environment, Part 261, *http://www.epa.gov/epahome/cfr40.htm* (accessed 25 Sept 2004).

85. "Recommended practices for standard and transmission-based precautions," in *Standards, Recommended Practices, and Guidelines* (Denver: AORN, Inc, 2004) 361-366.

86. "Hazard communication in the 21st century workplace," US Department of Labor, Occupational Safety and Health Administration, *http://www.osha.gov/dsg/hazcom/finalmsdsreport.html* (accessed 25 Sept 2004).

87. "Bloodborne pathogens and needlestick prevention," US Occupational Safety and Health Administration, *http://www.osha.gov/SLTC/bloodbornepathogens/index.html* (accessed 25 Sept 2004).

88. Joint Commission on Accreditation of Healthcare Organizations, "Crosswalk of 2003 standards for hospitals to 2004 leadership standards for hospitals," in *2004 Comprehensive Accreditation Manual for Hospitals: The Official Handbook* (Oakbrook Terrace, Ill: Joint Commission on Accreditation of Healthcare Organizations, 2003) LD.3.20.

Originally published June 1977, *AORN Journal, as* AORN "Recommended practices for cleaning and processing anesthesia equipment."

Revised March 1978; July 1982; March 1991.

Published as proposed recommended practices September 1994.

Revised; published November 1999, *AORN Journal.*

Reformatted July 2000.

Revised November 2004; published April 2005, *AORN Journal.*

Recommended Practices for Surgical Attire

The following recommended practices were developed by the AORN Recommended Practices Committee and have been approved by the AORN Board of Directors. They were presented as proposed recommended practices for comments by members and others. They are effective January 1, 2005.

These recommended practices are intended as achievable recommendations representing what is believed to be an optimal level of practice. Policies and procedures will reflect variations in practice settings or clinical situations, which will determine the degree to which the recommended practices can be implemented.

AORN recognizes the numerous types of settings in which perioperative nurses practice. These recommended practices are intended as guidelines adaptable to various practice settings. These practice settings include traditional ORs, ambulatory surgery units, physicians' offices, cardiac catheterization suites, endoscopy suites, radiology departments, and all other areas where operative and other invasive procedures may be performed.

Purpose

These recommended practices provide guidelines for attire worn within the semirestricted and restricted areas of the surgical environment. The human body is a major source of microbial contamination in this environment; therefore, scrub clothing is worn to promote a high level of cleanliness and hygiene within the surgical environment. These recommended practices are not intended to address sterile attire worn at the surgical field.

Recommended Practice I

All individuals who enter the semirestricted and restricted areas of the surgical suite should wear freshly laundered surgical attire intended for use only within the surgical suite.

1. Facility approved, clean, and freshly laundered surgical attire should be donned in a designated dressing area of the facility upon entry or re-entry to the facility.[1-3] If scrubs are worn into the institution from outside, they should be changed before entering semirestricted or restricted areas to minimize the potential for contamination (eg, animal hair, cross contamination from other uncontrolled environments).[4]

2. Surgical attire helps contain bacterial shedding and promotes environmental control.[1,5] Surgical attire made of reusable woven fabric or single-use, nonwoven fabric that is low-linting should be worn. Low-linting surgical attire that minimizes bacterial shedding and provides comfort, safety, and a professional appearance should be selected. As personnel move, friction between their bodies and clothing frees bacteria. Research indicates that chafing increases dispersal of body scurf into the environment.[5] If a two-piece pantsuit is worn, the top of the scrub suit should be secured at the waist, tucked into the pants, or fit close to the body. There is little evidence to support a preference for scrub pants over scrub dresses.

3. Surgical attire should be changed daily or whenever it becomes visibly soiled, contaminated, or wet.[2,4,6] Worn surgical attire should be placed in an appropriately designated container for washing or disposal and should not be hung or placed in a locker for wearing at another time. This promotes high-level cleanliness and hygiene within the practice setting. It has been reported that bacterial colony counts are higher when scrub clothing is removed, stored in a locker, and used again.[7-9]

4. Reusable woven or single-use, nonwoven attire should be appropriately placed in designated containers after use.[1,4,5]

5. Visibly soiled, contaminated, or wet surgical attire should be removed as soon as possible and replaced with fresh, clean surgical attire. Changing contaminated, soiled, or wet attire reduces the potential for cross-infection and protects personnel from prolonged exposure to potentially harmful bacteria.[4,5]

6. Surgical attire contaminated with visible blood or body fluids must remain at the facility and be laundered by the hospital or a hospital-contracted commercial laundry.[4,5,6,10] Controlled laundering of attire contaminated by blood or body fluids reduces the risk of transferring pathogenic microorganisms from the facility to the home or the general public.

7. Home laundering of surgical attire is not recommended.[4,6,10-15] Without clear evidence about the safety for patients, health care workers, and their family members, AORN does not support

the practice of home laundering of surgical attire. Reusable surgical attire, including cover jackets and cloth hats, should be laundered by a designated facility-approved and monitored commercial laundry after daily use.

Commercial laundries are required to follow strict guidelines[4,8,16-19] that incorporate

♦ proper and controlled water temperatures;

♦ use of detergents;

♦ use of oxidizing agents (eg, chlorine bleach) in specified and monitored concentrations;

♦ repeated changes of water; and

♦ dryer or iron and press drying temperatures that typically are not found in home laundry equipment.

Home laundering of surgical attire that is not visibly soiled is controversial, and there is no concrete evidence to either support or refute the practice. Surgical attire becomes soiled or contaminated with microorganisms during wear. Taking worn, soiled, or contaminated surgical attire into the home can result in the spread of contamination to the home environment.

AORN is aware that some provider facilities require personnel to launder scrub attire at home. Although AORN does not support this practice, steps should be taken to minimize contaminants to the home environment; therefore, laundering practices similar to regulations and professional standards for commercial laundries are recommended. When a facility requires home laundering of surgical attire, minimum criteria should be met.[4,8,16-18]

Suggested criteria for home laundering soiled surgical attire should include

♦ using an automatic washer and hot air dryer;

♦ using water temperature of 110° F to 125° F (43.33° C to 51.67° C) to facilitate microbial kill;

♦ using chlorine bleach (ie, sodium hypochlorite);

♦ using detergent according to manufacturer's instructions;

♦ laundering surgical attire in a separate load with no other items;

♦ laundering surgical attire as the last load after all other items have been laundered;

♦ washing hands immediately after placing laundry in the washing machine;

♦ keeping laundry items completely submerged during the entire wash and rinse cycle to facilitate removal of soil and microorganisms;

♦ avoiding placing hands or arms in the laundry or rinse water to keep items submerged;

♦ thoroughly cleaning the door and lid of the washing machine before removing the laundered attire to prevent reintroduction of contaminants on clean attire when removing it from the washing machine and before placing it in the dryer;

♦ using the highest drying setting possible that is safe for the material of attire construction; and

♦ promptly removing attire when dry to avoid desiccation of materials.

8. Laundered surgical attire should be protected from contamination during transfer and storage.[1,20] Freshly laundered surgical attire should be protected during transport to the practice setting.

9. The use of cover apparel should be determined by the individual practice setting. The value of cover apparel within the institution is unsubstantiated.[1,21-23] The use of cover apparel has been found to have little or no effect on reducing contamination, but it is used for practical enforcement and cost considerations. Donning fresh scrubs after each trip to other areas increases costs and is time-consuming. Laboratory coats or the use of cover gowns may provide a professional appearance, but they should be removed before entering a semirestricted or restricted area because they can be a source of contamination.[24] The decision on cover gowns depends on individual state regulatory rulings, the culture in each perioperative suite, and the manager's assessment of priorities.

10. Nonscrubbed personnel should wear long-sleeved jackets that are buttoned or snapped closed during use. Complete closure of the jacket avoids accidental contamination of the sterile field. Long-sleeved attire is advocated to prevent bacterial shedding from bare arms and is included in the Occupational Safety and Health Administration (OSHA) regulation for the use of personal protective equipment (PPE).[1,2]

11. Other garments should be contained completely within or covered by the surgical attire. Clothing that cannot be covered by the surgical attire should not be worn.

Recommended Practice II

Personnel should cover head and facial hair, including sideburns and necklines, when in the semi-restricted and restricted areas of the surgical suite.

1. A clean, low-lint surgical head cover or hood that confines all hair should be worn. Hair covers eliminate the possibility of hair or dandruff being shed onto surgical attire.[1,2,4,25] A bald or shaved head is covered to prevent shedding of squamous cells (ie, scurf).

2. The head cover or hood should be designed to minimize microbial dispersal. Hair acts as a filter when left uncovered and collects bacteria in proportion to its length, curliness, and oiliness.[1,25] Shedding from hair has been shown to affect surgical wound infection; therefore, complete coverage is necessary. Disposable bouffant and hood-style covers are preferred.[4] Skullcaps that fail to cover the side hair above the ears and hair at the nape of the neck should not be worn in the surgical suite. Net caps should not be used because they do not provide a barrier to dandruff and hair fallout.

3. Single-use headgear should be removed and discarded in a designated receptacle as soon as possible after daily use. Reusable hats or hoods should be laundered in a commercial laundry after each use.[2,4,16]

4. Contaminated headgear must be removed and laundered by the facility.[10]

Recommended Practice III

All individuals entering restricted areas of the OR suite should wear a mask when open sterile items and equipment are present.

1. A single surgical mask should be worn in surgical environments where open sterile supplies or scrubbed persons are located. A mask should fully cover both mouth and nose and be secured in a manner that prevents venting.[1,2,26] Masks are intended to contain and filter droplets of microorganisms expelled from the mouth and nasopharynx during talking, sneezing, and coughing.[27,28] Use of a double mask creates an impediment to breathing and does not increase filtration; therefore, this is unacceptable.[25,26]

Differences of opinion about whether masks should be worn exist in the literature. AORN recommends further research to determine changes in current practice.[29-31] In addition to possible surgical site contamination, blood exposure occurring on the face and neck of OR personnel is not uncommon; therefore, individual practice settings should develop policies based on OSHA and state-mandated recommendations for wearing masks.[32]

2. Masks should be removed carefully by handling only the ties, and they should be discarded immediately. Masks should not be saved by hanging them around the neck or tucking them into a pocket for future use. The filter portion of a surgical mask harbors bacteria collected from the nasopharyngeal airway. Handling this portion of the mask after use can transfer bacteria to the hands and initiate potential cross contamination.[1,2,33]

Recommended Practice IV

All personnel entering the semirestricted and restricted areas of the surgical suite should confine or remove all jewelry and watches.[2,34-37]

1. Rings should be removed from hands. These items may harbor organisms that cannot be removed during hand washing. Higher bacterial counts have been noted when jewelry is worn.

2. Other jewelry (eg, watches, earrings, bracelets, necklaces, piercings) should be removed or totally confined within the scrub attire. Although there is no evidence to demonstrate that other jewelry increases bacterial shedding, there is concern that jewelry could fall onto the sterile field or into the wound if not contained. Necklaces could contaminate the front of the sterile gown if not confined.[1]

Recommended Practice V

Fingernails should be kept short, clean, natural, and healthy.[2,35,38]

1. The subungual region harbors the majority of microorganisms found on the hand. Removing debris from fingernails requires the use of a nail cleaner under running water; additional effort is necessary for longer nails. The risk of

tearing gloves increases if fingernails extend past the fingertips. Long fingernails may cause injury when moving or positioning patients.[38]

Recent studies found no increase in microbial growth related to wearing freshly applied nail polish;[35,37] however, nail polish that is obviously chipped or worn longer than four days is associated with the presence of greater numbers of bacteria and has been associated with infections. Surgical conscience, therefore, must be a foremost behavior in individuals who choose to wear nail polish in the surgical setting.

2. Artificial nails should not be worn.[2,32,38-51] Studies show that artificial (eg, acrylic) nails on healthy hands increase the risk of surgical site infection. Artificial nails harbor organisms and prevent effective hand antisepsis. Higher counts of gram-negative microorganisms have been cultured from the fingertips of personnel wearing artificial nails than from personnel with natural nails, both before and after hand washing. Fungal growth occurs frequently under artificial nails as a result of moisture becoming trapped between the natural and artificial nail.[47-49]

Recommended Practice VI

Protective barriers must be made available to reduce the risk of exposure to potentially infectious materials.[34,52,53]

1. Gloves should be selected and worn as follows according to the task to be performed.[1]
   - Sterile gloves must be worn when performing sterile procedures.
   - Medical, nonsterile gloves are recommended for nonsterile activities.

2. Gloves should be changed between patient contacts or after contact with contaminated items when a task is complete. Surgical or examination gloves should be changed—not washed—between patient contacts. Hand hygiene should be performed after gloves are removed.[52-54] Gloves are worn to reduce gross contamination of the hands. Changing gloves between patient contacts and after completing a task reduces the risk of microorganism transmission. Disinfecting agents may cause glove deterioration. Research indicates that micro-

organisms are not always removed from gloves despite friction, use of cleansing agents, and drying. In addition, washing the glove may decrease the integrity of the glove.[50]

3. Protective eyewear, masks, or face shields must be worn when splashing or spraying is likely.[1,2,4,6,53,54] Masks should be worn, along with protective eyewear (eg, goggles, glasses with solid side shields, chin-length face shields) whenever eye, nose, or mouth contamination reasonably can be anticipated as a result of splashes, spray, or splatter of blood droplets or other potentially infectious materials.[53,54] Personal protective equipment is considered appropriate only if it prevents blood or other potentially infectious materials from contaminating an employee's work clothes, undergarments, skin, eyes, mouth, or other mucous membranes under normal conditions of use and for the duration of time for which the protective equipment will be used.[52]

4. Protective eyewear or face shields that become contaminated should be discarded or decontaminated promptly according to manufacturers' written instructions.[1,4,6,53] Failure to decontaminate or dispose of these items could result in contamination to the wearer.

5. Additional protective attire (eg, liquid-resistant aprons, gowns, shoe covers) should be worn when exposure to blood or potentially infectious materials is anticipated.[6] Protective barriers are worn to reduce the risk of exposure to blood, body fluids, or other liquids that may contain potentially infectious agents. There is evidence that supports the need for circulating personnel to wear PPE appropriate to the task being performed.[53,55,56]

6. Fluid-resistant shoe covers are considered part of PPE and must be worn when it can be reasonably anticipated that splashes or spills may occur. Foot attire has no proven significance in reducing the incidence of surgical site wound infections; the primary reason for its use is to facilitate sanitation.[1,57] If shoe covers are worn, they should be changed whenever they become torn, wet, or soiled, and they should be removed and discarded in a designated container before leaving the surgical area.[1,4]

7. Shoes worn within the surgical environment should be clean with no visible soiling and should provide protection.[1] Cloth or open-toe shoes do not offer protection against spilled liquids or sharp items that may be dropped or kicked. Shoes should have closed toes and low heels to minimize the risk of injury.[57,58]

Recommended Practice VII

Policies and procedures for surgical attire should be developed, reviewed periodically, and readily available in the practice setting. These policies and procedures should include, but not be limited to, definition of areas where surgical attire must be worn, appropriate attire within those defined areas, and the choice for the use of cover apparel outside the surgical suite.

1. These recommended practices should be used as guidelines for the development of policies and procedures within the practice setting. Policies and procedures establish authority, responsibility, and accountability and serve as operational guidelines. AORN's "Recommended practices for traffic patterns in the perioperative practice setting"[59] and "Recommended practices for surgical hand antisepsis and hygiene"[54] also should be consulted when developing policies and procedures. An introduction and review of policies and procedures should be included in the orientation and ongoing education of personnel to assist in the development of knowledge, skills, and attitudes that affect patient outcomes. Policies and procedures also assist in the development of quality assessment and improvement activities.

Glossary

Artificial nails: Substances or devices applied or added to the natural nails to augment or enhance the wearer's own nails. They include, but are not limited to, bonding, tips, wrappings, and tapes.

Cleaning: The physical removal of soil or organic material using water or mechanical action with or without detergent; cleaning removes rather than kills microorganisms.

Contaminated: The presence of pathogenic organisms (eg, blood, other potentially infectious material) on or in the material.

Cover gown: A garment, such as a laboratory coat, gown, or jacket, worn over surgical attire to prevent contamination.

Personal protective equipment: Personal protective equipment for standard precautions includes intact gloves, gowns, masks, and eye protection (eg, face shields, goggles, glasses with side shields).

Scrub attire: Additional sterile clothing worn to cover the surgical attire to present sterile boundaries during a sterile invasive procedure.

Scurf: A branlike desquamation of the epidermis.

Soiled: Worn or dirty, especially on the surface. Smirched or stained by body perspiration, body oils, or other substances.

Surgical attire: Nonsterile apparel designated for the OR practice setting that includes two-piece pantsuits, cover jackets, head coverings, shoes, masks, protective eyewear, and other protective barriers.

Restricted area: Includes the OR and procedure room, the clean core, and scrub sink areas. People in this area are required to wear full surgical attire and cover all head and facial hair, including sideburns, beards, and necklines.

Semirestricted area: Includes the peripheral support areas of the surgical suite and has storage areas for sterile and clean supplies, work areas for storage and processing of instruments, and corridors leading to the restricted areas of the surgical suite.

Unrestricted area: Includes a central point that is established to monitor the entrance of patients, personnel, and materials. Street clothes are permitted in this area, and traffic is not limited.

NOTES

1. D Fogg, "Infection prevention and control" in *Alexander's Care of the Patient in Surgery,* 12th ed, J C Rothrock, ed (St Louis: Mosby, 2003) 134-147.

2. Centers for Disease Control and Prevention, "Guideline for Prevention of Surgical Site Infection, 1999," *Infection Control and Hospital Epidemiology* 20 (April 1999) 250-278.

3. N L Belkin, "Use of scrubs and related apparel in health care facilities," *American Journal of Infection Control* 25 (October 1997) 401-404.

4. "Safe handling and biological decontamination of reusable medical devices in health care facilities and in nonclinical settings," ANSI/AAMI ST35:2003 (Arlington, Va: Association for the Advancement of Medical Instrumentation, 2003) 11-12; 51-57.

5. B M Anderson, N Solheim, "Occlusive scrub suits in operating theaters during cataract surgery: Effect on airborne contamination," *Infection Control Hospital Epidemiology* 23 (April 2002) 218-220.

6. "Regulations (Standards 29 CFR) Bloodborne pathogens—1910-1030," US Department of Labor, Occupational Safety and Health Administration, *http://www.osha-slc.gov/pls/oshaweb/owadisp.show_document?p_table=STANDARDS&p_id=10051* (accessed 22 May 2004) 15-16.

7. "Report to Congress on workers' home contamination study conducted under the Workers' Family Protection Act (29 USC 671A)" Centers for Disease Control and Prevention, National Institute for Occupational Safety and Health, *http://www.cdc.gov/niosh/contamin.html* (accessed 8 April 2002) 6.

8. A N Neely, M P Maley, "Survival of enterococci and staphylococci on hospital fabrics and plastic," *Journal of Clinical Microbiology* 38 (February 2002) 724-726.

9. I Callaghan, "Bacterial contamination of nurse's uniforms: A study," *Nursing Standard* 13 (Sept 23-29, 1998) 37-42.

10. Centers for Disease Control and Prevention, "Guidelines for environmental infection control in health-care facilities: Recommendations of CDC and the Healthcare Infection Control Practices Advisory Committee (HICPAC)," *Morbidity and Mortality Weekly Report* 52 (June 6, 2003) 27-28.

11. N Hawkes, "Infection Fear Over Nurses Who Wash Uniforms at Home," *The Times*, 30 June 2003, sec 2W.

12. Market and Opinion Research International, "Nurses' uniforms survey for JLA" (June 2003) 1-7.

13. N L Belkin, "Home laundering of soiled surgical scrubs: Surgical site infections and the home environment," *American Journal of Infection Control* 29 (February 2001) 58-64.

14. P Jurkovich, "Home versus hospital-laundered scrubs," *The American Journal of Maternal/Child Nursing* 29 (March/April 2004) 106-110.

15. L Spannraft, "Laundering scrubs at home," (Readers' Responses) *The American Journal of Maternal/Child Nursing* 23 (January/February 1998) 53.

16. D Barrie, "How hospital linen and laundry services are provided," *Journal of Hospital Infection* 27 (March 1994) 219-235.

17. D Fogg, "Body piercings in the OR; tabletop sterilizers; Joint Commission initiative; West Nile virus; home laundering" (Clinical Issues) *AORN Journal* 77 (February, 2003) 428-433.

18. J M Jaska, D L Fredell, "Impact of detergent systems on bacterial survival on laundered fabrics," *Applied and Environmental Microbiology* 39 (April, 1980) 743-748.

19. N L Belkin, "Surgical scrubs—Where we were, where we are going," *Today's Surgical Nurse* 20 (March/April 1998) 28-34.

20. L L McDonald, "Linen services," in *APIC Text of Infection Control and Epidemiology* (Washington, DC: Association for Professionals in Infection Control and Epidemiology, Inc, 2002) 75(1)-75(4).

21. H Kenny, E Lawson "The efficacy of cotton cover gowns in reducing infection in neutropenic patients: An evidence-based study," *International Journal of Nursing Practice* 6 (June 2000) 135-139.

22. J L Thigpen, "Responding to research: Realistic use of scrub clothes and cover gowns," *Neonatal Network* 9 (February 1991) 41-44.

23. C B Mailhot et al, "Cover gowns: Researching their effectiveness," *AORN Journal* 46 (September 1987) 482-490.

24. W Loh, VV Ng, J Holton, "Bacterial flora on the white coats of medical students," *Journal of Hospital Infection* 45 (January 2000) 65-68.

25. B Friberg et al, "Surgical area contamination—Comparable bacterial counts using disposable head and mask and helmet aspirator system, but dramatic increase upon omission of head-gear: An experimental study in horizontal laminar air-flow," *Journal of Hospital Infection* 47 (February 2001) 110-115.

26. N J Mitchell, S Hunt, "Surgical face masks in modern operating rooms—A costly and unnecessary ritual?" *Journal of Hospital Infection* 18 (July 1991) 239-242.

27. M G Romney, "Surgical face masks in the operating theatre: Re-examining the evidence," *Journal of Hospital Infection* 47 (April 2001) 251-256.

28. F McCluskey, "Does wearing a face mask reduce bacterial wound infection? A literature review," *British Journal of Theatre Nursing* 6 (August, 1996) 18-29.

29. N L Belkin "Surgical face masks in the operating theatre: Are they still necessary?" (Letters to the Editor) *Journal of Hospital Infection* 50 (March 2002) 233-235.

30. T G Tunevall, "Postoperative wound infections and surgical face masks: A controlled study," *World Journal of Surgery* 15 (May/June 1991) 383-387.

31. G A J Ayliffe, "Masks in surgery?" (Editorial) *The Journal of Hospital Infection* 18 (July 1991) 165-166.

32. Y Uehara et al, "Bacterial interference among nasal inhabitants: Eradication of *Staphylococcus aureus* from nasal cavities by artificial implantation of *Corynebacterium* sp." *Journal of Hospital Infection* 44 (February 2000) 127-133.

33. L Emsley, "Why wear surgical face masks?" *Nursing Times* 96 (July 2000) 38-39.

34. Centers for Disease Control and Prevention, "Guideline for hand hygiene in health-care settings: Recommendations of the Healthcare Infection Control Practices Advisory Committee and the HICPAC/SHEA/APIC/IDSA Hand Hygiene Task Force," *Morbidity and Mortality Weekly Report* 51, RR-16 (Oct 25, 2002) 29-33.

35. V A Arrowsmith et al, "Removal of nail polish and finger rings to prevent surgical infection," The Cochrane Database of Systematic Reviews 2 (2004) 1-16.

36. W E Trick et al, "Impact of ring wearing on hand contamination and comparison of hand hygiene agents in a hospital," *Clinical Infectious Disease* 36 (June 2003) 1383-1390.

37. E Edel et al, "Impact of a 5-minute scrub on the microbial flora found on artificial, polished, or natural fingernails of operating room personnel," *Nursing Research* 47 (January/February 1998) 54-59.

38. R L Moolenaar et al, "A prolonged outbreak of *Pseudomonas Aeruginosa* in a neonatal intensive care unit: Did staff fingernails play a role in disease transmission?" *Infection Control and Hospital Epidemiology* 21 (February 2000) 80-85.

39. C A Wynd, D E Samstag, A M Lapp, "Bacterial carriage on the fingernails of OR nurses," *AORN Journal* 60 (November 1994) 796-805.

40. R Baran, "Pathogen carriage in health care workers wearing nail cosmetics," *Dermatology Online Journal* 9, no 1 (2003) 17D.

41. C A Baumgardner et al, "Effects of nail polish on microbial growth of fingernails: Dispelling sacred cows," *AORN Journal* 58 (July 1993) 84-88.

42. A Jeanes, J Green, "Nail art: A review of current infection control issues," *Journal of Hospital Infection* 49 (October 2001) 139-142.

43. J Porteous, "Artificial nails: Very real risks," *Canadian Operating Room Nursing Journal* 20 (September 2002) 16-21.

44. L Saiman et al, "Banning artificial nails from health care settings," *American Journal of Infection Control* 30 (June 2002) 252-254.

45. M F Parry et al, "Candida osteomylitis and diskitis after spinal surgery: An outbreak that implicates artificial nail use," *Clinical Infectious Diseases* 32 (February 2001) 352-356.

46. S A Hedderwick et al, "Pathogenic organisms associated with artificial fingernails worn by healthcare workers," *Infection Control and Hospital Epidemiology* 21 (August 2000) 505-509.

47. D J Passaro et al, "Postoperative *Serratia marcescens* wound infections traced to an out-of-hospital source," *Journal of Infectious Diseases* 174 (April 1997) 992-995.

48. E H Winslow, A F Jacobson, "Can a fashion statement harm the patient?" *American Journal of Nursing* 100 (September 2000) 63-65.

49. J Pottinger, S Burns, C Manske, "Bacterial carriage by artificial versus natural nails," *American Journal of Infection Control* 17 (December 1989) 340-344.

50. "Make a 'revolutionary' change in hand hygiene," *Hospital Employee Health* 21 (February 2002) 13-24.

51. "CDC draft guidelines say no artificial nails," *Same-Day Surgery* 25 (August, 2001) 91.

52. B N Doebbeling et al, "Removal of nosocomial pathogens from the contaminated glove," *Annals of Internal Medicine* 109 (September 1988) 394-398.

53. B Goodner, *The OSHA Handbook: Interpretive Guidelines for the Bloodborne Pathogen Standard* (El Paso, Tex: Skidmore-Roth Publishing, Inc, 1993) 61-62.

54. "Recommended practices for surgical hand antisepsis/hand scrubs," in *Standards, Recommended Practices, and Guidelines* (Denver: AORN, Inc, 2004) 291-299.

55. "Occupational exposure to bloodborne pathogens; Final rule," *Federal Register* 56 (Dec 6, 1991) 64177.

56. S Hubbard et al, "Reducing blood contamination and injury in the OR: A study of the effectiveness of protective garments and OR procedures," *AORN Journal* 55 (January 1992) 194-201.

57. M O'Neale, "Used sponge exposure; processing peel packages; flash sterilization; protective arm attire; beverages in the OR" (Clinical Issues) *AORN Journal* 59 (February 1994) 504-506.

58. G Copp et al, "Footwear practices and operating room contamination," *Nursing Research* 36 (November/December 1987) 366-369

59. "Recommended practices for traffic patterns in the perioperative practice setting," in *Standards, Recommended Practices, and Guidelines* (Denver: AORN, Inc, 2004) 397-399.

Originally published March 1975, *AORN Journal,* as AORN "Standards for proper OR wearing apparel."

Format revision March 1978, July 1982.

Revised March 1984, March 1990.

Published as proposed recommended practices August 1994.

Revised November 1998; published December 1998.

Reformatted July 2000.

Revised November 2004; published February 2005, *AORN Journal.*

Recommended Practices for Sponge, Sharp, and Instrument Counts

The following recommended practices were developed by the AORN Recommended Practices Committee and have been approved by the AORN Board of Directors. They were presented as proposed recommended practices for comments by members and others. They are effective January 1, 2006.

These recommended practices are intended as achievable recommendations representing what is believed to be an optimal level of practice. Policies and procedures will reflect variations in practice settings and/or clinical situations that determine the degree to which the recommended practices can be implemented.

AORN recognizes the numerous settings in which perioperative nurses practice. These recommended practices are intended as guidelines that are adaptable to various practice settings. These practice settings include traditional operating rooms, ambulatory surgery centers, physicians' offices, cardiac catheterization suites, endoscopy suites, radiology departments, and all other areas where operative and other invasive procedures may be performed.

Purpose

These recommended practices provide guidance to perioperative registered nurses in performing sponge, sharp, and instrument counts in their practice settings. Counts are performed to account for all items and to lessen the potential for injury to the patient as a result of a retained foreign body. The expected outcome of primary importance to this recommended practice is outcome O2, "The patient is free from signs and symptoms of injury due to extraneous objects."[1] Complete and accurate counting procedures help promote optimal perioperative patient outcomes and demonstrate the perioperative practitioner's commitment to patient safety.

Legislation does not prescribe how counts should be performed, who should perform them, or even that they need to be performed. The law requires only that foreign bodies not be negligently left in patients.[2] The doctrine of res ipsa loquitur (ie, "the thing speaks for itself") is most applicable in cases involving retained foreign objects, rendering those litigations nearly indefensible.[2,3] Retained objects are considered a preventable occurrence, and careful counting and documentation can sig-

nificantly reduce, if not eliminate, these incidents.[4,5] The "captain of the ship" doctrine is no longer assumed to be true, and members of the entire surgical team can be held liable in litigation for retained foreign bodies.[6-11] All team members should be committed to and involved in establishing meaningful policies and procedures related to surgical counts.[12,13]

Recommended Practice I

Sponges should be counted on all procedures in which the possibility exists that a sponge could be retained.

1. Sponge counts should be performed
   - before the procedure to establish a baseline,
   - before closure of a cavity within a cavity,
   - before wound closure begins,
   - at skin closure or end of procedure, and
   - at the time of permanent relief of either the scrub person or the circulating nurse (although direct visualization of all items may not be possible).

2. Initial sponge counts should be performed and recorded, establishing a baseline for subsequent counts on all procedures in which the possibility exists that a sponge could be retained. Policies in the health care organization may identify situations in which this possibility does not exist and counts are not required.[14]

3. Accurately accounting for sponges throughout a surgical procedure should be a priority of the surgical team to minimize the risks of a retained sponge.[3,4,15,16] The Institute of Medicine has identified avoiding injuries from the care that is intended to help patients to be one of six aims to a better health care system.[17]

4. Established policies in the health care organization may define when additional counts must be performed or may be omitted (eg, cystoscopy, ophthalmology).[14] Closed claim studies conducted during the past 20 years have demonstrated that roughly two-thirds of reported cases of retained surgical items are attributed to sponges.[5,18-20] Although the majority of retained sponges are found in the abdomen and pelvis, there are reports in the

literature discussing retained sponges in the vagina, thorax, spinal canal, face, brain, and extremities.[5,21-27]

5. Sponges should be separated, counted audibly, and concurrently viewed during the count procedure by two individuals, one of whom should be a registered nurse circulator.[3,17,28] Concurrent verification of counts by two individuals lessens the risk of inaccurate counts. Separating sponges during the baseline count helps to determine whether a sponge has been added to or deleted from a sterilized package.[2,4,17,29] Use of a pocketed bag or other system for separating used sponges may facilitate visualization for counting. Separating sponges after use minimizes errors caused by sponges sticking together.

6. When additional sponges are added to the field, they should be counted at that time and recorded as part of the count documentation to keep the count current and accurate.[4]

7. Perioperative personnel should count all prepackaged sterile sponges for accuracy. Any package containing an incorrect number of sponges should be removed from the field, bagged, labeled, and isolated from the rest of the sponges in the OR. Containing and isolating the entire package helps reduce the potential for error in subsequent counts.[17]

8. Sponge counts should be conducted in the same sequence each time as defined by the facility. The counting sequence should be in a logical progression (eg, from large to small or from proximal to distal). A standardized count procedure, following the same sequence, assists in achieving accuracy, efficiency, and continuity among perioperative team members.[30] Studies in human error have shown that all errors involve some kind of deviation from routine practice.[31(p57)]

9. All sponges used during a surgical procedure should be x-ray-detectable. Radiopaque indicators facilitate locating an item presumed lost or left in the surgical field when a count discrepancy occurs. X-ray-detectable sponges should not be used as dressings. The use of x-ray-detectable sponges as surface dressings may invalidate subsequent counts if the patient

is returned to the OR. X-ray-detectable sponges used as dressings may appear as foreign bodies on postoperative x-ray studies.[29,32-34]

10. Only towels with radiopaque markers should be used in the wound. If towels are used in the open wound, they should be included in the count as miscellaneous items and should be easily distinguishable from other towels.[29,32,33]

11. Sponges should be left in their original configuration and should not be cut. Altering a sponge invalidates subsequent counts and increases the risk of a portion being retained in the wound.[16,22]

12. Nonradiopaque gauze dressing materials should be withheld from the field until the wound is closed or the case is completed. Keeping dressing materials separated from the actual counted sponges will help prevent intermingling with the sponges used in the procedure.[3]

13. All counted sponges should remain within the OR or sterile field during the procedure. Linen and waste containers should not be removed from the room until counts are completed and resolved. Confinement of all counted sponges to the OR helps eliminate the possibility of a count discrepancy.[17]

14. Counted sponges should not be used as postoperative packing. In certain circumstances, such as when counted sponges are intentionally used as packing and the patient leaves the OR with this packing in place, the number and types of sponges retained and the reason for the variation should be documented on the intraoperative record as correct and confirmed by the surgeon.[4,14,35] When the patient returns to surgery and the packed sponges are removed, the number and types should be reconciled with the number and types removed. The number and types removed should be noted in the current patient's record. The sponges removed should be isolated and not included in the counts for the subsequent procedure. The count on the subsequent procedure should be noted as correct after all sponges have been accounted for. If the sponges are removed in an area other than the OR, the number removed should be noted on the patient record.

15. Sponges should be removed from the OR at the end of the procedure. Removing sponges from the OR at the end of the procedure helps prevent potential count discrepancies during subsequent procedures.[17]

16. Contaminated sponges must be handled and disposed of according to the Bloodborne Pathogens Standard of the Occupational Safety and Health Administration (OSHA); AORN's "Recommended practices for environmental cleaning in the surgical practice setting"[36] and "Recommended practices for standard and transmission-based precautions in the perioperative practice setting"[37]; and facility policies and procedures. The use of leak-proof, tear-resistant containers and personal protective equipment (PPE) can help prevent environmental contamination and reduce the risk of personnel exposure to potentially infectious material.[36-38]

Recommended Practice II

Sharps and other miscellaneous items should be counted on all procedures.

1. Sharps and miscellaneous items (eg, vessel clip bars, vessel loops, umbilical and hernia tapes, vascular inserts, cautery scratch pads, trocar sealing caps) should be counted
   ♦ before the procedure to establish a baseline,
   ♦ before closure of a cavity within a cavity,
   ♦ before wound closure begins,
   ♦ at skin closure or end of procedure, and
   ♦ at the time of permanent relief of the scrub person and/or circulating nurse (although direct visualization of all items may not be possible).

2. Initial sharps counts should be performed and recorded on all procedures. Performing counts constitutes a primary and proactive injury-prevention strategy.[2] Counting sharps and miscellaneous items is not only important in preventing foreign body retention; the continuous accounting for these items can lessen injuries to those scrubbed in the sterile field. As many as 78% of reported needle-stick exposures occur to members of the surgical team.[39,40] Accurately accounting for sharps during a surgical procedure is a primary responsibility of the perioperative nurse and the surgical team members.

3. Sharps and miscellaneous items should be counted audibly and viewed concurrently by two individuals, one of whom should be a registered nurse circulator. Concurrent verification of counts by two individuals lessens the risk for count discrepancies.[2]

4. Additional sharps and miscellaneous items added to the field should be counted when added and recorded as part of the count documentation.

5. Suture needles should be counted and recorded according to the number marked on the outer package and verified by the scrub person when the package is opened.[41] Viewing each needle will help ensure an accurate needle count. Using empty suture packages to rectify a discrepancy in a closing needle count is not recommended.[42] The actual number of needles may not be the same as the number of empty packages.

6. The scrub person should be able to account for all sharps on the sterile field. Sharps remaining unconfined on the sterile field may be unintentionally introduced into the incision or dropped on the floor or may penetrate barriers.

7. Whenever possible, sharps must be handed to and from the surgeon on an exchange basis using a "neutral zone" or "hands-free" technique.[37,42] Passing sharps to the surgeon on an exchange basis will lessen the possibility of a lost sharp item and prevent injury to the surgical team members at the sterile field.[43]

8. Sharps counts should be conducted in the same sequence each time as defined by the facility. The counting sequence should be in a logical progression (eg, from large to small item size or from proximal to distal from the wound). A standardized count procedure, following the same sequence, assists in achieving accuracy, efficiency, and continuity among perioperative team members.[30] Studies in human error have shown that all errors involve some kind of deviation from routine practice.[31(p57)]

9. Members of the surgical team should account for sharps or other miscellaneous items that may have been broken or become separated

within the confines of the surgical site in their entirety. Breakage and/or separation of parts can occur during open as well as minimally invasive surgical procedures. Verification that all broken parts are present or accounted for helps prevent unintentional retention of a foreign body within the patient.[14,44-47]

10. Open sharps on the sterile field should be confined and contained. Used sharps on the sterile field should be kept in a disposable puncture-resistant container. Collecting used needles in a container helps ensure their containment on the sterile field and lessens the risk of injury to personnel at the sterile field.[36,37]

11. All counted sharps should remain within the OR and/or sterile field during the procedure. If a sharp is passed or dropped off the sterile field, the circulating nurse should retrieve it in a safe manner, show it to the scrub person, and isolate it from the field to be included in the final count. Linen or waste containers should not be removed from the OR until all counts are completed and resolved and the patient has been taken from the room. Confinement of all sharps to the OR helps minimize the possibility of a count discrepancy.[17]

12. Sharps must be handled according to the OSHA Bloodborne Pathogens Standard. Proper use, handling, and disposal of contaminated sharps help minimize the risk of exposure to bloodborne pathogens from patient to health care worker and from health care worker to patient.[38] AORN's "Recommended practices for standard and transmission-based precautions in the perioperative practice setting"[37] should be followed. Sharps should be disposed of according to AORN's "Recommended practices for environmental cleaning in the surgical practice setting."[36]

Recommended Practice III

Instruments should be counted for all procedures in which the likelihood exists that an instrument could be retained.

1. Instrument counts should be performed
   ♦ before the procedure to establish a baseline,
   ♦ before wound closure, and

   ♦ when feasible, at the time of permanent relief of the scrub person and/or circulating nurse.

   Instrument counts protect the patient by reducing the likelihood that an instrument will be retained in the patient. Instrument counts are a proactive injury-prevention strategy.[2] Retention of surgical instruments accounts for approximately one-third of retained item case reports.[5] Case studies demonstrate that many types and sizes of instruments have been found, ranging from small serrifine clamps to moderately sized hemostats (ie, 6 to 10 inches) to 13-inch-long retractors.[48,49]

2. Instruments should be counted audibly and viewed concurrently by two individuals, one of whom should be a registered nurse circulator. Concurrent verification of counts by two individuals assists in ensuring accurate counts.[2]

3. Instruments should be counted when sets are assembled for sterilization. This assembly count provides a basic reference for the instrument set and is not to be considered the initial count before the surgical procedure. A count performed outside the OR that is considered an initial count increases the number of variables that can contribute to a count discrepancy and unnecessarily extends responsibility to personnel not involved in direct patient care.[32]

4. Initial counts in the OR should be performed to establish a baseline for subsequent counts, including minimally invasive procedures (eg, laparoscopy, thoroscopy). The possibility of any incision being extended to allow for a more extensive procedure than anticipated supports the practice of performing an initial count for all procedures.

5. Individual pieces of assembled instruments (eg, suction tips, wing nuts, blades, sheathes) should be accounted for separately on the count sheet. Removable instrument parts can be purposefully removed or become loose and fall into the wound or onto or off the sterile field.[45]

6. When additional instruments are added to the field, they should be counted when added and recorded as part of the count documentation.

7. Members of the surgical team should account for instruments that may have been broken or become separated within the confines of the surgical site in their entirety. Breakage and/or separation of parts can occur during open as well as minimally invasive surgical procedures. Verification that all broken parts are present or accounted for helps prevent unintentional retention of a foreign body within the patient.[14,44-47]

8. Instrument counts should be conducted in the same sequence each time as defined by the organization. The counting sequence should be in a logical progression (eg, from large to small item size or from proximal to distal from the wound). A standardized count procedure, following the same sequence, assists in achieving accuracy, efficiency, and continuity among perioperative team members.[30] Studies in human error have shown that all errors involve some kind of deviation from routine practice.[31(p57)]

9. The final instrument count should not be considered complete until those instruments used in closing the wound (eg, malleable retractors, needle holders, scissors) are removed from the wound and returned to the scrub person.

10. All counted instruments should remain within the OR during the procedure until all counts are completed and resolved. If a counted instrument is passed or inadvertently dropped off the sterile field, the circulating nurse should retrieve it, show it to the scrub person, and isolate it from the field to be included in the final count.[38] Confinement of all counted instruments to the OR helps eliminate the possibility of a count discrepancy.[40]

11. All instruments should be accounted for and removed from the room during end-of-procedure cleanup. Accounting for all instruments facilitates inventory control and patient safety. Removing all instruments from the room helps avoid potential count discrepancies during subsequent procedures.[13]

12. Instrument sets should be standardized with the minimum variety and number of instruments needed for the procedure. Instruments that are not routinely used on procedures should be deleted from sets. Reducing the number and types of instruments and streamlining standardized sets improves ease and efficiency of counting.[29] Specialty instruments, if needed, can be opened and added to the count at the time of the procedure.[30]

13. Preprinted count sheets that are identical to the standardized sets should be used to record the counted items. Preprinted count sheets provide organization and efficiency, which are key to preventing unnecessary delays.[4] The circulating nurse should record only the number of instruments opened for the procedure. Additional instruments requested by the surgeon should be counted and added to the preprinted count sheet separately.[14]

14. Contaminated instruments must be handled according to the OSHA Bloodborne Pathogens Standard. Proper use and handling of contaminated instruments help minimize the risk of exposure to bloodborne pathogens from patient to health care worker and from health care worker to patient.[38] Contaminated instruments should be handled according to AORN's "Recommended practices for cleaning and caring for surgical instruments and powered equipment"[50] and "Recommended practices for cleaning and processing endoscopes and endoscope accessories,"[51] as well as the institution's policies and procedures.[45] Contaminated instruments may expose personnel to harmful pathogens.[46]

15. Alternative measures should be established to minimize the risk of retained instruments during procedures in which accurately accounting for instruments is not achievable (eg, anterior-posterior spinal procedures). These measures should include the use of an intraoperative x-ray, read by a radiologist, before the patient is discharged from the OR.

16. Organizations should define when instrument counts should be performed for pediatric patients. Instrument counts may be deferred when there is no perceived risk of retained instruments.

Recommended Practice IV

Additional measures for investigation, reconciliation, documentation, and prevention of retained surgical items should be taken.

1. When a discrepancy in the count(s) is identified, the surgical team is responsible for carrying out steps to locate the missing item.[4,13,45,51] Procedural steps include, but are not limited to,
   ◆ count discrepancy reported to surgeon and surgical team;
   ◆ procedure suspended, if patient's condition permits;
   ◆ manual inspection of the operative site;
   ◆ visual inspection of the area surrounding the surgical field, including floor, kick buckets, and linen and trash receptacles;
   ◆ if the patient's condition permits, intraoperative x-ray taken and read before patient leaves the OR or, if the patient's condition is unstable, an x-ray should be taken as soon as possible;
   ◆ documentation of all measures taken and outcomes on patient's record;
   ◆ reporting of incident following organization policy; and
   ◆ review of incident or near miss for cause, effect, and prevention.

2. The perioperative registered nurse circulator should inform and receive an acknowledgment from the surgeon and team as soon as a discrepancy in a surgical count (ie, sponge, sharps, instrument) is identified.[3,4,14,28,52]

3. The perioperative registered nurse circulator and scrub person should ask the surgeon to conduct a manual search of the wound to locate the missing item(s). The scrub person and perioperative registered nurse circulator should do a manual and visual search, respectively, of the sterile area surrounding the wound and the remainder of the sterile field. The perioperative registered nurse circulator should conduct a search of the nonsterile areas of the room in an attempt to locate the item(s).[3,18,20,45,52]

4. If the item is not recovered, an intraoperative x-ray should be taken before the final closure of the wound. It should be specified that the purpose of the x-ray is to rule out a retained foreign body (eg, needle, sponge, instrument). This x-ray should be read by a radiologist. Studies show greater accuracy when x-rays are read by a radiologist.[4,5,14,20,33] In the case of missing needles, there is no definitive evidence as to how effective x-rays are in detecting small suture needles. Studies done in recent years have demonstrated that needles 17 mm and smaller may not be consistently visible on an x-ray.[53,54]

5. Following organizational policy, documentation of a count discrepancy should include all the measures taken to recover the missing item and communications made regarding the outcome. Such documentation is considered sound professional practice and demonstrates that all reasonable efforts were made to protect the patient's safety.[2,4,17,34,48]

6. A critical investigation should be conducted of any patient safety incident process.[17(p157)] Error and near-miss reporting are the first steps to addressing error reduction.[55,56] The distraction-prone environment of the OR means that performing routine tasks, such as surgical counts, can be considered at risk for error.[13] Errors can be divided into two categories: those at the human interface in a complex system (ie, active), and those representing failed system design (ie, latent).[57] Elements of the root cause analysis tool should be considered in addressing the contributing causes (eg, human, process, system) and in identifying risks and preventive measures.[58] Multidisciplinary teams should be involved in the process of review and address any changes in policy that can improve patient safety.[17]

7. Additional measures should be established to minimize the risk of retained items in high-risk situations. The following situations have been identified through research to be of higher risk for retained foreign bodies:
   ◆ the emergent nature of a procedure,
   ◆ an unexpected change in the procedure, and
   ◆ patient obesity.[5]

8. Internal data from adverse events and near misses should be reviewed to identify high-risk situations within the organization. Health care organizations should identify conditions or situations that pose an increased risk for retained foreign bodies. Health care organizations should establish measures to be taken, in addition to a count, for identified high-risk situations. These measures should include an intraoperative x-ray for foreign body, read by a staff radiologist, before the patient leaves the OR. In

one study, three of 29 x-rays were read as negative when a retained sponge actually was present.[18] Therefore, x-ray alone may be insufficient to detect a retained item.

Recommended Practice V

Sponge, sharp, and instrument counts should be documented on the patient's intraoperative record by the registered nurse circulator.

1. The uniform perioperative nursing vocabulary should be used to document counts on the intraoperative patient record. The perioperative nursing vocabulary is a clinically relevant and empirically validated standardized nursing language. This standardized language consists of the Perioperative Nursing Data Set (PNDS) and includes perioperative nursing diagnoses, interventions, and outcomes. The expected outcome of primary importance to this recommended practice is outcome O2, "The patient is free from signs and symptoms of injury due to extraneous objects." This outcome falls within the domain of Safety (D1). The associated nursing diagnosis is X29, "Risk of injury." The associated interventions that may lead to the desired outcome may include (I93) "Performs required counts."[1]

2. Documentation of counts should include, but not be limited to,
   ♦ types of counts (ie, sponges, sharps, instruments, miscellaneous items) and number of counts;
   ♦ names and titles of personnel performing the counts;
   ♦ results of surgical item counts;
   ♦ notification of the surgeon;
   ♦ instruments intentionally remaining with the patient or sponges intentionally retained as packing;
   ♦ actions taken if count discrepancies occur;
   ♦ outcome of actions taken; and
   ♦ rationale if counts are not performed or completed as prescribed by policy.

3. Accurate documentation serves several purposes, including evidence of the patient's treatment, the basis of the plan of care, communication to all caregivers, protection from liability, and a link to reimbursement.[34,59] Documentation of nursing activities related to the patient's perioperative care provides an accurate picture of the nursing care administered and provides a mechanism for comparing actual versus expected outcomes.[60]

4. Justification for omission of counts in an emergency should be documented. Extreme patient emergencies may necessitate omission of counts to preserve a patient's life or limb. Documenting the omission and reasons for the variation provides a record of the occurrence and an alert to subsequent caregivers that the patient may be at an increased risk for a retained foreign body.[4]

Recommended Practice VI

Policies and procedures for sponge, sharps, and instrument counts should be developed, reviewed periodically, revised as necessary, and readily available in the practice setting.

1. These policies and procedures should include, but not be limited to,
   ♦ items to be counted,
   ♦ directions for performing counts (eg, sequence, item grouping),
   ♦ procedures in which baseline and/or subsequent counts may be exempt,
   ♦ alternative or additional safety measures for special circumstances,[5]
   ♦ nursing actions and procedures for count discrepancy reconciliation, and
   ♦ competency validation.

   Policies and procedures establish authority, responsibility, and accountability and serve as operational guidelines. Policies and procedures also assist in the development of patient safety, quality assessment, and quality improvement activities.[17] Nurses should collaborate with all members of the health care team to develop policies that address surgical counts.[13,14]

2. Policies and procedures should be written to include organ procurements. Counted items could be at risk for being retained and sent with the donated organ(s), retained in the donor, or left in the OR.

3. Practices, policies, and procedures are subject to change with the advent of new technologies.

4. An introduction and review of policies and procedures should be included in orientation and ongoing education of perioperative personnel to assist them in obtaining knowledge and developing skills and attitudes that affect patient outcomes.

Glossary

Instruments: Surgical tools or devices designed to perform a specific function, such as cutting, dissecting, grasping, holding, retracting, or suturing.

Sharps: Items with edges or points capable of cutting or puncturing through other items. In the context of surgery, items include, but are not limited to, suture needles, scalpel blades, hypodermic needles, electrosurgical needles and blades, and safety pins.

Sponges: Soft goods (eg, gauze pads, cottonoids, peanuts, dissectors, tonsil and laparotomy sponges) used to absorb fluids, protect tissues, or apply pressure or traction.

Minimally invasive surgery: Includes laparoscopy and other procedures that involve small incisions and endoscopic instrumentation performed in the OR.

Miscellaneous items: Includes vessel clip bars, vessel loops, umbilical and hernia tapes, vascular inserts, cautery scratch pads, trocar sealing caps, and any other small items that have the potential for being retained in a surgical wound.

Neutral zone (synonym: hands-free technique): A safe work practice control technique used to ensure that the surgeon and scrub person do not touch the same sharp instrument at the same time. This technique is accomplished by establishing a designated neutral zone on the sterile field and placing sharp items within the zone for transfer of the item between scrubbed personnel.

Near miss: An occurrence that could have resulted in an accident, injury, or illness but did not by chance, skillful management, or timely intervention.

Root cause analysis: A retrospective approach to error analysis that focuses on failures of system design as related to common root causes of adverse events.

NOTES

1. S C Beyea, ed, *Perioperative Nursing Data Set: The Perioperative Nursing Vocabulary,* second ed (Denver: AORN, Inc, 2002).

2. E K Murphy, "Operating room records, counts cause concern," (OR Nursing Law) *AORN Journal* 51 (June 1990) 1606-1612.

3. J Zuffoletto, "Nurses' vs surgeons' responsibility for sponge counts," (OR Nursing Law) *AORN Journal* 57 (June 1993) 1457-1458.

4. ECRI, "Sponge and instrument counts," (Risk Analysis, Surgery and Anesthesia 5) *Healthcare Risk Control* 4 (January 1996) 1-9.

5. A A Gwande et al, "Patient safety: Risk factors for retained instruments and sponges after surgery," *The New England Journal of Medicine* 348 (January 2003) 229-235.

6. E K Murphy, "'Captain of the ship' doctrine continues to take on water," (OR Nursing Law) *AORN Journal* 74 (October 2001) 525-528.

7. "Surgical nurses: Sponge count is strictly nurses' responsibility, court rules," *Legal Eagle Eye Newsletter for the Nursing Profession* 8 (September 2000) 2.

8. *Golinski v Hackensack Medical Center, Conley, Irani, Archer, Bruno, and Del Rosario,* 298 NJ Super 650; 690 A2d 147; 1997 NJ Super (New Jersey, 1997).

9. *Stafford v Molinoff and Halfen,* 228 AD2d 662; 645 NYS2d 313; 1996 NY App Div (New York, 1996).

10. *Ravi v Vaughn and Foxworthy v Athens-Limestone Hospital v Coates,* 662 So2d 218; 1995 (Alabama, 1995).

11. L E Rozovsky, F A Rozovsky, "The surgeon and the nurse share the blame: A case of a retained sponge," *Canadian Operating Room Nursing Journal* 9 (September/October 1991) 20-21.

12. A D Tammelleo, ed, "The surgeon's nondelegable responsibility for the sponge count," *The Regan Report on Nursing Law* 38 (July 1997) 2.

13. S C Beyea, "Counting instruments and sponges," (Patient Safety First) *AORN Journal* 78 (August 2003) 290-294.

14. J K Cherry, "Surgery: Foreign object retention," The Doctors Company, *http://www.thedoctors.com/risk /specialty/generalsurgery/J4219.asp* (accessed 8 Sept 2005).

15. E K Murphy, "Nurses' liability for inaccurate counts," (OR Nursing Law) *AORN Journal* 51 (April 1990) 1067-1069.

16. E K Murphy, "Liability for inaccurate counts; assistant circulators," (OR Nursing Law) *AORN Journal* 53 (January 1991) 157-161.

17. Institute of Medicine, *Crossing the Quality Chasm: A New Health System for the 21st Century* (Washington, DC: National Academy Press, 2001).

18. C W Kaiser et al, "The retained surgical sponge," *Annals of Surgery* 224 (July 1996) 79-84.

19. V C Gibbs, "Did we forget something? Retained surgical sponge," AHRQ Web M&M: Case and Commentary, *http://www.webmm.ahrq.gov/case.aspx ?caseID=27&searchStr=%22 retained+surgical+sponge %22+AND+Gibbs* (accessed 8 Sept 2005).

20. P R Lauwers, R H Van Hee, "Intraperitoneal gossypibomas: The need to count sponges," *World Journal of Surgery* 24 (May 2000) 512-527.

21. A P Zbar et al, "Gossypiboma revisited: A case report and review of the literature," *Journal of the Royal*

College of Surgeons of Edinburgh 43 (December 1998) 417-418.

22. B A Hemelt, M A Finan, "Abdominal sacral colpopexy resulting in a retained sponge: A case report," *The Journal of Reproductive Medicine* 44 (November 1999) 983-985.

23. S R Kim, H K Baik, Y W Park, "Retained surgical sponge presenting as a pelvic tumor after 25 years," *International Journal of Gynecology and Obstetrics* 82 (August 2003) 223-225.

24. H Nomori et al, "Retained sponge after thoracotomy that mimicked aspergilloma," *Annals of Thoracic Surgery* 61 (May 1996) 1535-1536.

25. J S Dhillon, A Park, "Transmural migration of a retained laparotomy sponge," *The American Surgeon* 68 (July 2002) 603-605.

26. R J Cruz et al, "Intracolonic obstruction induced by a retained surgical sponge after trauma laparotomy," (Case Reports) *Journal of Trauma* 55 (November 2003) 989-991.

27. R S McLeod, J M Bohnen, "Canadian Association of General Surgeons evidence based reviews in surgery 9: Risk factors for retained foreign bodies after surgery," *Canadian Journal of Surgery* 47 (February 2004) 57-59.

28. T Eskreis-Nelson, "Medical errors and the need for nurses' continuing education," (Nursing Case Law Update) *Journal of Nursing Law* 7 (2000) 49-59.

29. New York State Department of Health, "Retained surgical sponges," New York Patient Occurrence Reporting and Tracking System, *NYPORTS News & Alert* 11 (September 2002). Also available at *http://www.health.state .ny.us/nysdoh/hospital/nyports/annual_report/2000-2001 /news _and_alerts.htm* (accessed 8 Sept 2005).

30. D Fogg, "Retrieving flash sterilized items; occupational exposure to bloodborne pathogens; sponge, needle, and instrument counts," (Clinical Issues) *AORN Journal* 55 (April 1992) 1091-1093.

31. J Reason, "Safety in the operating theater—Part 2: Human error and organisational failure," *Quality and Safety in Health Care* 14 (February 2005) 56-60. Also available at *http://qhc.bmjjournals.com/cgi/search?and orexact- fulltext=and&resourcetype=1&disp _type=&sortspec =relevance&author1=reason&fulltext=&volume=14 &firstpage=* (accessed 8 Sept 2005).

32. ECRI, "Retained foreign object: Surgeon admits liability," *Operating Room Risk Management* (March 2003) 15-16.

33. R Gencosmanoglu, R Inceoglu, "An unusual cause of small bowel obstruction: Gossypiboma—Case report," *BMC Surgery* 3 (September 2003) 1-6. Also available at *http://www.biomedcentral.com/1471-2482 /3/6* (accessed 8 Sept 2005).

34. ECRI, "Locating 'lost' neurosurgical sponges, (Risk Analysis, Surgery and Anesthesia 5.1) *Healthcare Risk Control* 4 (January 1996) 1-2.

35. S Henry, "Damage control in 2001: Who, when, and how," *Trauma Quarterly* 15 (2002) 121-137.

36. "Recommended practices for environmental cleaning in the surgical practice setting," in *Standards, Recommended Practices, and Guidelines* (Denver: AORN, Inc, 2005) 361-366.

37. "Recommended practices for standard and transmission-based precautions in the perioperative practice setting," *Standards, Recommended Practices, and Guidelines* (Denver: AORN, Inc, 2005) 447-451.

38. Occupational Health and Safety Administration, "Occupational exposure to bloodborne pathogens; needlestick and other sharps injuries; final rule," *Federal Register* 66 (18 Jan 2001) 5317-5325. Also available at *http://www.osha.gov/pls/oshaweb/owadisp.show _document?p_table=FEDERAL _REGISTER&p_id=16265* (accessed 8 Sept 2005).

39. R Berguer, P J Heller, "Preventing sharps injuries in the operating room," *Journal of the American College of Surgeons* 199 (September 2004) 462-467.

40. J Perry, G Parker, J Jagger, "EPINet Report: 2001 percutaneous injury rates," *Advances in Exposure Prevention* 6 no 3 (2003) 32-36.

41. D Fogg, "Gas sterilizing medication; using wall suction for evacuating laser plumes; counting needles in multipacks," (Clinical Issues) *AORN Journal* 52 (August 1990) 408-412.

42. C Peterson, "Rectifying counts; neurostimulators; double gloving; reprocessing single-use devices; simultaneous counting," (Clinical Issues) *AORN Journal* 76 (September 2002) 510-515.

43. C Peterson, "Deep vein thrombosis; neutral zone; circulating and recovering; environmental controls; wound classifications; sterile field," (Clinical Issues) *AORN Journal* 79 (April 2004) 856-864.

44. L E Mendez, C Medina, "Late complication of laparoscopic salpingoophorectomy: Retained foreign body presenting as an acute abdomen," *Journal of the Society of Laparoendoscopic Surgeons* 1 (January/March 1997) 79-81.

45. ECRI, "Safe use and selection of trocars," (Risk Analysis, Surgery and Anesthesia 25) *Healthcare Risk Control* 4 (July 1999) 1-15.

46. E J Thomas, F A Moore, "The missing suction tip," AHRQ Web M&M: Case and Commentary, *http://www .webmm.ahrq.gov/case.aspx?caseID=37&search Str=%22spotlight+cases%22* (accessed 8 Sept 2005).

47. M Milanokov, S Dragan, N Miljkovic, "Broken blade in the knee: A complication of arthroscopic meniscectomy," *Arthroscopy: The Journal of Arthroscopic and Related Surgery* 18 (January 2002) 1-3.

48. A D Tammelleo, "Were nurses liable for clamp left in cardiac patient?" *The Regan Report on Nursing Law* 40 (July 1999) 1.

49. C Smith, "Surgical tools left in five patients," Seattle Post-Intelligencer, 8 Dec 2001, *http://seattlepi .nwsource.com/local/49883_error08.shtml* (accessed 8 Sept 2005).

50. "Recommended practices for cleaning and caring for surgical instruments and powered equipment," in *Standards, Recommended Practices, and Guidelines* (Denver: AORN, Inc, 2005) 395-403.

51. "Recommended practices for cleaning and processing endoscopes and endoscope accessories," in *Standards, Recommended Practices, and Guidelines* (Denver: AORN, Inc, 2005) 341-346.

52. "Retained foreign bodies: Reducing the risks," Self-Insurance Program: Risk Management and Loss Prevention (revised April 2004), University of Florida, *http://www.riskmanagementeducation.com/brochures/Retained%20Foreign%20Bodies.pdf* (accessed 8 Sept 2005).

53. C J Barrow, "Use of x-ray in the presence of an incorrect needle count," (Clinical Innovations) *AORN Journal* 74 (July 2001) 80-81.

54. M D Macilquham, R G Riley, P Grossberg, "Identifying lost surgical needles using radiologic techniques," *AORN Journal* 78 (July 2003) 73-78.

55. B A Liang, "The adverse event of unaddressed medical error: Identifying and filling holes in the healthcare and legal systems," Symposium: Patient Injury, Medical Errors, Liability and Reform, *The Journal of Law, Medicine and Ethics* 29 no 3–4 (Fall/Winter 2001) 346-368.

56. D Dunn, "Incident reports—Their purpose and scope," (Home Study) *AORN Journal* 74 (July 2003) 45-68.

57. H Wald, K G Shojania, "Root cause analysis," in *Making Health Care Safer: A Critical Analysis of Patient Safety Practices,* Agency for Healthcare Research and Quality (Evidence Report/Technology Assessment, Number 43, AHRQ Pub 01-E058). Also available at *http://www.ahrq.gov/clinic/ptsafety/pdf/ptsafety.pdf* (accessed 8 Sept 2005).

58. "Root cause analysis," VA National Center for Patient Safety, *http://www.patientsafety.gov/tools.html* (accessed 8 Sept 2005).

59. ECRI, "Perioperative documentation," (Risk Analysis, Surgery and Anesthesia 7) *Healthcare Risk Control* 4 (January 1996) 1-4.

60. "Recommended practices for documentation of perioperative nursing care," in *Standards, Recommended Practices, and Guidelines* (Denver: AORN, Inc, 2005) 321-323.

RESOURCES

Gic, J A. "Nursing and the law," in *Legal Medicine,* fifth ed (St Louis: Mosby, 2001) 128-136.

O'Connor, A; Coakley, F; Meng, M. "Imaging of retained surgical objects in the abdomen and pelvis," Department of Radiology, University of California, San Francisco, *http://www.radiology.ucsf.edu/instruction/abdominal/abdominal_ret_objects1.shtml* (accessed 8 Sept 2005).

Patterson, P. "How ORs decide when to count instruments," *OR Manager* 16 (April 2000) 1, 10, 12-14.

Rothrock, J C; Smith, D A. "Patient and environmental safety," in *Alexander's Care of the Patient in Surgery,* 12th ed, J C Rothrock, ed (St Louis: Mosby, 2003) 36-38.

Originally published May 1976, *AORN Journal,* as "Standards for sponge, needle, and instrument procedures." Format revision March 1978, July 1982.

Revised March 1984, March 1990.

Revised November 1995; published October 1996, *AORN Journal.*

Revised; published December 1999, *AORN Journal.* Reformatted July 2000.

Revised November 2005; published February 2006, *AORN Journal.*

Recommended Practices for High-Level Disinfection

The following recommended practices were developed by the AORN Recommended Practices Committee and have been approved by the AORN Board of Directors. They were presented as proposed recommended practices for comment to members and others. These recommended practices are effective January 1, 2005.

These recommended practices are intended to be achievable recommendations representing what is believed to be an optimal level of practice. Policies and procedures will reflect variations in practice settings or clinical situations that determine the degree to which recommended practices can be implemented.

AORN recognizes the various settings in which perioperative nurses practice. These recommended practices are intended to guide practice in these settings, including traditional ORs, ambulatory surgical units, physicians' offices, cardiac catheterization suites, endoscopy units, radiology departments, and all other areas where surgical and other invasive procedures may be performed.

Purpose

These recommended practices provide guidance for achieving high-level disinfection of instruments and equipment.

Recommended Practice I

Items to be disinfected should be categorized as critical, semicritical, and noncritical.

1. The Spaulding classification system, developed by Earle Spaulding in 1968, has withstood the passage of time and continues to be used today by infection control practitioners and others to determine the correct processing methods for preparing instruments and other items for patient use. According to the Spaulding system, the level of processing required is based on the nature of the item and the manner in which it is to be used.[1]

2. Items that enter sterile tissue or the vascular system are categorized as critical and should be sterile when used. Examples of critical items include
   - surgical instruments,
   - cutting endoscopic accessories that break the mucosal barrier and the endoscopes through which they are used,

- cardiac and urinary catheters,
- implants,
- needles, and
- ultrasound probes used in sterile body cavities.

   If critical items are contaminated with microorganisms, including bacterial spores, the risk of infection is substantial.[1-3]

   The Spaulding system does not consider problems with processing equipment that may be heat labile (eg, arthroscopic and laparoscopic endoscopes). New technologies make it easier to sterilize heat-labile items. Although sterilization of these endoscopes is preferred, there is no conclusive evidence that sterilization reduces patient infection risk more than high-level disinfection.[3-6] Practitioners affected by this controversy should consult and follow recommendations and guidelines developed by AORN, the Association for Professionals in Infection Control and Epidemiology, Inc (APIC), and the American Society for Gastrointestinal Endoscopy.[7-9] Telescopes are constructed of smooth, easily cleanable surfaces with no internal channels and few irregularities. Cleaning rather than the specific disinfection or sterilization procedure is the major factor determining the success or failure of reprocessing. Unless packaged and sterilized, critical items should be reprocessed immediately before use.

3. Items that come in contact with nonintact skin or mucous membranes are considered semicritical and should receive a minimum of high-level disinfection immediately before use. Examples of semicritical items include
   - respiratory therapy equipment,
   - anesthesia equipment,
   - bronchoscopes, and
   - gastrointestinal endoscopes.

   Unless packaged and sterilized, semicritical items (eg, endoscopes) should be reprocessed immediately before use. These items also may be sterilized. Intact mucous membranes generally provide a barrier to common bacterial spores but not to organisms such as tubercle bacilli and viruses.[1,2] Semicritical devices contaminated with hepatitis B virus (HBV), hepatitis C virus (HCV), HIV, or *Mycobacterium tuberculosis* (TB) should receive a minimum of high-level disinfection.[1] Research has demonstrated that high-level disinfectants inactivate these and other pathogens that may contaminate semicritical devices.[1] This practice is consistent with standard precautions, which presume that all patients potentially are infected.[1]

4. Items that come in contact only with intact skin are categorized as noncritical items and should receive intermediate-level disinfection, low-level disinfection, or cleaning. Examples of noncritical items include

   ♦ tourniquets and blood pressure cuffs,
   ♦ linens, and
   ♦ Mayo stands and other OR furnishings.

   Intact skin acts as an effective barrier to most organisms.[1]

5. Guidelines from APIC for inactivation of the Creutzfeldt-Jakob disease (CJD) agent should be observed.[10] When possible, disposable supplies should be used if a patient is thought to be infected with the CJD agent.[1] Critical and semicritical items or surfaces contaminated with the CJD agent require unique decontamination procedures because of an extremely resistant subpopulation of prions.[8] Although some discrepancies exist between studies, all studies show that these prions resist normal inactivation methods. Noncritical patient care items and surfaces have not been implicated in disease transmission.[1]

Recommended Practice II

Items should be thoroughly cleaned and decontaminated before disinfection.

1. Meticulous cleaning and decontamination should precede disinfection procedures. Particular attention should be given to complex medical devices with multiple pieces (eg, endoscopes) that have crevices, joints, lumens, ports, and channels because they are difficult to clean.[3] Cleaning and decontamination are the initial and most critical steps in breaking the chain of disease transmission. Debris, blood, mucous, fat, tissue, and organic matter will interfere with the action of the disinfectant. Microbial biofilms, collections of bacteria, and fungi existing in a multicellular matrix adhere to each other or to medical devices, particularly those with lumens, where they affect tissues

adjacent to virtually any medical device. Biofilms, as nidi of contamination, are difficult to remove and may serve as sources of bacterial toxin that can affect remote locations in the body. Friction or oxidizing chemicals must be used to remove biofilms. Initiating cleaning immediately after use reduces or eliminates the growth of biofilm-forming microorganisms.[11]

Adherence to a written cleaning protocol results in consistency of practice and facilitates the disinfection process.[3,8,12] According to the US Food and Drug Administration (FDA), manufacturers are obliged to provide users with adequate instructions for the safe and effective use of an instrument or device, including methods to clean and disinfect or sterilize the item if it is marked as reusable.[13,14]

2. Instruments to be disinfected should be cleaned according to AORN's "Recommended practices for cleaning and caring for surgical instruments and powered equipment"[15] and "Recommended practices for cleaning and processing endoscopes and endoscope accessories."[8] Cleaning processes to consider include

   ♦ pretreating with enzymatic agents;
   ♦ manual cleaning; and
   ♦ automated cleaning (eg, use of ultrasonic cleaner, washer/decontaminator, washer/sterilizer).

   Enzymatic pretreatment softens and breaks down dried blood and other organic material, but it does not decontaminate items. Cleaning physically removes deposits that were softened by the pretreatment. Detergents suited for manual cleaning have a neutral pH of seven and loosen and suspend soil when friction is applied. Ultrasonic cleaning uses cavitation to remove soil and foreign matter from hard-to-clean crevices, teeth, box-locks, and hinged areas.[12] Washer/decontaminators clean by spray force action and heat. Washer/sterilizers clean with a series of washes and rinses, followed by a steam sterilization cycle appropriate to load contents. More alkaline, low-sudsing detergents are used with automated equipment to compensate for the lack of friction and still loosen soil. Not all cleaning processes render items safe to handle after cleaning. Appropriate personal protective equipment (PPE) should be worn.

3. Chemicals used for cleaning and decontamination should be labeled for the cleaning process used and be
    ♦ able to breakdown organic and inorganic materials,
    ♦ able to prevent waterborne deposits,
    ♦ low foaming,
    ♦ free rinsing, and
    ♦ compatible with materials to be cleaned/decontaminated.[1,6]
    Organic and inorganic soils prevent contact of the disinfectant with all surfaces. Hard water ions (eg, calcium, magnesium) can cause deposits or scale formation. Excessive foaming does not produce the proper force of detergent solution impingement and may clog water pumps. Chemical manufacturers should supply data on standardized corrosion tests to determine material compatibility. Free rinsing is necessary to prevent residues from cleaning chemicals from remaining on instruments.[12]

4. Manufacturers' written instructions for use of chemical cleaners should be followed. Temperature, proper use, and dilution are important for efficient use of these products.[1,3,5]

5. Following the cleaning process, instruments should be rinsed and dried before being subjected to the disinfection process. Rinsing removes residual detergent from instruments and equipment. Drying prevents dilution of the disinfectant when instruments are placed in the solution and permits direct contact of all surfaces by the disinfectant.[1,3]

Recommended Practice III

Pasteurization should be used to achieve thermal high-level disinfection.

1. Items to be high-level disinfected using pasteurization should be placed inside the washer/pasteurizer chamber according to the manufacturer's written instructions. Medical washer/pasteurizers have wash, rinse, and pasteurization cycles. The wash cycle is accomplished either through a horizontal agitation method or a vertical rotational method, depending on the manufacturer's specifications, using warm water and detergent cleaning solution. The length of this cycle is determined by the manufacturer's written

instructions. At the conclusion of the wash and rinse cycles, the tank automatically drains in preparation for the pasteurization cycle. Pasteurization is achieved by immersing all devices in a hot water bath heated to 140° F to 212° F (60° C to 100° C) and held for 30 minutes.[16] Medical washer/pasteurizers may offer quality assurance data recorders that document the temperature of the pasteurizing bath and cycle time.

2. After processing, hang endoscopes in a vertical position to facilitate drying.[8]

Recommended Practice IV

An FDA-cleared agent should be used to achieve chemical high-level disinfection of medical devices.

1. Chemical high-level disinfection should be achieved by immersing an item for a specified period of time in a chemical agent that has been cleared by the FDA as a high-level disinfectant. These agents also are called chemical germicides. The FDA has primary responsibility for premarket review of safety and efficacy requirements for liquid chemical germicides intended for use on critical and semicritical devices.[9] A list of products that have been cleared for marketing by the FDA can be found on the FDA Center for Devices and Radiologic Health (CDRH) web site at http://www.fda.gov/cdrh/ode/germlab.html.[17]

2. Factors that influence efficacy of a chemical agent include, but may not be limited to,
    ♦ organic load present on the items to be disinfected;
    ♦ type and level of microbial contamination;
    ♦ precleaning, rinsing, and drying of the items before disinfection;
    ♦ active ingredients of the chemical agent;
    ♦ concentration of the chemical agent;
    ♦ exposure time to the chemical agent;
    ♦ physical configuration of the item;
    ♦ temperature and pH of the chemical agent;
    ♦ inorganic matter present;
    ♦ water hardness; and
    ♦ presence of surfactants.

3. Agents selected for chemical disinfection should be efficacious and compatible with the materials or items to be disinfected. Many disinfectants

are used in the practice setting (eg, glutaraldehyde, stabilized hydrogen peroxide, peracetic acid, orthophthalaldehyde). These agents are not interchangeable.[18] Items may be damaged by incompatible agents. An ideal high-level disinfectant should

- possess a broad spectrum of antimicrobial effectiveness,
- demonstrate rapid activity,
- possess material compatibility,
- be nontoxic,
- be odorless,
- have no disposal restrictions,
- possess prolonged reuse and shelf life,
- be easy to use,
- demonstrate resistance to organic material,
- be able to be monitored for concentration, and
- be cost effective.[17]

Emerging pathogens, such as *Cryptosporidium parvum,* human papilloma virus, rotavirus, Norwalk virus, *Helicobacter pylori, Escherichia coli 0157:H7,* multidrug-resistant TB, and nontuberculous mycobacteria (*M chelonae),* and prions are a growing concern for members of the public and infection control professionals. The susceptibility of each of these pathogens has been studied, and with the exception of *C parvum* and prions, all are susceptible to available chemical disinfectants and chemical sterilants.[5,19] Glutaraldehyde-resistant strains of *M chelonae* have been isolated in some automated endoscope reprocessors but have been found to be sensitive to other high-level disinfectants, such as orthophthaldehyde.[20,21]

4. Manufacturers' written instructions should be followed when preparing disinfectant solutions and calculating expiration dates. Most chemical disinfectants are effective for only a specific period of time.[18] Labels should indicate clearly the appropriate time for discarding solutions that may no longer be effective. Manufacturers' written instructions about the type of container used should be followed to ensure no interaction occurs between the container and the active ingredients of the disinfectant.[18]

5. A test strip or other FDA-cleared testing device specific for the disinfectant and minimum effective concentration (MEC) of the active ingredient should be used according to the manufacturer's written instructions for monitoring solution potency.[13,18] Testing devices may be available from manufacturers of individual products. If a solution falls below its MEC, it should be discarded, even if the designated expiration date has not been reached.

6. Items to be chemically disinfected should be completely immersed in the disinfectant solution according to manufacturers' written instructions and consistent with established infection control practice. Lumens and ports should be flushed and filled with the disinfectant and the entire item completely immersed for the designated exposure time. Disinfection of all surfaces can be achieved only if all surfaces of the items are in constant contact with the disinfecting solution. Flushing lumens and ports eliminates air pockets and facilitates contact of the disinfectant with internal channels.[1,3,5] Consult manufacturers' written instructions. If an automated endoscopic reprocessor (AER) is to be used for high-level disinfection, the AER manufacturer's written instructions should be congruent with the endoscope manufacturer's written instructions, or the endoscope should not be processed in the AER.

7. After being exposed to the disinfectant solution for the required exposure time, critical and semicritical items should be thoroughly rinsed with water according to the manufacturer's written instructions. Rinsing removes toxic and irritating residues that can result in tissue damage or staining.[19,21] Rinsing semicritical items with sterile water prevents potential recontamination that could result from tap water.[1] Semicritical items to be stored should be rinsed with either sterile water or tap water, followed by an alcohol rinse and forced-air drying. Use of an alcohol rinse and forced-air drying greatly reduces the possibility of contamination.[7] Endoscopes should be hung in a vertical position in a ventilated cabinet to facilitate drying and not stored in cases that cannot be cleaned and disinfected or sterilized.[7] Endoscopes that are packaged and sterilized should be reprocessed immediately before use.

8. Disposal of chemical disinfectants should be done in accordance with federal, state, and local regulations. State and local regulations may be more stringent than those imposed at

the federal level.[18] Personnel should know their obligations under state laws and local ordinances and use appropriate PPE when disposing of high-level disinfectants.

Recommended Practice V

Transportation of disinfected medical devices should be controlled.

1. Written policies and procedures should be in place to designate how critical and semicritical items are transported from the area where disinfection takes place to the point of use in patient care areas. Disinfected items should be transported to the point of use in a manner that preserves the processed status of the items.

Recommended Practice VI

A quality-control program should be established.

1. Documentation of high-level disinfection of medical devices should include, but not be limited to,
   ♦ date and time disinfection was performed;
   ♦ type of disinfectant used;
   ♦ test results indicating the solution used was at the proper concentration and within the expiration date;
   ♦ temperature of the disinfectant;
   ♦ load contents;
   ♦ submersion time;
   ♦ verification of rinsing of the disinfected item;
   ♦ name of the individual performing disinfection, rinsing, and transport; and
   ♦ a patient identifier, when applicable.[1,12,18]

2. Quality-control programs should be documented and should include, but not be limited to,
   ♦ orientation programs;
   ♦ competency assurance;
   ♦ continuing education;
   ♦ quality-control checks;
   ♦ investigation of adverse events, including outbreaks and exposures; and
   ♦ monitoring of solution replacement intervals.

Recommended Practice VII

Practice settings should provide a safe environment for personnel who are using chemical disinfectants.

1. Chemical disinfectants should be kept in covered containers with tight-fitting lids and used in well-ventilated areas according to manufacturers' written instructions and federal, state, and local regulations. Vapor generated from glutaraldehyde can be irritating to the respiratory tract and may aggravate pre-existing respiratory conditions. Glutaraldehyde should be used in well-ventilated areas or in freestanding or vented chemical fume hoods. The American Conference of Governmental Industrial Hygienists (ACGIH) recommends a ceiling limit of 0.05 parts per million (ppm) for occupational exposure to glutaraldehyde vapors. The Occupational Safety and Health Administration (OSHA) has established occupational exposure limits for several agents. No exposure limits have been established by OSHA for glutaraldehyde; however, OSHA can regulate exposure to glutaraldehyde and has recommended that the ACGIH limits be followed.[22]

2. Employers must provide employees with the information and training needed to protect themselves from chemical hazards in the workplace according to federal standards.[22] Employers must provide a written hazard communication program, hazard evaluation, hazardous materials inventory, materials safety data sheet (MSDS), labels on all containers of hazardous chemicals, and employee training. Employee training includes an explanation of the standard, identification of hazards and health effects, location of the written hazard communication program and MSDS, procedures to detect and measure contaminants, safe work practices, appropriate PPE, an explanation of labeling, and locations of spill kits and eyewash stations[7,22] in accordance with employees' right to know about hazards in the workplace.

3. The latest revision of the MSDS must be maintained on site and be readily accessible to personnel when they are in their work areas.[22] The MSDS provides users with valuable information abut toxicity, reactivity, required protective equipment and apparel, storage, and disposal of the material.[18]

4. When using chemical disinfectants, personnel should wear protective apparel that may include
   ♦ eyewear (eg, goggles, face shields);
   ♦ nitrile or butyl rubber gloves;

♦ masks (ie, to prevent contact with skin and not inhalation of fumes); and

♦ moisture-repellent or splash-proof skin protection (eg, gowns, jumpsuits, aprons).[23]

Chemical disinfectants can irritate or stain skin and mucous membranes.[19,21] Use of protective apparel decreases the potential for exposure to the chemical agent.[18]

Recommended Practice VIII

Policies and procedures for high-level disinfection should be written, reviewed periodically, and readily available in the practice setting.

1. These recommended practices should be used to guide policy and procedure development addressing high-level disinfection within the practice setting. Policies and procedures establish authority, responsibility, and accountability and serve as operational guidelines.

2. Introduction to and review of policies and procedures should be included in the orientation and ongoing education of personnel to help develop knowledge, skills, and attitudes that affect patient care and occupational safety. Policies and procedures also may guide performance improvement activities.

Glossary

Automated endoscope reprocessor (AER): A unit for mechanical cleaning, disinfecting, and rinsing of flexible endoscopes.

Bioburden: The microbiologic load or the number of contaminating organisms in the product before sterilization.[16]

Biofilm: A microbial mass attached to a surface in a liquid.

Cavitation: A process by which high-frequency energy causes microscopic bubbles to form, become unstable, and implode, thus creating minute vacuum areas that draw particles of debris from crevices in instruments.[12]

Chemical disinfectant/germicide: A generic term for a government-registered agent that destroys microorganisms. Germicides are classified as sporicides, general disinfectants, sanitizers, and others.

Critical item: Instruments or other objects that are introduced directly into the human body either into or in contact with the bloodstream or normally sterile areas of the body.

Decontamination: Any physical or chemical process that serves to reduce the number of microorganisms on any inanimate object to render that object safe for subsequent handling.

Disinfection: A process that destroys some forms of microorganisms, excluding bacterial spores.

Free-rinsing: Ability to be removed without leaving residue.

High-level disinfection: A process that destroys all microorganisms with the exception of some bacterial spores. High-level disinfectants have the capability of inactivating HBV, HCV, HIV, and TB. High-level disinfectants do not inactivate the virus-like prion thought to cause CJD.

Hospital disinfectant: A chemical germicide with label claims for effectiveness against *Salmonella, Staphylococcus,* and *Pseudomonas.* Hospital disinfectants may be low-, intermediate-, or high-level disinfectants.

Intermediate-level disinfection: A process that inactivates *Mycobacterium tuberculosis,* vegetative bacteria, most viruses, and most fungi but does not necessarily kill bacterial spores.

Low-level disinfection: A process that kills most bacteria, some viruses, and some fungi but that cannot be relied on to kill resistant microorganisms, such as tubercle bacilli or bacterial spores.

Minimum effective concentration: The minimum concentration of a liquid chemical germicide that achieves the claimed microbicidal activity as determined by dose-response testing.

Nidus; pl nidi: A focus of infection; or the coalescence of small particles that is the beginning of a solid deposit.

Noncritical: Instruments or items that come in contact with the patient but, in most instances, only with unbroken skin.

Pasteurization: A process developed by Louis Pasteur of heating milk, wine, or other liquids to between 140° F and 212° F (60° C to 100° C) for approximately 30 minutes to kill or significantly reduce the number of pathogenic and spoilage organisms.[16]

Personal protective equipment (PPE): Specialized equipment or clothing used by health care workers to protect themselves from direct exposure to patients' blood, tissue, or body fluids that may be infectious. Personal protective equipment may include gloves, gowns, liquid-resistant aprons, head and foot coverings, face shields or masks, eye protection, and ventilation devices (eg, mouthpieces, respirator bags, pocket masks).

NOTES

1. W A Rutala, "APIC guideline for selection and use of disinfectants," *American Journal of Infection Control* 24 (August 1996) 313-342.

2. J J Perkins, *Principles and Methods of Sterilization in Health Sciences*, second ed (Springfield, Ill: Charles C. Thomas, 1980) 328-329.

3. M S Favaro, W W Bond, "Chemical disinfection of medical and surgical materials," in *Disinfection, Sterilization, and Preservation*, fifth ed, S S Block ed (Philadelphia: Lippincott Williams & Wilkins, 2001) 881-917.

4. A E Cowen, "The clinical risks of infection associated with endoscopy," *Canadian Journal of Gastroenterology* 15 (May 2001) 321-331.

5. W A Rutala, D J Weber, "Disinfection of endoscopes: Review of new chemical sterilants used for high-level disinfection," *Infection Control and Hospital Epidemiology* 20 (January 1999) 69-76.

6. D W Hobson, L A Seal, "Evaluation of a novel, rapid-acting sterilizing solution at room temperature," *American Journal of Infection Control* 29 (October 2000) 370-375.

7. C J Alvarado, M Reichelderfer, "APIC guideline for infection prevention and control in flexible endoscopy," *American Journal of Infection Control* 28 (April 2000) 138-155.

8. "Recommended practices for cleaning and processing endoscopes and endoscope accessories," in *Standards, Recommended Practices, and Guidelines* (Denver: AORN, Inc, 2004) 261-266.

9. D B Nelson et al, "Multi-society guideline for reprocessing flexible gastrointestinal endoscopes," *Infection Control and Hospital Epidemiology* 24 (July 2003) 532-537.

10. W A Rutala, D J Weber, "Creutzfeldt-Jakob disease: Recommendations for disinfection and sterilization," *Healthcare Epidemiology* 32 (May 1, 2001) 1348-1356.

11. D W Morck, M E Olson, H Ceri, "Microbial biofilms: Prevention, control, and removal," in *Disinfection, Sterilization, and Preservation*, fifth ed, S S Block ed (Philadelphia: Lippincott Williams & Wilkins, 2001) 675-683.

12. American Society for Healthcare Central Service Professionals of the American Hospital Association, *Training Manual for Health Care Central Service Technicians* (San Francisco: Jossey-Bass, 2001) 61-173.

13. C S Lin, J Fuller, E S Mayhall, "Federal regulation of liquid chemical germicides by the US Food and Drug Administration," in *Disinfection, Sterilization, and Preservation*, fifth ed, S S Block ed (Philadelphia: Lippincott Williams & Wilkins, 2001) 1293-1301.

14. "Procedures for performance standards development" in *Code of Federal Regulations (CFR)* 21: Food and Drugs, Part 861 (Washington, DC: US Government Printing Office, 2004) 176-178.

15. "Recommended practices for cleaning and caring for surgical instruments and powered equipment," in *Standards, Recommended Practices, and Guidelines* (Denver: AORN, Inc, 2004) 309-317.

16. S S Block, "Definition of terms" in *Disinfection, Sterilization, and Preservation*, fifth ed, SS Block ed (Philadelphia: Lippincott Williams & Wilkins, 2001) 19-28.

17. "Device evaluation information: FDA-cleared sterilants and high-level disinfectants with general claims for processing reusable medical and dental devices, March 2003)," US Food and Drug Administration, Center for Devices and Radiological Health, *http://www.fda.gov/cdrh/ode/germlab.html* (accessed 25 Aug 2004).

18. *Chemical Sterilants and High-level Disinfectants: A Guide to Selection and Use* (Arlington, Va: Association for the Advancement of Medical Instrumentation, 2000) 1-38.

19. S Fraud, J Y Maillard, A D Russell, "Comparison of the mycobactericidal activity of orthophthaldehyde, gluteraldehyde and other dialdehydes by a quantitative suspension test," *Journal of Hospital Infection* 48 (July 2001) 214-221.

20. G McDonnell, D Pretzer, "New and developing antimicrobials," in *Disinfection, Sterilization, and Preservation*, fifth ed, SS Block ed (Philadelphia: Lippincott Williams & Wilkins, 2001) 431-443.

21. W A Rutala, D J Weber, "New disinfection and sterilization methods," *Emerging Infectious Diseases* 7 (March/April 2001) 348-353.

22. Occupational Safety and Health Administration, Department of Labor, "Toxic and hazardous substances, hazard communication standard," Title 29 6, Parts 1910.1000 to end, 29CFR1910.1200 (Washington, DC: US Government Printing Office, July 1, 1999) 461-469.

23. "Hospital eTool—HealthCare wide hazards module: Glutaraldehyde," US Department of Labor, Occupational Safety and Health Administration, *http://www.osha.gov/SLTC/etools/hospital/hazards/glutaraldehyde/glut.html* (accessed 25 Aug 2004).

RESOURCES

Phillips, N F. *Berry & Kohn's Operating Room Technique*, 10th ed (St Louis: Mosby, 2004).

Rothrock, J C ed. *Alexander's Care of the Patient in Surgery*, 12th ed (St Louis: Mosby-Year Book, 2003).

Originally published August 1980, *AORN Journal*, as AORN "Recommended practices for sterilization and disinfection."

Format revision July 1982; revised February 1987.

Revised October 1992 as "Recommended practices for disinfection"; published as proposed recommended practices September 1994 as "Recommended practices for chemical disinfection."

Revised November 1998 as "Recommended practices for high-level disinfection"; published March 1999, *AORN Journal.*

Revised November 2004; published February 2005, *AORN Journal.*

Recommended Practices for Documentation of Perioperative Nursing Care

The following recommended practices were developed by the AORN Recommended Practices Committee and have been approved by the AORN Board of Directors. They were presented as proposed recommended practices for comment by members and others. They are effective January 1, 2000.

These recommended practices are intended as achievable recommendations representing what is believed to be an optimal level of practice. Policies and procedures will reflect variations in practice settings and/or clinical situations that determine the degree to which the recommended practices can be implemented.

AORN recognizes the numerous types of settings in which perioperative nurses practice. These recommended practices are intended as guidelines adaptable to various practice settings. These practice settings include traditional ORs, ambulatory surgery units, physicians' offices, cardiac catheterization suites, endoscopy suites, radiology departments, and all other areas where operative and other invasive procedures may be performed.

Purpose

These recommended practices provide guidelines to assist perioperative nurses in documenting nursing care in the perioperative practice setting. Documentation using the nursing process should be completed for each surgical and other invasive procedure. The nursing process is a formalized systematic approach to providing and documenting patient care. Perioperative documentation is essential for the continuity of goal-directed care and for comparing achieved patient outcomes to expected patient outcomes.

Recommended Practice I

The patient's record should reflect the perioperative patient's plan of care, including assessment, diagnosis, outcome identification, planning, implementation, and evaluation.

1. Documentation should include information about the status of the patient, nursing diagnoses and interventions, expected patient outcomes, and evaluation of the patient's response to perioperative nursing care. The nursing process provides the governing framework for documenting perioperative nursing care. When the nursing process is used in perioperative practice settings, it demonstrates the critical-

thinking skills practiced by the nurse in caring for the surgical patient.[1]

2. The patient's record should reflect an assessment (ie, physical, psychosocial, cultural, spiritual) performed by the perioperative nurse before surgical or other invasive procedures. A documented assessment forms a baseline for developing nursing diagnoses and planning patient care. Continuing this assessment throughout each subsequent phase of the patient's care (ie, intraoperative, postoperative) contributes to continuity of care.[2]

3. The patient's record should reflect the plan of care. The planning process begins when the perioperative nurse identifies nursing interventions that will address the patient's actual or potential risk for health problems (ie, nursing diagnoses). Documentation facilitates communication among health care team members, promotes continuity of care, and serves as a legal record of care provided.[3] Identifying desired patient outcomes that are individualized, prioritized, measurable, realistic, and obtainable aids in developing the plan of care.[4]

4. The patient's record should specify what nursing interventions were performed and when, where, and by whom during each phase of perioperative care.[5] The implementation process is a result of assessment and planning using nursing judgment and critical thinking skills. The goals of nursing interventions are to prevent potential patient injury or complications and to intervene/treat actual patient problems. Documenting nursing interventions promotes continuity of patient care and improves communication between health care team members.[6]

5. The patient's record should reflect a continuous evaluation of perioperative nursing care and the patient's response to applied nursing interventions. The nursing process directs perioperative nurses to evaluate the effectiveness of nursing interventions toward attaining desired patient outcomes. The evaluation process provides information for continuity of care, performance improvement activities, perioperative nursing research, and risk management. Documentation provides a mechanism for comparing actual versus expected outcomes.[7]

6. Perioperative documentation should include, but not be limited to,

- identification of persons providing perioperative patient care (ie, name, title, signature of person responsible for the care);
- description of patient's overall skin condition on arrival and discharge from the perioperative suite;
- perioperative patient care planning, including baseline physical, emotional, psychosocial, and cultural data;
- presence and/or disposition of sensory aids and prosthetic devices (eg, eyewear, hearing aids, denture, artificial limbs);
- placement of electrosurgical unit (ESU) dispersive pad and identification of the ESU and setting used during the surgical procedure;
- use of temperature-regulating devices, including identification of the unit and documentation of the patient's body temperature before and after discharge from the perioperative suite;
- placement of electrocardiogram electrodes, blood pressure cuff, oximetry and temperature probes, and other invasive and monitoring devices;
- patient positioning and/or repositioning devices and supports, including immobilization devices used during the surgical procedure;
- placement of tourniquet cuffs, including identification of the unit, pressure settings, and inflation and deflation times;
- location of skin prep, including prep solution used;
- use of lasers, including identification of the unit, name of surgeon and support staff members, type of laser used, surgical procedure, the lens used, length of time laser was used, and the wattage;
- use of intraoperative x-rays and fluoroscopy and protective devices used (if any);
- patient specimens and cultures taken during the surgical procedure;
- location and type of drains, catheters, wound packing, casting material, and dressings used;
- placement and location of implants (eg, medical devices, synthetic and biologic grafts, tissue, bone), including the name of the manufacturer or distributor, lot and serial numbers, type and size of implant, and expiration dates as appropriate, and other information required by the US Food and Drug Administration;
- placement of radioactive implants, including the time, number, location, and type of radioactive material placed in the patient;
- administration of blood or blood products, medications, irrigation solution, and other solutions to the patient during the perioperative period;
- wound classification;
- anesthesia classification and mode of anesthesia provided;
- documentation of sponge, sharp, and instrument count outcomes as appropriate;
- time of patient discharge, patient status at discharge, patient disposition, and method of transfer;
- any significant or unusual occurrences pertinent to perioperative patient outcomes;
- communication with family members or significant others during the surgical procedure; and
- patient/family teaching provided.

Documentation of all nursing activities performed is legally and professionally important for clear communication, collaboration between health care team members, and continuity of patient care.[8]

Recommended Practice II

Policies and procedures for documenting perioperative nursing care should be written, reviewed periodically, revised as necessary, and be readily available within the practice setting.

1. These recommended practices should be used as guidelines for developing policies and procedures for documentation within the perioperative practice setting. Documentation policies and procedures establish authority, responsibility, and accountability and serve as operational guidelines. An introduction and review of documentation policies and procedures should be included in the orientation and ongoing education of personnel to assist them in obtaining knowledge and developing skills and competencies that will influence perioperative patient outcomes.

2. Every perioperative practice setting uses a formal system of documentation of patient care. Although the method of documenting perioperative nursing care varies among practice settings, documentation forms should include, but not be limited to, the following:

- ◆ operative record,
- ◆ preoperative patient checklist,
- ◆ nurses' notes,
- ◆ flow sheets,
- ◆ care plans,
- ◆ implant records, and
- ◆ laser logs.

The methods selected for documenting perioperative nursing care will be based on the facility's overall philosophy of documentation and record keeping.

NOTES

1. C S Ladden, "Concepts basic to perioperative nursing," in *Alexander's Care of the Patient in Surgery,* 11th ed, M H Meeker, J C Rothrock, eds (St Louis: Mosby, Inc, 1999) 7, 12-13; J Gill et al, "Incorporating nursing diagnosis and King's theory in the OR documentation," *Canadian Operating Room Nursing Journal* (March/April 1995) 10-11; K Blais, "Perioperative nursing process," in *Perioperative Nursing Principles and Practice,* second ed, S S Fairchild, ed (Boston: Little, Brown & Co, 1996) 271-272, 284; L J Atkinson, N H Fortunato, *Berry & Kohn's Operating Room Technique,* eighth ed (St Louis: Mosby-Year Book, Inc, 1996) 23, 53, 437, 447.

2. Ladden, "Concepts basic to perioperative nursing," 12; Gill et al, "Incorporating nursing diagnosis and King's theory in the OR documentation," 10-14; J Palmerini, "Developing a comprehensive perioperative nursing documentation form," *AORN Journal 63* (January 1996) 239-247; Blais, "Perioperative nursing process," 271-272, 274; L C A Simunek, "Legal and ethical dimensions of perioperative nursing practice," in *Perioperative Nursing Principles and Practice,* second ed, S S Fairchild, ed (Boston: Little, Brown & Co 1996) 390-394; Atkinson, Fortunato, *Berry & Kohn's Operating Room Technique,* 23, 30-31, 53.

3. Atkinson, Fortunato, *Berry & Kohn's Operating Room Technique,* 53-55, 424; Ladden, "Concepts basic to perioperative nursing," 3-19; B J Gruendemann, B Fernsebner, *Comprehensive Perioperative Nursing, Volume I: Principles* (Boston: Jones and Bartlett Publishers, 1995) 95.

4. Ladden, "Concepts basic to perioperative nursing," 8; Blais, "Perioperative nursing process," 271-285; Atkinson, Fortunato, *Berry & Kohn's Operating Room Technique,* 21-31.

5. Gruendemann, Fernsebner, *Comprehensive Perioperative Nursing, Volume I: Principles,* 95, 308; Ladden, "Concepts basic to perioperative nursing," 12; Blais, "Perioperative nursing process," 280; Atkinson, Fortunato, *Berry & Kohn's Operating Room Technique,* 55, 269, 276, 424.

6. Palmerini, "Developing a comprehensive perioperative nursing documentation form," 241; Simunek, "Legal and ethical dimensions of perioperative nursing practice," 391, 394; Atkinson, Fortunato, *Berry & Kohn's Operating Room Technique,* 27-31, 53, 55; S Null, D Richter-Abt, J Kovac, "Development of a perioperative nursing diagnoses flow sheet," *AORN Journal* 61 (March 1995) 57.

7. Gruendemann, Fernsebner, *Comprehensive Perioperative Nursing, Volume I: Principles,* 95; L K Groah, *Perioperative Nursing,* third ed (Stamford, Conn: Appleton & Lange, 1996) 304, 314; Atkinson, Fortunato, *Berry & Kohn's Operating Room Technique,* 24, 30-31, 53, 55, 546; Ladden, "Concepts basic to perioperative nursing," 12, 13; Palmerini, "Developing a comprehensive perioperative nursing documentation form," 241-242; Blais, "Perioperative nursing process," 272, 283.

8. Gruendemann, Fernsebner, *Comprehensive Perioperative Nursing, Volume I: Principles,* 95; Atkinson, Fortunato, *Berry & Kohn's Operating Room Technique,* 55, 424.

Originally published March 1982, *AORN Journal.*
Format revision July 1982.
Revised March 1987.
Revised September 1991.
Revised November 1995; published June 1996.
Revised; scheduled for publication January 2000, *AORN Journal.*
Reformatted July 2000.

Recommended Practices for Electrosurgery

The following recommended practices were developed by the AORN Recommended Practices Committee and have been approved by the AORN Board of Directors. They were presented as proposed recommended practices for comment to members and others. These recommended practices are effective January 1, 2005.

These recommended practices are intended as achievable recommendations representing what is believed to be an optimal level of practice. Policies and procedures will reflect variations in practice settings and/or clinical situations that determine the degree to which the recommended practices can be implemented.

AORN recognizes the various settings in which perioperative nurses practice. These recommended practices are intended as guidelines adaptable to various practice settings. These practice settings include traditional ORs, ambulatory surgery units, physician's offices, cardiac catheterization laboratories, endoscopy suites, radiology departments, and all other areas where surgery may be performed.

Purpose

These recommended practices provide guidance to perioperative nurses in the use and care of electrosurgical equipment. Proper care and handling of electrosurgical equipment is essential to patient and personnel safety. Electrosurgery is used routinely to cut, coagulate, dissect, fulgurate, ablate, and shrink body tissue with high frequency (ie, radio frequency) electrical current. Ultrasonic dissectors dissect tissue by vibration. Vessel sealing devices use a combination of pressure and heat to permanently occlude vessels. These recommended practices address all of these technologies and do not endorse any specific product.

Recommended Practice I

Personnel selecting the electrosurgical unit (ESU) and accessories for purchase or use should make decisions based on safety features to minimize risks to patients and personnel.

1. Equipment selected should include technology to detect stray current that could result in patient injury and to alert the user of this condition. Electrosurgical units are high-risk equipment. Historically, the most frequently reported patient injury

has been a skin injury (eg, burn) at the dispersive electrode site.[1] The risk of this type of injury has been minimized through advances in dispersive pad design (eg, nondrying conductive material, dual-contact dispersive electrodes) and the use of return electrode contact quality monitoring.[2] Minimum safety standards for ESU systems have been developed by the Association for the Advancement of Medical Instrumentation and approved by the American National Standards Institute.[3]

2. Equipment should be designed to minimize the risk of alternate site injuries. These injuries can result from use of ground-referenced (ie, spark-gap) ESUs that allow electrical current to seek alternate pathways to complete the circuit.[3,4] The use of isolated (ie, solid-state) ESUs has minimized this risk.

3. Equipment should be designed to minimize the risk of capacitive coupling injuries. During minimally invasive procedures, alternate site injuries have resulted from insulation failure and capacitive coupling.[4,5-11] These injuries are very serious and have increased in number with the increased use of laparoscopic surgery.[12] The use of active electrode monitoring has minimized these risks.[13-17]

4. Equipment should be designed to minimize unintentional activation that could result in patient and personnel injury. Audible activation tones minimize this risk.[3,18,19]

5. Electrosurgical accessories selected should be compatible with the equipment and other accessories. Injuries have resulted when equipment intended for bipolar use is inserted into monopolar connectors and, subsequently, inadvertently activated.[20] Appropriate matching and use of accessories minimizes this risk.

6. Electrosurgical technology continues to evolve, changing the way in which surgical hemostasis is achieved. It is the responsibility of each facility to stay abreast of evolving technology and its impact on patient care and safety.

Recommended Practice II

Personnel should demonstrate competence in the use of the ESU and accessories.

1. Personnel working with electrosurgery equipment should be knowledgeable about the principles of electrosurgery, risks to patients and personnel, measures to minimize these risks, and corrective actions to employ in the event of a fire or injury. Electrosurgical equipment and accessories have been associated with numerous fires and patient injuries.[1,11,21,22] The National Fire Protection Association has identified ESUs as high-risk equipment, warranting training and retraining of personnel.[23] Personnel should be instructed in the proper operation, care, and handling of the ESU and accessories before use.[23] Initial education on the underlying principles of electrosurgical safety provides direction for personnel in providing a safe environment. Additional, periodic educational programs provide reinforcement of principles of electrosurgery and new information on changes in technology, its application, compatibility of equipment and accessories, and potential hazards.

2. Administrative personnel should assess and document annual competency of personnel in the safe use of the ESU and accessories according to hospital and department policy. Incorrect use can result in serious injury to patients and personnel. A regular competency assessment provides a record that personnel have a basic understanding of electrosurgery, its risks, and appropriate corrective action to take in the event of a fire or injury. This knowledge is essential to minimize the risks of misuse of the equipment and providing a safe environment of care.

Recommended Practice III

The ESU and accessories should be used according to manufacturers' written instructions.

1. Instructions for ESU use, warranties, and a manual for maintenance and inspections should be obtained from the manufacturer and be readily available to users.[23] Equipment manuals assist in developing operational, safety, and maintenance guidelines, as well as serve as a reference for appropriate use.[23]

2. Each type of ESU has specific manufacturer's written operating instructions to be followed for safe operation of the unit. A brief set of clearly readable operating instructions should be readily accessible with each system.[24] These instructions should be placed on or attached to each ESU for reference.

3. Accessories should be used, handled, cleaned, and processed according to manufacturers' instructions.

Recommended Practice IV

The ESU system should be used in a manner that minimizes the potential for injuries.

1. The ESU should be securely mounted on a shelf or tip-resistant cart. The ESU electrical cord should be adequate in length and flexibility to reach the electrical outlet without stress or the use of an extension cord.[25] Applying tension on the electrical cord increases the risk that it will become disconnected, frayed, or move the equipment, which may result in injuries to patients and personnel.

2. The ESU should be tested before initial use, inspected periodically, and receive preventive maintenance by a designated individual responsible for equipment maintenance (eg, bioengineering services personnel).[26] Personnel should visually inspect the ESU and test the return electrode contact monitor before each use (eg, attempt to use the device with the dispersive electrode not connected).[25,27,28] The manufacturer's written precautions should be followed for the safety of the patient and personnel involved in the procedure.

3. An ESU that is not working properly or is damaged should be removed from service immediately and reported to the designated individual responsible for equipment maintenance (eg, bioengineering services personnel). Each ESU should be assigned an identification or serial number. This number allows designated personnel to track function problems and document maintenance performed on individual ESUs.[29]

4. Safety/warning alarms should be operational at all times. Lights should be operational and visible. Audible activation indicator(s) and alarms should be present and loud enough to be heard above other sounds in the OR. The volume of the

activation indicator should be maintained at an audible level to immediately alert personnel when the ESU is activated inadvertently.[3,18,19]

5. The ESU should be protected from spills. Fluids should not be placed on top of the ESU. Fluids entering the ESU can cause unintentional activation or device failure. Liquids seeping into the ESU pose an electrical hazard. Personnel should encase the ESU foot pedal in a clean, impervious cover when there is a potential for fluid spills.

6. The operator should confirm the power settings before activation. Settings should be based upon the manufacturer's written instructions and the intended application. The ESU should be operated at the lowest effective power setting to achieve the desired effect. If the operator requests a continual increase in power, personnel should check the entire ESU and accessories circuit, beginning with checking the dispersive electrode. If a single-use electrode is used, it should be replaced, not repositioned.[30] Prolonged current at high power can cause patient injury. The most common cause for ineffective coagulation and cutting is high impedance at the dispersive electrode.[30] Replacing the dispersive electrode provides an opportunity to examine the electrode and the patient's skin condition.

7. After use, personnel should turn off the ESU, clean all reusable parts, and inspect these parts according to the manufacturer's written instructions.

Recommended Practice V

The electrical cords and plugs of the ESU should be handled in a manner that minimizes the potential for damage and subsequent patient injuries.

1. The ESU should be placed near the sterile field, and the cord should reach the wall or column outlet without stress on the cord and without blocking a traffic path.[25] Stress on the cord may cause damage to the cord, posing an electrical hazard. The cord should be free of kinks, knots, and bends that could damage the cord or cause leakage, current accumulation, and overheating of the cord's insulation.

2. The ESU plug, not the cord, should be held when it is removed from the outlet. Pulling on the cord may cause cord breakage, which poses a fire hazard.

3. The ESU and cord should be kept away from fluids. Fluids dripping into the ESU or connections cause an electrical hazard.

Recommended Practice VI

The active electrode should be used in a manner that minimizes the potential for injuries.

1. The active electrode should be connected directly into a designated receptacle on the ESU. If an adapter is used, it should be approved by the manufacturers of both the ESU and the accessory and not compromise the ESU's safety features. Incomplete circuitry, unintentional activation, and incompatibility of the active electrode to the ESU may result in patient and personnel injuries.[19,20]

2. The active electrode should be visually inspected at the surgical field, before use, to identify any apparent damage to the cord or hand piece (eg, impaired insulation).[25] Insulation failure allows an alternate pathway for current to leave the electrode. Additional information about use of electrosurgery for endoscopic procedures can be found in the AORN "Recommended practices for endoscopic minimally invasive surgery."[31]

3. If securing the active electrode cord to the drapes, plastic or another nonconductive material should be used. The cord should not be coiled. This minimizes the risk of patient or staff member injury from conduction of stray current.

4. Active electrodes should not be used in the presence of flammable agents, including vapors (eg, antimicrobial skin prep or hand antisepsis agents, tinctures, defatting agents, collodian, petroleum-based lubricants, phenol, aerosol adhesives, uncured methyl methacrylate).[29,32] Opened suture packages containing alcohol should be removed from the sterile field as soon as possible.[19,32] Ignition of flammable substances by active electrodes has

caused fires and patient injuries.[19,32-39] Alcohol-based skin prep agents are particularly hazardous because the surrounding hair or fabric can become saturated. Pooling can occur in body folds and crevices (eg, umbilicus, sternal notch). Vapors can become trapped under an incise drape or surgical drapes. This has led to fires and patient injuries.[37-39] Using nonflammable prep agents eliminates this risk.[19,32,34,38]

5. The active electrode should be placed in a clean, dry, well-insulated safety holster when not in use to minimize the risk of injury from unintentional activation. Injuries have resulted when the active electrode has been left lying on the patient between uses.[18] Electrodes that do not fit in the holster should be placed in a designated location with tips away from flammable material (eg, drapes). When battery-powered, hand-held cautery is used, the protective cap should be reapplied when the cautery is not in use, thus preventing inadvertent pressure on the activation button.[40]

6. The active electrode tips should be securely seated into the hand piece. A loose tip may cause a spark or burn to tissue contacting the exposed, noninsulated section of the tip.[41] Tips should be used according to the manufacturer's instructions and not be altered (eg, bent) unless specified by the manufacturer. If insulation is desired, it should be acquired from a medical device manufacturer. Fires and patient injuries have resulted when insulating sheaths have been made from inappropriate material (eg, rubber catheters).[42,43]

7. The active electrode tip should be cleaned frequently, away from the incision, to remove eschar. Eschar buildup on the active electrode tip impedes the desired current flow, causing the entire unit to function less effectively and serving as a fuel source, which can lead to fires.[42] Debris on the electrode tip can tear tissue and cause rebleeding.[1] Abrasive electrode cleaning pads are commercially available for noncoated electrodes. Electrosurgical tips also are available with a special coating that minimizes eschar buildup.

8. Sponges used close to the active electrode tip should be moist to prevent unintentional ignition. Active electrodes should not be cleaned with a dry sponge. Fires have resulted from ignition of dry sponges near the incision site and when they are used to clean the active electrode.[34,44-46]

9. The active electrode should not be used in the presence of intestinal gases. These gases contain hydrogen and methane, which are highly flammable. Fires and patient injuries have occurred.[47-51]

10. The active electrode should not be used in an oxygen-enriched environment.[22,52] Caution should be exercised during surgery on the head and neck near combustible anesthetic gases. The active electrode should be used as far from the oxygen source as possible. The lowest practical level of oxygen should be administered to the patient. When administering oxygen in an open system (eg, nasal prongs), drapes should be tented or a scavenging system used to prevent buildup of oxygen under the drapes. Fires, including airway fires, have resulted from the active electrode sparking in the presence of concentrated oxygen.[22,52-58]

11. If the active electrode is being used in a fluid-filled cavity, the fluid used should be an electrically inert, near isotonic solution (eg, dextran 10, dextran 70, glycine 1.5%, sorbitol, mannitol) unless the manufacturer of the equipment instructs otherwise.[1,59-63] Using an electrolyte solution instead of a nonconductive medium may render the active electrode less effective. Subsequent increases in the power setting have resulted in burns at the dispersive (ie, return) electrode site.[1,64]

12. If the active electrode becomes contaminated, it should be disconnected from the ESU. This minimizes the risk of unintentional activation and reduces the potential for patient and personnel injuries.

13. When battery-powered, hand-held cautery units are used, the batteries should be removed before disposal of the cautery unit. Inadvertent activation after disposal has caused fires.[40,65] Batteries are hazardous waste.

14. Personnel should be prepared to immediately extinguish flames should they occur. Saline or water should be available on the sterile field. A carbon dioxide (CO_2) fire extinguisher should be readily available.[19,66] This type of fire extinguisher

can extinguish fires involving cloth and paper, and it is safe to use in the presence of electrical current. Fire blankets should not be used in the OR.[19] Using a fire blanket on a patient traps the fire around the patient. Fire blankets should be used only on conscious fire victims who can roll and pinpoint the location of the fire under the blanket so responders can extinguish the fire by vigorously patting the blanket at the identified site. If a fire blanket is present in the OR, staff members may assume it is safe for patient use, thereby placing the patient at further risk. Fire blankets will burn if used in oxygen-enriched atmospheres.

Recommended Practice VII

When monopolar electrosurgery is used, a dispersive electrode should be used in a manner that minimizes the potential for injuries.

1. The patient's skin condition should be assessed and documented before and after ESU use. The most frequently reported patient injury from electrosurgery has been tissue damage (eg, burn) at the dispersive electrode site.[25] With advances in technology in return electrode monitors and increased use of laparoscopy, this may be changing to other types of injuries (eg, direct coupling, capacitive coupling); however, burns at the site of the dispersive electrode continue to occur. Preoperative and postoperative assessments allow evaluation of the patient's skin condition for possible injuries.

2. Dispersive electrodes should be compatible with the ESU.

3. Single-use dispersive electrodes should be used according to the manufacturer's written instructions for safe operation; in addition to instructions on the electrode package, additional instructions may be located in the box of electrode packages.

   ◆ Electrodes should be an appropriate size for the patient (eg, neonate, infant, pediatric, adult) and not altered (eg, cut, folded). Using the appropriately sized dispersive electrode is important for preventing patient injuries. Using a large dispersive electrode prevents concentration of current and minimizes the potential for electrosurgical injuries.[28,30]

◆ Personnel should verify that the electrode is intact; conductive gel, if present, is moist; and the manufacturer's expiration date has not been reached.[28,30]

◆ The conductive and adhesive surfaces of the electrode should be placed on clean, dry skin, over a large, well-perfused muscle mass on the surgical side, and close to the surgical site. Muscle is a better conductor of electricity than adipose tissue.[28,30]

◆ Electrodes should not be placed over bony prominences, scar tissue, hairy surfaces, or areas distal to tourniquets and pressure points.[28,30] Fatty tissues, tissue over bone, scar tissue, and hair can impede electrosurgical return current flow. High impedance leads to heating of the tissue, arcing to the tissue under the dispersive electrode, and subsequent burns.[67] Burns have resulted when electrodes have been positioned over hairy surfaces.[68] Hair removal may be necessary. Adequate tissue perfusion cannot be assured if the dispersive electrode is placed distal to tourniquets or over scar tissue.

◆ The electrode should not be placed over an implanted metal prosthesis.[1] The tissue over prostheses contains scar tissue, which impedes return of the electric current. Although there has been no reported injury from superheating of the implant causing a tissue burn, this is a theoretical risk; therefore, it is prudent to avoid placing a dispersive electrode on the patient's skin over the site of a metal implant or prosthesis.

◆ Avoid placing the dispersive electrode over a tattoo, many of which contain metallic dyes. Although there have been no reported electrosurgery injuries from dispersive electrodes placed over tattoos, superheating of the tissue has occurred during magnetic resonance imaging;[69,70] therefore, it is prudent to avoid this site when possible.

◆ The single-use dispersive electrode should maintain uniform body contact. Potential problems include tenting, gaping, and moisture, all of which interfere with adhesion to the patient's skin. Injuries have been associated with inadequate adhesion of the dispersive electrode.[71-73]

◆ The single-use dispersive electrode should be placed on the patient after final positioning for the surgical procedure to prevent buckling of the electrode and to maintain good skin contact with the electrode. If any tension is applied to the dispersive electrode cord or if the surgical team repositions the patient, personnel should reassess the integrity of the dispersive electrode, its contact with the patient's skin, and its connection to the ESU. If the patient is repositioned, personnel should verify that the dispersive electrode remains in full contact with the patient's skin to avoid burns resulting from inadequate contact with the dispersive electrode.

♦ The dispersive electrode should be removed carefully. Skin injuries can result when the adhesive border pulls on the skin during electrode removal.[74] Holding the adjacent skin in place and peeling the dispersive electrode back slowly will avoid denuding the surface of the skin.

4. Large, reusable, capacitive-coupled return electrode systems should be used according to manufacturers' written instructions for safe operation in conjunction with a compatible ESU.

♦ These electrodes are inappropriate for patients under 25 lbs. A patient injury has been reported when the electrode was used on a smaller patient.[75]

♦ When using a reusable, capacitive-coupled return electrode, personnel should ensure adequate contact (ie, weight-bearing area) with the patient and use minimal materials between the pad and patient. Thick foam, gel pads, and extra linen increase the distance between the patient and electrode and should not be used. Some complex patient positioning also decreases contact between the skin and the electrode. Distance and barriers between the patient and electrode increase impedance, which can result in an alternate site injury.[76]

♦ Personnel should verify that no small metal material (eg, snaps on gowns) is in contact with the patient's skin. Current can concentrate at the site of metal contact. Snaps on patient gowns have resulted in patient injuries when the capacitive-coupled return electrode was used.[77]

5. Dispersive electrodes should be kept dry and protected from seeping or pooling of fluids under the dispersive electrode.[30] Liquids may prevent the electrode from adequately contacting the skin. These solutions also can cause skin injury from prolonged skin exposure.

6. There should be no contact between the patient and metal devices that could offer potential alternate return paths for the electrical current (eg, OR beds, stirrups, positioning devices, safety strap buckles). Patient monitoring electrodes (eg, electrocardiogram, oximetry, fetal) should be placed as far away from the surgical site as possible. Alternate pathway burns have been reported at electrocardiogram (ECG) electrode sites and temperature probe entry sites with ground-referenced electrosurgery units.[4]

7. The patient's metal jewelry should be removed if it is within the activation range of the active electrode. Metallic jewelry, including that used in body piercing, presents a potential risk of burn from directed current (ie, active electrode touching it), heat conducted before an electrode cools, and leakage current. Eliminating metal near the activation site minimizes this risk. Although there may be other reasons for removal of all patient jewelry (eg, risk of swelling, theft), the risk of an alternative site injury from stray current is negligible.[78] When using a reusable, capacitive-coupled return electrode, all of the patient's metal jewelry should be removed. Small metal objects touching the return electrode can concentrate current and result in patient injury.[77] Eliminating contact with metal minimizes this risk.

8. If multiple ESUs are used simultaneously during a surgical procedure, the applicable instructions from the manufacturer should be followed. Compatibility of equipment and proper functioning of corresponding electrode monitoring systems should be verified with the manufacturer. Separate dispersive electrodes should be used for each ESU. Personnel should place the dispersive electrodes as close as possible to their respective surgical sites and ensure that single-use dispersive electrodes do not overlap.

9. Two dispersive electrodes should be used in unique situations when high impedance is reasonably anticipated (eg, very obese patients) or

during prolonged application of current at high power settings (eg, ablation).[30,64] Users should refer to the manufacturer's recommendations for these applications.

Recommended Practice VIII

Personnel should take special precautions when using the ESU during endoscopic procedures.

1. Personnel should understand the risks of electrosurgery during endoscopic procedures. Electrosurgical injuries are caused by direct coupling of current, insulation failure, and capacitive coupling. Direct coupling is caused by the surgeon touching the laparoscopic active electrode to another anatomic structure. This can cause necrosis of underlying tissue. Insulation failure of the laparoscopic electrode can be caused by trauma during use or reprocessing. Current leaves the electrode through this alternate pathway. This can cause serious patient injury, particularly when the injury is internal. Capacitively coupled radio frequency currents can cause undetected burns to nearby tissue and organs outside the endoscope's viewing field. Severe patient injuries have resulted.[7,9,11,79]

2. Endoscopic trocar cannula systems should meet safety criteria established for the practice setting. When an all-metal system is used, capacitive current is safely dispersed through the greater surface area provided by the chest or abdominal wall, thereby reducing current concentration. Metal cannula systems are best for the port of electrosurgical instruments.[6,11,79,80] An all-plastic system is another alternative. Using this system, the capacitor is the patient, which minimizes the concern of concentrated capacitively coupled current;[81] however, a risk of direct coupling injuries remains. Hybrid trocar (ie, combination plastic and metal) systems should not be used.[1,5,11,80] Each trocar and cannula can act as an electrical conductor, thereby inducing an electrical current from one to the other, which could cause capacitive coupling injuries.

3. Personnel should verify that the insufflation gas is nonflammable (ie, carbon dioxide). An intra-abdominal fire has occurred when a carbon dioxide-oxygen mixture was attached inadver-

tently to an insufflator rather than the intended carbon dioxide tank.[82]

4. All electrodes should be examined for impaired insulation before use. Insulation failure of electrodes caused by trauma during use or reprocessing provides an alternate pathway for the electrical current to leave the active electrode. Some insulation failures are not visible. This has resulted in serious patient injuries.[4,6,11,13-15,17,79,80] These injuries may be outside the endoscope's visual field. Use of active electrode shielding and monitoring minimizes the risks of insulation failure and capacitive coupling injuries.[4,6,11,13-15,17,79,80]

5. When active electrode monitoring is not used, additional precautions should be employed to minimize the risks associated with insulation failure and direct and capacitive coupling.
   - The lowest power setting that achieves the desired result should be selected, and
   - the low-voltage cutting waveform setting should be selected whenever clinically feasible.

   Lower power settings for both cut and coagulation reduce the likelihood of insulation failure and capacitive-coupling injuries. Lower power settings also minimize damage from direct coupling when the active electrode is activated while in close proximity to another metal device inserted in an adjacent trocar port.[6]

6. The active electrode should not be activated until it is in close proximity to the tissue; this minimizes the risk of contacting unintended tissue.[6,11] Activating the electrode when it is not in very close proximity to the targeted tissue increases the risk of capacitive coupling. Capacitance is reduced during closed-circuit activation.

7. Patients should be taught to immediately report any signs or symptoms of infection, excessive pain, bleeding, or inability to void. Symptoms of a laparoscopic electrosurgical injury can occur days after discharge from the perioperative setting and may include infection from an injured intestinal tract. Lower gastrointestinal bleeding and inability to void may be early manifestations of a bowel injury.[11] Patients should understand what symptoms to look for and report to ensure prompt treatment that minimizes the adverse outcome.[79]

Recommended Practice IX

Personnel should take special precautions when using the ESU with patients who have pacemakers, internal cardioverter-defibrillators (ICDs), or other electrical implants.

1. Patients with pacemakers should be continuously monitored (ie, minimally, ECG, peripheral pulse) during electrosurgery use. Electrosurgery can interfere with both the pacemaker's circuitry and function and create ECG artifact.[1,83] Monitoring the peripheral pulse provides a mechanism to evaluate peripheral perfusion in the presence of ECG artifact. Although modern pacemakers are designed to be shielded from radio frequency current, they are subject to interference during electrosurgery use.[1,83,84] For patients with pacemakers, personnel should take additional precautions, which include, but are not limited to,

    ♦ checking with the pacemaker manufacturer or the patient's cardiologist regarding its function during use of electrosurgery and discussing reprogramming the pacemaker to an asynchronous mode during surgery;

    ♦ having a pacemaker programmer unit (or magnet if appropriate for the type of pacemaker) available to place the pacemaker in an asynchronous mode;

    ♦ having a defibrillator immediately available for emergencies during surgery;

    ♦ keeping all electrosurgical cords and cables away from the pacemaker and its leads;

    ♦ using bipolar electrosurgery whenever possible;

    ♦ using the lowest possible power setting on the electrosurgical generator;

    ♦ if monopolar electrosurgery is deemed necessary, ensuring that the distance between the active and dispersive electrodes is as short as possible (place both electrodes as far away from the pacemaker as possible, and ensure that the current path does not pass through the vicinity of the patient's heart or the implanted pacemaker device);[1,83] and

    ♦ having the proper functioning of the pacemaker evaluated by an individual trained in the use of the pacemaker programmer immediately postoperatively.

    The patient's pacemaker may interpret radio frequency from electrosurgery as cardiac activity and inhibit the pacemaker from initiating a heartbeat. This can result in life-threatening arrhythmia. Reprogramming demand pacemakers to an asynchronous mode protects the patient from this risk. A magnet placed over the pacemaker is effective in temporarily placing some models of pacemaker in asynchronous mode. Other models require the use of a pacemaker programmer unit.[83] Monopolar electrical current seeks a ground through the patient's body. This ground may be through the pacemaker wire, which can result in inadvertent reprogramming of the pacemaker, permanent damage to the pacemaker, or an electrical burn in the heart; therefore, having a programmer and defibrillator readily available is advisable. Short bursts of energy also minimize the risk of injury. Placing as much distance as possible between both the active and dispersive electrode and the pacemaker encourages the energy to return to the ESU through the dispersive electrode, rather than the pacemaker wire. There is a risk of reprogramming or damage to the pacemaker, so evaluation of the pacemaker is warranted.

2. Precautions for a patient with an ICD should include

    ♦ preoperatively obtaining a cardiology consultation to evaluate the correct functioning of the ICD and determine the risks associated with temporarily deactivating the ICD intraoperatively;

    ♦ having a defibrillator immediately available;

    ♦ having the ICD device deactivated by trained personnel before the ESU is activated—using electrosurgery on a patient with an activated ICD may trigger an electrical shock to the patient;[85]

    ♦ having continuous ECG and peripheral pulse monitoring;

    ♦ using bipolar electrosurgery as an alternative whenever possible;

    ♦ if monopolar electrosurgery is deemed necessary, ensuring that the distance between the active and dispersive electrodes is as short as possible (place both electrodes as far away from the ICD as possible, and ensure that the current path from the surgical site to the dispersive electrode does not pass through the vicinity of the patient's heart or the implanted ICD);[83,85] and

♦ immediately postoperatively, having the correct functioning of the ICD verified by an expert in electrophysiology.

3. Precautions for patients with other electric stimulators (eg, bone growth, cochlear implants) should include the following.

♦ Use bipolar electrosurgery as an alternative whenever possible. If monopolar electrosurgery is deemed necessary, ensure that the distance between the active and dispersive electrodes is as short as possible, place both electrodes as far away from the stimulator and wire as possible, and ensure that the current path from the surgical site to the dispersive electrode does not pass through the vicinity of the stimulator or lead wire.

♦ In the presence of a cochlear implant, use bipolar electrosurgery at least 1 cm away from the implant.[22]

♦ Immediately postoperatively, have the proper functioning of the device verified by a trained individual.

4. Precautions for patients with an implantable mechanical pump (eg, morphine, Baclofen) should include

♦ using bipolar electrosurgery as an alternative whenever possible, and

♦ immediately postoperatively, having the proper functioning of the pump verified by an individual trained in the programming of the pump.

Recommended Practice X

Bipolar active electrodes (including vessel occluding devices) should be used according to manufacturers' written instructions.

1. Unlike the monopolar ESU, bipolar technology incorporates an active (ie, efferent) electrode and a return (ie, afferent) electrode into a two-poled instrument, such as forceps or scissors.[5,22,86] Current flows only through the tissue contacted between two poles of instruments; thus, the need for a dispersive grounding pad is eliminated.[86] This also eliminates the chance of stray or alternate pathways for current flow.[86] The bipolar ESU provides precise hemostasis at the surgical site without stimulation or current spread to nearby body structures.[86]

2. Connection of a bipolar active electrode to a monopolar receptacle may activate current, causing a short circuit. Plugs should be differentiated to prevent misconnections of active and inactive electrodes.[20] Molded, fixed-positioned pin placement bipolar cords also are available.

Recommended Practice XI

Ultrasonic electrosurgical devices function differently from monopolar active electrodes and should be used according to manufacturers' written instructions.

1. When using an ultrasonic electrosurgical device, a dispersive electrode is not necessary. An ultrasonic device has a generator that produces electrical energy that is sent to the hand piece, where it is converted into mechanical energy. This energy is transmitted through a hand piece to a blade or probe that can be used for sharp or blunt dissection, coagulation, or breaking apart of tissue, without damage to adjacent tissues. Some ultrasonic dissectors incorporate an aspirator to remove tissue or fluids from the surgical field. Because no electrical current enters the tissue, current does not need to be returned to the generator by a dispersive electrode.[87]

2. Inhalation of aerosols generated by an ultrasonic electrosurgical hand piece should be minimized by implementing control measures that include, but are not limited to, the use of

♦ smoke evacuation systems, and

♦ wall suctions with in-line filters, which are only appropriate for a minimal amount of aerosol (aerosols generated using ultrasonic electrosurgery are within the respirable range and include blood, blood by-products, and tissue).[88]

3. Biomedical personnel should routinely inspect ultrasonic electrosurgical equipment to reduce the potential for equipment malfunction.

Recommended Practice XII

Argon enhanced coagulation (AEC) technology poses unique risks to patient and personnel safety and should be used according to manufacturers' written instructions.

1. All safety measures for monopolar electrosurgery should be used when using AEC technology. The AEC unit uses monopolar alternating current delivered to the tissue through ionized argon gas.[89,90] The risks of monopolar electrosurgery are present. Additional risks are associated with application of argon gas. Precautions should be taken to minimize these risks.

2. Air should be purged from the argon gas line and electrode by activating the system before use after moderate delays between activations and between uses.[89-90] Argon gas pressure exceeds venous pressure in the circulating system, and application to bleeding vessels has resulted in gas emboli in open surgical procedures.[91,92] Activating without adequately purging may present the greatest risk of embolism when operating in an open cavity.[89,90]

3. The coagulation or blended cutting current, which contains coagulation, should be used. The coagulation waveform seals the venous blood vessels, minimizing the risk of gas emboli entering the blood stream. Purging the argon gas line prevents delays in coagulation and reduces the potential for the operator to move the hand piece, thus minimizing the risk of gas embolism.[89,90]

4. The argon gas flow should be limited to the lowest level possible. Argon gas flow is most likely to be directed to tissue without simultaneous coagulation when the initiation of ionization of the argon gas is delayed due to air bubbles in the argon gas line.[89,90]

5. The electrode should not be placed in direct contact with tissue and should be moved away from the patient's tissue after each activation.[89,90] There is a risk of gas emboli when the active electrode is placed in direct contact with tissue.

6. Personnel using the AEC technology should be knowledgeable about signs, symptoms, and treatment of venous emboli.

7. Patient monitoring should include devices that are considered effective for early detection of gas emboli (eg, end-tidal carbon dioxide).[89,90]

Recommended Practice XIII

When using the AEC unit with endoscopic procedures, personnel should follow the manufacturer's written instructions and recommendations for use.

1. When using the AEC unit during endoscopic procedures, personnel should
   - follow all safety measures identified for AEC technology,
   - flush the patient's intraabdominal cavity with several liters of CO_2 between extended activation periods,[93]
   - use endoscopic CO_2 insufflators equipped with audible and visual overpressurization alarms that cannot be deactivated.[93]

The AEC system acts as a secondary source of pressurized argon gas that can cause the patient's intraabdominal pressure to rise rapidly and exceed venous pressure, possibly creating argon-enriched gas emboli formation. This has resulted in gas emboli.[93] Using the lowest argon gas flow setting, purging the active electrode and argon gas line of air according to the manufacturer's recommendations, and flushing the intraabdominal cavity with several liters of CO_2 between extended periods of deactivation reduces the potential for argon gas emboli formation.[93]

Recommended Practice XIV

Exposure to smoke plume generated during electrosurgery should be minimized.

1. Inhalation of smoke generated by electrosurgery should be minimized by implementing control measures that include, but are not limited to, the use of
   - smoke evacuation systems and
   - wall suction with in-line filters, which is only appropriate for a minimal amount of plume.

Smoke plume generated from electrosurgery is the same as laser plume. This smoke has been found to contain toxic gases and vapors (eg benzene, hydrogen cyanide, formaldehyde); bioaerosols, including blood fragments; and viruses. In high concentrations, the smoke causes ocular and upper respiratory tract irritation in health care personnel.[94] The smoke generated from electrosurgery contains chemical by-products.[94,95] The National Institutes of Occupational Safety and Health recommends that smoke evacuation systems be used to reduce potential acute and chronic health risks to patients and personnel.[94] The Occupational Safety and Health Administration (OSHA) has no separate standard related to surgical smoke. The OSHA addresses such safety hazards in the General Duty Clause and Bloodborne Pathogen Standard.[95]

2. Smoke evacuation systems and accessories should be used according to manufacturers' written instructions. Health care facilities should consult AORN's "Recommended practices for product selection in perioperative practice settings" to assist in selecting a smoke evacuation system.[96] When a smoke evacuation system is used, the suction wand should be placed as close to the source of the smoke as possible. This will maximize smoke capture and enhance visibility at the surgical site.

Recommended Practice XV

Health care facilities' policies and procedures for electrosurgery must be in compliance with the Safe Medical Devices Act of 1990.

1. If patient or personnel injuries or equipment failures occur, the ESU and the active and dispersive electrodes should be handled in accordance with the Safe Medical Devices Act of 1990, amended in March 2000.[97] Device identification, maintenance and service information, and adverse event information should be included in the report from the practice setting. Retaining the ESU, the active and dispersive electrodes, and packaging allows for a complete systems check to determine electrosurgical system integrity.

Recommended Practice XVI

Policies and procedures for electrosurgery should be developed, reviewed periodically, revised as necessary, and readily available in the practice setting.

1. Policies and procedures for electrosurgery should include, but are not limited to,
   - safety features required on ESUs;
   - equipment maintenance programs;
   - supplemental safety monitors required;
   - equipment checks before initial use;

- reporting and impounding malfunctioning equipment;
- preoperative, intraoperative, and postoperative patient assessments;
- precautions during use;
- reporting of injuries;
- ESU sanitation; and
- documentation.

2. Documentation should include, but not be limited to,
   - electrosurgical system identification serial number,
   - range of settings used,
   - dispersive electrode placement and patient's skin condition before and after electrosurgery, and
   - adjunct electrical devices used (eg, ultrasonic scalpel, bipolar forceps).

Documentation of details of the electrosurgical equipment and supplies allows for retrievable information for investigation into an adverse event.

3. These recommended practices should be used as guidelines for the development of policies and procedures in the perioperative practice setting. Policies and procedures establish authority, responsibility, and accountability within the facility. They also serve as operational guidelines.

4. An introduction and review of policies and procedures for electrosurgery should be included in orientation and ongoing education of personnel to assist in the development of knowledge, skills, and attitudes that affect surgical patient outcomes. Policies and procedures also assist in the development of quality assessment and improvement activities.

5. Information about adverse patient outcomes and near misses associated with electrosurgery should be collected, analyzed, and used for performance improvement as part of the institution-wide performance improvement program. To evaluate the quality of patient care and formulate plans for corrective action, it is necessary to maintain a system of evaluation. Quality improvement standards for perioperative nurses that may be used for evaluating electrosurgical safety have been published.[98]

Glossary

Active electrode: The electrosurgical unit (ESU) accessory that directs current flow to the surgical site (eg, pencils, various tips).

Active electrode monitoring: A dynamic process of searching for insulation failures and capacitive coupling during monopolar surgery. If the monitor detects an unsafe level of stray energy, it signals the generator to deactivate.

Argon enhanced coagulation: Radio frequency coagulation from an electrosurgical generator that is capable of delivering monopolar current through a flow of ionized argon gas.

Bioengineering services personnel: Those individuals in an institution who are trained and qualified to check, troubleshoot, and repair medical equipment.

Bipolar electrosurgery: Electrosurgery in which current flows between two tips of a bipolar forceps that is positioned around tissue to create a surgical effect. Current passes from the active electrode of one tip of the forceps through the patient's desired tissue to the dispersive electrode of the other forceps' tip—thus completing the circuit without entering another part of the patient's body. No dispersive electrode is required.

Capacitance: Ability of an electrical circuit to transfer an electrical charge from one conductor to another, even when separatedby an insulator.

Capacitive coupling: Transfer of electrical current from the active electrode through intact insulation to adjacent conductive items (eg, tissue, trocars).

Capacitively coupled return electrode: A large, nonadhesive return electrode placed close to and forming a capacitor with the patient, returning electrical current from the patient back to the ESU.

Current: A movement of electrons analogous to the flow of a stream of water.

Direct coupling: The contact of an energized metal active electrode tip with another metal instrument or object within the surgical field.

Dispersive electrode: The accessory that directs electrical current flow from the patient back to the electrosurgical generator—often called the patient plate, return electrode, inactive electrode, or grounding pad.

Electrosurgery: The cutting and coagulation of body tissue with a high frequency (ie, radio frequency) current.

Electrosurgical accessories: For the purposes of this document, electrosurgical accessories are defined as the active electrode with tip(s), dispersive electrode, adapters, and connectors to attach these devices to the generator.

Electrosurgical unit: For the purposes of this document, the ESU includes the generator that produces the high frequency current waveform that is delivered to tissues, the foot switch with cord (if applicable), the electrical plug, cord, and connections.

Eschar: Charred tissue residue.

Generator: The machine that produces radio frequency waves (eg, ESU, power unit).

Ground-referenced electrosurgical unit: A system in which electrical current is sent to the patient and follows the path of least resistance back to the ground. This technology, which no longer is manufactured, produces high frequency, high voltage current and sometimes is referred to as a "spark gap" unit.

Insulator: A material that does not conduct electricity.

Insulation failure: Damage to the insulation of the active electrode that provides an alternate pathway for the current to leave that electrode as it completes the circuit to the dispersive electrode.

Isolated electrosurgical unit: A system in which electrical current is sent to the patient and selectively returns and is grounded through the generator.

Monopolar electrosurgery: Electrosurgery in which only the active electrode is in the surgical wound, and the electrical current is directed through the patient's body, received by the dispersive pad, and transferred back to the generator, completing the monopolar circuit.

Oxygen-enriched environment: Atmosphere containing more than 23% oxygen, frequently occurring in the oropharynx, trachea, lower respiratory tract, and near the head and neck during administration of oxygen to the patient.

Return electrode contact quality monitoring: A dynamic monitoring circuit measuring impedance of the dispersive return electrode. If the dispersive electrode becomes compromised, the circuit inhibits the ESU's output.

Ultrasonic scalpel: A cutting/coagulation device that converts electrical energy into mechanical energy, providing a rapid ultrasonic motion.

Vessel sealing device: Bipolar technology that fuses collagen and elastin in the vessel walls and permanently obliterates the lumen of the vessel.

NOTES

1. "Electrosurgery," (Operating Room Risk Management) *ECRI* (January 1999) 7.

2. "Electrosurgical units," *Health Devices* 27 (March 1998) 93-96.

3. ANSI/AAMI, "Electrosurgical devices," HF18: 2001, 1-26.

4. R C Odell, "Pearls, pitfalls, and advancements in the delivery of electrosurgical energy during laparoscopy," *Problems in General Surgery* 19 no 2 (2002) 5-17.

5. "Laparoscopic electrosurgery risks," (Operating Room Risk Management) *ECRI* (May 1999) 1-11.

6. "Guidance section: Ensuring monopolar electrosurgical safety during laparoscopy," *Health Devices* 24 (January 1995) 20-27.

7. J T Bischoff et al, "Laparoscopic bowel injury: Incidence and clinical presentation," *The Journal of Urology* 161 (March 1999) 888-890.

8. B J Carroll, M Birth, E H Phillips, "Common bile duct injuries during laparoscopic cholecystectomy that result in litigation," *Surgical Endoscopy* 12 (April 1998) 310-314.

9. K A Kern, "Malpractice litigation involving laparoscopic cholecystectomy: Cost, cause, and consequences," *Archives of Surgery* 132 (April 1997) 392-398.

10. R D Tucker, C E Platz, S K Landas, "A laparoscopic complication? A medical legal case analysis. Part I," *Journal of Gynecologic Surgery* 11 no 2 (1995) 113-121.

11. M P Wu et al, "Complications and recommended practices for electrosurgery in laparoscopy," *The American Journal of Surgery* 179 (January 2000) 67-73.

12. *Laparoscopic Injury Study* (Rockville, Md: Physician Insurers Association of America, August 2000) 1-5.

13. "Evaluation of electroscope electroshield system," (Guidance Article) *Health Devices* 24 (January 1995) 11-19.

14. V Dennis, "Implementing active electrode monitoring: A perioperative call," *Surgical Services Management* 7 (April 2001) 32-38.

15. R D Tucker, C R Voyles, S E Silvis, "Capacitive coupled stray currents during laparoscopic and endoscopic electrosurgical procedures," *Biomedical Instrumentation and Technology* 26 (July/August 1992) 303-311.

16. T G Vancaillie, "Active electrode monitoring: How to prevent unintentional thermal injury associated with monopolar electrosurgery at laparoscopy," *Surgical Endoscopy* 12 (August 1998) 1009-1012.

17. C R Voyles, R D Tucker, "Education and engineering solutions for potential problems with laparoscopic monopolar electrosurgery," *The American Journal of Surgery* 164 (July 1992) 56-62.

18. "Burns and fires from electrosurgical active electrodes," (Hazard Update) *Health Devices* 22 (August-September 1993) 421-422.

19. "Fires in the operating room," (Healthcare Hazard Control) *ECRI* (February 2003) 1-10.

20. "Misconnection of bipolar electrosurgical electrodes," (Hazard Report) *Health Devices* 24 (January 1995) 34-35.

21. National Fire Protection Association, *NFPA 99: Standard for Health Care Facilities*, sec D.5.2.1 (Quincy, Mass: NFPA International, 2002) 200.

22. T L Smith, J M Smith, "Electrosurgery in otolaryngology-head and neck surgery: Principles, advances, and complications," *The Laryngoscope* 111 (May 2001) 769-780.

23. National Fire Protection Association, *NFPA 99: Standard for Health Care Facilities*, sec D.5.2.5 (Quincy, Mass: NFPA International, 2002) 200.

24. National Fire Protection Association, *NFPA 99: Standard for Health Care Facilities*, sec D.5.2.3 (Quincy, Mass: NFPA International, 2002) 200.

25. National Fire Protection Association, *NFPA 99: Standard for Health Care Facilities*, sec D.7.3 (Quincy, Mass: NFPA International, 2002) 203.

26. National Fire Protection Association, *NFPA 99: Standard for Health Care Facilities*, sec D.5.3.1 (Quincy, Mass: NFPA International, 2002) 200.

27. National Fire Protection Association, *NFPA 99: Standard for Health Care Facilities*, sec D.5.3.3 (Quincy, Mass: NFPA International, 2002) 200.

28. "Electrosurgery checklist," (Operating Room Risk Management) *ECRI* (January 1999) 1.

29. Joint Commission on Accreditation of Health Care Organizations, *2003 Hospital Accreditation Standards*, section EC.2.10.3 (Oakbrook Terrace, Ill: Joint Commission Resources, 2003) 236.

30. "ESU burns from poor dispersive electrode site preparation," (Hazard Update) *Health Devices* 22 (August-September 1993) 423.

31. "Recommended practices for endoscopic minimally invasive surgery," in *Standards, Recommended Practices and Guidelines* (Denver: AORN, Inc, 2004) 267-271.

32. National Fire Protection Association, *NFPA 99: Standard for Health Care Facilities*, sec C.13.1.3.2.2 (Quincy, Mass: NFPA International, 2002) 182.

33. T D Datta, "Flash fire hazard with eye ointment," (Letters to the Editor) *Anesthesia and Analgesia* 63 (July 1984) 700-701.

34. "The patient is on fire! A surgical fires primer," (Guidance) *Health Devices* 21 (January 1992) 19-34.

35. "Medical devices: Reclassification of polymethylmethacrylate (PMMA) bone cement," *Federal Register* 67 (July 17, 2002) 46852-46855.

36. MAUDE database (Feb 2, 2000), 9610726-2000-00003; (Aug 30, 2002), 435173 (Washington, DC: Center for Devices and Radiological Health).

37. S J Barker, J S Polson, "Fire in the operating room: A case report and laboratory study," *Anesthesia and Analgesia* 93 (October 2001) 960-965.

38. "Fire hazard created by the misuse of DuraPrep solution," (Hazard Report) *Health Devices* 27 (November 1998) 400-401.

39. MAUDE database (July 31, 1995), 32071; (Sept 12, 1997) 119838; (March 21 2002), 384493; (April 15, 2002), 1720159-2002-00032 (Washington, DC: Center for Devices and Radiological Health).

40. "Fire caused by improper disposal of electrocautery units," (Hazard Report) *Health Devices* 23 (March 1994) 98.

41. "Alternate-site burns from improperly seated electrosurgical pencil active electrodes," (Hazard Report) *Health Devices* 29 (January 2000) 24-27.

42. "Ignition of debris on active electrosurgical electrodes," (Hazard Report) *Health Devices* 27 (September-October 1998) 367-370.

43. Center for Devices and Radiological Health, MAUDE database (May 7, 2002), 393590.

44. MAUDE database (Aug 23, 2002), 441523 (Washington, DC: Center for Devices and Radiological Health).

45. R A Ortega, "A rare cause of fire in the operating room," *Anesthesiology* 89 (December 1998) 1608.

46. D K Wood, R Hollis, "Thermal cautery causes a gauze pad fire," (Letters) *JAMA* 270 (Nov 17, 1993) 2299-2300.

47. Y Y Bonnet et al, "Explosion of intestinal gas during surgery," *Annales Francaises d'Anesthesie et de Reanimation* 2 no 6 (1983) 431-435.

48. E Gross, O Jurim, M Krausz, "Diathermy-induced gas explosion in the intestinal tract," *Harefuah* 123 no 1-2 (1992) 12-13, 71-72.

49. F S Joyce, T N Rasmussen, "Gas explosion during diathermy gastrotomy," *Gastroenterology* 96 (February 1989) 530-531.

50. E B Soussan et al, "Bowel explosion with colonic perforation during argon plasma coagulation for hemorrhagic radiation-induced proctitis," *Gastrointestinal Endoscopy* 57 (March 2003) 412-413.

51. E Zinsser, et al "Bowel gas explosion during argon beam coagulation," (Unusual Cases and Technical Notes) *Endoscopy* 31 (May 1999) S26.

52. "Electrosurgical airway fires still a hot topic," *Health Devices* 25 (July 1996) 260-261.

53. J A Bennett, M Agree, "Fire in the chest," *Anesthesia and Analgesia* 78 (February 1984) 406.

54. "$40 million sought after electrosurgery burn death," *Biomedical Safety and Standards* 15 (December 1995) 170.

55. W K Chee, J L Benumof, "Airway fire during tracheostomy: Extubation may be contraindicated," *Anesthesiology* 89 (December 1998) 1576-1578.

56. R J Greco et al, "Potential dangers of oxygen supplementation during facial surgery," *Plastic Reconstructive Surgery* 95 (May 1995) 978-984.

57. M J Lucarelli, B N Lemke, "Monopolar electrosurgical flash fire," *Ophthalmic Surgery and Lasers* 29 (March 1998) 249-250.

58. K F Mattucci, C J Militana, "The prevention of fire during oropharyngeal electrosurgery," *Ear, Nose and Throat Journal* 82 (February 2003) 107-109.

59. A M J Michels, S Stott, "Explosion of tracheal tube during tracheostomy," (Correspondence) *Anaesthesia* 49 (December 1994) 1104.

60. R J Reyes et al, "Supplemental oxygen: Ensuring its safe delivery during facial surgery," *Plastic and Reconstructive Surgery* 95 (April 1995) 924-928.

61. J W Thompson et al, "Fire in the operating room during tracheostomy," *Southern Medical Journal* 91 (March 1998) 243-247.

62. E S Wegrzynowicz et al, "Airway fire during jet ventilation for laser excision of vocal cord papillomata," (Case Reports) *Anesthesiology* 76 (March 1992) 468-469.

63. P T J Wilson, U Igbaseimokumo, J Martin, "Ignition of the tracheal tube during tracheostomy," (Correspondence) *Anaesthesia* 49 (August 1994), 734-735.

64. "Skin burns resulting from the use of electrolyte distention/irrigation media during electrosurgery with a rollerblation electrode," (Hazard Report) *Health Devices* 27 (June 1998) 233-235.

65. MAUDE database (Oct 9, 2002), 421908 (Washington, DC: Center for Devices and Radiological Health).

66. National Fire Protection Association, *NFPA 99: Standard for Health Care Facilities*, sec C.13.4.43.4 (Quincy, Mass: NFPA International, 2002) 186.

67. MAUDE database (March 31, 2003) 2110898-2003-00006 (Washington DC: Center for Devices and Radiological Health). Also available at *http://www.accessdata.fda.gov/scripts/cdrh/cfdocs/cfMAUDE/Detail.cfm?MDRFOI__ID=474982* (accessed 24 Sept, 2004).

68. MAUDE database (March 31, 2004) 2110898-2004-00006 (Washington DC: Center for Devices and Radiological Health). Also available at *http://www.accessdata.fda.gov/scripts/cdrh/cfdocs/cfMAUDE/Detail.CFM?MDRFOI__ID=523194* (accessed 24 Sept 2004).

69. M Vahlensieck, "Tattoo-related cutaneous inflammation (burn grade I) in a mid-field MR scanner," (Letters to the Editor) *European Radiology* 10 (January 2000) 197.

70. W A Wagle, M Smith, "Tattoo-induced skin burn during MR imaging," (On the AJR Viewbox) *American Journal of Roentgenology* 174 (June 2000) 1795.

71. MAUDE database (October 15, 2003) 2110898-2003-00016 (Washington DC: Center for Devices and Radiological Health). Also available at *http://www.accessdata.fda.gov/scripts/cdrh/cfdocs/cfMAUDE/Detail.cfm?MDRFOI__ID=495428* (accessed 24 Sept 2004).

72. MAUDE database (November 25, 2003) 1643264-2003-00066 (Washington, DC: Center for Devices and Radiological Health). Also available at *http://www.accessdata.fda.gov/scripts/cdrh/cfdocs/cfMAUDE/Detail.cfm?MDRFOI__ID=499965* (accessed 24 Sept 2004).

73. MAUDE database (February 16, 2004) 2110898-2004-00004 (Washington DC: Center for Devices and Radiological Health). Also available at *http://www.accessdata.fda.gov/scripts/cdrh/cfdocs/cfMAUDE/Detail.cfm?MDRFOI__ID=516905* (accessed 24 Sept 2004).

74. "Skin lesions from aggressive adhesive on electrosurgical return electrode pads," *Health Devices* 24 (April 1995) 159-161.

75. MAUDE database (June 24, 2002), 401617 (Washington, DC: Center for Devices and Radiological Health).

76. "MegaDyne Mega 2000 return electrode," *Health Devices* 29 (December 2000) 445-460.

77. MAUDE database (May 16, 2002), 396295; (July 6, 2002), 286226 (Washington, DC: Center for Devices and Radiological Health).

78. "Allowing patients to wear jewelry during surgical (and electrosurgical) procedures," *Health Devices* 26 (November 1997) 441-443.

79. G J Harrell, D R Kopps, "Minimizing patient risk during laparoscopic electrosurgery," *AORN Journal* 67 (June 1998) 1194-1205.

80. T G Vancaillie, "Electrosurgery at laparoscopy: Guidelines to avoid complications," *Gynaecological Endoscopy* 3 (1994) 143-150.

81. P D Willson et al, "Port site electrosurgical (diathermy) burns during surgical laparoscopy," *Surgical Endoscopy* 11 (June 1997) 653-654.

82. P E Greilich, N B Greilich, E G Froelich, "Intraabdominal fire during laparoscopic cholecystectomy," *Anesthesiology* 83 (October 1995) 871-874.

83. J L Atlee, A D Bernstein, "Cardiac rhythm management devices (Part II): Perioperative management," *Anesthesiology* 95 (December 2001) 1492-1506.

84. M A Rozner, R J Nishman, "Electrocautery-induced pacemaker tachycardia: Why does this error continue?" (Correspondence) *Anesthesiology* 96 (March 2002) 773-774.

85. "Electrosurgery on patients with implantable cardioverter-defibrillators,"(Talk to the Specialist) *Health Devices* 31 (February 2002) 74.

86. National Fire Protection Association, *NFPA 99: Standard for Health Care Facilities*, sec D.6.7.3 (Quincy, Mass: NFPA International, 2002) 202.

87. S D McCarus, "Physiologic mechanisms of the ultrasonically activated scalpel," *The Journal of American Association of Gynecologic Laparoscopists* 3 (August 1996) 601-608.

88. D E Ott, E Moss, K Martinez, "Aerosol exposure from an ultrasonically activated (harmonic) device," *Journal of American Association of Gynecologic Laparoscopists* 5 (February 1998) 29-32.

89. K Matthews, "Argon beam coagulation: New directions in surgery," *AORN Journal* 56 (November 1992) 885-896.

90. "Risk analysis: Argon-enhanced coagulation," (Hospital Risk Control) *ECRI* (January 1991) 1-3.

91. N Stojeba et al, "Possible venous argon gas embolism complicating argon gas enhanced coagulation during liver surgery," *Acta Anaesthesiologica Scandinavica* 43 (September 1999) 866-867.

92. F Veyckemans, I Michel, "Venous gas embolism from an argon coagulator," *Anesthesiology* 85 (August 1996) 443-444.

93. "Fatal gas embolism caused by overpressurization during laparoscopic use of argon enhanced coagulation," (Hazard Report) *Health Devices* 23 (June 1994) 257-259.

94. "Control of smoke from laser/electric surgical procedures," DHHS (NIOSH) publication 96-128 (Atlanta: National Institute for Occupational Safety and Health, September 1996).

95. "Laser/electrosurgery plume," US Department of Labor, Occupational Safety and Health Administration (Feb 13, 2002), *http://www.osha.gov/SLTC/laserelectrosurgeryplume* (accessed 25 April 2003).

96. "Recommended practices for product selection in perioperative practice settings," in *Standards, Recommended Practices, and Guidelines* (Denver: AORN, Inc, 2004) 347-350.

97. "Medical device reporting: Manufacturer reporting, importer reporting, user facility reporting, distributor reporting," *Federal Register* 65 (Jan 26, 2000) 4112-4121.

98. "Quality and performance improvement standards for perioperative nursing," in *Standards, Recommended Practices, and Guidelines* (Denver: AORN, Inc, 2004) 187-196.

Originally published March 1985, *AORN Journal.*

Revised April 1991; revised July 1993.

Revised November 1997; published January 1998, *AORN Journal.* Reformatted July 2000.

Revised November 2003; published February 2004, *AORN Journal.*

Revised November 2004; published March 2005, *AORN Journal.*

Recommended Practices for Cleaning and Processing Endoscopes and Endoscope Accessories

The following recommended practices were developed by the AORN Recommended Practices Committee and have been approved by the AORN Board of Directors. They were presented as proposed recommended practices for comments by members and others. They are effective January 1, 2003.

These recommended practices are intended as achievable recommendations representing what is believed to be an optimal level of practice. Policies and procedures will reflect variations in practice settings and/or clinical situations that determine the degree to which the recommended practices can be implemented.

AORN recognizes the numerous different settings in which perioperative nurses practice. These recommended practices are intended as guidelines adaptable to various practice settings. These practice settings include traditional ORs, ambulatory surgery units, physicians' offices, cardiac catheterization suites, endoscopy suites, radiology departments, and all other areas where operative and other invasive procedures may be performed.

Purpose

These recommended practices provide guidelines to assist personnel in the care, cleaning, decontamination, maintenance, handling, storage, and sterilization and/or disinfection of flexible and rigid endoscopes and related accessories. Use of these recommended practices will assist personnel in providing a safe environment for patients and health care workers. These recommended practices are based on the most current literature and thinking at the time of their development. They should be used to develop policies and procedures for care of endoscopes and accessories in the practice setting. As new information becomes available, perioperative nurses should consult with infection control professionals and epidemiologists to review and revise procedures as appropriate.

Recommended Practice I

Personnel should demonstrate competency in the use, care, and processing of endoscopes and related equipment.

1. Each facility should develop a system for measuring and documenting personnel competency.[1]

Personnel working with endoscopes and endoscopic accessories should demonstrate competency commensurate with their responsibilities. Education programs should be specific to the type and design of endoscopes used and the procedures performed in the facility. Manufacturers' specific instructions for endoscope care and use will be an important component of the education program. Personnel should be required to demonstrate competency periodically and when new endoscopic equipment and/or accessories are introduced into the practice setting. Educational activities should be documented and maintained on file in the facility.[2]

2. Personnel should practice standard and transmission-based/expanded precautions during endoscopy procedures and when handling and processing contaminated endoscopes and related equipment.[3] Standard precautions include the use of personal protective equipment. Personal protective equipment reduces the risk of direct exposure to blood, body fluids, or other fluids that may contain potentially infectious microorganisms.[4]

Recommended Practice II

Endoscopes and related equipment should be inspected at all stages of handling.

1. Endoscopes and related equipment should be inspected for integrity, function, and cleanliness at the following times:
   - before use,
   - during the procedure,
   - after the procedure,
   - immediately after decontamination, and
   - before disinfection or sterilization.

   Visual inspection helps personnel detect structural damage, loss of function, and/or gross soil that may impact further processing and/or patient outcomes.[5]

2. Damaged and/or soiled endoscopes and/or accessories should be removed from service. A damaged instrument that has been used should be considered contaminated and treated accordingly, using the appropriate level of precaution to protect personnel from exposure to potentially harmful microorganisms.[6]

Recommended Practice III

Endoscopes and related equipment should be tested before use and used according to manufacturers' instructions.

1. Pressure (ie, leak) tests should be performed on used flexible fiber-optic endoscopes with leak testing capabilities before they are immersed in cleaning solutions or water. Leaks in either the covering or one or more of the inside channels can be determined by the presence of air bubbles when air pressure is applied to the inside of the insertion tube. If using a leak test system not requiring water, follow manufacturers' instructions. Unless otherwise specified in manufacturers' instructions, a damaged endoscope should not be submerged. If damage is detected, the endoscope should be removed from service before it is cleaned, and the manufacturer should be consulted for directions regarding further action to be taken. If the pressure test identifies interstitial space damage to a fiber-optic endoscope, the endoscope requires repair. An endoscope being returned to the manufacturer for repair is considered a contaminated medical device and should be labeled accordingly for shipping. The endoscope must be packaged in impervious material and labeled with a biohazard symbol for transport. The biohazard label will act as a warning of potentially infectious material. Refer to Occupational Safety and Health Administration regulations for preventing exposure to bloodborne pathogens for specific information on labeling contaminated equipment being shipped for repair.[7]

2. Insulated endoscopic accessories/related equipment should be tested for insulation failure. Test kits are available commercially to assist with this process. Visual inspection may not be sufficient to detect minute breaks in insulating materials. Damaged equipment should be removed from service immediately to prevent patient injury, such as burns and/or other tissue injury. Pre-use testing and proper use of endoscopes, endoscopic accessories, and related equipment minimize the risk for adverse patient outcomes.[8]

Recommended Practice IV

Endoscopes and related equipment should be cleaned and decontaminated immediately after use, following manufacturers' written instructions.

1. Endoscopes and their accessories should be cleaned and processed according to the manufacturers' specific instructions. Flexible endoscopes, by virtue of the body cavities in which they are used, acquire high levels of microbial contamination during each use.[9] More health care associated infection outbreaks have been associated with contaminated endoscopes than with any other medical device.[10] Use of proper protocols reduces the risk for adverse patient outcomes, prevents damage to the lenses and fiber-optic components of the instruments, and helps prevent delays by avoiding unnecessary malfunction.[11]

2. Endoscopes, endoscopic accessories, and related equipment should be disassembled and cleaned manually, using mechanical friction when possible. Endoscopes and related equipment are considered contaminated after use. Immediate cleaning reduces the formation of thick masses of cells and extracellular materials known as biofilms.[12] Biofilms are microbial masses that attach to surfaces that are immersed in liquids. After they have formed, sterilizing/disinfecting agents must penetrate the agent-resisting biofilms before killing microorganisms within the biofilms. Immediate decontamination is necessary to protect patients and personnel and to prevent transmission of potentially infectious microorganisms. Flexible endoscopes that have crevices, joints, and internal channels may be more difficult to clean and sterilize or disinfect than rigid instruments that have flat surfaces. Removing gross soil from narrow internal channels and lumens may be difficult.

3. Manufacturers' written instructions for cleaning endoscopes should be followed. A sample cleaning protocol follows.[13]
   ♦ Wash the insertion tube of the endoscope with an enzymatic detergent solution using a soft cloth or sponge. Follow the manufacturers' written instructions when selecting and using an enzymatic detergent for cleaning. Appropriate dilution of the enzymatic

product helps preserve the life of the endoscope. Abrasive or corrosive solutions may damage the surfaces of endoscopes and contribute to corrosion and degradation.[14]

♦ Remove all detachable parts (eg, hoods, valves, water bottle) and soak in the enzymatic detergent solution. Enzymes assist in degrading biofilms.

♦ Open all ports during the cleaning process.

♦ Irrigate internal suction/biopsy channels of flexible endoscopes with copious amounts of enzymatic detergent and tap water to soften, moisten, dilute, and remove organic soils (eg, blood, feces, respiratory secretions).[15]

♦ Brush accessible channels to remove particulate matter. Reusable cleaning brushes require thorough cleaning and sterilization/disinfection after each use.[16] Disposable cleaning brushes are available commercially.

♦ Clear the air-water channel with forced air.

♦ Gently wipe/brush the tip of the endoscope to remove any debris or tissue that might be lodged around the air-water outlet. Do not abrade the tip or lens of the endoscope.

♦ Clean detached parts in enzymatic solution. Brush irregular surfaces to remove all organic debris.

♦ Rinse the endoscope and all parts thoroughly to remove residual debris and cleaning agents.

♦ Thoroughly dry the endoscope, channels, and removable parts. For internal channels of flexible endoscopes, complete all of the following steps:
  – flush with either sterile or tap water,
  – flush with a 70% to 90% alcohol solution, and
  – dry with forced air.

♦ Discard the enzymatic detergent solution after each use. This solution has no antimicrobial properties and may allow microbial growth.[17]

Recommended Practice V

Endoscopes should be sterilized or disinfected according to the AORN "Recommended practices for sterilization in perioperative practice settings,"[18] the AORN "Recommended practices for high-level disinfection,"[19] and the "APIC guideline for infection prevention and control in flexible endoscopy."[20]

1. According to the Spaulding classification system published in 1968 and still used today,[21] endoscopes, accessories, and related equipment entering sterile tissue or the vascular system should be sterilized before use. Endoscopes contacting only mucous membranes and/or nonintact skin require only high-level disinfection. Some endoscopes are heat-labile and cannot be sterilized expeditiously. Even with emerging sterilization technologies, endoscope sterilization may not be possible. ☞ Presently, there is no conclusive evidence that sterilization of these endoscopes reduces patient infection risk.[22] Nevertheless, some infection control experts continue to suggest that endoscopes entering sterile tissue or the vascular system be sterilized or receive a minimum of high-level disinfection with a US Food and Drug Administration (FDA)-cleared liquid sterilant/disinfectant.[23]

2. A protocol should be used for high-level disinfection of endoscopes. A sample protocol follows.

♦ Select a disinfectant/sterilant that has no deleterious effects on the items to be sterilized. Follow manufacturers' warnings regarding specific agents that may cause functional damage to the endoscope.

♦ Completely immerse the endoscope, accessories, and related equipment in the disinfecting solution. Flush all channels with disinfectant solution. Contact with all surfaces, including internal channels, is necessary for disinfection. Replace any endoscope that cannot be immersed completely.[24] Follow manufacturers' instructions for product use and contact time unless documented studies suggest otherwise.

♦ If an automatic endoscope reprocessor is used, clean endoscopes manually before using the automatic endoscope reprocessor. Attach all endoscope channels to the unit according to manufacturers' instructions. Failure to do so will result in disinfection failure because the disinfectant/sterilant may not be exposed to all surfaces of the endoscope.[25] Obtain information from the manufacturer regarding efficacy testing. Design flaws have compromised the effectiveness of some automatic endoscope reprocessors. Bacterial biofilms have been found after processing. Not all endoscope products can be processed successfully in all automatic endoscope reprocessors.[26] Contact the manufacturer of the endoscope and the automatic endoscope reprocessor to determine product compatibility.

♦ After high-level disinfection and/or processing in an automatic endoscope reprocessor (AER) before storage, rinse endoscopes, including internal channels, with sterile water followed by a rinse with 70% to 90% ethyl or isopropyl alcohol, and dry with forced air. This process reduces the potential for recontamination by waterborne microorganisms.[27]

♦ Sterilize or disinfect the water bottle, cap, and tubing used for intraprocedural flush solution at least daily and preferably after each use. Sterile water, as opposed to tap water, should be used for procedures.

♦ After processing, hang endoscopes in a vertical position to facilitate drying. Store them in a manner that protects them from contamination.[28]

♦ Endoscopes removed from the OR for use in other practice environments in the facility should be processed immediately before use and transported in a manner that preserves the sterilization/disinfection status of the endoscope.

3. Unless packaged and sterilized, endoscopes should be processed immediately before use. If a "just in time" sterilization system is used, the processed equipment should be used immediately upon completion of the processing cycle. This equipment may not be stored for later use. Likewise, high-level disinfection of endoscopes should occur immediately before use. Endoscopes and related equipment are considered medical devices and surgical instruments. They represent a risk to patients if they are not processed correctly. Failed or improperly performed cleaning procedures may result in disinfection failure with outbreaks of infection. Numerous infections have been transmitted via gastrointestinal endoscopy and bronchoscopy. Clinical manifestations ranged from symptomatic colonization to death. One multistate investigation found that 23.9% of bacterial cultures from the internal channels of 71 gastrointestinal endoscopes grew more than 100,000 bacterial

colonies after all disinfection/sterilization procedures and before use on the subsequent patient.[29]

4. Endoscopic accessories (eg, biopsy forceps, cytology brushes) that enter sterile tissue or the vascular system should be sterile. These devices are invasive and carry a higher risk of patient infection. These accessories often are difficult to clean and sterilize. Disposable accessories may be safer, more efficient, and more economic.[30] Biopsy forceps technology continues to evolve. Practitioners should remain knowledgeable about new technologies and select products that are both safe and cost effective.

Recommended Practice VI

Policies and procedures for cleaning and processing endoscopes, endoscope accessories, and related equipment should be developed, reviewed regularly, revised as necessary, and readily available in the practice setting.

1. Emerging technology and a proliferation of FDA-cleared sterilization/disinfection processes and products present a continuing challenge to perioperative nurses. Perioperative nurses and others should consult with knowledgeable infection control professionals when developing and reviewing/revising policies and procedures for endoscope, accessory, and related equipment cleaning and processing. Perioperative nurses should collaborate with infection control professionals to monitor and validate infection control practices. Infection control professionals can identify necessary prospective surveillance.

2. Policies and procedures should establish authority, responsibility, and accountability for endoscope care, cleaning, and processing and should be based on current literature and thinking in the infection control and patient safety arenas. Orientation and ongoing education activities for personnel should include an introduction to and/or review of policies and procedures to be applied in the practice setting. Compliance with policies and procedures helps develop/reinforce knowledge, skills, and attitudes that affect patient outcomes. Policies and procedures also may be an integral part of continuous quality assessment and improvement activities.

Glossary

Biofilm: Thick masses of cells and extracellular materials that protect embedded microorganisms; microbial masses that attach to surfaces submerged in water.

Cleaning: A process using friction, detergent, and water to remove soil, including organic debris; the process by which any type of soil, including organic material, is removed. Cleaning is accomplished with detergent, water, and scrubbing action.

Decontamination: Any physical or chemical process that serves to reduce the number of microorganisms on any inanimate object to render that object safe for subsequent handling; the process by which contaminants are removed, either by hand cleaning or mechanical means, using specific solutions capable of rendering the blood and debris harmless and removing them from the surface of an object or instrument.

Disinfection: A process that destroys some forms of microorganisms, excluding bacterial spores; a process that kills most forms of microorganisms on inanimate surfaces.

High-level disinfection: A process that destroys all microorganisms with the exception of high numbers of bacterial spores. High-level disinfectants have the capability of inactivating the hepatitis B virus, HIV, and *Mycobacterium tuberculosis.* High-level disinfectants do not inactivate the virus-like prion that causes Creutzfeldt-Jakob disease.

Personal protective equipment: Specialized equipment or clothing used by health care workers to protect themselves from direct exposure to patients' blood, tissue, or body fluids. Personal protective equipment may include gloves, gowns, fluid-resistant aprons, head and foot coverings, face shields or masks, eye protection, and ventilation devices (eg, mouth pieces, respirator bags, pocket masks).

Sterilization: The complete elimination of all forms of microbial life, including spores.

NOTES

1. Joint Commission on Accreditation of Healthcare Organizations, "Management of human resources," in *Comprehensive Accreditation Manual for Hospitals: The Official Handbook* (Oakbrook Terrace, Ill: Joint Commission on Accreditation of Healthcare Organizations, 2002) HR-8 to HR-15.

2. *Ibid;* K A Ball, *Endoscopic Surgery* (St Louis: Mosby, 1997) 23-25.

3. J S Garner, the Hospital Infection Control Practices Advisory Committee, "Guideline for isolation precautions in hospitals," *Infection Control and Hospital Epidemiology* 17 (January 1966) 53-80; "Recommended practices for standard and transmission-based precautions in the perioperative practice setting," in *Standards, Recommended Practices, and Guidelines* (Denver: AORN, Inc, 2002) 321-325.

4. "Occupational exposure to bloodborne pathogens; Final rule," *Federal Register* 56 (Dec 6, 1991) 64177.

5. C J Alvarado, M Reichelderfer, "APIC guideline for infection prevention and control in flexible endoscopy," *American Journal of Infection Control* 28 (April 2000) 145; Ball, *Endoscopic Surgery,* 100, 116; B J Ott, C J Gostout, "Endoscopic maintenance and repairs," *Gastrointestinal Endoscopy Clinics of North America* 3 (July 1993) 559-569.

6. Alvarado, Reichelderfer, "APIC guideline for infection prevention and control in flexible endoscopy,"145; Ott, Gostout, "Endoscopic maintenance and repairs," 559-569.

7. "Occupational exposure to bloodborne pathogens; Final rule," 64180.

8. Alvarado, Reichelderfer, "APIC guideline for infection prevention and control in flexible endoscopy," 145; Ball, *Endoscopic Surgery,* 100.

9. N S Chu, M Favero, "The microbial flora of the gastrointestinal tract and the cleaning of flexible endoscopes," *Gastrointestinal Endoscopy Clinics of North America* 10 (April 2000) 233-244.

10. D H Spach, F E Silverstein, W E Stamm, "Transmission of infection by gastrointestinal endoscopy and bronchoscopy," *Annals of Internal Medicine* 118 (Jan 15, 1993) 117-128; D J Weber, W A Rutala, A J DiMarino, "The prevention of infection following gastrointestinal endoscopy: The importance of prophylaxis and reprocessing," in *Gastrointestinal Diseases: An Endoscopic Approach,* ed A J DiMarino, S B Benjamen (Thorofare, NJ: Slack, Inc, 2002) 87-106; D J Weber, W A Rutala, "Lessons from outbreaks associated with bronchoscopy," *Infection Control and Hospital Epidemiology* 22 (July 2001) 403-408.

11. Weber, Rutala, "Lessons from outbreaks associated with bronchoscopy," 403-408; Ball, *Endoscopic Surgery,* 100; Spach, Silverstein, Stamm, "Transmission of infection by gastrointestinal endoscopy and bronchoscopy," 117-128.

12. J W Costerton, P S Stewart, E P Greenberg, "Bacterial biofilms: A common cause of persistent infections," *Science* 284 (May 21, 1999) 1318-1322; R M Donlan, "Biofilms: A source of infection?" in *Disinfection, Sterilization and Antisepsis: Principles and Practices in Healthcare Facilities,* ed W A Rutala (Washington, DC: Association for Professionals in Infection Control and Epidemiology, Inc, 2001) 219-226; C Johansen, P Falholt, L Gram, "Enzymatic removal and disinfection of bacterial biofilms," *Applied and Environmental Microbiology* 63 (September 1997) 3724-3728.

13. Alvarado, Reichelderfer, "APIC guideline for infection prevention and control in flexible endoscopy," 144-145.

14. *Ibid,* 144; Ball, *Endoscopic Surgery,* 87-90; D Fogg, "Infection control," in *Alexander's Care of the Patient in Surgery,* 11th ed, M H Meeker, J C Rothrock eds (St Louis: Mosby, 1999) 111; "Recommended practices for cleaning and caring for surgical instruments and powered equipment," in *Standards, Recommended Practices, and Guidelines* (Denver: AORN, Inc, 2002) 267-275.

15. Alvarado, Reichelderfer, "APIC guideline for infection prevention and control in flexible endoscopy," 144-145; Ball, *Endoscopic Surgery,* 87.

16. Alvarado, Reichelderfer, "APIC guideline for infection prevention and control in flexible endoscopy," 145.

17. *Ibid,* 152.

18. "Recommended practices for sterilization in perioperative practice settings," in *Standards, Recommended Practices, and Guidelines* (Denver: AORN, Inc, 2002) 333-342.

19. "Recommended practices for high-level disinfection," in *Standards, Recommended Practices, and Guidelines* (Denver: AORN, Inc, 2002) 211-216.

20. Alvarado, Reichelderfer, "APIC guideline for infection prevention and control in flexible endoscopy," 138-155.

21. C A Lawrence, S S Block, eds, *Disinfection, Sterilization, and Preservation* (Philadelphia: Lea and Febiger, 1968) 517-531; Alvarado, Reichelderfer, "APIC guideline for infection prevention and control in flexible endoscopy," 145-146.

22. S Burns et al, "Impact of variation in reprocessing invasive fiberoptic scopes on patient outcomes," (Abstract) *Infection Control and Hospital Epidemiology* 17 5 pt 2 (May 1996) P42; H A Fuselier, Jr, C Mason, "Liquid sterilization versus high level disinfection in the urologic office," *Urology* 50 no 3 (1997) 337-340; L F Muscarella, "High-level disinfection or 'sterilization' of endoscopes?" *Infection Control and Hospital Epidemiology* 17 (March 1996) 183-187.

23. W A Rutala, APIC Guidelines Committee, "APIC guideline for selection and use of disinfectants," *American Journal of Infection Control* 24 (August 1996) 313-342; Alvarado, Reichelderfer, "APIC guideline for infection prevention and control in flexible endoscopy," 146, 152.

24. Alvarado, Reichelderfer, "APIC guideline for infection prevention and control in flexible endoscopy," 144-145, 152; Spach, Silverstein, Stamm, "Transmission of infection by gastrointestinal endoscopy and bronchoscopy," 121.

25. Alvarado, Reichelderfer, "APIC guideline for infection prevention and control in flexible endoscopy," 144-145; M F Reichert, J K Schultz, "Infection control with endoscopes," in *Disinfection, Sterilization, and Preservation,* fifth ed, S S Block, ed (Philadelphia: Lippincott

Williams & Wilkins, 2001) 967-977; Weber, Rutala, DiMarino, "The prevention of infection following gastrointestinal endoscopy: The importance of prophylaxis and reprocessing," 87-106; Weber, Rutala, "Lessons from outbreaks associated with bronchoscopy," 403-408; Centers for Disease Control and Prevention, "Bronchoscopy-related infections and pseudoinfections—New York, 1996 and 1998," *Morbidity and Mortality Weekly Report* 48 (July 9, 1999) 557-560; M Sorin et al, "Nosocomial transmission of imipenem-resistant *Pseudomonas aeruginosa* following bronchoscopy associated with improper connection to the STERIS system 1 processor," *Infection Control and Hospital Epidemiology* 22 (July 2001) 409-413.

26. *Ibid.*

27. Alvarado, Reichelderfer, "APIC guideline for infection prevention and control in flexible endoscopy," 152; W A Rutala, D J Weber, "Water as a reservoir of nosocomial pathogens," *Infection Control and Hospital Epidemiology* 18 (September 1997) 609-616; Spach, Silverstein, Stamm, "Transmission of infection by gastrointestinal endoscopy and bronchoscopy," 121; Weber, Rutala, DiMarino, "The prevention of infection following gastrointestinal endoscopy: The importance of prophylaxis and reprocessing," 87-106.

28. Alvarado, Reichelderfer, "APIC guideline for infection prevention and control in flexible endoscopy," 152; Ball, *Endoscopic Surgery,* 116; Rutala, APIC Guidelines Committee, "APIC guideline for selection and use of disinfectants," 319.

29. Spach, Silverstein, Stamm, "Transmission of infection by gastrointestinal endoscopy and bronchoscopy," 117-128; D J Weber, W A Rutala, "Environmental issues and nosocomial infections," in *Prevention and Control of Nosocomial Infections,* third ed, R P Wenzel, ed (Baltimore: Williams & Wilkins, 1997) 491-514; Weber, Rutala, DiMarino, "The prevention of infection following gastrointestinal endoscopy: The importance of prophylaxis and reprocessing," 87-106; Weber, Rutala, "Lessons from outbreaks associated with bronchoscopy," 403-408.

30. Alvarado, Reichelderfer, "APIC guideline for infection prevention and control in flexible endoscopy," 145, 152.

Originally published February 1993, *AORN Journal.*
Revised November 1997; published January 1998.
Reformatted July 2000.
Revised; published February 2003, *AORN Journal.*

Recommended Practices for Endoscopic Minimally Invasive Surgery

The following recommended practices were developed by the AORN Recommended Practices Committee and have been approved by the AORN Board of Directors. They were presented as proposed recommended practices for comment to members and others. These recommended practices are effective January 1, 2005.

These recommended practices are intended as achievable recommendations representing what is believed to be an optimal level of practice. Policies and procedures will reflect variations in practice settings or clinical situations that determine the degree to which the recommended practices can be implemented.

AORN recognizes the numerous types of settings in which perioperative nurses practice. These recommended practices are intended to provide guidance for various practice settings. These practice settings include traditional ORs, ambulatory surgery units, physicians' offices, cardiac catheterization suites, endoscopy suites, radiology departments, and all other areas where operative and other invasive procedures may be performed.

Purpose

Endoscopic minimally invasive surgery (MIS) has evolved from a diagnostic modality to a widespread surgical technique. This evolution occurred in response to the reported benefits of endoscopic surgery compared to the benefits of conventional surgical procedures for patients. These recommended practices provide guidance to help perioperative personnel reduce risks to patients during endoscopic surgery. Benefits to the patient include reduced pain, faster healing, decreased length of hospital stay, and quicker return to normal life. The primary benefit to the hospital is financial, resulting from the decreased length of stay.

The perioperative nursing vocabulary is a clinically relevant and empirically validated standardized language. This standardized language consists of the Perioperative Nursing Data Set (PNDS) and includes perioperative nursing diagnoses, interventions, and outcomes. The expected outcomes of primary import to these recommended practices fall into two categories: freedom from injury during the perioperative period and maintenance/improvement of baseline physiological status. Specifics will be found in the documentation section.

Recommended Practice I

Potential patient injuries and complications associated with endoscopic MIS should be identified, and practices that reduce the risk of injuries and complications should be established.

1. The perioperative nurse should understand the goals and objectives of endoscopic MIS. Nursing knowledge, technological skills, and a thorough preoperative patient assessment provide the basis for establishing an appropriate plan of care for a patient undergoing endoscopic surgery.[1]

2. Patient monitoring during laparoscopic procedures should include measurement of the patient's
   - electrocardiogram,
   - end tidal carbon dioxide (CO_2),
   - noninvasive blood pressure,
   - oxygen saturation, and
   - temperature.

   Although endoscopic procedures are minimally invasive, using CO_2 for insufflation increases the risk of hypercarbia, subcutaneous emphysema, pulmonary embolism, pneumoscrotum, and hypothermia. End tidal CO_2 is closely monitored to detect the onset of hypercarbia, and the patient is observed for subcutaneous emphysema.[2] Carbon dioxide insufflation is one cause of hypothermia and is one contributing factor to thermal loss, along with irrigation, room temperature, exposed body surface, procedure length, and patient age and medical condition. The higher the flow of the CO_2, the lower the temperature of the gas,[3] but the incidence of hypothermia during endoscopic surgery has been reported to be similar to that of open surgery.[4,5] Additionally, endoscopic surgery presents a risk of limited visibility, which may result in undetected and uncontrolled bleeding.[6]

3. Specific positioning devices should be provided to secure the patient and provide safety in accordance with AORN's "Recommended practices for positioning the patient in the perioperative practice setting."[7] Exaggerated positioning may be used during endoscopic surgery to displace intracavity organs or enhance visibility for the surgical team. Positioning devices should be readily available before the patient is moved onto the OR bed.

4. Patients undergoing endoscopic procedures should be prepped and draped for an open procedure when applicable. It may be necessary to convert to an open procedure at any time. Prior preparation reduces anesthesia time and increases OR efficiency.[8] Prior preparation will facilitate conversion to an open procedure should that become necessary.[8] Instruments and supplies for an open procedure should be readily available. When it is necessary to convert to an open procedure, the conversion should be accomplished efficaciously.

5. Instruments that enter sterile body cavities are classified as critical items and should be sterile when used.[9] Endoscopes and endoscopic instruments (eg, biopsy forceps, graspers) used for endoscopic surgery should be processed according to AORN's "Recommended practices for cleaning and processing endoscopes and endoscope accessories."[10] Endoscopes and accessories to be sterilized should be packaged before sterilization or be processed immediately before use.

6. Illuminated endoscopic light cords should not be allowed to remain in contact with drapes, patients' skin, personnel's skin, or any flammable material. The heat from light cords or endoscopes may cause drapes to burn. Turning off light sources when they are not in use and holding cords away from drapes or placing them on a moist towel helps prevent burns and fire.[11] Complete all cable connections before activating the source. Place the source on standby when disconnecting cables. Drape the patient only when all flammable prep solutions have fully dried.[12]

7. In practice settings where technology for sterilization of endoscopes is not available, endoscopes and other heat-sensitive items should receive high-level disinfection immediately before each use. Refer to AORN's "Recommended practices for cleaning and processing endoscopes and endoscope accessories" for appropriate protocols.[10] The availability and use of disinfectants in the health care field is dynamic, and manufacturers' recommendations should be followed. As newer disinfectants become available, selection should be guided by information in the scientific literature.

Recommended Practice II

Potential patient injuries and complications associated with the distention media used during endoscopic MIS should be identified, and practices that reduce the risk of injuries and complications should be established.

1. The perioperative nurse should demonstrate competence in CO_2 insufflation and management of its risks.

   ♦ Carbon dioxide is the most commonly used insufflation gas because it is readily absorbed by the body and excreted by the lungs, does not support combustion, and is commonly available.[13]

   ♦ Carbon dioxide insufflators should be filtered with a single-use hydrophobic filter that is compatible with the insufflator and impervious to fluids. A hydrophobic filter helps prevent gas cylinder contaminants from flowing through the insufflator into the surgical cavity, prevents backflow of abdominal fluids and particulates that could contaminate the insufflator, and prevents cross contamination. When the filter is compatible with the insufflator, it does not interfere with flow rate. The flow of contaminants occurs more readily when the volume of remaining gas in the cylinder is low. Replacing the primary cylinder before the gas level is low helps prevent contamination of the sterile field by particulate matter.[13] Cylinders with nonferrous internal surfaces and surfaces incapable of creating residual material that could escape during the gaseous phase of delivery may be helpful in preventing the transfer of particulate matter.

   ♦ The cylinder should be checked to verify that the gas is CO_2. Only medical grade CO_2 should be used.

   ♦ The CO_2 cylinder should be replaced as needed. A second CO_2 cylinder should be readily available for each procedure. Methods of monitoring the level of remaining gas in the cylinder include

     – observing the insufflator gas cylinder gauge level,

     – monitoring the refill history, and

     – tracking cylinder use.

♦ The insufflator should be elevated above the level of the surgical cavity. Insufflator pressures should be monitored throughout the procedure, and the insufflator tubing should be disconnected from the trocar cannula before personnel deactivate the insufflator. When the pressure on the patient side is higher than at the insufflator connecting point, body fluid or gas is allowed to flow up the trocar cannula through the insufflation tubing and into the insufflator. This may result in cross contamination or damage to the insufflating device.[13]

♦ The insufflator and insufflation tubing should be flushed with gas before personnel connect the tubing to the cannula (eg, Verres needle). Flushing removes residual air from tubing, reducing the risk of air embolism. It also determines whether residues are present inside the insufflator.[13]

2. The perioperative nurse should demonstrate competence in fluid insufflation and management of its risks.

♦ Resectoscopes have been used for urologic procedures for many years. Since the 1950s, glycine 1.5% has been used as a cavity-distention medium for urologic procedures, primarily transurethral resection of the prostate (TURP), in which the resectoscope is used.[14] A complication sometimes observed with the use of glycine is TURP syndrome, which is caused by excessive absorption of the irrigating solution. Exposed blood vessels from tissue removal and elevated pressure being applied to the distention fluid enables intravasation (ie, distention fluid flows into the vascular system).[14,15] Physiological outcomes that can result from excessive fluid absorption include
  – cardiac overload,
  – cerebral edema,
  – dilutional hyponatremia, and
  – water intoxication.[14,16]
  Comparable symptoms can occur in women undergoing hysteroscopic surgery with distention fluids.

♦ Some gynecological procedures resect or ablate abnormal tissue using cutting or coagulating monopolar current. Procedures might include

  – endometrial ablation,
  – evaluation of infertility,
  – intrauterine assessment,
  – removal of intrauterine fibroids, and
  – removal of polyps.
  Cavity distention, often with irrigating fluids, provides a broader visual field. Irrigation fluids help clear the field of blood and debris.[17] Only electrically inert (ie, nonconductive), near-isotonic solutions should be used for uterine irrigation when monopolar electrosurgical current is used. Instead of energy being focused on the tissue, conductive solutions diffuse the energy, resulting in decreased tissue effect.

♦ Perioperative nurses should implement safety measures to minimize fluid-related patient complications during hysteroscopy procedures.
  Selection of distention fluid. When electrosurgical energy is to be used, only non-conductive, salt-free solutions should be used.[11] Media for cavity distention include
  – CO_2 gas;
  – dextran 70;
  – glycine;
  – isotonic electrolytic solution (eg, normal saline, Ringer's lactate);
  – mannitol;
  – sorbitol; and
  – water.
  Fluid deficit monitoring. Fluid deficit is the difference between the volume of fluid infused and the volume recovered.[18] This deficit should be monitored to determine how much fluid is being absorbed by the patient (ie, fluid intravasation). Dilutional hyponatremia is associated with intravasation. Rapid influx of hypotonic fluid increases circulation of free water and reduces the extracellular sodium concentration.[19] As a general rule, serum sodium falls 10 millimoles per L for every liter of hypotonic fluid absorbed.[19] The critical volume of intravasation before symptoms are exhibited is not predictable.[20] The American Association of Gynecological Laparoscopists suggests that 750 mL of fluid absorption implies impending excessive intravasation and completion of the procedure should be planned.[21] Fluid deficit amount

should be reported to the anesthesia care provider and surgeon at regular intervals during the procedure.

Fluid pressure monitoring and control. The ideal pressure at which fluid is delivered to the cavity is believed to be at or below the patient's mean arterial pressure.[18] There are four basic types of fluid delivery/monitoring systems.

- Gravity-fed systems deliver fluid at a rate and pressure dependent on the difference between height of the bag and the OR bed, the inner bore of the tubing, how tightly the endoscope sheath fits into the cavity, and the aperture of the outflow valve.[17]
- Automated gravitational systems maintain pressure and outflow control.
- Automated pressure systems deliver fluid at a constant pressure and release return flow when the internal pressure reaches a specified level.
- Automated roller pump systems measure fluid inflow by counting rotations on a pump roller or deliver fluid at a constant, pressure-regulated flow rate maintained by a pressure transducer. Fluid is extracted by a self-contained vacuum system. Fluid deficit is calculated on weight of the fluid infused versus the weight of the fluid returned.[18]

Procedure length. Fluid absorption increases with increased length of the procedure. Safe completion of procedures in an expedient manner (ie, one hour or less) can help limit complications from fluid absorption. Complications from fluid overload are less likely to occur and postoperative recovery time may be decreased with shorter anesthetic and procedure times.[18]

Recommended Practice III

Potential patient injuries and complications associated with electrosurgery used during endoscopic MIS should be identified, and practices that reduce the risk of injuries and complications should be established.

1. Perioperative team members should continuously monitor the functioning of equipment and the integrity of endoscopic instruments to ensure that hazards are minimized. Electrosurgical injuries are caused by insulation failure, direct coupling of current, and capacitive coupling. Equipment

should be used according to manufacturers' written instructions. Perioperative team members should continuously monitor the functioning of equipment and the integrity of endoscopic instruments to ensure that hazards are minimized.

- Insulation failure of the laparoscopic active electrode can be caused by trauma during reprocessing and provides an alternate pathway for the current to leave the electrode. Current leaves the electrode at the point of insulation failure as opposed to the tip of the electrode as intended. This can cause significant tissue damage and serious patient injury, particularly when the injury is internal and not immediately recognized. Routine visual inspection may reveal small cracks or mechanical damage. Use of disposable devices will not guarantee elimination of insulation failure because the quality of the insulation material may be less than that of a reusable item.[22]
- Direct coupling is caused by touching the active electrode to an anatomic structure other than the one intended. Three potential problems arise from direct coupling.
  - Metal-to-metal sparking can cause necrosis of underlying tissue.
  - Metal-to-metal sparking can cause frequency demodulation. The demodulated current results in lower frequency, which can result in neuromuscular stimulation noted by muscular twitching.
  - Metal-to-metal sparking may cause current flow to unintended sites. The density of the current determines the amount of tissue damage. A large point of contact will have low current density, and no tissue damage would be expected. A small point of contact will have high current density, and significant tissue damage is possible.[23]
- Capacitive coupling is caused by stray currents being transferred from one conductor to another with no insulation break. This occurs when magnetic fields are produced around the current-carrying, active electrode. When radio-frequency currents flow through an electrode, the flow may initiate stray currents onto other nearby conductors even though the insulation on the electrode and its wires are intact. Three common equipment arrangements may lead to significant amounts of stray current causing capacitive coupling.

– Active electrodes are placed through metal cannulae.
– Active electrodes are housed through operative laparoscopes.
– Active electrodes are used through metal suction irrigators.[24]

Capacitive-coupled, radio-frequency currents may cause undetected burns to nearby structures outside the endoscope's viewing area. Alternative-site burns can be severe and may damage tissue. These burns are particularly dangerous to hollow organs and may lead to undetected perforation with subsequent infection and possible death.[25] Use of active electrode monitoring devices minimizes the risk of undetected insulation failure, direct coupling, and capacitive coupling.

2. Electrical cords and plugs should be handled in a manner that minimizes the potential for damage and subsequent patient injuries. Equipment should be placed near the sterile field, with cords reaching the wall or column outlet without stress on a cord or blocking a traffic path. Stress on cords may cause damage to the cord, posing an electrical hazard. Cords should be free of kinks, knots, and bends that could damage the cord or cause leakage, current accumulation, and overheating of the cord's insulation. The internal parts of the connectors should be inspected for the appearance of shiny metal. If the presence of char debris is noted, the cord should be removed from use. Cords should be kept away from fluids. Fluids dripping onto the cord or connections cause electrical hazards.

Recommended Practice IV

Reusable endoscopic instruments should be processed according to AORN's recommended practices using methods that reduce the risk of personnel injury.

1. Perioperative personnel involved with endoscopic procedures should practice according to AORN's "Recommended practices for standard and transmission-based precautions in the perioperative practice setting."[26] Endoscopic surgery is referred to as *minimally invasive*. This terminology may lead to a false sense of security when considering potential hazards. This false sense of security may result in a less diligent use of standard precautions. Those performing the procedure and those who clean and process instruments and accessory equipment should wear personal protective equipment (PPE).[27]

2. Endoscopic surgery should be performed in a manner that minimizes perioperative personnel's exposure to blood and body fluids, droplets, noxious fumes, gases, or smoke. Smoke and laser plume should be evacuated throughout the procedure with appropriate smoke evacuation equipment. The release of gas, electrosurgical smoke, and laser plume during endoscopic surgery may expose surgical team members to blood products, fluid, and cellular debris. Smoke evacuation systems provide protection and reduce the risk of exposure to potentially infectious or toxic agents. Spontaneous sparking may result if electrosurgical smoke is allowed to accumulate in large amounts. AORN's "Recommended practices for electrosurgery"[28] and "Recommended practices for laser safety in practice settings"[29] should be used when selecting a smoke evacuation system.

3. Cleaning methods should minimize splashing, spraying, splattering, and droplet generation to minimize risk of exposure to blood or body fluids. Using standard precautions (eg, wearing gowns, gloves, goggles or face shields) helps protect employees. Standard precautions should include use of protective barriers or PPE, such as
   ♦ eye protection (eg, face shields, goggles, glasses with side shields);
   ♦ gowns; and
   ♦ intact gloves.

   Leg coverings, shoe covers, and other PPE may be used when indicated. Exposure to potentially infectious material is reduced by use of these products.

4. Disposable, reusable, and reposable instruments should be used according to manufacturers' recommendations. To ensure that the device is assembled correctly and will perform as intended after processing and reassembly, manufacturers' recommendations should include clear, understandable instructions for processing that include guidelines for

♦ assembly and disassembly,

♦ cleaning,

♦ routine user testing, and

♦ sterilization.

Products should not be purchased or used unless such information is provided.

Manufacturers are required by the US Food and Drug Administration to supply detailed instructions for processing reusables. Reposable instruments have a reusable component and a single-use or limited-use component. Adhering to AORN's "Recommended practices for cleaning and caring for surgical instruments and powered equipment"[30] and "Recommended practices for cleaning and processing endoscopes and endoscope accessories."[10] will minimize the risk of personnel injury associated with cleaning endoscopes and related equipment.

5. Sharps should be handled, processed, and stored in a manner that reduces the risk of injury to employees. Transporting reusable sharp instruments in containers that allow instrument handles to be immediately accessible to staff members minimizes risk of injury. Disposing of singe-use sharp instruments as regulated medical waste complies with state and federal guidelines.[27]

Recommended Practice V

Endoscopic instruments and equipment should meet performance and safety criteria established by the practice setting.

1. Written information regarding safety, testing methods, warranties, maintenance, and inspections for all endoscopic equipment should be obtained from the manufacturer. Endoscopic equipment manuals provide guidelines for developing operating, safety, and maintenance practices. Proper inspection, testing, use, and processing of equipment reduces the risk of adverse outcomes or damage to equipment.[27]

2. Each piece of endoscopic equipment (eg, camera system, monitor, insufflator) should be assigned an identification number. Identification numbers allow for inspections and tracking equipment problems.

3. Monitors should be positioned for good visibility for surgical team members and secured to carts or ceiling mounts. Good visibility is essential for patient care. Securing the monitors prevents injury to patients and personnel as well as equipment damage.[11]

4. All endoscopic equipment, including cameras, light sources, and videocassette recorders (VCRs) should be checked before use. Correct control settings should be labeled on equipment and on a quick reference chart attached to the equipment. When practical, equipment should be standardized so that systems are interchangeable.[11] Standardization of equipment allows for interchangeability in the event of equipment malfunction. To promote patient safety without delays during surgical procedures, all equipment should function correctly.

5. Endoscopic trocars should meet safety criteria established for the practice setting. The most frequent catastrophic patient injury involves trocars. Organ and vessel trauma may occur from excessive use of pressure during trocar insertion. When an all-metal system is used, capacitive current is safely dispersed through the metal anchor and the greater surface area provided by the chest or abdominal wall, thereby reducing current concentration. Metal cannula systems are best for the electrosurgical instrument port.[31] An all-plastic system is another alternative. Using this system, the capacitor is the patient, which minimizes the risk of concentrated capacitive-coupled current.[31] A risk of direct coupling injuries, however, remains. Hybrid trocars (ie, metal trocars with plastic anchors) are not recommended due to the unsafe dispersion of electrical energy.[31,32] Each trocar and cannula can act as an electrical conductor, inducing an electrical current from one to the other. This could result in capacitive-coupling injuries.

6. Fiber-optic light cords or cables should be long enough to reach from the surgical field to the equipment without undue stress. The cord should be inspected for broken light bundles before use. Broken light bundles will diminish the transmission of light and decrease visibility. A backup cord should be available. Tension increases the risk that the cords and fiber-optic cables will become disconnected or break, thereby creating a safety hazard for patients and

personnel. Having sterile backup cords readily available decreases surgical delays.[11]

7. Robotic devices may be used to hold and manipulate the laparoscope under the physician's guidance. The movement is voice activated or is managed by hand-held controls or a foot pedal. The robotic arm maintains the laparoscope in proper orientation, maximizing visualization and providing stable images. The laparoscope attaches to the robotic positioning arm with a magnetic coupling device. A sterile drape covers the arm to maintain a sterile field. The control system allows the operator to move the arm for exact positioning of the laparoscope.[33] All robotic equipment should be checked before use. Problematic issues identified with robotics include, but are not limited to,

 ♦ insufficient white balancing, which can cause the robot to misread the marker;
 ♦ limitation of the surgeon's movement due to positioning of the robotic arm; and
 ♦ a potential for conversion to an open procedure or need for a human camera assistant.[33]

Recommended Practice VI

Personnel should demonstrate competency in the use of endoscopic surgical equipment in the practice setting.

1. Perioperative personnel should demonstrate competence in the use of endoscopic surgical equipment before use. Instruction and return demonstration in proper usage minimizes the risk of injury and extends the life of the equipment.

2. Perioperative practitioners should be knowledgeable about advancing instrumentation, dissection and hemostasis, computer-assisted technologies (eg, voice recognition software, robotics), and camera technologies that simplify endoscopic MIS and expand its application (Table 1). Technology is continually evolving. Ongoing advances will need to be monitored and competencies, including skills validation, updated to reflect those advances.

3. Perioperative practitioners should be knowledgeable about procedural advances that simplify endoscopic MIS and that can expand its application (Table 2).

Recommended Practice VII

Perioperative nursing care for patients experiencing endoscopic MIS should be documented in the patient's record.

1. Documentation should be consistent with AORN's "Recommended practices for documentation of perioperative nursing care."[34]

2. The PNDS[35] should be used when documenting perioperative nursing care. Use of standardized nomenclature will facilitate data capture and analysis for safe, quality patient care. Documentation should include safety parameters implemented during MIS. The following PNDS outcomes are expected to be met with this recommended practice.
 ♦ O2—The patient is free from signs and symptoms of injury caused by extraneous objects.[35 (p85-90)]
 ♦ O4—The patient is free from signs and symptoms of electrical injury.[35 (p94-95)]
 ♦ O10—The patient is free from signs and symptoms of infection.[35 (p105-117)]
 ♦ O13—The patient's fluid, electrolyte, and acid-base balances are consistent with or improved from baseline levels established preoperatively.[35 (p123-127)]

 The PNDS should be referred to for identification of specific nursing diagnoses and nursing interventions.[35]

3. Information about adverse patient outcomes related to endoscopic MIS should be collected and analyzed as part of a facility-wide quality management program. To monitor the quality of patient care and formulate recommendations for changes, it is necessary to maintain a system of evaluation. Quality improvement standards for perioperative nurses that can be used for evaluating endoscopic surgery have been published.[36]

Recommended Practice VIII

Policies and procedures for endoscopic surgery should be developed, reviewed periodically, and readily available in the practice setting.

Table 1

TECHNOLOGICAL ADVANCES IN ENDOSCOPIC MINIMALLY INVASIVE SURGERY

The use of endoscopic surgery has increased exponentially during the past 10 years. Previously lengthy and difficult procedures now are being performed endoscopically. Advances in instrumentation, dissection and hemostasis techniques, and camera technologies have simplified surgical procedures and expanded application of the minimally invasive surgical approach. Following are examples of some of these advances.

Instrumentation advances
- Optical trocars allow for direct visualization when dissecting through layers of the abdominal wall into the peritoneum.[1]
- Blunt-tipped trocars (eg, open Hasson technique) prevent insufflation leakage. An inflatable balloon on the trocar sheath and a compressed sponge collar form an external seal.[1]
- Converterless trocars eliminate the need for adapters or converters when using different diameter instruments.[1]
- Built-in flush ports clean instruments of blood and debris.[1]
- One-handed control rotation wheels rotate instrument shafts.[1]
- Smaller instruments (eg, 2 mm) allow use of miniscopes.[1]

Dissection and hemostasis advances
- Electrosurgical instruments enhance cutting and hemostatic techniques.
- Ultrasonic energy delivered through a vibrating blade creates friction heat that denatures tissue proteins and forms a coagulum.[1]
- High-pressure fluid streams deflect accurately to cleave tissue planes.[1]
- Warming systems avoid potential hypothermia.[1]
- Tripolar cutting forceps have been developed to grasp, coagulate, and transect tissue using bipolar electrosurgery.[1]
- Argon beam coagulators have been adapted for laparoscopic hemostasis.[1]
- Carbon dioxide lasers are being used for ablation of pulmonary bullae.[2]

- Organ entrapment systems have been developed for removal of organs (ie, a plastic and nylon sack can be introduced, opened, and the organ placed inside for retrieval).[3]
- Morcellation techniques (ie, fragmenting tissue into small pieces that then are suctioned out through the barrel of a morcellator).[3]

Equipment advances
- Laparoscopic smoke evacuation has improved visibility.
- Digital documentation recorders allow procedures to be recorded.
- Digital flat panel monitors provide improved images and more flexibility in mounting positions.
- Robotic endoscope holders and positioners provide stability and improved motor control.
- Voice activation is used to control devices.
- Integrated ORs control the environment through touch-screen technologies.

Camera advances
- High resolution cameras using digital-signal processing and minimum illumination provide a distortion-free image.[1]
- Videotape endoscopes have video chips at the tip, thereby placing the camera in the surgical field.[1]
- Three-dimensional endoscopes offer depth perception to facilitate instrument manipulation and accurate internal structure interpretation.[4]

NOTES
1. J A Cadeddu et al, "Advances in laparoscopic instrumentation," Contemporary Urology *(October 1997) 14-24.*
2. M Benner et al, "Thoracoscopic laser ablation of pulmonary bullae," The Journal of Thoracic and Cardiovascular Surgery *107 (July 1993) 883-890.*
3. D A Urban et al "Organ entrapment and renal morcellation: Permeability studies," The Journal of Urology *150 (December 1993) 1792-1794.*
4. D H Birkett, L G Josephs, J Este-McDonald, "A new 3-D laparoscope in gastrointestinal surgery," Surgical Endoscopy *8 (December 1994) 1448-1451.*

1. These policies and procedure should include, but not be limited to,
   - documentation of identification numbers, settings used, and volume of gas;
   - equipment maintenance programs;
   - guidelines for equipment processing; and
   - staff member competency requirements.

2. These recommended practices should be used as guidelines for developing policies and procedures within the practice setting. Policies and procedures establish authority, responsibility, and accountability and serve as operational guidelines. An introduction to reviewing the policies and procedures should be included in

Table 2

PROCEDURAL ADVANCES IN ENDOSCOPIC MINIMALLY INVASIVE SURGERY (MIS)

Like other technologies, procedural advances in MIS are ongoing. Improved technology, enables an ever-growing cadre of MIS procedures within surgical specialty areas. The following represent some of the advances in various surgical specialties.

General surgery

Procedures include mediastinoscopy, an early entry into the MIS field; laparoscopic cholecystectomy; appendectomy; small bowel resection; bariatric procedures; gastrectomy; splenectomy; hernia repair; Nissen fundoplication; thymectomy; various biopsies; node sampling; and others.

▪ Carbon dioxide insufflation is the standard for providing visualization of abdominal structures and offering safe pneumoperitoneum.[1]

▪ Gasless laparoscopic procedures are performed to overcome adverse effects of pneumoperitoneum without altering cardiac function.[1]

▪ Abdominal walls can be elevated by means of a subcutaneous lifting system of curved blades suspended from a mechanical arm attached to a rigid pillar. The arm then is elevated as far as necessary to obtain optimal exposure.[2]

▪ Hand-assisted laparoscopic surgery has been introduced for use in laparoscopic-assisted splenectomy and colorectal procedures. The hand can be used as a retractor, dissector, and tactile sensor.[3]

Gynecological surgery

Initially, diagnostic procedures were performed, but with time, surgical procedures were performed, including abdominal wall lifting, gasless procedures, and robotics. Combination approaches blend the use of laparoscopy and vaginal approaches for laparoscopy-assisted hysterectomy.[4]

▪ Endometrial ablation now is performed via hysteroscopy for menorrhagia.

▪ In the 1980s, methods were developed including neodimium: yttrium-aluminum-garnet (Nd-YAG) laser ablation, transcervical resection of the endometrium, and rollerball electrocoagulation of the endometrium.[5]

▪ In the 1990s, techniques improved, including balloon heating, intrauterine instillation of heated saline, endometrial laser thermal therapy using a diode laser, global three-dimensional bipolar ablation, punctual vaporization, photodynamic endometrial ablation, microwave endometrial ablation, radio frequency procedures, menostat, and cryotherapy. Discussion of single methods or comparison of two methods can be found in the literature.[5-8]

Orthopedic surgery

Procedures began as diagnostic and were limited primarily to the knee. Procedures now are both diagnostic and surgical. Shoulder, elbow, and ankle arthroscopy now are commonplace. Less commonly performed are hip and wrist arthroscopy.[9]

▪ Lasers have been used to shrink stretched capsular tissues of the shoulder. When heated to the appropriate temperature, the tissue contracts.[9]

▪ Articular tissue also can be replaced by various methods, including abrasion arthroplasty; harvesting the patient's own articular cartilage, growing it, and reinjecting it; and mosaicplasty, which consists of taking cores of bone with articular cartilage attached and impacting them into predrilled holes in arthritic areas.[9]

Ear, nose, and throat surgery

Visualization of the larynx was the first reported procedure. Procedural advances now include tumor removal, polyp removal, encephalocele repair, cerebrospinal fluid leak repair, septal reconstruction, pituitary surgery, and others.[10]

▪ Equipment advances such as the progression from distally lighted endoscopes, to telescopic rod lens systems, to flexible fiber-optic systems have led to enhanced visualization. Brushings, washings, and biopsies can be taken from the upper lobes of the lungs.[11]

▪ Microscopically controlled laryngoscopy allows for vocal cord procedures.

▪ Laser surgery allows for precise excision of lesions of the larynx, trachea, and bronchi.[11]

▪ Endoscopic sinus procedures relieve sinus obstruction.[10]

Urological surgery

Cystoscopy was the first urologic procedure using MIS. Now, this often is performed as an office procedure. Urological MIS procedures now include endoscopic nephrectomy, hand-assisted nephrectomy, and transperitoneal laparoscopic nephrectomy. Additionally, balloon insufflation has been used as a dissection technique in the upper retroperitoneal space allowing for nephrectomy, tumor nephrectomy, nephropexy, renal cyst marsupialization, and renal biopsy.[12]

Cardiovascular/thoracic surgery

Videotape assistance first was used for closed chest internal mammary artery harvests and congenital heart defect procedures.[13] Videotape-assisted thoracic surgery provides for more complete exploration than traditional mediastinotomy and allows better access for biopsies.

Table 2, *continued*

PROCEDURAL ADVANCES IN ENDOSCOPIC MINIMALLY INVASIVE SURGERY (MIS)

■ Mitral valve replacement has advanced to using videotape-directed, voice-activated, robotically-controlled cameras.[13]

■ Computer-enhanced instrumentation allows for endoscopic coronary artery bypass grafting.[14]

■ The first human laparoscopically-assisted aorto-bifemoral bypass was completed in 1993. With the development of clamps, forceps, and best approaches, the procedure is performed entirely laparoscopically today.[15]

■ Endoscopic subfascial perforator ligation is performed for chronic venous insufficiency with results similar to open procedures and without the concomitant morbidity and mortality.[16]

Plastic surgery

■ Endoscopically-assisted plastic surgery was introduced in the mid 1980s.[17]

■ Procedures evolving during the 1990s include forehead lifts, full facelifts, corrugator muscle resection, breast augmentation, carpal tunnel release, reconstructive breast surgeries, facial fracture reduction, and various muscle harvesting procedures.[17]

Neurosurgery

■ The earliest reported endoscopic neurosurgery was performed in 1910 when two children were treated for hydrocephalus by endoscopic coagulation of the choroids plexus.[18]

■ By 1960, technological advances allowed for additional endoscopic procedures, such as fenestration, biopsy, partial or total removal of cystic lesions; partial or total removal of tumors; evacuation of intracerebral or subdural hematomas; spinal excision of herniated discs; and carpal tunnel release.[18]

■ Endoscopically-assisted procedures include aneurysm excision and repair, acoustic neuroma removal, and transsphenoidal pituitary surgery.[18]

NOTES

1. A Vezakis et al, "Randomized comparison between low-pressure laparoscopic cholecystectomy and gasless laparoscopic cholecystectomy," Surgical Endoscopy 13 (September 1999) 890-893.

2. A Alijani, A Cushier, "Abdominal wall lift systems in laparoscopic surgery: Gasless and low pressure systems," Seminars in Laparoscopic Surgery 8 (March 2001) 53-62.

3. Y Miura et al, "Gasless hand-assisted laparoscopic surgery for colorectal cancer," Diseases of the Colon Rectum 44 (June 2001) 896-898.

4. M Canestrelli et al, "The new techniques of gynaecologic laparoscopy: Gasless, open Hasson, optic trocar," Panminerva Medica 41(December 1999) 371-374.

5. O R Kochli "Endometrial ablation in the year 2000—Do we have more methods than indications?" in Contributions to Gynecology and Obstetrics vol 20 (Basel, Switzerland: Karger, 2000) 90-120.

6. O Taskin et al, "Long-term histopathologic and morphologic changes after thermal endometrial ablation," Journal of the American Association of Gynecologic Laparoscopists 9 (May 2002) 186-190.

7. F D Loffer, "Three-year comparison of thermal balloon and rollerball ablation in treatment of menorrhagia," Journal of the American Association of Gynecologic Laparoscopists 8 (February 2001) 48-54.

8. M Pellicano et al, "Hysteroscopic transcervical endometrial resection versus thermal destruction for menorrhagia: A prospective randomized trial on satisfaction rate," American Journal of Obstetrics and Gynecology 187 (September 2002) 545-550.

9. G K Miller "Operative arthroscopy into the next century," Comprehensive Therapy 24 (August 1998) 383-387.

10. D W Kennedy, M Roth, "Functional endoscopic sinus surgery," in Otorhinolaryngology: Head and Neck Surgery, 15th ed, J J Ballenger, J B Snow, eds (Baltimore: Williams & Wilkins, 1996) 173-181.

11. J B Snow, J A Schild, "Introduction to peroral endoscopy," in Otorhinolaryngology: Head and Neck Surgery, 15 ed, J J Ballenger, J B Snow, eds (Baltimore: Williams & Wilkins, 1996) 1189-1199.

12. J J Rassweiler et al, "Retroperitoneal laparoscopic nephrectomy and other procedures in the upper retroperitoneum using a balloon dissection technique," European Urology 25 (1994) 229-236.

13. W R Chitwood, L W Nifong, "Minimally invasive videoscopic mitral valve surgery: The current role of surgical robotics," Journal of Cardiac Surgery 15 (January/February 2000) 61-75.

14. V Falk et al, "Total endoscopic off-pump coronary artery bypass grafting," The Heart Surgery Forum 3 (February 2000) 29-31.

15. Y M Dion, C R Gracia, O Hartung, "Laparoscopic vascular surgery," in Surgical Laparoscopy, second ed, K A Zucker, ed (Baltimore: Lippincott Williams & Wilkins, 2001) 709-719.

16. W Schum, W S Thomas, "Endoscopic technique for subfascial perforating vein interruption," in Surgical Laparoscopy, second ed, K A Zucker, ed (Baltimore: Lippincott Williams & Wilkins, 2001) 720-726.

17. P Giovanoli, M Frey "The history of endoscopy in plastic and reconstructive surgery up to video assisted microsurgery," in Endoscopy and Microsurgery, M Frey, ed (New York: Springer-Verlag Wein, 2001) 1-4.

18. J Caemaert "Endoscopic neurosurgery," in Operative Neurosurgical Techniques: Indications, Methods, and Results, vol 1, fourth ed, H Schmidek, ed (Philadelphia: WB Saunders, 2000) 535-570.

orientation and ongoing educational sessions to help personnel develop the appropriate knowledge, skills, and attitudes that affect patient care. Policies and procedures also assist in developing quality assurance and improvement activities.

3. Policies and procedures for equipment must be in compliance with the Safe Medical Devices Act (SMDA) of 1990, as well as facility-specific policies and procedures.[37] If patient or personnel injuries or equipment failures occur, the laparoscopic equipment and associated attachments must be handled in accordance with the SMDA. Device identification, maintenance and service information, and adverse event information should be included in the report from the practice setting.[38]

4. Policies and procedures must comply with the Standards of Privacy and Security of the Health Insurance Portability and Accountability Act of 1996 for the protection of health information. In addition, these policies and procedures should take into account applicable state laws, as well as applicable national and professional standards. These policies and procedures should cover not only the disclosure of information but also access to and use of databases, including, but not limited to, digital pictures and patient information. Policies and procedures should be revised as needed to account for any changes or amendments to applicable laws, rules, and standards.[39]

Glossary

Capacitive coupling: Transfer of electrical current from the active electrode through intact insulation to adjacent conductive items (eg, tissue, trocars).

Capacitors: Two conductors separated by an insulator (eg, insulated active electrode, trocar cannula); instrument for storing electricity.

Critical item: Instruments or objects that are introduced directly into the human body, either into or in contact with the blood stream or normally sterile areas of the body; an item that enters sterile tissue or the vascular system.

Demodulation: The operation on a previously modulated wave in such a way that it will have substantially the same characteristics as the original modulating wave.

Dilutional hyponatremia: A decrease in the serum sodium level due to intravasation of fluids, which dilute the soluble components of the serum.

Direct coupling: Touching the laparoscopic active electrode to another surgical field.

Endoscopic minimally invasive surgery (MIS): Surgical techniques that use endoscopic approaches rather than dissection.

High-level disinfection: A process that kills all microorganisms with the exception of high numbers of bacterial spores; using an Environmental Protection Agency-registered agent that kills vegetative bacteria, tubercle bacilli, some spores, fungi, and lipid and non-lipid viruses given appropriate concentration, submersion, and contact time. Manufacturers' recommendations may differ.

Hypertonic: Having a greater osmotic pressure (ie, higher solute concentration) than a reference solution. If a cell is surrounded by a hypotonic solution, osmotic pressure tends to force the water out of the cell, and the cell shrinks.

Hyponatremia: An abnormally low concentration of sodium ions in circulating blood.

Hypotonic: Having a lower osmotic pressure (ie, lower solute concentration) than a reference solution. If a cell is in a hypotonic solution, osmotic pressure tends to force the water into the cell, and the cell swells.

Hydrophobic insufflation filter: An in-line filter that retains a high percentage of particulates greater than a specified size. The hydrophobic media protects against fluid backflow into the insufflation gas.

Hysteroscopy: Endoscopic visualization of the uterine cavity and tubal orifices.

Insufflate: To blow into; to fill any cavity or orifice of the body.

Insufflation: The act or instance of insufflating.

Intravasation: The entrance of foreign material into a blood vessel.

Invasive procedures: Surgical entry into tissues, cavities, or organs.

Light cord: A cable of fiber-optic filaments used to transport light to the surgical field.

Morcellation: The process of fragmenting tissue into small pieces.

Osmole: The standard unit of osmotic pressure; the molecular weight of a solute, in grams, divided by the number of ions or particles into which it dissociates in solution.

Osmosis: The passive movement of fluid through a semipermeable membrane from a region of lower solute concentration to a region of higher solute concentration.

Osmotic pressure: The tendency and rate of water to move across a semipermeable membrane toward a region of higher solute concentration.

Reposable: An instrument that has limited use or an instrument with a combination of reusable and disposable components.

Solute: A dissolved substance suspended within a solution.

Solution: A homogeneous mixture of two or more compounds.

NOTES

1. "Standards of perioperative clinical practice," in *Standards, Recommended Practices, and Guidelines* (Denver: AORN, Inc, 2004) 181-183.

2. J L Flowers, K A Zucker, R W Bailey, "Complications," in *Laparoscopic Surgery,* ed G H Ballantyne, P F Leahy, I M Modlin (Philadelphia: WB Saunders, Co, 1994) 78-82.

3. K A Ball, "Surgical modalities," in *Alexander's Care of the Patient in Surgery,* 12th ed, J C Rothrock, D A Smith, D R McEwen, eds (St Louis: Mosby, 2003) 41-96.

4. A J Luck et al, "Core temperature changes during open and laparoscopic colorectal surgery," *Surgical Endoscopy* 13 (May 1999) 480-483.

5. E Berber et al, "Intraoperative thermal regulation in patients undergoing laparoscopic vs open surgical procedures," *Surgical Endoscopy* 15 (March 2001) 281-285.

6. R M Colver, "Laparoscopy: Basic technique, instrumentation, and complications," *Surgical Laparoscopy & Endoscopy* 2 (March 1992) 3540.

7. "Recommended practices for positioning the patient in the perioperative setting," in *Standards, Recommended Practices, and Guidelines* (Denver: AORN, Inc, 2004) 341-346.

8. K A Ball "Implementing and evaluation patient care," in *Endoscopic Surgery* (St Louis: Mosby-Year Book, Inc, 1997) 41-49.

9. W A Rutala, 1994-1996 APIC Guidelines Committee "APIC guideline for selection and use of disinfectants," *American Journal of Infection Control* 24 (August 1996) 313-342.

10. "Recommended practices for cleaning and processing endoscopes and endoscope accessories," in *Standards, Recommended Practices, and Guidelines* (Denver: AORN, Inc, 2004) 261-266.

11. K A Ball "Basic endoscopic equipment," in *Endoscopic Surgery* (St Louis: Mosby-Year Book, Inc, 1997) 111-139.

12. "The patient is on fire! A surgical fires primer," *ECRI Health Devices* 12 (January 1992) 21.

13. "Entry of abdominal fluids into laparoscopic insufflator," *ECRI Health Devices* 21(May 1992) 181.

14. O Istre, "Fluid balance during hysteroscopic surgery," *Current Opinions in Obstetrics and Gynecology* 9 (August 1997) 219-225.

15. R H Harrison, J S Boren, J R Robison, "Dilutional hyponatremic shock: Another concept of the transurethral prostatic resection reaction," *Journal of Urology* 75 (January 1956) 95-110.

16. D Gravenstein "Transurethral resection of the prostrate (TURP) syndrome: A review of the pathophysiology and management," *Anesthesia Annals* 84 (February 1997) 438-446.

17. S L Corson "Hysteroscopic fluid management," *The Journal of the American Association Gynecological Laparoscopists* 4 (May 1997) 375-379.

18. K L Bennett, C Ohrmundt, J A Malone, "Preventing intravasation in women undergoing hysteroscopic procedures," *AORN Journal* 64 (November 1996) 792-799.

19. K B Isaacson, "Complications of hysteroscopy," *Obstetrics and Gynecology Clinics of North America* 26 (March 1999) 39-51.

20. D M Morrison, "Management of hysteroscopic surgery complications," *AORN Journal* 69 (January 1999) 194-209.

21. F D Loffer et al, "Hysteroscopic fluid monitoring guidelines," *The Journal of American Association of Gynecological Laparoscopists* 7 (February 2000) 167-168.

22. R C Odell, "Electrosurgery principles and safety issues," *Clinical Obstetrics and Gynecology* 38 (September 1995) 610-621.

23. S Rohlf, "Electrosurgical safety considerations for minimally invasive surgery," *Minimally Invasive Surgical Nursing* 9 (Spring 1995) 26-29.

24. R D Tucker, C R Voyles, "Laparoscopic electrosurgical complications and their precautions," *AORN Journal* 62 (July 1995) 51-71.

25. W Ming-Ping et al, "Complications and recommended practices for electrosurgery in laparoscopy," *American Journal of Surgery* 179 (January 2000) 67-73.

26. "Recommended practices for standard and transmission-based precautions in the perioperative practice setting," in *Standards, Recommended Practices, and Guidelines* (Denver: AORN, Inc, 2004) 361-366.

27. K A Ball, "Care and maintenance of instruments," in *Endoscopic Surgery* (St Louis: Mosby-Year Book, Inc, 1997) 83-110.

28. "Recommended practices for electrosurgery," in *Standards, Recommended Practices, and Guidelines* (Denver: AORN, Inc, 2004) 245-260.

29. "Recommended practices for laser safety in practice settings," in *Standards, Recommended Practices, and Guidelines* (Denver: AORN, Inc, 2004) 319-324.

30. "Recommended practices for cleaning and caring for surgical instruments and powered equipment," in *Standards, Recommended Practices, and Guidelines* (Denver: AORN, Inc, 2004) 309-317.

31. T G Vancaillie, "Electrosurgery at laparoscopy: Guidelines to avoid complications," *Gynaecological Endoscopy* 3 (Spring 1994) 143-150.

32. K A Ball, "Endoscopic instruments," in *Endoscopic Surgery* (St Louis: Mosby-Year Book, Inc, 1997) 51-82.

33. K Omote et al, "Self-guided robotic camera control for laparoscopic surgery compared with human camera control," *The American Journal of Surgery* 177 (April 1999) 321-324.

34. "Recommended practices for documenting perioperative nursing care," in *Standards, Recommended Practices, and Guidelines* (Denver: AORN Inc, 2004) 241-243.

35. S C Beyea, ed, *Perioperative Nursing Data Set: The Perioperative Nursing Vocabulary,* second ed (Denver: AORN, Inc, 2002).

36. "Quality improvement standards for perioperative nursing," in *Standards, Recommended Practices, and Guidelines* (Denver: AORN, Inc, 2004) 187-196.

37. US Food and Drug Administration, "Medical devices; Device tracking: Final rule and request for comments," *Federal Register* 58 (Aug 16, 1993) 43442–43450.

38. M A Heller, *Guide to Medical Device Regulation,* vol 2 (Washington DC: Thompson Publishing, 1998) Appendix 2000; 366.

39. "Standards for privacy of individually identifiable health information; Final rule," *Federal Register* 164 (Aug 14, 2002) 53183-53273.

RESOURCES

Ballantyne, G H. *Atlas of Laparoscopic Surgery* (Philadelphia: WB Saunders, 2000).

Eubanks, S; Swanstrom, L. *Mastery of Endoscopic and Laparoscopic Surgery* (Philadelphia: Lippincott Williams & Wilkins, 2000).

Talamini, M. *Advances in Minimally Invasive Surgery* (Philadelphia: Lippincott Williams & Wilkins, 2001).

Zucker, K. *Surgical Laparoscopy,* second ed, K A Zucker, ed (Baltimore: Lippincott Williams & Wilkins, 2001).

Originally published as proposed recommended practices February 1994, *AORN Journal.*

Revised November 1998; published February 1999, *AORN Journal.*

Reformatted July 2000.

Revised November 2004; published March 2005, *AORN Journal.*

Recommended Practices for Environmental Cleaning in the Surgical Practice Setting

The following recommended practices were developed by the AORN Recommended Practices Committee and have been approved by the AORN Board of Directors. They were presented as proposed recommended practices for comments by members and others. They are effective January 1, 2003.

These recommended practices are intended as achievable recommendations representing what is believed to be an optimal level of practice. Policies and procedures will reflect variations in practice settings and/or clinical situations that determine the degree to which the recommended practices can be implemented.

AORN recognizes the numerous types of settings in which perioperative nurses practice. These recommended practices are intended as guidelines adaptable to various practice settings. These practice settings include traditional ORs, ambulatory surgery units, physicians' offices, cardiac catheterization suites, endoscopy suites, radiology departments, and all other areas where operative and other invasive procedures may be performed.

Purpose

These recommended practices provide guidance for environmental cleaning in the surgical practice setting. Conscientious application of these recommended practices should result in a clean environment for surgical patients. These recommended practices should be carried out in a manner that minimizes health care workers' and patients' exposure to potentially infectious microorganisms. All patients potentially are infected with bloodborne and other pathogens. All surgical procedures, therefore, must be considered potentially infectious, and the same environmental cleaning protocols must be implemented for all procedures.

Recommended Practice I

Patients should be provided a safe, clean environment.

1. Cleaning should be performed on a regular basis to reduce the amount of dust, organic debris, and microbial load in surgical environments.[1] Operating rooms should be cleaned before and after each surgical procedure and at the end of each day. Cleaning also may be necessary during any surgical procedure (see recommende practice II). Environmental cleaning is a team effort involving surgical personnel and environmental services personnel. The ultimate responsibility for ensuring a clean surgical environment rests with perioperative nurses. Administrative personnel should ensure that environmental cleaning practices comply with the standards established for the practice setting.[2]

2. All horizontal surfaces in the OR (eg, furniture, surgical lights, equipment) should be damp dusted before the first scheduled surgical procedure of the day with a clean, lint-free cloth moistened with an Environmental Protection Agency (EPA)-registered hospital disinfectant.[3] Equipment from areas outside the OR should be damp dusted before being brought into the OR. Dust and lint are deposited on horizontal surfaces. Proper cleaning of these surfaces helps reduce airborne contaminants that may travel on dust and lint.[4]

3. For subsequent surgical procedures, between-procedure cleaning is performed. Preparation of the OR should include visual inspection for cleanliness before case carts, supplies, and instrument sets are brought into the room. Although the level of contamination that can influence surgical site infection rates is not known, a clean surgical environment will reduce the number of microbial flora present.[5]

4. If at all possible, latex-sensitive patients should be scheduled as the first procedure of the day. It is difficult to remove all traces of latex proteins when latex products have been used during the previous procedure. For additional information about latex-sensitive patients, consult the "AORN latex guideline."[6]

Recommended Practice II

During surgical procedures, contamination should be confined and contained within the immediate vicinity of the surgical field to the degree possible.

1. Spills of contaminated debris (eg, blood, tissue, body fluids) in areas outside the surgical field should be removed as promptly as possible. Prompt cleanup and decontamination of

potentially infectious materials helps maintain a safe, clean surgical environment.[7] When cleaning spills of blood or other potentially infectious material (OPIM), use gloves and other personal protective equipment (PPE) as appropriate to the task. It is unknown which patients may harbor harmful pathogens. Use of PPE protects health care workers from direct exposure to potentially infectious microorganisms.[8]

2. Small (ie, less than 10 mL) spills should be cleaned and disinfected using a soft, absorbent, low-linting cloth and either an intermediate-level germicide (ie, germicides that are EPA-registered for hospital use and have a tuberculocidal claim) or an EPA-registered germicide product having a label claim for HIV and/or hepatitis B virus.[9] The selected product should be used at the recommended dilution and for the full contact time. Sodium hypochlorite (ie, chlorine bleach) in a 1:100 dilution may be used for small spills (eg, blood, OPIM) on nonporous surfaces.

3. Spills containing large amounts (ie, greater than 10 mL) of blood and OPIM should be cleaned first using a disposable absorbent material followed by application of the selected germicidal product. Used cleaning materials, including the absorbent material, should be discarded in biohazard-labeled containers. For large spills, a 1:10 dilution of sodium hypochlorite may be added to the spill before cleanup.[10]

4. A fresh solution of sodium hypochlorite for cleanup and disinfection should be prepared daily for maximum effectiveness. Even when stored in a covered, dark, plastic container, a chlorine solution may lose up to 50% of its disinfecting capability during a 30-day period. Solutions of sodium hypochlorite should be labeled, dated, and discarded after 24 hours. If used for cleaning instruments and other metal surfaces, sodium hypochlorite may cause pitting and/or other damage to those surfaces; therefore, it is preferable to use a readily available EPA-registered hospital-grade disinfectant with a tuberculocidal claim for noncritical items and environmental surfaces.[11] Alcohol is not recommended for cleaning large environ-

mental surfaces.[12] For chemical spills, consult the appropriate material safety data sheet for the chemical(s) in question.

5. Contaminated disposable patient care items should be discarded in leak-proof, tear-resistant, labeled containers to prevent exposure of personnel to items potentially contaminated with infectious microorganisms and to prevent contamination of the surgical environment.[13]

6. People handling contaminated items should wear gloves, gowns, and/or other protective attire as appropriate to the task.

7. Contaminated items should not leave the OR unless necessary for patient care. All blood, tissue, and body-fluid specimens should be placed in leak-proof containers for health care workers' protection. The exterior surfaces of specimen containers received from the surgical field should be cleaned with an EPA-registered hospital-grade disinfectant before leaving the surgical environment. Inanimate objects (eg, laboratory slips, x-rays, patient charts) contaminated with blood, tissue, or body fluids may expose health care workers to bloodborne pathogens. Items that cannot be discarded and replaced with noncontaminated items (eg, x-rays, patient records) should be placed in a protective covering when possible.[14] Items that can be discarded and replaced with noncontaminated items (eg, laboratory requisitions) should be handled accordingly.

Recommended Practice III

After each surgical procedure, a safe, clean environment should be reestablished. Disposable items should be disposed of according to local, state, and federal regulations and in accordance with the AORN "Recommended practices for environmental responsibility in the practice setting."[15] Reusable items should be processed according to the policies and procedures of the surgical practice setting.

1. Patient transport vehicles, including nondisposable straps and attachments, should be cleaned after use with a cloth moistened with an EPA-registered hospital-grade germicidal agent. Transport vehicles are considered

contaminated through patient contact.[16] Consult manufacturers' instructions and safety advisories when using EPA-registered low- to intermediate-level germicides.

2. Avoid unnecessarily exposing neonates to disinfectant residue on environmental surfaces. Do not use phenolics or any other chemical germicide to disinfect bassinets or incubators. If a disinfectant solution is used, prepare the solution in concentrations as directed by the manufacturer. After disinfection, rinse the disinfected surface(s) with water.[17]

3. Operating room equipment and furniture that are visibly soiled should be cleaned with an EPA-registered hospital-grade germicidal agent at the end of each surgical procedure. High-level disinfectants are not recommended for environmental surfaces.[18] Walls, doors, surgical lights, and ceilings should be spot cleaned if soiled with blood, tissue, or body fluids. Anesthesia equipment should be cleaned according to the AORN "Recommended practices for cleaning and processing anesthesia equipment."[19] Mechanical friction should be used when cleaning. Effective cleaning depends on the scrubbing action. Equipment and furniture used for surgical procedures are considered contaminated through contact with patients and OPIM, including blood.

4. Visibly soiled areas on the floor should be cleaned using a new or freshly laundered mop head and an EPA-registered hospital-grade germicidal agent. Unless the germicidal agent is changed after each use, the mop head should be dipped into the solution only when it is clean and before the mopping activity is begun. A used/soiled mop head should not be redipped into the solution. If the floor is grossly soiled so as to necessitate redipping the mop into the solution, the solution should be discarded after use and a fresh solution mixed for additional mopping activity. Soiled mop handles should be cleaned with the EPA-registered germicide or discarded according to the type of contamination present. Floor cleaning removes soil, organic debris, and dust. For end-of-procedure cleaning, it is only necessary to clean a 3-ft to 4-ft perimeter around the

surgical field when it is visibly soiled. The area cleaned should be extended as necessary to adjacent visibly soiled areas. The OR bed should be moved to check for any items (eg, sponges, instruments) that may be concealed under the bed. For daily terminal cleaning, the entire floor should be cleaned, including the area under the OR bed. There is no scientific evidence to support cleaning the entire floor after each procedure.[20]

5. Disposable items contaminated with blood and/or tissue that would release blood or other infectious materials in a liquid or semiliquid state if compressed or items that are caked with dried blood or OPIM must be placed in closable, leak-proof containers or bags that are color coded, labeled, or tagged for easy identification as biohazardous waste. These containers or bags should be transported in washable carts or vehicles. If there is a likelihood or even a possibility that the containers or bags could leak, the transport container must be covered.[21] State regulations for transport and disposal of regulated waste should be consulted. State regulations may be more stringent than federal regulations, and if so, supersede federal regulations. Contaminated disposable items are placed in leak-proof containers to prevent exposure of personnel to blood, tissue, and/or body fluids and to prevent contamination of the environment. Color coding and/or labeling alert personnel and others to the presence of items potentially contaminated with infectious microorganisms, prevent exposure of personnel to infectious waste, and prevent contamination of the environment.[22] Disposable items may include gowns and gloves; procedural drapes; suction tubing, liners, and canisters; and opened and used supplies. Disposable items that do not release blood or other infectious material in a liquid or semi-liquid state if compressed or that are not caked with dried blood or OPIM are considered non-infectious and should be placed in a separate receptacle designated for noninfectious waste. Again, state regulations should be consulted.

6. All used, disposable sharps (eg, needles, scalpels, staples/stapling devices, electrosurgical

tips, pins) are considered infectious waste. They must be placed in designated puncture-resistant containers that have a biohazard label. Puncture wounds from used sharp items expose personnel to potentially infectious microorganisms.[23]

7. Reusable items contaminated with blood and/or tissue that would release blood or other infectious materials in a liquid or semiliquid state if compressed or items that are caked with dried blood or OPIM must be placed in closable, leak-proof containers or bags that are color coded, tagged, or labeled as infectious. These containers should be transported in closed washable carts or vehicles. Contaminated reusable items are placed in leak-proof containers to prevent exposure of personnel to blood, tissue, and/or body fluids and to prevent contamination of the environment. Color coding and/or labeling alert personnel and others to the presence of items potentially contaminated with infectious microorganisms, prevent exposure of personnel to infectious waste, and prevent contamination of the environment.[24] Reusable items may include procedural drapes, gowns, and other items. Reusable items that do not release blood or other infectious material in a liquid or semiliquid state if compressed or that are not caked with dried blood or OPIM are considered noninfectious. These items should be cleaned, decontaminated, and processed according to facility policy. As with disposables, any state regulations governing cleaning and processing of reusables should be consulted and followed.

8. If a reusable suction system is used, suction contents should be disposed of according to local, state, and/or federal regulations. Engineering controls (eg, specialized liquid waste management systems) and PPE should be used as appropriate to protect the health care worker if emptying, cleaning, and disinfecting the equipment is required. Any item that has been in contact with blood, tissue, or body fluids potentially is contaminated with infectious microorganisms.[25]

9. Until contaminated surgical instruments, basins, trays, and other items are decontaminated, people handling these items must wear appropriate PPE to reduce the risk of exposure

to bloodborne or other potentially infectious microorganisms.[26]

Recommended Practice IV

Surgical procedure rooms and scrub/utility areas should be terminally cleaned daily.

1. Operating rooms in which procedures may be performed, regardless of whether they are used, should be terminally cleaned once during each 24-hour period during the regular work week. A clean surgical environment will reduce the number of microbial flora present.[27]

2. Mechanical friction and an EPA-registered agent are used to clean equipment and areas that should include, but are not limited to,
   ♦ surgical lights and external tracks;
   ♦ fixed and ceiling-mounted equipment;
   ♦ all furniture and equipment, including wheels, casters, step stools, foot pedals, telephones, and light switches;
   ♦ hallways and floors;
   ♦ handles of cabinets and push plates;
   ♦ ventilation faceplates;
   ♦ horizontal surfaces (eg, tops of counters, sterilizers, fixed shelving);
   ♦ substerile areas;
   ♦ scrub/utility areas; and
   ♦ scrub sinks.[28]
   Refillable liquid soap dispensers are not recommended. Refillable liquid soap dispensers can become contaminated and serve as reservoirs for microorganisms.[29]

3. Operating room floors should be wet-vacuumed with an EPA-registered hospital-grade disinfectant after the last scheduled procedure of the day or at least once during a 24-hour period. Terminal cleaning in the surgical practice setting reduces the number of microorganisms, dust, and organic debris present in the surgical environment.[30]

4. Cleaning equipment should be disassembled, cleaned with an EPA-registered facility-approved agent, and dried before storage. Equipment is cleaned to prevent growth of microorganisms during storage and to prevent subsequent contamination of the surgical practice setting.[31]

Recommended Practice V

All areas and equipment in the surgical practice setting should be cleaned according to an established schedule.

1. Areas and equipment to be cleaned should include, but are not limited to,
   - ducts and filters, including high-efficiency particulate air filters;
   - air-conditioning equipment;
   - return ventilation and heating grills;
   - recessed ceiling tracks (eg, overhead lighting tracks);
   - closets, cabinets, and shelves;
   - storerooms;
   - sterilizers, warming cabinets, and refrigerators;
   - ice machines;
   - walls and ceilings; and
   - offices, lounges, lavatories, and locker rooms.
   A clean environment will reduce the number of microorganisms present.[32]

Recommended Practice VI

Policies and procedures for environmental cleaning should be written, reviewed annually, and readily available in surgical practice settings.

1. These recommended practices should be used as guidelines for the development of policies and procedures in surgical practice settings. Policies and procedures establish authority, responsibility, and accountability and serve as operational guidelines. The AORN recommended practices that deal with environmental cleaning should be consulted when developing those policies and procedures. An introduction to and review of policies and procedures should be included in the orientation and ongoing education of personnel to assist in the development of knowledge, skills, and attitudes that affect patient outcomes. Policies and procedures also assist in the development of continuous quality assessment/improvement activities.

Glossary

Cleaning: The process by which any type of soil, including organic material, is removed. Cleaning is accomplished with detergent, water, and scrubbing action.

Confine and contain: A principle that recommends prompt cleanup of items contaminated with blood, tissue, or body fluids.

Contaminated: The presence of potentially infectious pathogenic microorganisms on animate or inanimate objects.

Decontamination: A process that removes contaminating infectious agents and renders reusable medical products safe for handling.

Disinfection: A process that kills most forms of microorganisms on inanimate surfaces.

End-of-procedure cleaning: Cleaning that is performed at the end of one surgical procedure and before the start of another surgical procedure in the same room.

Exogenous: From a source other than the patient (eg, personnel, equipment, the environment, instruments, supplies).

Facility-approved agent: A microorganism-killing agent registered with the EPA. The EPA classifies germicides as sporicides, general disinfectants, hospital disinfectants, detergents, sanitizers, and others.

High-level disinfection: A process that kills all microorganisms with the exception of high numbers of bacterial spores.

Intermediate-level disinfection: A process that kills *Mycobacterium tuberculosis,* vegetative bacteria, most viruses, and most fungi but does not necessarily kill bacterial spores.

Low-level disinfection: A process that kills most bacteria and some viruses and fungi but cannot be relied on to kill resistant microorganisms such as *Mycobacterium tuberculosis* or bacterial spores.

Organic debris: Blood, tissue, and body fluids.

Personal protective equipment (PPE): Specialized equipment or clothing used by health care workers to protect themselves from direct exposure to patients' blood, tissue, or body fluids that may include gloves, gowns, liquid-resistant aprons, head and foot coverings, face shields or masks, eye protection, and ventilation devices (eg, mouth pieces, respirator bags, pocket masks).

Reusable: Any product or piece of equipment intended by the manufacturer for multiple uses. As appropriate to each item, the manufacturer is to provide instructions for reprocessing, care, and/or maintenance of the item.

Terminal cleaning: Cleaning that is performed at the completion of surgical practice settings' daily surgery schedules. Terminal cleaning is performed in surgical procedure rooms and scrub/utility areas and includes, but is not limited to, surgical lights and external tracks; fixed and ceiling-mounted equipment; all furniture, including wheels and casters; equipment; handles of cabinets and push plates; ventilation faceplates; horizontal surfaces (eg, tops of counters, sterilizers, fixed shelving); the entire floor; kick buckets; and scrub sinks.

Used items: Items that are opened for a surgical procedure that may or may not have come in contact with a patient's blood, tissue, or body fluids.

NOTES

1. A J Mangram et al, "Guideline for prevention of surgical site infection, 1999," *Infection Control and Hospital Epidemiology* 20 (April 1999) 247-280; J S Garner, the Hospital Infection Control Practices Advisory Committee, "Guideline for isolation precautions in hospitals," *Infection Control and Hospital Epidemiology* 54 (January 1996) 54-80; D Fogg, "Infection control," in *Alexander's Care of the Patient in Surgery,* 11th ed, M H Meeker, J C Rothrock, eds (St Louis: Mosby, 1999) 149-150; L Rhyne, B C Ulmer, L Revell, "Monitoring and controlling the environment," in *Patient Care During Operative and Invasive Procedures* (Philadelphia: W B Saunders Co, 2000) 158-161.

2. Mangram et al, "Guideline for prevention of surgical site infection, 1999," 261; Rhyne, Ulmer, Revell, "Monitoring and controlling the environment," 158-161.

3. Mangram et al, "Guideline for prevention of surgical site infection, 1999," 261.

4. P Wells, "'Confine and contain' approach to OR cleanup," *AORN Journal* 25 (January 1977) 61-62; Rhyne, Ulmer, Revell, "Monitoring and controlling the environment," 158-161; R Berguer et al, "Preparing the operating room," in *ACS Surgery: Principles and Practice,* ed D W Wilmore et al (New York: WebMD Corp, 2002) 595-596.

5. *Ibid;* American College of Surgeons Committee on Control of Surgical Infections of the Committee on Pre- and Postoperative Care, *Manual on Control of Infection in Surgical Patients,* second ed (Philadelphia: JB Lippincott Co, 1984) 281.

6. "AORN latex guideline," in *Standards, Recommended Practices, and Guidelines* (Denver: AORN, Inc, 2004) 103-118.

7. "Occupational exposure to bloodborne pathogens; Final rule," *Federal Register* 56 (Dec 6, 1991) 64177.

8. *Ibid.*

9. Centers for Disease Control, "Guidelines for prevention of transmission of human immunodeficiency virus and hepatitis B virus to health-care and public-safety workers," *Morbidity and Mortality Weekly Report* 38 (June 23, 1989) 16-17; W A Rutala, "APIC guideline for selection and use of disinfectants," *American Journal*

of Infection Control 24 (August 1996) 327; L Sehulster, R Y W Chinn, "Guidelines for environmental infection control in health-care facilities," *Morbidity and Mortality Weekly Report* 52, Part 10 (June 6, 2003); D J Weber et al, "The effect of blood on the antiviral activity of sodium hypochlorite, a phenolic, and a quaternary ammonium compound," *Infection Control and Hospital Epidemiology* 20 (December 1999) 821-827.

10. *Ibid.*

11. R J Sharbaugh, "Decontamination: Principles of disinfection," in *Sterilization Technology for the Health Care Facility,* second ed, M Reichert, J H Young, eds (Gaithersburg, Md: Aspen Publishers, 1997) 23.

12. M S Favero, W W Bond, "Chemical disinfection of medical and surgical materials," in *Disinfection, Sterilization, and Preservation,* fifth ed, S S Block, ed (Philadelphia: Lippincott Williams & Wilkins, 2001) 904; Rutala, "APIC guideline for selection and use of disinfectants," 326, 332; Centers for Disease Control and Prevention, "Guideline for environmental infection control and prevention in healthcare facilities, 2001."

13. "Occupational exposure to bloodborne pathogens; Final rule," 64178.

14. *Ibid,* 64176-64180.

15. "Recommended practices for environmental responsibility," in *Standards, Recommended Practices, and Guidelines* (Denver: AORN, Inc, 2002) 245-249.

16. L K Groah, *Perioperative Nursing,* third ed (Stamford, Conn: Appleton & Lange, 1996) 161.

17. Rutala, "APIC guideline for selection and use of disinfectants," 332; Centers for Disease Control and Prevention, "Guideline for environmental infection control and prevention in healthcare facilities, 2001"; American Academy of Pediatrics, the American College of Obstetricians and Gynecologists, *Guidelines for Perinatal Care,* fourth ed (Elk Grove Village, Ill: American Academy of Pediatrics, the American College of Obstetricians and Gynecologists, 1997) 272.

18. Groah, *Perioperative Nursing,* third ed, 160; Mangram et al, "Guideline for prevention of surgical site infection, 1999," 261; Favero, Bond, "Chemical disinfection of medical and surgical materials," 895-896; "Occupational exposure to bloodborne pathogens; Final rule," 64177; Rutala, "APIC guideline for selection and use of disinfectants," 334.

19. "Recommended practices for cleaning and processing anesthesia equipment," in *Standards, Recommended Practices, and Guidelines* (Denver: AORN, Inc, 2002) 195-198.

20. Groah, *Perioperative Nursing,* third ed, 159-160; Mangram et al, "Guideline for prevention of surgical site infection, 1999," 261.

21. "Occupational exposure to bloodborne pathogens; Final rule," 64175-64180.

22. *Ibid.*

23. *Ibid.*

24. *Ibid.*

25. *Ibid,* 64176; Groah, *Perioperative Nursing,* third ed, 151.

26. "Occupational exposure to bloodborne pathogens; Final rule," 64176-64177.

27. Mangram et al, "Guideline for prevention of surgical site infection, 1999," 261; Groah, *Perioperative Nursing,* third ed, 160-161; Wells, "'Confine and contain' approach to OR cleanup," 63.

28. Groah, *Perioperative Nursing,* third ed, 160-161; Berguer et al, "Preparing the operating room," 596.

29. L K Archibald et al, "*Serratia marcescens* outbreak associated with extrinsic contamination of 1% chlorxylenol soap," *Infection Control and Hospital Epidemiology* 18 (October 1997) 704-709; L A Grohskopf et al, "*Serratia liquefaciens* bloodstream infections from contamination of epoetin alfa at a hemodialysis center," *The New England Journal of Medicine* 344 (May 17, 2001) 1496.

30. Mangram et al, "Guideline for prevention of surgical site infection, 1999," 261; Groah, *Perioperative Nursing,* third ed, 160.

31. Groah, *Perioperative Nursing,* third ed, 161.

32. *Ibid;* Berguer et al, "Preparing the operating room," 596.

Originally published June 1975, *AORN Journal,* as "Recommended practices for sanitation in the surgical practice setting."

Format revised March 1978; March 1982; July 1982.

Revised April 1984; November 1988; December 1992.

Revised June 1996; published October 1996, *AORN Journal.*

Reformatted July 2000.

Revised; published December 2002, *AORN Journal.*

Recommended Practices for Environmental Responsibility

The following recommended practices were developed by the AORN Recommended Practices Committee and have been approved by the AORN Board of Directors. They were presented as proposed recommended practices in June 1997 for comment by AORN members and others.

These recommended practices are intended as achievable recommendations representing what is believed to be an optimal level of nursing practice. Policies and procedures will reflect variations in practice settings and/or clinical situations that determine the degree to which the recommended practices can be implemented.

AORN recognizes the numerous different settings in which perioperative nurses practice. These recommended practices are intended as guidelines adaptable to various practice settings. These practice settings include traditional ORs, ambulatory surgery units, physicians' offices, cardiac catheterization suites, endoscopy suites, radiology departments, and all other areas where operative and other invasive procedures may be performed.

Purpose

These recommended practices provide guidelines to help personnel undertake measures to reduce the environmental impact in their practice settings. Personnel should become ecologically sensitive and advocate changes that reduce the quantity of waste generated while maintaining quality patient care and worker safety. The appropriate committees in the practice setting should review all practices for waste management to reduce the risk of infection, facilitate regulatory compliance and resource conservation, and promote cost containment.

Recommended Practice I

Personnel should actively promote and participate in resource conservation.

1. Resource conservation measures, including but not limited to those of water and electricity, should be incorporated into daily practice.

Personnel preserve the environment by minimizing the use of material resources needed to complete a particular task.[1]

2. Water conservation measures should be implemented during surgical hand scrub times. Water should not run continuously and be wasted during surgical hand scrub procedures. Use automated or foot- or knee-operated faucets on scrub sinks to allow water to run only when the hands and arms are wet or rinsed. Place signs that encourage water conservation near scrub sinks.

3. Energy-efficient electrical equipment, lights, and appliances should be installed and used. Occupancy sensors should be installed in certain areas of the practice setting to control lighting based on the presence or absence of personnel and patients. Saving electricity minimizes air pollution caused by electric generation and reduces cost.[2]

4. Energy conservation measures should be determined in each practice setting in collaboration with facility management personnel. Collaborative efforts to conserve energy will help create an energy-efficient facility.[3]

Recommended Practice II

Surgical supplies should be opened only when there is reasonable certainty they will be used during the procedure.

1. Sterile supplies that are opened and not used should be evaluated for potential reprocessing, recycling, or use in areas where sterility is not required. Sterile supplies that are opened and not used are wasted resources.

2. Personnel should be aware of cost containment measures. The variety and number of supplies needed for each procedure should be kept to a minimum. Physician preference lists should be kept up-to-date. Implantable devices should be opened only when the desired specifications are known and announced by the surgeon.[4] Cost-containment measures that minimize waste provide economic benefits without compromising quality of care.

3. Use of standardized procedure packs should be considered. Use of standardized packs may

reduce personnel time for supply handling, consolidate storage space needs, facilitate inventory control, encourage standardization, reduce waste, and be cost-effective for facilities.[5]

4. Industry should participate in resource conservation by developing better packaging methods and product designs. Better packaging methods and product design can minimize the use of materials.[6]

Recommended Practice III

Single use and reusable products should be selected and used with consideration for the environment during the entire lifetime of products.

1. Patient and health care worker safety should be primary concerns when considering reprocessing single-use items. Alternative product utilization may provide cost savings and help minimize environmental impact. If a facility chooses to reprocess a single-use item, the facility assumes full liability for the product.[7]

2. Health care facilities should use AORN's "Recommended practices for product selection in perioperative practice settings" to evaluate, on an individual basis, the advantages and disadvantages of using single-use products, reusable products, or both.[8] The decision to purchase single-use or reusable products can be difficult for health care facilities who are trying to reduce both disposal costs and high labor costs related to the maintenance of reusable products.[9] When evaluating product performance, comfort, and cost, consideration should be given to the availability of resources or specific environmental issues in the geographic location of the health care facility (eg, clean water supply availability, limitations on disposal of solid waste).

3. The incineration of products that may release environmentally persistent hazardous chemicals should be minimized. Burning products containing mercury, or other heavy metals, and/or plastics, including polyvinylchloride (PVC), can release contaminants that are persistent in the environment and bioaccumulative in humans and other animals. Heavy metals can be neurotoxic; burning PVC can create dioxins that are endocrine disrupting agents.[10]

Recommended Practice IV

An efficient segregation program for infectious and noninfectious waste should be developed and implemented according to AORN's "Recommended practices for environmental cleaning in the surgical practice setting."

1. Personnel involved in managing medical waste should receive adequate training in the safe handling and disposal of infectious waste. When handling waste, personnel should wear personal protective equipment (PPE) and follow AORN's "Recommended practices for environmental cleaning in the surgical practice setting." Carefully managed infectious waste helps reduce costs.[11]

2. Infectious waste should be segregated from noninfectious waste in the general waste stream. Color-coded, labeled bags should be used to visually segregate infectious waste from noninfectious waste.[12] Segregating waste at the point of generation reduces volume, cost, and the risk of unnecessary personnel exposure.[13]

Recommended Practice V

Blood, body fluids, disinfectant solutions, and other hazardous materials should be disposed of in accordance with local, state, and federal recommendations and with concern for the environment.

1. Health care facilities should comply with waste disposal regulation. In choosing the method for disposal of infectious waste, the most cost-effective, environmentally sensitive method should be selected from among the alternatives. Treatment methods should be chosen with respect to the practice setting in accordance with local, state, and federal regulations. Waste disposal regulations minimize risk of personnel exposure to blood and body fluids.[14] Compliance with regulations and laws is mandatory and supersedes any professional or voluntary standard.[15]

2. When handling blood, body fluids, disinfectant solutions, or other hazardous materials, PPE should be used according to AORN's "Recommended practices for environmental cleaning in

the surgical practice setting," AORN's "Recommended practices for high-level disinfection," and OSHA requirements. Facility-supplied PPE protects personnel from potential exposure when used. Educating staff members regarding PPE use helps avoid potentially hazardous situations for personnel and for the facility.[16] Fluid containers with blood, body fluids, disinfectant solutions, and other hazardous wastes should be handled with extreme care. Fluid containers should be

♦ impermeable to moisture;
♦ resistant to puncture, rupture, or tears under normal conditions; and
♦ sealed for transport to prevent leakage.

Recommended Practice VI

Recycling programs should be an integral part of health care facilities' policies and procedures.

1. Personnel should explore recycling opportunities and encourage their health care facility administrators to support recycling efforts. All personnel play vital roles in recycling programs. Education programs are necessary to inform staff members of their respective responsibilities.[17] Items that may be part of recycling programs include, but are not limited to,
   ♦ plastic,
   ♦ disposable wrappers,
   ♦ paper,
   ♦ cardboard,
   ♦ glass, steel and aluminum cans, and
   ♦ batteries.

2. Manufacturers should be encouraged to identify product materials that are recyclable. Many surgical products can be recycled to reduce the amount of waste in landfills. Recycling reduces the amount of virgin resources that must be used. Uniform labeling of medical items would identify the components of surgical products. Perioperative personnel have extensive interactions with industry representatives and are in a unique position to participate in recycling programs. They have significant purchasing power, and manufacturers want to meet their customers' needs. Opportunities for recycling should be an expressed need, and personnel should consider products made from recycled materials when making purchasing decisions. Personnel can

contact resource groups for information about getting involved in collecting medical supplies and equipment for donation to nonprofit health care organizations overseas.

Recommended Practice VII

Sterilization of items in health care facilities should be accomplished with steam sterilization as the method of choice. Alternative methods include low-temperature sterilization technologies (eg, gas plasma or mixed chemical plasma), liquid sterilization (eg, peracetic acid), or ethylene oxide (EO) sterilization.

1. Ethylene oxide should be used only when other sterilization methods are unavailable or incompatible with instrumentation/materials. Exposure to ethylene oxide (EO) creates an occupational health hazard.[18] Acute exposure can cause headache, nausea, vomiting, disorientation, respiratory distress, and death. Direct contact with liquid EO causes chemical burns. Long-term exposure to EO may be carcinogenic, mutagenic, or may cause neurologic disease.[19]

2. Manufacturers should be encouraged to design products that can be steam sterilized. Costs of sterilization using EO and other gas or liquid alternatives are much higher than steam sterilization. Sterilization cycles are longer with EO than with steam and other alternative methods.[20] Ethylene oxide is still needed to sterilize some items with long lumens, complex hinges, or made of certain materials.

Recommended Practice VIII

Policies and procedures regarding environmental protection should be written in accordance with local, state, and federal regulations; reviewed periodically; and be readily available within the perioperative practice setting.

1. These policies and procedures should include, but not be limited to,
   ♦ resource conservation,
   ♦ management of medical waste from generation to disposal, and
   ♦ recycling.

   These recommended practices should be used as guidelines to develop policies and procedures. Policies and procedures establish authority, responsibility, and accountability and serve as operational guidelines.

2. An introduction and review of policies and procedures should be included in orientation and ongoing education of personnel to assist in developing knowledge, skills, and attitudes that affect patient outcomes. Policies and procedures also assist in the development of continuous quality improvement activities. Additionally, ongoing education regarding advances in recycling is recommended.

Glossary

Infectious waste: Medical waste (eg, blood, body fluids, sharps) that is capable of producing infectious diseases.[21]

Regulated medical waste: Sharps (both used and unused), cultures and stocks of infectious agents, carcasses and bedding of animals inoculated with infectious agents, select isolation waste from patients having diseases caused by so-called Class 4 etiologic agents, pathological waste, and human blood.[22]

Segregation: Separation of infectious waste from other types of medical waste at the point at which materials become waste.

Source reduction: Reduction of solid waste by minimizing packaging and materials of construction.

Waste stream: Flow of discarded materials and fluids that eventually return to the land, water system, and air.

NOTES

1. P R O'Leary, P W Walsh, R K Ham, "Managing solid waste," *Scientific American* 259 (December 1988) 37.

2. US Environmental Protection Agency, *Light Brief* (Washington, DC: US Environmental Protection Agency, June 1992) 7000.

3. *Ibid.*

4. L J Atkinson, N H Fortunato, *Berry & Kohn's Operating Room Technique,* eighth ed (St Louis: Mosby-Yearbook, Inc, 1996) 434.

5. Atkinson, Fortunato, *Berry & Kohn's Operating Room Technique,* eighth ed, 556.

6. O'Leary, Walsh, Ham, "Managing solid waste," 37.

7. Atkinson, Fortunato, *Berry & Kohn's Operating Room Technique,* eighth ed, 554-556.

8. "Recommended practices for product selection in perioperative practice settings," in *Standards, Recom-*
mended Practices, and Guidelines (Denver: AORN, Inc, 2004) 347-350.

9. L Souhrada, "Reusables revisited as medical waste adds up," *Hospitals* 62 (Oct 20, 1988) 82; M Wagner, "Environment, cost concerns spur new interest in reusables," *Modern Healthcare* 20 (May 14, 1990) 46.

10. R Reeder, *The Case Against Mercury: Diagnosis, Treatment, and Alternatives* (Washington, DC: The Terrine Institute, 1995); J Thornton et al, "Hospitals and plastics: Dioxin prevention and medical waste incinerators," *Public Health Reports,* vol III (July/Aug 1996) 298-313.

11. M F Fay et al, "Medical waste: The growing issues of management and disposal," *AORN Journal* 51 (June 1990) 1508; W M Wagner, "Hospital waste and the future: Managing infectious waste in the OR," *Today's OR Nurse* 13 (April 1991) 26.

12. R D Barlow, "Medical waste becomes monster in cost-cutting fight," *Hospital Materials Management* 16 (December 1991) 10.

13. Fay et al, "Medical waste: The growing issues of management and disposal," *AORN Journal* 51 (June 1990) 1508.

14. A Furlong, "Powders added to body fluids facilitate waste handling," *Hospital Materials Management* 16 (October 1991) 2; Wagner, "Hospital waste and the future: Managing infectious waste in the OR," 26.

15. T J Loving, "Infectious waste: Doing your best for the environment, your employees and your bottom line," *Journal of Healthcare Materiel Management* 10 (August 1992) 39.

16. G L Nohrianni, "Glutaraldehyde overexposure: Myth or reality? One hospital-wide study," *Journal of Healthcare Materiel Management* 10 (July 1992) 34.

17. P Patterson, "Nurse sets up project to recycle OR waste," *OR Manager* 7 (August 1991) 1.

18. V M Steelman, "Ethylene oxide: The importance of aeration," *AORN Journal* 55 (March 1992) 773; P E Haney, B A Raymond, L C Lewis, "Ethylene oxide: An occupational health hazard for hospital workers," *AORN Journal* 51 (February 1990) 480.

19. Steelman, "Ethylene oxide: The importance of aeration," 778; Haney, Raymond, Lewis, "Ethylene oxide: An occupational health hazard for hospital workers," 485; Atkinson, Fortunato, *Berry & Kohn's Operating Room Technique,* eighth ed, 226.

20. Steelman, "Ethylene oxide: The importance of aeration," 775; Atkinson, Fortunato, *Berry & Kohn's Operating Room Technique,* eighth ed, 226.

21. W A Rutala, R L Odette, G P Samsa, "Management of infectious waste by US hospitals," *Journal of the American Medical Association* 262 (Sept 22-29, 1989) 1636.

22. W A Rutala, W A C G Mayhall. "SHEA position paper: Medical waste," *Infection Control and Hospital Epidemiology* 13 (January 1992) 38-48.

RESOURCES

Bisson, C I; McRae, G; Shaner, H. *An Ounce of Prevention—Waste Reduction Strategies for Health Care Facilities.* Chicago: American Society for Health Care Environmental Services of the American Hospital Association, 1993.

Freed, D. "Medical waste quality monitoring: Changing employee behavior." *Journal of Healthcare Materiel Management* 8 (February/March 1990) 20-30.

Hedrick, E R. "Infectious waste management: Will science prevail?" *Infection Control and Hospital Epidemiology* 9 (November 1988) 488-490.

Keene, J H. "Medical waste: A minimal hazard." *Infection Control and Hospital Epidemiology* 12 (November 1991) 682-685.

McVeigh, P. "OR nursing and environmental ethics, medical waste reduction, reuse and recycling." *Today's OR Nurse* 15 (January/ February 1993) 13-18.

Rutala, W A; Weber, D J. "Infectious waste: Mismatch between science and policy." *The New England Journal of Medicine* 32S (Aug 22, 1991) 578-581.

Spry, C, et al. "A report on infectious and noninfectious surgical waste disposal and its relation to the overall waste problem." *AORN Journal* 53 (April 1991) 905-916.

Tieszen, M E; Gruenberg, J C. "A quantitative, qualitative, and critical assessment of surgical waste: Surgeons venture through the trash can." *Journal of the American Medical Association* 267 (May 27, 1992) 2765-2768.

Originally published October 1993, *AORN Journal.*

Revised November 1997.

Reformatted July 2000.

Recommended Practices for Selection and Use of Surgical Gowns and Drapes

The following recommended practices were developed by the AORN Recommended Practices Committee and have been approved by the AORN Board of Directors. They were presented as proposed recommended practices for comments by members and others. They are effective January 1, 2003.

These recommended practices are intended as achievable recommendations representing what is believed to be an optimal level of practice. Policies and procedures will reflect variations in practice settings and/or clinical situations that determine the degree to which the recommended practices can be implemented.

AORN recognizes the numerous types of settings in which perioperative nurses practice. These recommended practices are intended as guidelines adaptable to various practice settings. These practice settings include traditional ORs, ambulatory surgery units, physician's offices, cardiac catheterization suites, endoscopy suites, radiology departments, and all other areas where operative and other invasive procedures may be performed.

Purpose

These recommended practices provide guidelines for evaluation, selection, and use of surgical gowns and drapes. These products should provide a safe, effective means of protecting patients and health care personnel during use. Patients are at risk of contamination from both endogenous and exogenous microorganisms. Health care workers are at risk of contamination from a variety of bloodborne pathogens that can be contracted via exposure to patients' blood and body fluids. The barrier quality required of surgical gowns and drapes varies according to the planned use of the product and its anticipated exposure to blood and body fluids.

Recommended Practice I

Surgical gowns and drapes should be evaluated according to the AORN "Recommended practices for product selection in perioperative practice settings."[1]

1. Materials selected for construction of surgical gowns and drapes should be safe, meet identified needs, and promote patient and personnel safety.

2. Selection of gown and drape products for use in the practice setting should be based on criteria specific to the products' function and use. Surgical gowns and drapes are constructed of either single-use or reusable materials. Each of these has advantages and disadvantages. Further, in each of the two categories, design and performance characteristics vary. This variation stems from trade-offs in cost, comfort, and the amount of barrier protection provided. Both single-use and reusable gowns and drapes often are reinforced to improve their barrier quality. Reinforcements may consist of additional layers of the same material or layers of different material(s).[2]

Recommended Practice II

Materials used for surgical gowns and drapes should be resistant to penetration by blood and other body fluids as necessitated by their intended use.

1. Perioperative managers and purchasing agents should obtain from manufacturers data verifying that materials used in gowns and drapes are protective barriers against the transfer of microorganisms, particulates, and fluids to minimize strike-through and the potential for personnel contamination. Microorganisms can be transferred through barrier materials by wicking of fluids and/or pressure or leaning on a flooded area of the product. Mechanical action such as pressure can result in both liquid and dry penetration of microbes if the pressure exceeds the maximum level of resistance that the material provides.[3]

2. Surgical gowns should be selected for use according to the barrier quality of the item and the wearers' anticipated exposure to blood and body fluids in accordance with the Occupational Safety and Health Administration guidelines for use of personal protective equipment.[4] Short procedures during which there is little or no anticipated exposure to blood or body fluids can be completed successfully using a surgical gown with minimal barrier protection. As the complexity and length of the planned procedure increases, there may be increased potential for exposure to bloodborne pathogens, and it would be prudent to select a gown with greater barrier capability.

Recommended Practice III

Surgical gowns and drapes should maintain their integrity and be durable.

1. Surgical gowns and drapes should have an acceptable quality level (ie, be free of holes/defects).

2. Surgical gowns and drapes should be resistant to tears, punctures, and abrasions. The inability to withstand tears, punctures, and abrasions may allow for passage of microorganisms, particulates, and fluids between sterile and nonsterile areas and expose patients to exogenous organisms. Health care workers may be exposed to bloodborne pathogens. Reusable materials should be inspected visually to determine their integrity before use.[5] Reusable textiles should be patched with heat-sealed patches of the same quality material as the item to which they are applied. If the item is of a single-ply material, a patch need only be applied to one side of the item. Patches must allow for penetration and removal of sterilant while maintaining the integrity of the barrier quality of the item. The percentage of exposed surface that can be patched is dependent on the sterilization method and the number of layers of patched textile.[6] Areas covered by heat-sealed patches on woven textiles should be examined carefully before the fabric is used. The patched area should maintain the original barrier properties each time the product is used. Patches of any kind should never be stitched to woven barrier materials as a method of repairing holes. Stitching creates permanent holes that reduce the barrier quality of the item.[7]

3. Surgical gowns and drapes should be low-linting. Barrier materials used for surgical gowns and drapes should be as lint-free as possible. Lint particles are disseminated into the environment where bacteria attach to them. This bacteria-carrying lint may settle in surgical sites and wounds with a resultant increase in postoperative patient complications.[8]

4. Seams of barrier materials should be evaluated to determine their capability to minimize either penetration or passage of potential contaminants. Many surgical gown seams have little or no barrier property. If wicking or pressure on a seam causes liquid transfer between sterile and unsterile surfaces, one or both sides may become contaminated.[9]

Recommended Practice IV

Materials used for surgical gowns and drapes should be appropriate to the method(s) of sterilization.

1. To achieve a sterile product, the sterilizing agent must contact all surfaces of the item to be sterilized. Common sterilization methodologies include
   - radiation,
   - steam, and
   - ethylene oxide.

   The primary methodologies used in health care facilities are steam and ethylene oxide. Most facilities have neither the capability of nor access to radiation as a means of sterilization.

2. Tightly woven reusable textiles will lose their protective barrier quality after repeated processing. Manufacturers' written instructions for handling, the suggested number of processings, and the useful life of barrier materials should be provided and followed. A system should be established to track the number of processings for each item. This tracking should include, but not be limited to, the number of wash cycles and sterilization processings to which the textile product is subjected. Repeated processing ultimately will diminish the protective barrier ability of reusable textiles; however, items constructed of reusable textiles should continue to meet the original barrier quality level throughout the manufacturer-recommended life cycle (ie, number of processings) for the textile. The user facility should monitor the barrier quality of reusable textiles at intervals while the product is in service. Purchasers of reusable textile gowns and/or drapes should obtain from the manufacturer instructions for testing the material to document the ongoing barrier quality of the item(s) for the entire useful life of the item(s).[10] Products that no longer meet the manufacturer-stated barrier level should be downgraded to a nonprotective category and used accordingly.

3. Unused, single-use surgical gowns and drapes should not be resterilized unless manufacturers provide specific written instructions for reprocessing or the US Food and Drug Administration (FDA) regulations are followed. Surgical gowns and drapes intended for single use may not sterilize adequately, may be damaged during the sterilization process, or may retain toxic residues.[11] If a health care facility chooses to reprocess single-use items, including gowns and drapes, the FDA considers the facility to be the manufacturer of the item(s) and, as such, the facility is subject to the same stringent regulations as the original manufacturer of the item.[12]

Recommended Practice V

Surgical gowns and drapes should resist combustion.

1. Gowns and drapes selected for use should be consistent with accepted flammability standards that will provide the safest environment for patients and health care workers.[13] Specific standards for surgical materials have not been developed. All materials used in the surgical environment will burn given the right conditions.

2. Barrier materials are made of natural and/or synthetic fibers and may be flammable, needing only a combination of heat, fuel, and oxygen to ignite.[14] Care should be taken when gowns and drapes are exposed to light and heat sources, electrosurgical devices, lasers, and other power equipment. Materials ignite and burn at various rates. Even materials said to be flame-resistant might burn or melt when subjected to intense heat or an oxygen-rich environment.[15] Some materials not only ignite more easily than others but also may burn more rapidly.

Recommended Practice VI

Surgical gowns and drapes should be comfortable and contribute to maintaining the wearer's desired body temperature.

1. Surgical gowns and drapes should be free of toxic ingredients and allergens. Patients and/or health care workers may experience untoward reactions to toxic ingredients and/or allergens, ranging from mild discomfort to anaphylactic collapse.

2. Surgical drapes should have limited memory and be flexible enough to conform loosely to the patient's contour, allow for placement and unhampered manipulation of surgical instruments, and appropriately drape related equipment.[16] Surgical gowns should have limited memory and be flexible enough to conform loosely to the wearer's body while at the same time protect the wearer from contamination from blood and body fluids.

3. Surgical gowns and drapes should have the ability to maintain an isothermic environment for patients and health care workers. People vary in their ability to tolerate heat and cold. Thermal comfort exists when a balance occurs between the heat the human body loses and the heat the body generates. Care must be taken to avoid hypothermia or hyperthermia in surgical patients. Normothermic or near-normothermic patients may have a more favorable postoperative course.[17]

Recommended Practice VII

Surgical gowns and drapes selected for use should have a favorable cost-benefit ratio.

1. Surgical gowns and drapes should not be selected on the basis of cost only. Nor should cost be the primary consideration when making a selection. In today's economic environment, however, it is imperative that after providing for patient and provider safety, fiscal factors be considered. Careful selection of the appropriate gowns and drapes for the practice setting will contribute to the fiscal soundness of the provider facility.[18] A lesser-priced product that fails consistently is not cost effective because additional volume will be required to replace the defective or poorly performing item(s).

2. Surgical gowns and drapes are considered medical devices, and failure of these devices is subject to medical device reporting requirements according to the Safe Medical Devices Act of 1990[19] (SMDA) and/or the FDA voluntary Problem Reporting Program. This voluntary program provides users with a mechanism for reporting events that do not meet the strict reporting criteria of the SMDA. Reports should be filed by

telephone at (800) 638-6725. Consistent failure of a surgical gown or drape product should be reported to the manufacturer and the FDA. Any strike-through constitutes a threat of exposure to potentially harmful bloodborne pathogens.

Recommended Practice VIII

Policies and procedures for selecting and using surgical gowns and drapes should be developed, reviewed regularly, revised as necessary, and readily available in the practice setting.

1. These recommended practices should be used as guidelines when developing policies and procedures. Written policies and procedures establish authority, responsibility, and accountability. They serve as operational guidelines in the practice setting. Other AORN recommended practices addressing packaging systems, sterilization, creating and maintaining a sterile field, and surgical attire also should be consulted when developing policies and procedures for the selection and use of surgical gowns and drapes.

2. Orientation and ongoing education activities for personnel should include an introduction to and/or review of policies and procedures to be applied in the practice setting. Compliance with policies and procedures helps develop and reinforce knowledge, skills, and attitudes that affect patient outcomes. Policies and procedures also may be an integral part of continuous quality assessment and improvement activities.

Glossary

Barrier material: Material that minimizes or retards the penetration of microorganisms, particulates, and fluids.

Heat-sealed patch: A patch of the same textile with an adhesive back applied to reusable textiles containing a hole or tear with high-intensity heat.

Isothermic environment: The surroundings, conditions, or influences that affect maintaining an equal temperature.

Nonwoven material: A manufactured sheet, web, or batt of directionally or randomly oriented fibers or filaments, natural or man-made, excluding paper and paper products, that are woven, knotted, tufted, or stitch bonded and have not been converted into yarns. Nonwovens are bonded to each other by friction and/or cohesion and/or adhesion. They are designed as single-use materials.

Strike-through: Penetration of microorganisms, particulates, or fluids through a barrier material.

Useful life: The anticipated life of a product, such as a woven material. Useful life is affected by the number of sterilization processing and washing cycles a product can endure and yet maintain an acceptable barrier capability.

Wicking: Absorption of a liquid by capillary action along a thread or through the material.

Woven material: Fabric constructed from yarns made of natural or synthetic fibers or filaments that are woven together to form a web in a repeated interlocking pattern.

NOTES

1. "Recommended practices for product selection in perioperative practice settings," in *Standards, Recommended Practices, and Guidelines* (Denver: AORN, Inc, 2004) 347-350.

2. K K Leonas, R S Jinkins, "The relationship of selected fabric characteristics and the barrier effectiveness of surgical gown fabrics," *American Journal of Infection Control* 25 (February 1997) 16-23; *Selection of Surgical Gowns and Drapes in Health Care Facilities* (Arlington, Va: Association for the Advancement of Medical Instrumentation, 2000) 4-12.

3. *Ibid.*

4. "Occupational exposure to bloodborne pathogens; Final rule," *Federal Register* 56 (Dec 6, 1991) 640004-64182; N L Belkin, "A historical review of barrier materials," *AORN Journal* 76 (October 2002) 648-653.

5. *Processing of Reusable Surgical Textiles for Use in Health Care Facilities* (Arlington, Va: Association for the Advancement of Medical Instrumentation, 2000) 23-28.

6. *Ibid,* 27-28; American Society for Healthcare Central Service Professionals of the American Hospital Association, *Training Manual for Central Service Technicians,* third ed (Chicago: American Hospital Association, 1997) 136.

7. *Ibid.*

8. *Processing of Reusable Surgical Textiles for Use in Health Care Facilities,* 24; *Selection of Surgical Gowns and Drapes in Health Care Facilities,* 16-17; C Edmiston et al, "Airborne particulates in the OR environment," *AORN Journal* 69 (June 1999) 1169-1183.

9. J Pournoor, "New scientific tools to expand the understanding of aseptic practices," *Surgical Services Management* 6 (April 2000) 28-32; J W Smith et al, "Determination of surgeon-generated gown pressures during various surgical procedures in the operating room," *American Journal of Infection Control* 23 (August 1995) 238; E A McCullough, "Methods for determining the barrier efficacy of surgical gowns," *American Journal of Infection Control* 21 (December 1993) 368; I D Learmonth, "Prevention of infec-

tion in the 1990s," *Orthopedic Clinics of North America* 24 (October 1993) 736; K W Altman et al, "Transmural surgical gown pressure measurements in the operating theater," *American Journal of Infection Control* 19 (June 1991) 147.

10. *Selection of Surgical Gowns and Drapes in Health Care Facilities,* 17, 18, 23; *Processing of Reusable Surgical Textiles for Use in Health Care Facilities,* 14, 24, 25; D Fogg, "Infection control," in *Alexander's Care of the Patient in Surgery,* 11th ed, M H Meeker, J C Rothrock, eds (St Louis: Mosby, 1999) 145.

11. *Good Hospital Practice: Steam Sterilization and Sterility Assurance* (Arlington, Va: Association for the Advancement of Medical Instrumentation, 1994) 9.

12. *Ibid;* "Reuse of single-use devices," (Clinical Issues) *AORN Journal* 73 (May 2001) 957-966; "AORN guidance statement: Reuse of single-use devices," in *Standards, Recommended Practices, and Guidelines* (Denver: AORN, Inc, 2002) 113-119.

13. *Selection of Surgical Gowns and Drapes in Health Care Facilities,* 15, 16, 18; "Standard for the flammability of clothing textiles," in *Code of Federal Regulations (CFR)* 16: Commercial Practices, Part 1610 (Washington, DC: US Government Printing Office, 2001) 608-616; "Standard for the flammability of vinyl plastic film," in *Code of Federal Regulations (CFR)* 16: Commercial Practices, Part 1611 (Washington, DC: US Government Printing Office, 2001) 622-630.

14. *Ibid;* J R Sommers, "Flammability standards for surgical drapes and gowns: Past, present, and future," *Surgical Services Management* 4 (February 1998) 41-44; *Fire Safety in the Perioperative Setting* (Woodbury, Conn: Ciné-med, 2000) Videotape; "Surgical fires in the OR," ORRM 2 (1992).

15. *Ibid;* "Recommended practices for laser safety in practice settings," in *Standards, Recommended Practices, and Guidelines* (Denver: AORN, Inc, 2002) 277-281.

16. *Selection of Surgical Gowns and Drapes in Health Care Facilities,* 13, 14.

17. *Ibid;* A C Meling et al, "Effects of preoperative warming on the incidence of wound infection after clean surgery: A randomised controlled trial," *The Lancet* 358 (Sept 15, 2001) 876-880; Agency for Healthcare Research and Quality, University of California, San Francisco-Stanford Evidence-Based Practice Center, *Making Healthcare Safer: A Critical Analysis of Patient Safety Practices* (Rockville, Md: Agency for Healthcare Research and Quality, US Department of Health and Human Services, 2001) 231-234; A Kurz, D I Sessler, R Lenhardt, "Perioperative normothermia to reduce the incidence of surgical-wound infection and shorten hospitalization," *The New England Journal of Medicine* 334 (May 9, 1996) 1209-1215.

18. *Selection of Surgical Gowns and Drapes in Health Care Facilities,* 19.

19. *Safe Medical Devices Act of 1990,* sec 519 (21 USC 360); "Medical device reporting," in *Code of Federal Regulations (CFR)* 21: Food and Drugs, Part 803 (Washington, DC: US Government Printing Office, 2002) 38-55; "Medical devices: Reports of corrections and removals," in *Code of Federal Regulations (CFR)* 21: Food and Drugs, Part 806 (Washington, DC: US Government Printing Office, 2002) 55-58.

Originally published February 1988, *AORN Journal.*
Revised March 1992.
Revised November 1995; published March 1996, *AORN Journal.*
Reformatted July 2000.
Revised; published January 2003, *AORN Journal.*

Recommended Practices for
Surgical Hand Antisepsis/Hand Scrubs

The following recommended practices were developed by the AORN Recommended Practices Committee and have been approved by the AORN Board of Directors. They were presented as proposed recommended practices for comment to members and others. These recommended practices are effective January 1, 2004.

These recommended practices are intended as achievable recommendations representing what is believed to be an optimal level of practice. Policies and procedures will reflect variations in practice settings and/or clinical situations that determine the degree to which the recommended practices can be implemented.

AORN recognizes the numerous types of settings in which perioperative nurses practice. These recommended practices are intended as guidelines adaptable to various practice settings. These practice settings include traditional ORs, ambulatory surgery units, physicians' offices, cardiac catheterization suites, endoscopy suites, radiology departments, and all other areas where operative and other invasive procedures may be performed.

Purpose

Microorganism transfer from the hands of health care workers to patients is an important factor in health care-associated (ie, nosocomial) infections and has been recognized since the observations of Semmelweis and others more than 100 years ago.[1] Skin is a major potential source of microbial contamination in the surgical environment. Hand hygiene is a critical step in preventing infections and the spread of infections, is of critical importance for the entire health care team, and remains the most effective and least expensive measure to prevent the transmission of microorganisms and health care-associated infections. It is the single most important step in the prevention of infections.[2] The term *general hand hygiene* refers to decontamination of the hands by one of two methods—hand washing with either an antimicrobial or plain soap and water, or use of an antiseptic hand rub.[3]

The term *surgical hand antisepsis* refers to the antiseptic surgical scrub or antiseptic hand rub performed before donning sterile attire preoperatively. Although scrubbed members of the surgical team wear sterile gloves, the skin of their hands and forearms should be cleaned preoperatively to significantly reduce the number of microorganisms. The

moist environment underneath surgical gloves can promote microorganism proliferation on the hands of the wearer. Both surgical and examination gloves can fail during a procedure. Choice of surgical hand antiseptic/scrub agents should be limited to those that are US Food and Drug Administration (FDA) compliant, have a documented ability to kill organisms immediately upon application, provide antimicrobial persistence to reduce regrowth of microorganisms, and have a cumulative effect over time.[3] The purpose of surgical hand antisepsis/hand scrubs is to

- ◆ remove debris and transient microorganisms from the nails, hands, and forearms;
- ◆ reduce the resident microbial count to a minimum; and
- ◆ inhibit rapid rebound growth of microorganisms.

Perioperative nursing vocabulary

The perioperative nursing vocabulary is a clinically relevant and empirically validated standardized language. This standardized language consists of the Perioperative Nursing Data Set and includes perioperative nursing diagnoses, interventions, and outcomes. The expected outcome of primary importance to this recommended practice is outcome 10 (O10), "The patient will be free of signs and symptoms of infection."[4]

Recommended Practice I

All personnel should practice general hand hygiene.

1. Hand hygiene immediately before and after patient contact remains the most cost-effective and simplest measure for health care workers to prevent cross contamination in the health care setting.[5] General hand hygiene should be performed before and after patient contact, after removing gloves, any time there is a possibility that there has been contact with blood or other potentially infectious materials, before and after eating, and after using a restroom.[3] Wearing gloves is not a substitute for hand hygiene.[6] Hands are a major source of transient flora and, therefore, a major vector of cross contamination in health care. Health care workers should avoid contact with surfaces that are potentially contaminated, such as equipment and other inanimate objects in the patient care setting (see

"Recommended practices for standard and transmission-based precautions").[7]

2. Fingernails should be kept short, clean, and healthy. The subungual region harbors the majority of microorganisms found on hands. Removal of debris underneath fingernails requires the use of a disposable, single-use nail cleaner under running water. Additional effort may be necessary for longer nails. The risk of tearing gloves can increase if fingernails extend past the fingertips. Long fingernails may cause patient injury during the moving or positioning process.[8-12] Ideal nail length has been described as not extending beyond the fingertips.[13] Polish, if used, should not be chipped. Studies have found no increase in microbial growth related to wearing freshly applied nail polish, but chipped nail polish may support the growth of larger numbers of organisms on fingernails.[3,9,12] There is concern, however, that individuals who spend considerable time and money on maintaining their nails may be less inclined to perform a vigorous surgical scrub to protect their nails. If this occurs, there could be a detrimental effect of bacterial growth on the hands, not from the polish itself, but from a change in hygienic practices. Available data indicate that nail polish that has been obviously chipped or worn for more than four days harbors greater numbers of bacteria.[9,12] This time frame may suggest a guide for changing polish so that nails remain well manicured. Individuals who choose to wear nail polish in the surgical setting should be guided by surgical conscience.[8,9,12]

3. Artificial nails should not be worn.[3] The variety and amount of potentially pathogenic bacteria cultured from the fingertips of personnel wearing artificial nails is greater than from the fingertips of personnel with natural nails, both before and after hand washing.[13-16] Numerous state boards of cosmetology report that fungal growth occurs frequently under artificial nails as a result of moisture becoming trapped between the natural and artificial nail.[8,17-19]

4. Cuticles, hands, and forearms should be free of open lesions and breaks in skin integrity. Open lesions and breaks in skin integrity increase the risk of patient and surgical team member infec-

tion. Cuts, abrasions, exudative lesions, and hangnails tend to ooze serum, which may contain pathogens. Broken skin permits microorganisms to enter the various layers of skin, providing deeper microbial breeding grounds.[8,17,20]

5. Rings, watches, and bracelets should be removed before performing hand hygiene. During hand hygiene, rings, watches, and bracelets may harbor microorganisms or inhibit their removal. Allergic skin reactions (eg, irritation) have been observed as a result of hand soaps, antimicrobial agents, residual chemicals, or glove powder accumulating under jewelry.[8,21,22] Removal of all jewelry from the hands and forearms permits full skin contact with the chosen surgical hand antimicrobial agent. The risk of infection from transient microorganisms increases exponentially in relation to the number of rings worn. A recent study found that there was no increase in reported microbial counts on the hands of personnel who removed rings before work.[23] Ring wearing has been associated with up to a 10-fold increase in median skin microorganism count (ie, bioload).[23]

6. Lotions, if used, should be chosen based on infection control practices, approved by infection control professionals, and compatible with the hand antimicrobial agent and gloves used. Lotions should be packaged in nonrefillable containers that are discarded when empty.[3] Skin moisturizing products can prevent drying, discomfort, and dermatitis and may help reduce bacterial shedding from the skin.[24,25] The use of moisturizing products in health care facilities should be examined and incorporated in a formalized and standardized manner into policies, procedures, and practices.[26] Petroleum-based products may weaken latex gloves, causing increased permeability.[27] Anionic-based lotions (ie, many over-the-counter products) that commonly are available on the market and used in health care facilities can neutralize the cumulative antimicrobial activity of chlorhexidine gluconate and chloroxylenol, ingredients that are found in many antimicrobial hand antiseptic products.[3,28] Always check with the manufacturer of the skin care product to verify that it is indeed compatible with the chosen hand antiseptic agent.

7. If hands are soiled visibly, wash them as soon as possible with plain or antimicrobial soap and water as follows.
   ♦ Wet hands with warm water.
   ♦ Apply soap to the hands according to the manufacturer's written instructions, if given.
   ♦ Rub hands together vigorously for at least 15 seconds, covering all surfaces of the hands and fingers. Pay particular attention to areas often overlooked (ie, the backs of the hands, fingertips, the thumb and inner web).[29]
   ♦ Rinse hands with warm water and dry thoroughly with a disposable towel.
   ♦ Use towel to turn off the faucet.[3]

   Alcohol-based hand rubs are not appropriate for use when hands are visibly dirty or contaminated with proteinaceous materials (eg, blood, saliva) because these hand rubs do not remove soil or debris.[3]

8. If hands are not soiled visibly, an alcohol-based hand rub may be used for routine decontamination of hands.[3] Degerming with an alcohol-based hand rub is more effective than washing with soap and water and requires much shorter exposure time. Data indicate that the use of an alcohol-based agent may increase overall compliance with hand hygiene.[30-32] When relatively small amounts of proteinaceous material are present (ie, nonvisible soiling), alcohol may reduce viable bacterial counts on hands more rapidly than plain or antimicrobial soap.[3] Follow manufacturers' written directions for product application.[3] Alcohol-impregnated towelettes, if used in the facility, should have the Centers for Disease Control and Prevention's (CDC's) recommended volume and percentage of alcohol (ie, 60% to 95%). Lesser concentrations may be only comparable to soap and water.[3]

9. To improve adherence to general hand-hygiene recommendations among personnel working in busy patient care environments, an appropriate alcohol-based agent should be available in convenient locations (eg, wall, bedside). Individual, disposable, pocket-sized containers may be carried by health care providers.[3,31-34] Specific regulations may limit placement of alcohol-based products because of fire hazard considerations. Consult applicable local, state, and federal regulations for specific direction.

Recommended Practice II

An FDA-compliant, surgical hand antiseptic agent (ie, surgical hand scrub/rub) approved by the facility's infection control personnel should be used for all surgical hand antisepsis/hand scrubs.

1. The surgical hand antiseptic agent should
   ♦ significantly reduce microorganisms on intact skin;
   ♦ contain a nonirritating, antimicrobial preparation;
   ♦ be broad spectrum;
   ♦ be fast acting; and
   ♦ have a persistent effect.[35]

   An antimicrobial ingredient is intended to kill microorganisms. A characteristic of certain hand antiseptic agents that sets them apart from plain soap is their ability to bind with the stratum corneum of the skin, resulting in persistent chemical activity. Organisms can proliferate in the moist environment underneath gloves. Surgical gloves may become damaged during procedures, placing both the wearer and patient at risk. In appropriate concentrations (ie, 60% to 95%), alcohols provide the most rapid and greatest reduction in microbial counts on skin but have no persistent activity. Persistent antimicrobial activity, measured in hours, helps decrease rebound microbial growth after surgical hand antisepsis.[3] Cumulative effect is a progressive decrease in the number of microorganisms over time, usually measured in days, after repeated applications of product. According to the CDC, alcohol-based preparations containing 0.5% to 1% chlorhexidine gluconate have persistent and cumulative activity that, in certain studies, has equaled or exceeded that of chlorhexidine gluconate-containing detergents.[3,36-39]

2. Product selection for surgical hand antisepsis should follow AORN's recommended practices for product selection.[40] Infection control professionals, managers, and end users should be involved in the trial and selection of surgical hand antiseptic agents. Options should be included for individuals with product sensitivities. If an alcohol-based product is selected, the product should meet FDA requirements as outlined in the Tentative Final Monograph (TFM) for Health-Care Antiseptic Drug Products or be the

subject of a new drug approval (NDA) process or an abbreviated new drug approval process (ANDA).[35] The FDA requires that products for surgical hand scrubs provide a one-log reduction on day one, a two-log reduction on day two, a three-log reduction on day five, and show persistent activity for at least six hours on each of the three test days.[35]

3. Infection control professionals and committees should review the data provided by manufacturers to ensure that the surgical hand antisepsis agents chosen comply with current FDA testing and labeling criteria. Testing should be performed by an independent, FDA-approved testing laboratory employing standard methods as published by ASTM International.

4. Whenever possible, containers of surgical hand antisepsis agents should be placed in areas that facilitate ease of access and use by health care staff members while complying with local, state, and federal guidelines and/or regulations. New products continue to enter the market, and practitioners should consult manufacturers' scientific data when selecting products for use.

5. Surgical hand antisepsis agents should be stored in clean, closed containers. Single-use containers are recommended and should be discarded when empty. Reusable containers, if used, should be washed and dried thoroughly before refilling. Do not top off reusable containers. Refilling before cleaning or topping off dispensers with surgical hand antiseptic agents may cause contamination and could contribute to the spread of potentially harmful microorganisms.[11] Dispensers should function for long periods without becoming occluded or obstructed.[41]

6. Alcohol-based products are flammable and should be stored away from high temperatures, sparking devices, or flames. Reports about alcohol-based hand rubs in Europe, where alcohol-based rubs have been in clinical use for years, indicate few fires.[42] There has been a recent report of one fire associated with an alcohol-based hand rub in the United States.[43] Containers should be designed to minimize spilling, leaking, and evaporation because alcohols are

extremely volatile. The National Fire Protection Agency does not specifically address alcohol-based sanitizers, and the judgment falls to the local authority having jurisdiction. Consideration must be given to location of use, mounting location (eg, near light switches, egress hallways, emergency exits), volume and size of individual dispensing units, bulk storage conditions and location, frequency of use, and the specific medical benefits of the chosen product. Further studies are underway to determine true flammability and improved safety in containers.[33,44-46] The American Society of Healthcare Engineers states that it is permissible to install 1.2-L containers of alcohol-based hand rub in egress corridors.[47] Additional information may be found at http://www.cdc.gov/handhygiene/firesafety/default.htm. Check for individual state regulations.

Recommended Practice III

Surgical hand antisepsis/hand scrub should be performed before donning sterile gloves for surgical or other invasive procedures. Use of either an FDA-compliant, antimicrobial surgical scrub agent intended for surgical hand antisepsis or an FDA-compliant, alcohol-based antiseptic hand rub with documented persistent and cumulative activity that has been approved for surgical hand antisepsis is acceptable.[3]

1. Rings, watches, and bracelets should be removed before beginning the surgical hand antisepsis/scrub procedure (see recommended practice I, number 5).

2. Hands should be washed with plain or antimicrobial soap and running water immediately before beginning the surgical hand antisepsis/scrub (see recommended practice I, number 7).

3. Each surgical hand antisepsis/scrub procedure should follow a standardized protocol established and approved by the health care facility and the manufacturer's written directions for use, regardless of method. A standardized protocol should be adopted for each method used in the facility. Table 1 provides a summary of directives for general hand hygiene and surgical hand antisepsis.

Recommended Practice IV

Surgical hand antisepsis/hand scrub using an FDA-compliant, traditional antimicrobial scrub agent should include a standardized hand scrub procedure that follows the manufacturer's written directions for use and is approved by the health care facility.

1. A traditional, standardized, surgical hand antisepsis scrub procedure should include, but may not be limited to, the following.

   ♦ Wash hands and forearms with soap and running water immediately before beginning the surgical scrub.

   ♦ Clean the subungual areas of both hands under running water using a disposable nail cleaner.

   ♦ Rinse hands and forearms under running water.

   ♦ Dispense the approved antimicrobial scrub agent according to the manufacturer's written directions.

   ♦ Apply the antimicrobial agent to wet hands and forearms. Some manufacturers may recommend using a soft, nonabrasive sponge.

   ♦ Visualize each finger, hand, and arm as having four sides. Wash all four sides effectively. Repeat this process for opposite fingers, hand, and arm.

   ♦ Repeat this process if directed to do so by the manufacturer's written directions for use.

   ♦ Avoid splashing surgical attire.

   ♦ For water conservation, turn water off when it is not directly in use, if possible.

   ♦ Hold hands higher than elbows and away from surgical attire.

   ♦ Discard sponges, if used, in appropriate containers.

   ♦ In the OR, dry hands and arms with a sterile towel before donning a sterile surgical gown and gloves.

   Although the skin never can be rendered sterile, it can be made surgically clean by reducing the number of microorganisms.[17] A short, prescrub wash can loosen surface debris and transient microorganisms.[8] Subungual areas that are cleaned improperly can harbor microorganisms.[3,8,12] The mechanical action associated with hand scrubbing removes

Table 1

GENERAL HAND HYGIENE AND SURGICAL HAND ANTISEPSIS DIRECTIVES	
TOPIC	*ACTION*
General hand hygiene	
Visible soil	Wash hands with plain or antimicrobial soap and water.
No visible soil	Sanitize hands with an alcohol-based hand rub or wash with plain or antimicrobial soap and water.
Surgical hand antisepsis	
Visible soil/no visible soil	Wash hands with soap and water, then use either a US Food and Drug Administration (FDA) compliant, antimicrobial scrub agent or an FDA-compliant, alcohol-based antiseptic hand rub agent that is cleared for surgical hand antisepsis and provides persistent and cumulative activity.

microorganisms. This can be accomplished by rubbing the skin with or without a sponge to produce friction. With the addition of a facility-approved soap, which acts as a surfactant, transient and some resident microorganisms can be lifted and flushed away under running water.[17] Surgical hand antisepsis/hand scrubs are effective only if all surfaces are exposed to the mechanical cleaning and chemical antisepsis processes.[8,17] Hands and forearms should be held higher than the elbows and away from surgical attire to prevent contamination and allow water to run from the clean to the less clean area down the arm.[8,17] Appropriate disposal of sponges, if used, prevents cross contamination of the surgical scrub sink area. A sterile gown cannot be put on over wet or damp surgical attire without resultant potential contamination of the gown by strike-through moisture.[17]

2. A traditional, standardized, anatomical, timed method or a counted stroke method may be used for surgical hand antisepsis/hand scrubs. The degree of microbial reduction necessary

for effective prophylaxis of surgical wound infections has not been characterized fully. The advantages of a shorter scrub time include less skin trauma, greater water conservation, and actual OR time savings. European and Australian studies have evaluated scrub times between two and six minutes, concluding that with specific products, scrub times of three to four minutes are as effective as five-minute scrubs.[3,20] Facilities are encouraged to follow scrub agent manufacturers' written directions for use when establishing policies and procedures for scrub times.[3,20,48-52]

3. The use of a brush for surgical hand antisepsis/ hand scrubs is not necessary for adequate reduction of bacterial counts.[3] Skin damage from scrubbing with brushes can lead to an increased number of gram-negative bacteria and *Candida*.[18,53] Scrubbing with a brush is associated with an increase in skin cell shedding.[53-55]

4. General hand hygiene should be performed immediately after surgical gloves are removed and before any further activities are undertaken.

Recommended Practice V

Surgical hand antisepsis/hand rub with an FDA-compliant, alcohol-based surgical hand rub product should follow a standardized application according to the manufacturer's written directions for use.[3]

1. Alcohol-based solutions reduce bacterial counts on hands more rapidly than do antimicrobial soaps or detergents in the majority of experimental in vivo and in vitro models.[3] Alcohol hand-hygiene products alone kill more organisms than any product on the market but offer no appreciable persistence or cumulative effect. Use of a combination of active ingredients (eg, alcohol and chlorhexidine gluconate) to achieve both rapid reduction of microbial counts and the persistence and cumulative effect needed to prevent microbial regrowth is desirable. Randomized trials demonstrate better compliance with a surgical hand antisepsis protocol using an alcohol-based hand rub agent than with the traditional surgical scrub protocol.[56-59]

2. A standardized protocol for alcohol-based surgical hand rubs should follow manufacturers' written instructions and include, but may not be limited to, the following.
   ♦ Wash hands and forearms with soap and running water immediately before beginning the surgical hand antisepsis procedure.
   ♦ Clean the subungual areas of both hands under running water using a nail cleaner.
   ♦ Rinse hands and forearms under running water.
   ♦ Dry hands and forearms thoroughly with a paper towel.
   ♦ Dispense the manufacturer-recommended amount of the surgical hand rub product.
   ♦ Apply the product to the hands and forearms, following the manufacturer's written directions. Some manufacturers may require the use of water as part of the process.
   ♦ Rub thoroughly until dry.
   ♦ Repeat the product application process if indicated in the manufacturer's written directions.
   ♦ In the OR, don a sterile surgical gown and gloves.

3. General hand hygiene should be performed immediately after surgical gloves are removed and before any further activities are undertaken.

Recommended Practice VI

Policies and procedures for surgical hand antisepsis should be developed, reviewed periodically, and readily available in the practice setting.

1. Policies and procedures for surgical hand antisepsis should include, but may not be limited to,
   ♦ identifying facility-approved, FDA-compliant, surgical hand antisepsis agents;
   ♦ defining the duration of surgical hand antisepsis procedures; and
   ♦ establishing standardized protocols for each hand antisepsis method used.

   To provide optimal effect, antimicrobial-containing products should be chosen from the FDA's product category defined as surgical hand antisepsis agents.[35] Contact times should follow manufacturers' written directions for optimum efficacy. Policies for general hand hygiene and surgical hand antisepsis should be established in conjunction with infection control practitioners and meet the particular needs of the practice setting. AORN's "Recommended practices for surgical attire" should be consulted when developing guidelines.[60]

2. Education regarding surgical hand antisepsis products and protocols should be ongoing and systematic for all personnel in the perioperative setting.

3. Recommended practices should be used as guidelines for developing policies and procedures in the practice setting. Policies and procedures establish authority, responsibility, and accountability and serve as operational guidelines. Introduction and review of policies and procedures should be included in orientation and ongoing education of personnel to assist in the development of knowledge, skills, and attitudes that affect patient outcomes. Policies and procedures also assist in developing quality assessment and improvement activities.

Glossary

Alcohol-based hand rub: "An alcohol-containing preparation designed for application to the hands for reducing the number of viable microorganisms on the hands. In the United States, such preparations usually contain 60% to 95% alcohol."[3(p3)]

Alcohol-based preparations: Products used for general hand hygiene and/or surgical hand antisepsis. Appropriate products (ie, alcohol-based products) may be used as an alternative to the traditional surgical hand scrub using detergent-based antiseptic agents. These alcohol-based products do not remove soil; therefore, application of these products for surgical hand antisepsis must be preceded by a soap and water wash.

Anatomical timed scrub or counted stroke scrub method: An anatomical scrub method that uses a prescribed number of strokes or specified amount of time for scrubbing each surface of the fingers, hands, and arms.

Antimicrobial soap: Soap containing an FDA-compliant antiseptic agent.

Antiseptic agent: Antimicrobial substance applied to the skin to reduce the log number of microbial flora. Examples include alcohols,

chlorhexidine, chlorine, hexachlorophene, iodine, parachloroxylenol, quaternary ammonium compounds, and triclosan.

Artificial nails: Substances or devices applied or added to the natural nails to augment or enhance the wearer's own nails. They include, but are not limited to, bondings, tips, wrappings, and tapes.

Cumulative effect: A progressive decrease over time, usually measured in days, in the number of microorganisms present after repeated applications of a product.

Hand antisepsis: Refers to either hand wash or hand rub using an antiseptic agent.

Hand hygiene: A generic term that applies to hand washing with either a plain or antimicrobial soap or use of an alcohol-based, antiseptic hand rub product.

In vitro: Outside the living body and in an artificial environment.

In vivo: In the living body of a plant or animal.

Persistence: Prolonged or extended antimicrobial activity, usually measured in hours, that prevents or inhibits the regrowth of microorganisms after application of the product.

Resident microorganisms: Microorganisms considered to be permanent residents of the skin and not readily removed by hand washing.

Stratum corneum: The outermost layer of the epidermis. The cells of the stratum corneum are rough and jagged and contain myriad niches in which bacteria dwell.

Subungual: Under the nail (eg, fingernail).

Surgical hand antisepsis: "Antiseptic hand wash or antiseptic hand rub performed preoperatively by surgical personnel to eliminate transient bacteria and reduce resident hand flora. Antiseptic detergent preparations often have persistent antimicrobial activity."[3(p4)] Previously known as surgical hand scrub.

Surgical hand antiseptic agent: An FDA-compliant product that is a broad-spectrum, fast-acting, and nonirritating preparation containing an antimicrobial ingredient designed to significantly reduce the number of microorganisms on intact skin. Surgical hand antiseptic agents demonstrate both persistent and cumulative activity.

Transient microorganisms: Microorganisms isolated from the skin. Such microorganisms are of concern because they can be transmitted readily on hands unless removed by mechanical friction and soap and water hand washing or use of a hand rub agent.

US Food and Drug Administration compliant: Refers to an agent that meets the testing and labeling criteria outlined by the FDA in the TFM for Health-Care Antiseptic Drug Products, a NDA, or an ANDA. The process required depends on the components, concentration, and mixture of ingredients used in the individual product. Both persistence and cumulative effect are critical to providing optimum product effectiveness and patient safety. When following the FDA over-the-counter TFM process, there is no specific clearance or letter of approval from the FDA; however, the FDA requires all studies and product labeling to meet the TFM criteria and remain on file for their review.[35]

Vector: An organism that transmits a pathogen.

Waterless antiseptic agent: "An antiseptic agent that does not require use of exogenous water. After applying such an agent, the hands are rubbed together until the agent has dried."[3(p4)]

Notes

1. L Mody et al, "Introduction of a waterless alcohol-based hand rub in a long-term care facility," *Infection Control and Hospital Epidemiology* 24 (March 2003) 165-171.

2. D Pittet, "Improving adherence to hand hygiene practice: A multidisciplinary approach," *Emerging Infectious Diseases* 7 (March/April 2001) 234-240.

3. Centers for Disease Control and Prevention, "Guidelines for hand hygiene in health-care settings, Recommendations and reports," *Morbidity and Mortality Weekly Report* 51 (RR-16) (Oct 25, 2002).

4. S C Beyea, ed, *Perioperative Nursing Data Set,* second ed (Denver: AORN Inc, 2002).

5. S Hugonnet, D Pittet, "Hand hygiene—beliefs or science?" *Clinical Microbiology and Infection* 6 (July 2000) 350-356.

6. P B Graves, C L Twomey, "The changing face of hand protection," *AORN Journal* 76 (August 2002) 248-258.

7. "Recommended practices for standard and transmission-based precautions in the perioperative practice setting," in *Standards, Recommended Practices, and Guidelines* (Denver: AORN, Inc, 2003) 345-349.

8. N F Phillips, *Berry & Kohn's Operating Room Technique,* tenth ed (St Louis: Mosby, 2004).

9. C A Baumgardner et al, "Effects of nail polish on microbial growth of fingernails," *AORN Journal* 58 (July 1993) 84-88.

10. D Fogg, "OR attire; endoscopic equipment; artificial nails and chewing gum in the OR; monitoring patients," (Clinical Issues) *AORN Journal* 54 (August 1991) 335-339.

11. E L Larson, "APIC guideline for handwashing and hand antisepsis in health care settings," *American Journal of Infection Control* 23 (August 1995) 251-263.

12. C A Wynd, D E Samstag, A M Lapp, "Bacterial carriage on the fingernails of OR nurses," *AORN Journal* 60 (November 1994) 796-805.

13. R L Moolenaar et al, "A prolonged outbreak of *Pseudomonas aeruginosa* in a neonatal intensive care unit: Did staff fingernails play a role in disease transmission?" *Infection Control and Hospital Epidemiology* 21 (February 2000) 80-85.

14. E Edel et al, "Impact of a 5-minute scrub on the microbial flora found on artificial, polished, or natural fingernails of operating room personnel," *Nursing Research* 47 (January/February 1998) 54-59.

15. S A McNeil et al, "Effects of hand cleansing with antimicrobial soap or alcohol-based gel on microbial colonization of artificial fingernails worn by health care workers," *Clinical Infectious Diseases* 32 (February 2001) 367-372.

16. S A Hedderwick et al, "Pathogenic organism associated with artificial fingernails worn by healthcare workers," *Infection Control and Hospital Epidemiology* 21 (August 2000) 505-509.

17. D M Fogg, "Infection prevention and control," in *Alexander's Care of the Patient in Surgery,* 12th ed, J C Rothrock, ed (St Louis: Mosby, 2003) 97-158.

18. J Pottinger, S Burns, C Manske, "Bacterial carriage by artificial versus natural nails," *American Journal of Infection Control* 17 (December 1989) 340-344.

19. A Mangram et al, "Guideline for prevention of surgical site infection, 1999," *Infection Control and Hospital Epidemiology* 20 (April 1999) 250-278.

20. S M Wheelock, S Lookinland, "Effect of surgical hand scrub time on subsequent bacterial growth," *AORN Journal* 65 (June 1997) 1087-1098.

21. M F Fay, "Hand dermatitis: The role of gloves," *AORN Journal* 54 (September 1991) 451-467.

22. D M Salisbury et al, "The effect of rings on microbial load of health care workers' hands," *American Journal of Infection Control* 25 (February 1997) 24-27.

23. W E Trick et al, "Impact of ring wearing on hand contamination and comparison of hand hygiene agents in a hospital," *Clinical Infectious Diseases* 36 (June 2003) 1383-1390.

24. A T Lane, S S Drost, "Effects of repeated application of emollient cream to premature neonates' skin," *Pediatrics* 92 (September 1993) 415-419.

25. G S Hall, C A Mackintosh, P N Hoffman, "The dispersal of bacteria and skin scales from the body after showering and after application of a skin lotion," *Journal of Hygiene* 97 (October 1986) 289-298.

26. E L Larson et al, "Changes in bacterial flora associated with skin damage on hands of health care personnel," *American Journal of Infection Control* 26 (October 1998) 513-521.

27. R D Jones et al, "Moisturizing alcohol hand gels for surgical hand preparation," *AORN Journal* 71 (March 2000) 584-599.

28. C Marino, M Cohen, "Washington state hospital survey 2000: Gloves, handwashing agents, and moisturizers," *American Journal of Infection Control* 29 (December 2001) 422-424.

29. E Pinney, "Hand washing," *British Journal of Perioperative Nursing* 10 (June 2000) 328-331.

30. D Pittet et al, "Effectiveness of a hospital-wide programme to improve compliance with hand hygiene," *The Lancet* 356 (Oct 14, 2000) 1307-1312.

31. S Hugonnet, T V Perneger, D Pittet, "Alcohol-based handrub improves compliance with hand hygiene in intensive care units," *Archives of Internal Medicine* 162 (May 13, 2002) 1037-1043.

32. S Harbarth et al, "Interventional study to evaluate the impact of an alcohol-based hand gel in improving hand hygiene compliance," *Pediatric Infectious Disease Journal* 21 (June 2002) 489-495.

33. F Myers, S Parini, "Hand hygiene: Understanding and implementing the CDC's new guideline," *Nursing Management* 34 (April 2003) 1-14.

34. D Pittet, "Promotion of hand hygiene: Magic, hype, or scientific challenge," *Infection Control and Hospital Epidemiology* 23 (March 2002) 118-119.

35. "Topical antimicrobial drug products for over-the-counter human use; tentative final monograph for health-care antiseptic drug products," in *Code of Federal Regulations* (CFR) 21: Food and Drugs, Parts 333 and 369 (Washington, DC: US Government Printing Office, 1994) 31402-31452.

36. M L Rotter, "Hand washing and hand disinfection," in *Hospital Epidemiology and Infection Control,* second ed, C G Mayhall, ed (Philadelphia: Lippincott Williams & Wilkins, 1999).

37. A Rosenberg, S D Alatary, A F Peterson, "Safety and efficacy of the antiseptic chlorhexidine gluconate," *Surgery, Gynecology & Obstetrics* 143 (November 1976) 789-792.

38. E J Lowbury, H A Lilly, G A Ayliffe, "Preoperative disinfection of surgeons' hands: Use of alcoholic solutions and effects of gloves on skin flora," *British Medical Journal* 4 (Nov 16, 1974) 369-372.

39. G Mulberrry et al, "Evaluation of a waterless, scrubless chlorhexidine gluconate/ethanol surgical scrub for antimicrobial efficacy," *American Journal of Infection Control* 29 (December 2001) 377-382.

40. "Recommended practices for product selection in perioperative practice settings," in *Standards, Recommended Practices, and Guidelines* (Denver: AORN, Inc, 2004) 347-350.

41. C Kohan et al, "The importance of evaluating product dispensers when selecting alcohol-based handrubs," *American Journal of Infection Control* 30 (October 2002) 373-375.

42. A F Widmer, "Replace hand washing with use of a waterless alcohol hand rub?" *Clinical Infectious Diseases* 31 (July 2000) 136-143.

43. K A Bryant, J Pearce, B Stover, "Flash fire associated with the use of alcohol-based antiseptic agent," (Letter) *American Journal of Infection Control* 30 (June 2002) 256-257.

44. G Pugliese, J Bartley, T Lundstrom, "Alcohol-based handwashing agents: A clash with regulators or opportunity for a common-sense approach?" *Infection Control Today* 7 no 2 (2003) 1-4.

45. J M Boyce, M L Pearson, "Low frequency of fires from alcohol-based hand rub dispensers in healthcare facilities," *Infection Control and Hospital Epidemiology* 24 (August 2003) 618-619.

46. W M Wagner, "Double-edged sword: Managing the potential fire hazards posed by alcohol-based hand cleaning products," *Health Facilities Management* 16 (June 2003) 47-50.

47. "Alcohol based hand rubs," HospitalConnect.com, http://www.hospitalconnect.com/ashe/currentevent/abhi.html (accessed 29 Dec 2003).

48. L J Pereira, G M Lee, K J Wade, "An evaluation of five protocols for surgical handwashing in relation to skin condition and microbial counts," *Journal of Hospital Infection* 36 (May 1997) 49-65.

49. M O'Shaughnessy et al, "Optimum duration of surgical scrub-time," *British Journal of Surgery* 78 (June 1991) 685-686.

50. B Rehork, H Ruden, "Investigations into the efficacy of different procedures for surgical hand disinfection between consecutive operations," *Journal of Hospital Infection* 19 (October 1991) 115-127.

51. J R Babb, J G Davies, G A J Ayliffe, "A test procedure for evaluating surgical hand disinfection," *Journal of Hospital Infection* 18 no B suppl (June 1991) 41-49.

52. V Hingst et al, "Evaluation of the efficacy of surgical hand disinfection following a reduced application time of 3 instead of 5 min," *Journal of Hospital Infection* 20 (February 1992) 79-86.

53. K Kikuchi-Numagami et al, "Irritancy of scrubbing up for surgery with or without a brush," *Acta Dermato-Venereologica* 79 (May 1999) 230-232.

54. E L Larson et al, "Alcohol for surgical scrubbing?" *Infection Control and Hospital Epidemiology* 11 (March 1990) 139-143.

55. P D Meers, G A Yeo, "Shedding of bacteria and skin squames after handwashing," *Journal of Hygiene* 81 (August 1978) 99-105.

56. J J Parienti et al, "Hand-rubbing with an aqueous alcoholic solution vs traditional surgical hand-scrubbing and 30-day surgical site infection rates," *JAMA* 288 (Aug 14, 2002) 722-727.

57. E L Larson et al, "Comparison of different regimens for surgical hand preparation," *AORN Journal* 73 (February 2001) 412-432.

58. D Pittet, "Compliance with hand disinfection and its impact on hospital-acquired infections," *Journal of Hospital Infection* 48 no A suppl (August 2001) S40-S46.

59. B J Gruendemann, N B Bjerke, "Is it time for brushless scrubbing with an alcohol-based agent?" *AORN Journal* 74 (December 2001) 859-871.

60. "Recommended practices for surgical attire," in *Standards, Recommended Practices, and Guidelines* (Denver: AORN, Inc, 2003) 215-219.

Originally published May 1976, *AORN Journal,* as "Recommended practices for surgical hand scrubs."

Revised March 1978, July 1982, May 1984, October 1990.

Published as proposed recommended practices August 1994.

Revised November 1998; published April 1999, *AORN Journal.* Reformatted July 2000.

Revised November 2003; published February 2004, *AORN Journal.*

Recommended Practices for Safe Care Through Identification of Potential Hazards in the Surgical Environment

The following recommended practices were developed by the AORN Recommended Practices Committee and have been approved by the AORN Board of Directors. They are effective January 1, 2003.

These recommended practices are intended as achievable recommendations representing what is believed to be an optimal level of practice. Policies and procedures will reflect variations in practice settings and/or clinical situations that determine the degree to which the recommended practices can be implemented.

AORN recognizes the numerous types of settings in which perioperative nurses practice. These recommended practices are intended as guidelines adaptable to various practice settings. These practice settings include traditional ORs, ambulatory surgery units, physicians' offices, cardiac catheterization suites, endoscopy suites, radiology departments, and all other areas where operative and other invasive procedures may be performed.

Purpose

These recommended practices provide guidelines for the implementation of safe care to patients and assist in the identification of potential hazards in the practice setting. They are not intended to cover aspects of perioperative patient care addressed in other recommended practices.

Recommended Practice I

Potential hazards associated with patient transport/ transfer activities should be identified, and safe practices should be established.

1. The patient always should be attended by appropriate personnel during transport and transfer. Patient needs should be assessed by an RN before transport to determine the necessary skill level of transport personnel. Many patient care problems can occur during transport. Observation and assessment by a registered professional nurse allows for identification of potential problems and implementation of appropriate interventions.[1]

2. When selecting the appropriate transport vehicle, design features to be considered include, but are not limited to,
   - locking devices on wheels;
   - protective devices such as safety straps and side rails and for cribs rails high enough to prevent a standing child from falling out;
   - stable, adjustable IV poles or stands;
   - holding devices for oxygen tanks;
   - positioning capabilities;
   - controls that are easy to operate and within reach of the operator;
   - maneuverability;
   - sufficient size;
   - removable head and foot boards;
   - mattress stabilizing devices;
   - easily cleanable surfaces; and
   - a rack or shelf to hold monitoring equipment.

   These design features promote safety and help prevent injury to patients and staff members during transport.[2]

3. The transporter should demonstrate competency in operating transport equipment. Demonstrated competency in operating transport equipment is necessary to prevent harm to the patient and operator.[3]

4. An adequate number of staff members should be available to ensure patient and staff member safety during transport/transfer activities. Individual patient assessment will dictate the number of staff members needed.[4] A minimum of four staff members is needed to move an adult who is unable to assist with transfer.[5]

   To promote the safety of patients and staff members, patient movement devices may be useful. If mechanical devices are not available, extra personnel may be needed. Safety devices include, but are not limited to,
   - roller devices,
   - hoists, and/or
   - slides.[6]

5. Specific needs of the patient should be assessed and appropriate interventions implemented during the transport phase.[7] Safety measures to be implemented during transport/ transfer activities should include, but are not limited to,
   - locking wheels on the transport vehicle and the patient's bed during transfer activities;
   - elevating side rails and using safety straps;
   - hanging and securing IV containers away from the patient's head;

♦ protecting the patient by giving special attention to the head, arms, and legs;

♦ ensuring that one staff member remains at the head of the patient transport vehicle;

♦ pushing the transport vehicle with the patient's feet first, avoiding rapid movement through hallways and when turning corners;

♦ maintaining integrity and function of IV infusions, indwelling catheters, tubes, drainage systems, and monitoring equipment; and

♦ obtaining appropriate skilled assistance and specific instructions for the patient with special needs.

Locking wheels, raising the side rails, and securing safety straps prevent the patient from falling. Securing IV containers prevents container breakage and subsequent patient injury.[8] Maintaining proximity to the patient's head provides access to the patient's airway in case of respiratory distress or vomiting. Rapid movements can cause patient disorientation, nausea and vomiting, and dizziness.[9]

6. Scheduled preventive maintenance and repair should be performed on all transport vehicles. Preventive maintenance and repair promote proper functioning.[10]

Recommended Practice II

Potential hazards associated with controlling patient temperature should be identified, and safe practices should be established.

1. Body temperature should be monitored and maintained as close to normothermic as possible during the preoperative period. Overheating due to excessive use of warming devices and inappropriate monitoring of body core temperature can result in passive hyperthermia. Monitoring and maintaining body temperature during the preoperative phase has a significant impact on the patient's risk for the following:

♦ myocardial ischemia,
♦ cardiac morbidity,
♦ surgical site infection,
♦ surgical bleeding, and
♦ patient discomfort.[11]

Skin temperature monitoring has limitations. Core temperature monitoring (ie, esophageal or tympanic membrane) is the preferred measure-

ment technique for anesthetized patients. Passive hyperthermia does not result from thermoregulatory intervention and can be treated easily by discontinuing active warming devices and removing excessive insulation on the patient.

The increase in body temperature during malignant hyperthermia results from an enormous increase in metabolic heat produced by internal and skeletal muscles.[12] The "AORN malignant hyperthermia guideline" should be used to develop protocols for addressing malignant hyperthermia.[13]

2. Direct contact of the patient's skin with plastic surfaces should be avoided. When used, temperature-regulating devices should be placed in an effective and safe manner and monitored during the surgical procedure. Any heat-regulating device should be used according to the manufacturer's recommendations. Thermal burns or pressure necrosis may occur when using temperature-regulating devices. Unless temperature-regulating blankets are designed to be placed next to patients' skin, a thin cloth covering is needed to protect surgical patients.[14]

3. Measures to prevent hypothermia should begin in the preoperative phase and continue into the postoperative phase. Perioperative nursing interventions include

♦ applying warm blankets upon the patient's arrival in the surgical area and after sterile drapes are removed;

♦ limiting the amount of skin surface exposed during positioning and skin preparation;

♦ limiting time between prepping of the skin and draping;

♦ preventing surgical drapes from becoming wet;

♦ adjusting the room temperature;

♦ monitoring patient temperature to avoid overheating;

♦ using heat-maintenance devices (eg, caps, blankets, leggings, warming units);

♦ warming irrigation or infusion solutions; and

♦ humidifying the airway.

The anesthetized patient loses heat intraoperatively and is unable to restore body heat through the normal mechanism of shivering or increased muscle activity. Hypothermia occurs during the immediate preoperative phase and continues throughout the postoperative phase.

Factors that contribute to perioperative hypothermia include, but are not limited to,

♦ decreased metabolic heat production,
♦ increased environmental heat loss,
♦ redistribution of heat within the body,
♦ induced inhibition of thermoregulation during surgical procedures,[15]
♦ patient's age,
♦ patient's physical status,
♦ type of anesthesia used,
♦ body fat, and
♦ length and type of surgical procedure.[16]

Preventative measures protect the patient from heat loss due to radiation, conduction, and/or evaporation.[17]

4. Skin integrity should be inspected before, periodically during (when possible), and after using devices such as ice packs, temperature-regulating blankets, and heat lamps. Individuals vary in their ability to tolerate heat and cold. Conditions that predispose patients to injury include age, immobility, body fat, open wounds, broken skin, edematous areas, abscesses, peripheral vascular disease, confusion or unconsciousness, nerve injuries, and/or regional anesthesia.[18]

5. Irrigation/infusion solutions should be warmed or cooled to the temperatures appropriate for the surgical need. Fluids should be heated or cooled in devices intended for that purpose. Microwaves and autoclaves should not be used as warming devices. Microwaves do not heat uniformly, cannot be monitored, and are not designed for medical use. Appropriate temperatures of irrigation/infusion solutions can help prevent hypothermia or hyperthermia during surgical procedures. Devices designed to heat or cool fluids have been tested, calibrated, and validated to promote safety. Microwaves and autoclaves do not distribute heat evenly and cannot be monitored.[19]

Recommended Practice III

Potential hazards associated with medication use in the practice setting should be identified, and safe practices should be established.[20]

1. Medication use in the OR should be governed by the following five rights:

♦ right patient,
♦ right medication,
♦ right dose,
♦ right time, and
♦ right route.

2. The perioperative nurse should confirm any/all verbal orders by repeating the entire order using a digit-by-digit technique (ie, one-two as opposed to twelve) to reduce the chance of error. The order should be documented in the patient's chart as soon as it is feasible. Verbal orders should be taken from physicians or licensed qualified anesthesia care providers only.

3. Medications should be stored in a safe manner. Medications having similar names and/or labels should be physically separated in the storage area. Medications not likely to be used in the practice setting should be removed from the area. Full package inserts should be available for all medications used in the practice setting. When obtaining and preparing medications for administration, labels should be checked three times to determine that the right medication has been selected for use. Check the label

♦ upon procurement from storage and/or the pharmacy,
♦ when preparing and drawing the medication into a syringe or other administration device, and
♦ when placing the medication on the sterile field or transferring it to the anesthesia care provider for administration.

4. The patient's identity should be verified by checking his or her identification band before administering any medication. During the intraoperative phase of care, the circulating nurse and anesthesia care provider should check the patient's identification band concurrently along with the patient's chart to determine patient identity. If the patient is able, he or she should be asked to state his or her name. Patient identification should be verified before the patient enters the OR, before induction of anesthesia, and before any medication is administered either from within the sterile field or outside the sterile field. If medication is to be administered after the procedure has begun and the patient identification band cannot be visualized (eg, due to positioning or draping), the

circulating nurse and anesthesia care provider may verify the patient's identity based on previous identification with the identification band and the patient's record. This process should be documented on the patient record.

5. To the extent possible, medications should be used in the strengths, dilutions, and/or dosages commercially available from the manufacturer. Strength, dilution, and dosage calculation charts should be immediately available in the OR at all times. Any medication calculation should be checked and verified by the RN and at least one other licensed, qualified individual before administration.

6. Medications should be delivered to the sterile field in an aseptic manner. Medications should not be poured on the sterile field unless the medication container is designed specifically for that purpose. Rubber stoppers should not be removed for the purpose of pouring the medication. Wipe the top of the stopper with an antiseptic agent according to facility policy and use the appropriate transfer devices (eg, syringe/needle, vial spike, filter straw) when delivering the medication to and mixing medication on the sterile field.

7. When medication is placed on the sterile field, the circulating nurse and scrub person should verify the medication label concurrently and audibly before and after the medication is placed on the field. Each person should view the label and verify the medication name, strength, dosage, and expiration date. When medication is procured for administration by the anesthesia care provider, the circulating nurse and anesthesia care provider should read the medication label aloud when the medication is transferred to the anesthesia care provider for administration.

8. Medications and/or containers (eg, syringes, medicine cups, basins) should be labeled at all times, both on and off the sterile field. A single medication should be prepared, delivered to the sterile field, and labeled by the scrub person before a second medication is prepared. The scrub person and circulating nurse should verify the labeled medication on the field concurrently, noting the medication name, strength, and dosage. The method of labeling may be determined by the facility. Sterile labels also are available commercially. All solutions on the sterile field, including medications, saline, and/or water, should be labeled. Original medication/solution containers and delivery devices should be kept in the OR for reference until the conclusion of the procedure. Any unlabeled solution or medication, either on or off the sterile field, should be discarded.

9. If there is a change in either scrub or circulating personnel at any time during a procedure, all medications and their labels, both on and off the sterile field, should be noted and verified concurrently by entering and exiting personnel.

10. When a medication is handed to the surgeon for administration, the name, strength, dilution, and/or dosage should be announced aloud so that all team members are aware of the medication being administered. As with verbal orders, use a digit-by-digit technique (ie, one-two as opposed to twelve) to announce strength, dilution, and/or dosage to decrease the potential for error.

Recommended Practice IV

Potential hazards associated with chemicals used in the practice setting should be identified, and safe practices should be established for their use.

1. According to Occupational Safety and Health Administration (OSHA) regulations, potential hazards related to chemicals present in the practice setting must be identified, and employees must be notified. These chemicals include, but are not limited to,
   - disinfectants and sterilants;
   - skin prepping, degreasing, and adhesive agents;
   - environmental cleaning agents;
   - chemotherapeutic (eg, cytotoxic) agents;
   - tissue preservatives; and
   - methyl methacrylate.

   The OSHA "Hazard communication standard," or "right-to-know" directive, states that every employee must be informed of the hazards associated with chemicals present in the work setting. Chemicals that are potentially hazardous to employees also may present hazards to patients. Periodic review of chemicals used will help determine whether decreased amounts of hazardous chemicals could be used.[21]

2. Personnel should read and follow all instructions provided on the container label or found on the material safety data sheet (MSDS) provided by the manufacturer of the chemical. The MSDS must be readily accessible within the practice setting. In accordance with the OSHA "Hazard communication standard," MSDS information for every potentially hazardous chemical must be available to employees. This information includes identification of hazards, precautions or special handling needed, signs and symptoms of toxic exposure, and first aid treatments for exposure.[22]

3. Chemicals should not be combined unless safe outcomes can be ensured. Do not combine mixing chemicals either intentionally or inadvertently. Mixing chemicals can result in unsafe substances. Chemical mixtures can be unstable and caustic in a variety of ways.[23]

4. Chemotherapeutic agents should be handled properly during preparation and administration. Specific handling techniques can minimize spread of contaminants and exposure for patients and health care workers.[24]

5. Personnel exposed to cytotoxic agents should have regular health evaluations to prevent overexposure. Accrued evidence does not indicate mutagenicity, carcinogenicity, and teratogenicity when exposure to antineoplastic agents is limited by proper precautions; however, medical surveillance of personnel continually exposed to these cytotoxic agents will aid in early detection of any exposure should it occur. Personnel continually exposed to these cytotoxic agents should have scheduled health evaluations, and exposure frequency should be reported to the employee's physician.[25]

Recommended Practice V

Potential hazards associated with the use of electrical equipment in the practice setting should be identified, and safe practices should be established.

1. Staff members should demonstrate competence in using electrical equipment in the practice setting. All electrical equipment should be inspected before use. Inspection should include, but not be limited to,

- checking outlets and switch plates for damage,
- checking power cords and plugs for fraying or other damage, and
- inspecting (ie, by a biomedical technician or electrical safety officer) new equipment before it is introduced into the practice setting.

Damaged power cords or outlets can result in excessive current being delivered to the patient and/or staff members. Biomedical technicians or electrical safety officers can determine whether electrical equipment is safe for the intended use in the practice setting.[26]

2. Device cord length should be appropriate for the intended use of the equipment. Extension cords should be avoided. Cords that do not lie flat produce a potential for tripping or accidental unplugging of the equipment. Use of extension cords can result in excessive current leakage and/or electrical system overload.[27]

3. Line isolation monitoring systems or ground fault interrupting systems should provide for continuous monitoring of current leakage. Systems that monitor current leakage and ground integrity reduce the hazards of shock, cardiac fibrillation, or burns produced by electrical current flowing through the patient's body to ground.[28]

Recommended Practice VI

Potential environmental hazards that affect patient care should be identified, and safe practices should be established.

1. Floors should be clean, dry, unobstructed, and in good repair. Floor traction can be impaired and injuries can occur when floors are not clean and well maintained.[29]

2. Air exchanges in the OR should adhere to guidelines established by the Centers for Disease Control and Prevention and the American Institute of Architects (AIA). All air should be filtered with appropriate filters as recommended by the AIA.[30] A number of devices used in the OR produce smoke, plume, or aerosols, which may be harmful. Additional sources of air contamination in the OR include power equipment, electrosurgical units, lasers, ultrasonic scalpels, other high-speed devices,

and people. Adequate air exchange assists in reducing the level of air contamination and in controlling odors and noxious vapors.[31]

3. Staff members should demonstrate knowledge about the use, handling, storage, and disposal of gas cylinders. Multiple hazards can occur with improper handling of gas cylinders. An unsupported cylinder can act as a projectile if the cylinder is knocked over and the neck is broken. Gas cylinders should be stored in a well-ventilated room in a holder or rack. Securing cylinders with a chain-like device prevents the cylinders from falling out of the holder or rack. Gas leaks can occur if valves are not closed properly.[32]

4. Lighting should be in working order and adequate for
   ♦ illuminating the surgical field,
   ♦ monitoring the patient, and
   ♦ performing perioperative duties.
   Adequate lighting is necessary to perform the planned invasive procedure and to evaluate the patient.

5. In case of power failure, a source of light from a circuit separate from the usual supply should be available. The operating light should be equipped with an automatic switch to the emergency power source for use if the usual power fails.[33]

Recommended Practice VII

Polices and procedures related to the identification of potential hazards and establishment of safe practices should be developed, reviewed periodically, revised as necessary, and available to staff members in the practice setting.

1. These recommended practices should be used as guidelines for developing polices and procedures within the practice setting. When developing polices and procedures related to the identification of potential hazards, applicable local, state, and federal regulations also should be considered. The AORN recommended practices that deal with traffic patterns, environmental cleaning, skin preparation of patients, sterilization, high-level disinfection, use of the pneumatic tourniquet, anesthesia equipment, electrosurgery, radiation safety, and laser safety also should be considered.

2. Policies and procedures establish authority, responsibility, and accountability and serve as operational guidelines. Introduction and review of policies and procedures should be included in orientation and ongoing education of personnel to assist in the development of knowledge, skills, and attitudes that affect patient care. Policies and procedures also assist in the development of performance activities.

Glossary

Ground-fault circuit interrupter: A device that senses a significant flow of leakage current and interrupts the flow of electricity to prevent electric shock.

Hypothermia: A decrease in core body temperature to a level below the normothermic range.

Line isolation monitor: A device used to continuously monitor an ungrounded power system that is isolated from the commercial power supply received from the utility company. Isolated, ungrounded power systems may allow leakage currents, also known as hazard currents, to flow from the power system to ground. This leakage current may flow through a person's body and present a shock hazard to that person. Standards for the maximum allowed leakage current have been established. The line isolation monitor displays the calculated level of leakage current and sounds an alarm if the current exceeds the predetermined level.

Passive hyperthermia: The result of heating a patient excessively to a core body temperature exceeding normal values.

Teratogenicity: The ability of a substance to cause development of abnormal structures in an embryo or fetus if the individual is exposed to that substance during pregnancy.

Warming device: A device designed for this purpose is used in the perioperative setting to assist with the control of body temperature. Generally, this device is used to prevent hypothermia.

NOTES
1. J A Kneedler, G H Dodge, eds, *Perioperative Patient Care: The Nursing Perspective,* third ed (Boston: Jones and Bartlett Publishers, Inc, 1994) 211-227; C Spry, *Essentials of Perioperative Nursing,* second ed (Gaithersburg, Md: Aspen Publishers, Inc, 1997) 127-128, 235-236.

2. Kneedler, Dodge, eds, *Perioperative Patient Care: The Nursing Perspective,* third ed, 215-216; Spry, *Essentials of Perioperative Nursing,* second ed, 128.

3. Kneedler, Dodge, eds, *Perioperative Patient Care: The Nursing Perspective,* third ed, 215-222.

4. *Ibid,* 215, 216.

5. *Ibid,* 226.

6. *Ibid,* 292-293, 307-308.

7. Spry, *Essentials of Perioperative Nursing,* second ed, 236-237.

8. Kneedler, Dodge, eds, *Perioperative Patient Care: The Nursing Perspective,* third ed, 215-217.

9. Spry, *Essentials of Perioperative Nursing,* second ed, 302.

10. Kneedler, Dodge, eds, *Perioperative Patient Care: The Nursing Perspective,* third ed, 295.

11. S M Frank et al, "Temperature monitoring practices during regional anesthesia," *Anesthesia and Analgesia* 88 (February 1999) 373-377; L K Groah, *Perioperative Nursing,* third ed (Standford, Conn: Appleton and Lange, 1996) 238.

12. D I Sessler, "Temperature monitoring," in *Anesthesia,* fourth ed, R D Miller, ed (New York: Churchill Livingstone, 1994) 1379-1380.

13. "AORN malignant hyperthermia guideline," in *Standards, Recommended Practices, and Guidelines* (Denver: AORN, Inc, 2002) 71-79.

14. Groah, *Perioperative Nursing,* third ed, 315-317; Sessler, "Temperature monitoring," 1374-1375.

15. B Bissonnette, "Temperature monitoring in pediatric anesthesia," *International Anesthesiology Clinics* 30 (Summer 1992) 69-70, 74; M E Goldberg et al, "Do heated humidifiers and heat and moist exchangers prevent temperature drop during lower abdominal surgery?" *Journal of Clinical Anesthesia* 4 (January/ February 1992) 16-24.

16. M Hind, "An investigation into factors that affect oesophageal temperature during abdominal surgery," *Journal of Advanced Nursing* 19 (March 1994) 457-464.

17. A C Guyton, J E Hall, "Body temperature, temperature regulation, and fever," in *Textbook of Medical Physiology,* ninth ed (Philadelphia: W B Saunders Co, 1995) 912-914; Hind, "An investigation into factors that affect oesophageal temperature during abdominal surgery," 457, 461-462; Sessler, "Temperature monitoring" 1369-1370, 1373-1375.

18. E M Bernthal, "Inadvertent hypothermia prevention: The anesthetic nurse's role," *British Journal of Nursing* 8 (Jan 14-27, 1999) 17-25; Hind, "An investigation into factors that affect oesophageal temperature during abdominal surgery," 457-464.

19. S S Moore et al, "The role of irrigation in the development of hypothermia during laparoscopic surgery," *American Journal of Obstetrics and Gynecology* 176 (March 1997) 598-602.

20. "AORN guidance statement—Safe medication practices in perioperative practice settings," *AORN Journal* 75 (May 2002) 1008-1009.

21. Occupational Safety and Health Administration, Department of Labor, "Toxic and hazardous substances, hazard communication standard," *Federal Regulations,* Title 29 6, Parts 1910.1000 to end, 29CFR1910.1200 (Washington, DC: US Government Printing Office, July 1, 1999) 461-469.

22. *Ibid,* 461-462, 468-470, 472.

23. "Chemical hazards in the hospital," *Health Devices* 9 (October 1980) 320.

24. S M Gullo, "Safe handling of antineoplastic drugs: Translating the recommendations into practice," *Oncology Nursing Forum* 15 no 5 (1988) 596-598; M J Saurel-Cublzolles, N Job-Spira, M Estryn-Behar, "Ectopic pregnancy and occupational exposure to antineoplastic drugs," *The Lancet* 341 (May 8, 1993) 1169-1171.

25. Gullo, "Safe handling of antineoplastic drugs: Translating the recommendations into practice," 596-598.

26. Occupational Safety and Health Administration, "Electrical standards for construction: Final rule," *Federal Register* 51 (July 11, 1986) 25331.

27. D Fecteau, "Patient and environmental safety," in *Alexander's Care of the Patient in Surgery,* 11th ed, M H Meeker, J C Rothrock, eds (St Louis: Mosby, Inc, 1994) 24.

28. *Ibid,* 25; G B Buczko, W P S McKay, "Electrical safety in the operating room," Canadian Journal of Anesthesia 34 (May 1987) 315-322.

29. Fecteau, "Patient and environmental safety," 22.

30. A J Mangram et al, "Guideline for prevention of surgical site infection," *American Journal of Infection Control* 27 (April 1999) 97-132; American Institute of Architects Academy of Architecture for Health, *1996-1997 Guidelines for Design and Construction of Hospitals and Health Care Facilities* (Washington, DC: The American Institute of Architects Press, 1996) 57-60.

31. "Aerosol safety in the OR: Help staff breathe easier," *Materials Management in Health Care* 4 (August 1995) 32-34; Fecteau, "Patient and environmental safety," 23, 26-28; B C Ulmer, "Air quality in the operating room," *Surgical Services Management* 3 (March 1997) 18-21.

32. Kneedler, Dodge, *Perioperative Patient Care: The Nursing Perspective,* third ed, 130.

33. N Fortunato, *Berry & Kohn's Operating Room Technique,* ninth ed (St Louis: Mosby, 2000) 156; R Brown, "There is a science to the elimination of darkness," *Journal of Operating Research* 2 (August 1982) 11, 21-23, 38-41.

Originally published February 1988, *AORN Journal.*

Revised March 1992.

Revised November 1995; published March 1996, *AORN Journal.*

Reformatted July 2000.

Revised; published March 2003, *AORN Journal.*

Recommended Practices for Cleaning and Caring for Surgical Instruments and Powered Equipment

The following recommended practices were developed by the AORN Recommended Practices Committee and have been approved by the AORN Board of Directors. They were presented as proposed recommended practices for comment by members and others. These recommended practices are effective January 1, 2002.

These recommended practices are intended as achievable recommendations representing what is believed to be an optimal level of practice. Policies and procedures will reflect variations in practice settings and/or clinical situations that determine the degree to which the recommended practices can be implemented.

AORN recognizes the numerous types of settings in which perioperative nurses practice. These recommended practices are intended as guidelines adaptable to various practice settings. These practice settings include traditional ORs, ambulatory surgery units, physicians' offices, cardiac catheterization suites, endoscopy suites, radiology departments, and all other areas where operative and other invasive procedures may be performed.

Purpose

These recommended practices provide guidelines to assist perioperative nurses in decontaminating, cleaning, maintaining, handling, storing, and/or sterilizing surgical instruments and powered equipment. These recommended practices are general recommendations as it is impossible to make a recommendation for each instrument. These recommended practices complement AORN's "Recommended practices for sterilization in perioperative practice settings."[1] Perioperative nurses should consult this document to assist in providing a safe environment for the patient. The appropriate committees in the practice setting should review all practices related to care and handling of surgical instruments and powered equipment.

Recommended Practice I

Surgical instruments and powered equipment should be cleaned, handled, and used according to manufacturers' instructions.

1. Manufacturers' instructions provide direction for care, cleaning, handling, and correctly using surgical instruments and powered equipment. Proper care, cleaning, and handling

helps safeguard instruments' function and effectiveness. Using instruments according to their intended use reduces the likelihood of procedure delay, patient/personnel injury, infections caused by instrument damage or malfunction, and/or costly repairs.[2]

Recommended Practice II

Instruments should be kept free of gross soil during surgical procedures.

1. Instruments should be wiped with sponges moistened with sterile water. Corrosion, rusting, and pitting occur when blood and debris are allowed to dry in or on surgical instruments.[3]

2. Lumened instruments should be irrigated with sterile water. Cannulated or lumened instruments may become obstructed with organic material. Irrigating instruments with sterile water helps remove residue. Saline causes deterioration of instrument surfaces and should not be used.[4]

Recommended Practice III

Effective and timely decontamination of instruments should be performed in a manner that minimizes risk to those performing the task.

1. All instruments opened on the sterile field require decontamination.

2. Personal protective attire should be worn by personnel when decontaminating instruments. Personal protective equipment can prevent contaminated blood and body fluids from coming in contact with personnel involved in decontamination. Protective attire is designed to protect the skin, mucous membranes, and eyes from exposure to blood, body fluids, and other infectious materials.[5]

3. Instruments should be prepared for decontamination after use. Instruments should be taken apart and arranged in an orderly fashion in mesh-bottom trays so that all surfaces are exposed to the action of an automated cleaner, if used. The following activities should be completed:
   - open instrument box locks;
   - place heavy retractors and/or other heavy instruments on the bottom or in a separate tray;

- place scissors, lighter-weight instruments, and microsurgical instruments on top;
- separate all reusable sharp instruments from general instruments; and
- cover instruments with a damp towel, at a minimum, to prevent drying during transportation to the decontamination area.[6]

An enzymatic soak solution, spray, gel, or foam may be used for these and other hard-to-clean instruments during transport.[7] Corrosion, rusting, and pitting occur when blood and debris are allowed to dry in or on surgical instruments.[8] Cannulated or lumened instruments may become obstructed with organic material.[9]

4. In the decontamination area, automated and/or manual cleaning methods of equal effectiveness should be used for decontaminating instruments.[10] The following methods may be used for decontamination.

- *Washer/sterilizer:* The washer/sterilizer processes instruments through several cycles, including cold water prerinse, high-temperature wash with alkaline detergent, neutralizing cycle, final rinse, and sterilization.
- *Ultrasonic cleaner:* Ultrasonic cleaners facilitate removal of small particles and debris from instrument crevices through a process called cavitation.[11] Ultrasonic energy is passed through a water bath, creating bubbles that implode. The process of implosion creates a suction action that pulls debris away from instrument surfaces. When using an ultrasonic cleaning process, follow manufacturers' instructions for detergent selection and proper use, care, and maintenance of the ultrasonic unit.[12] When using an ultrasonic cleaning process
  - combine only instruments made of similar metals in the ultrasonic cleaner to avoid ion transfer, which may result in instrument etching and pitting;
  - avoid placing chrome-plated instruments in the unit because the mechanical vibrations can cause the plating to flake; and
  - close the lid of the ultrasonic cleaner or cover it to prevent aerosolization of contaminants.

- *Washer/decontaminator:* A washer/decontaminator may use a single chamber for rinsing, cleaning, and drying or may use multiple chambers—one for each phase of the cycle. These phases may include
  - an initial cool water rinse to remove protein debris,
  - an enzymatic soak,
  - a wash with detergent,
  - an ultrasonic cleaning,
  - a sustained hot water rinse,
  - a liquid chemical germicide rinse, and
  - a drying cycle.[13]
  Sequencing and number of stages may vary among manufacturers.
- *Manual cleaning:* Although automated methods are preferred, instruments may be washed manually in a manner that protects personnel who are handling the instruments.

5. Personnel should wear protective attire as described in AORN's "Recommended practices for surgical attire."[14] Instruments, with the exception of powered equipment, should be submerged in warm water with appropriate detergent and cleaned and rinsed while completely submerged. Aerosolization of contaminants, splashing of infectious material, and injury from sharp objects is possible when manual cleaning is performed. Protective attire worn by personnel involved in manual cleaning of instruments is designed to protect the skin and mucous membranes from exposure to blood, body fluids, and other infectious materials.[15]

Manufacturers' instructions and AORN's "Recommended practices for product selection in perioperative practice settings" should be followed for detergent selection and proper use, care, and maintenance of instruments.[16] Following manufacturers' instructions decreases the possibility of selecting detergents that may be harmful to instruments. For example, abrasives can damage the protective surfaces of instruments, contribute to corrosion, and impede sterilization.[17]

Recommended Practice IV

Surgical instruments should be checked for function after cleaning. Those with moving parts may require lubrication according to manufacturers' instructions.

1. Water-soluble lubricants should be applied to those instruments that require lubrication. Instruments should be cleaned before the lubricant is applied. Cleaning, particularly ultrasonic cleaning, removes lubricants from instruments. Lubricants decrease friction between working surfaces. Unless otherwise specified, lubricants should be water soluble to allow steam penetration during sterilization; oil-based products cannot be penetrated.[18]

Recommended Practice V

Instruments that have come in contact with prions should be treated according to a specific prion-deactivation protocol.

1. Creutzfeldt-Jakob disease (CJD) is a rare and fatal disease of the central nervous system. Creutzfeldt-Jakob disease is known as a "slow viral infection" and is caused by agents commonly known as "unconventional viruses" (ie, prions).[19] The CJD-causing prion is an isoform of a normal protein concentrated in brain tissue. Prions, in general, are resistant to a number of standard disinfection and sterilization procedures, including steam sterilization, exposure to dry heat, ethylene oxide gas, and chemical disinfection using alcohol, formaldehyde, or glutaraldehyde.[20]

2. Tissue varies in its degree of infectivity, depending on prion content:
   ◆ high-infectivity tissue (ie, central nervous system tissue, brain dura mater, spinal cord, eye [cornea]);
   ◆ medium-infectivity tissue (ie, cerebrospinal fluid, lymph node, spleen, pituitary gland, tonsil); and
   ◆ low- or no-infectivity tissue (ie, blood, including serous exudate and leukocytes; bone marrow; heart, lung, liver, kidney; thyroid, adrenal, thymus glands; skin, peripheral nerves, skeletal muscle, adipose tissue, intestines; prostate, testes, semen; placenta, vaginal secretions, milk; tears, nasal mucous, sputum).[21]

3. Information about prions, prion infectivity, and decontamination is evolving. For updates, consult the Centers for Disease Control and Prevention and the World Health Organization, as well as material published by experts in the field.

4. General measures for cleaning instruments and the environment when prion disease is known or suspected should include the following steps.[22]
   ◆ Keep instruments moist until they are cleaned and decontaminated.
   ◆ Clean instruments as soon as possible after use to minimize drying of tissue, blood, and body fluids on the instruments.
   ◆ Avoid mixing instruments used on low- or no-infectivity tissues with those used on high- or medium-infectivity tissues.
   ◆ Prepare reusable items used on high-infectivity tissues for reuse only after specific decontamination methods have been used (ie, see number six below).
   ◆ Decontaminate instruments by the methods that follow before processing them in an automated processor. After being used for CJD-infected instruments, automated washers or other equipment should be run through an empty cycle before any further routine use.[23]
   ◆ Cover work surfaces with disposable impermeable material that can be removed and incinerated after the procedure. Clean and spot decontaminate underlying surfaces with a 1:10 dilution of sodium hypochlorite (ie, bleach). Use routine hospital decontamination procedures for surface decontamination.[24]
   ◆ Be familiar with and observe safety guidelines when working with hazardous chemicals such as sodium hydroxide and bleach.[25]
   ◆ Follow manufacturers' recommendations regarding care and maintenance of equipment.

5. Guidelines vary regarding the recommended method for decontaminating equipment and/or instruments that have come into contact with high-infectivity tissue of patients with known or suspected CJD.[26] Disposable instrumentation should be used as much as possible and then incinerated. This is the most unambiguous method for ensuring that there is no risk of residual infectivity.[27]

6. The ability to adequately clean instruments after contact with high-infectivity tissue of a patient known or suspected to have CJD determines subsequent decontamination procedures.
   ◆ Reusable critical or semicritical devices exposed to high-infectivity tissue from a patient known or suspected to have CJD that

can be adequately cleaned should be kept moist between the time of exposure and subsequent decontamination and cleaning.[28]

♦ After thorough cleaning, if the item is heat and moisture tolerant, steam autoclave at 134° C (272° F) for 18 minutes in a prevacuum sterilizer or at 121° C (250° F) for 60 minutes in a gravity displacement sterilizer.[29]

♦ Reusable critical or semicritical devices that are difficult to clean should be discarded or decontaminated initially by steam autoclaving at 132° C to 134° C (270° F to 272° F) for 18 minutes in a prevacuum sterilizer or at 121° C (250° F) for 60 minutes in a gravity displacement sterilizer. Alternatively, items may be soaked for 60 minutes in 1 Normal sodium hydroxide. After one hour, rinse, clean, and sterilize as above.[30]

♦ Items that are impossible to clean should be discarded.[31]

♦ Use of power drills or saws should be avoided if they are likely to come into contact with high-infectivity tissue. Power drills and saws by their very nature and design are difficult to clean and too expensive to discard.

7. Critical instruments used on high-infectivity tissue from a patient known or suspected to have CJD that permit only low-temperature sterilization (ie, ethylene oxide or hydrogen peroxide gas plasma) should be discarded.[32]

8. Flash sterilization should not be used for reprocessing instruments contaminated with high-infectivity tissue from a patient known or suspected to have CJD.[33]

9. Devices that have been contaminated with medium-, low-, or no-infectivity tissue may be cleaned and disinfected or sterilized using conventional protocols of heat, chemical sterilization, or high-level disinfection. When a device is contaminated with tissue or body fluids that are not deemed high-infectivity and the device can be cleaned effectively, the probability of infection transmission appears to be so low that it would not be measurable.[34]

10. After initial deactivation of the prion by the methods described in number six above, instruments should be decontaminated and sterilized in the usual fashion. When a potentially contaminated device can be cleaned and prion/tissue load decreased or physically removed, the probability of infection transmission is reduced significantly.[35]

11. A protocol for caring for instruments exposed to prions should be developed and followed by all personnel in the facility. Use of a defined protocol helps protect patients and health care workers from pathogen transmission. A summary of the preceding information is presented in Table 1.

Recommended Practice VI

Surgical instruments should be inspected and prepared for storage and/or sterilization after decontamination.

1. Instruments should be inspected for
   ♦ cleanliness;
   ♦ proper functioning and alignment;
   ♦ corrosion, pitting, burrs, nicks, and cracks;
   ♦ sharpness of cutting edges;
   ♦ loose set pins;
   ♦ wear and chipping of inserts and plated surfaces; and/or
   ♦ any other defects.[36]

2. Instruments in disrepair should be labeled and taken out of service until properly replaced or repaired. Inspection provides evidence of thorough cleaning and ensures that all organic materials have been removed. Inspection also provides evidence of proper functioning of all instruments. Instruments in poor working condition are hazardous to patients and personnel.[37]

3. Instruments to be stored after decontamination/sterilization should be dried thoroughly. Thoroughly drying instruments helps prevent rust formation. Proper storage provides protection from unnecessary damage.[38]

4. Instruments with removable parts should be disassembled when placed in trays designed for sterilization. Ring-handled instruments should be secured in a manner that retains them in an open position. Sterilization can be achieved only if the sterilizing agent contacts all instrument surfaces. Careful placement of instruments in the sterilization tray/container facilitates this process.[39]

Table 1

CARE OF INSTRUMENTS EXPOSED TO THE CREUTZFELDT-JAKOB DISEASE PRION[1]			

High-infectivity tissue

Item/device[2]	Cleanable	Heat/moisture stable	Disposition
Critical/semicritical instruments	If easily cleanable	If yes	1) Thoroughly clean with detergent germicide. 2) Decontaminate using one of the following methods. ♦ Autoclave at 134° C (272° F) in prevacuum sterilizer for 18 minutes. ♦ Autoclave at 121° C (250° F) in gravity sterilizer for 60 minutes. ♦ Immerse in 1 Normal sodium hydroxide for 60 minutes at room temperature followed by steam sterilization at 121° C (250° F) in gravity sterilizer for 30 minutes. 3) Thoroughly clean, wrap, and sterilize by conventional methods.
		If no	Discard.
	If difficult to clean	If yes	1) Discard, or decontaminate initially using one of the following methods. ♦ Autoclave at 134° C (272° F) in prevacuum sterilizer for 18 minutes. ♦ Autoclave at 121° C (250° F) in gravity sterilizer for 60 minutes. ♦ Immerse in 1 Normal sodium hydroxide for 60 minutes at room temperature followed by steam sterilization at 121° C (250° F) in gravity sterilizer for 30 minutes. 2) Thoroughly clean, wrap, and sterilize by conventional methods.
		If no	Discard.
	If impossible to clean	n/a	Discard.
Noncritical instruments	If cleanable	n/a	1) Clean according to routine procedures. 2) Disinfect with a 1:10 dilution of sodium hypochlorite or 1 Normal sodium hydroxide using the solution least damaging to the item. 3) Continue processing according to routine procedures.
	If noncleanable	n/a	Discard.
Environmental surfaces	n/a	n/a	1) Cover surface with disposable, impermeable material. 2) Incinerate material after use. 3) Disinfect surface with 1:10 dilution of sodium hypochlorite. 4) Wipe entire surface using routine facility decontamination procedures for surface decontamination.

Medium-, low-, or no-infectivity tissue

Item/device	Cleanable	Heat/moisture stable	Disposition
Critical/semicritical/noncritical instruments	Cleanable	n/a	Clean, disinfect, and sterilize according to routine procedures.
	Noncleanable		Discard.
Environmental surfaces	n/a	n/a	1) Cover surfaces with disposable, impermeable material. 2) Dispose of material according to facility policy after use. 3) Disinfect surface with Occupational Safety and Health Administration-recommended agent for decontamination of blood-contaminated surfaces (eg, 1:10 or 1:100 dilution of sodium hypochlorite).

NOTES

1. M S Favero, W W Bond, "Chemical disinfection of medical and surgical materials," in Disinfection, Sterilization, and Preservation, *fifth ed, S S Block, ed (Philadelphia: Lippincott Williams & Wilkins, 2001) 910-913; W A Rutala, D J Weber, "Creutzfeldt-Jakob disease: Recommendations for disinfection and sterilization,"* Healthcare Epidemiology *32 (May 1, 2001) 1348-1356; "WHO infection control guidelines for transmissible spongiform encephalopathies," World Health Organization, http://www.who.int/emc-documents/tse/whocdscsraph2003c.html (accessed 20 Nov 2001).*

2. E H Spaulding, "Chemical disinfection of medical and surgical materials," in Disinfection, Sterilization, and Preservation, *ed C A Lawrence, S S Block (Philadelphia: Lea & Febiger, 1968) 517-531.*

5. Delicate and sharp instruments should be protected according to manufacturers' instructions. Damage to delicate and sharp instruments can render them ineffective.[40]

6. Instrument containers should be designed to allow for sterilization of the contents. The size and design of instruments, distribution of density in the set, risk of personnel injury when lifting, and capability to achieve sterilization should determine instrument set weight. Information provided by the container manufacturer should describe size and design of instruments to be sterilized in the container and the correct loading configuration to facilitate sterilization of the contents. Container contents can be sterilized only if the sterilant can contact all instrument surfaces. Poor weight distribution of instruments can cause damage to neighboring instruments. Excessive tray weight can increase the chances of personnel injury.[41]

Recommended Practice VII

Powered equipment and any attachments should be decontaminated after use, lubricated, assembled, tested, and sterilized according to manufacturers' instructions.

1. Powered equipment should be cleaned and decontaminated thoroughly after use. Personnel should adhere to the following guidelines when cleaning and decontaminating powered equipment and attachments.
   ♦ Remove blades after use and dispose of them in proper sharps containers.
   ♦ Inspect air hoses, batteries, attachments, and power cords for damage or wear.
   ♦ Attach air hoses to hand pieces during cleaning.
   ♦ Use manufacturer-recommended detergent/germicide for cleaning.
   ♦ Do not immerse or place powered equipment and/or air hoses in automated or ultrasonic cleaners.
   ♦ Wipe air hoses with a clean, damp cloth using detergent/germicidal solution.
   ♦ Wipe all traces of detergent/germicide and excess fluids from the equipment and attachments.
   ♦ Dry the outer surfaces of the powered equipment and attachments with lint-free towels.[42]

2. Organic debris left on powered equipment hinders the sterilization process and may interfere with proper functioning.[43] Following manufacturers' instructions reduces the possibility of selecting detergents that may damage equipment. For example, abrasives will damage protective surfaces of powered equipment, contribute to corrosion, and impede sterilization. Permanent damage may result if fluid enters the internal mechanisms of powered equipment. Improper cleaning may result in damage to powered equipment, an inability to sterilize, and patient injury and/or infection.[44]

3. Powered equipment and attachments should be lubricated according to manufacturers' instructions.[45] Proper lubrication of powered equipment is essential for proper functioning. Following manufacturers' instructions will help prolong equipment life. Lubricants decrease friction between working surfaces. Lubricants should be used as specified. Although not recommended for routine instruments, some manufacturers recommend oil-based lubricants for powered equipment as opposed to other instruments. Extended sterilization exposure times often are necessary. Manufacturers' instructions should be followed carefully.

4. Powered equipment and attachments should be packaged and sterilized according to manufacturers' instructions.
   ♦ Disassemble powered equipment before sterilization.
   ♦ Protect delicate parts of the equipment.
   ♦ Coil air hoses loosely when packaged for sterilization.
   ♦ Consult manufacturers' instructions to determine sterilization parameters for powered equipment, batteries, and attachments.[46]

5. Sterilization depends on contact of the sterilant with all surfaces of the equipment.[47] Sterilization cycles required to sterilize powered equipment vary and may exceed preset sterilizer times and temperatures.[48]

6. Prevacuum steam sterilization is the preferred method for sterilizing powered equipment and attachments because it removes entrapped air and allows for rapid air removal and steam

penetration into the internal portions of the equipment. Ethylene oxide gas and low-temperature hydrogen peroxide gas plasma should be used only if the instrument cannot withstand the heat or moisture of steam sterilization. Ethylene oxide and low-temperature hydrogen peroxide gas plasma sterilization should be used according to the sterilizer and equipment manufacturer's instructions.[49]

7. Powered equipment and attachments should be inspected, tested, and used according to manufacturers' instructions. Personnel should adhere to the following guidelines when inspecting, testing, and using powered equipment, electrical cords for powered equipment, batteries, and attachments.

   ♦ Affix attachments to the units and test before use.
   ♦ Place trigger handles in the safety position when changing attachments.
   ♦ Use medical-grade compressed air or compressed dry nitrogen (ie, 99% pure) to operate air equipment.
   ♦ Use only grounded outlets if the powered equipment is operated with electrical cords.
   ♦ Use manufacturers' instructions to determine the correct pressure settings in pounds per square inch to operate equipment.[50]

   Testing the equipment or device before use can decrease the chance of injury.[51] Improperly seated attachments can be thrown from the equipment with great force and cause injury to patients and personnel. Accidental activation of powered equipment also can cause injury. Use of impure gases to run powered equipment may result in equipment damage and/or patient injury. Using excessive pressure can damage equipment and exert great stress on air hoses. Unless pressure is set with the equipment running, incorrect pressures may result. Underpressurized equipment may not perform in the designated manner.

8. Powered equipment instructions vary among manufacturers. Becoming familiar with the manufacturers' instructions assists in correct use of the equipment. Improperly functioning powered equipment can injure both patients and personnel.

Recommended Practice VIII

Policies and procedures regarding the care and cleaning of surgical instruments and powered equipment should be developed, reviewed at regular intervals, and readily available in the practice setting.

1. These recommended practices should be used as guidelines for developing policies and procedures in the practice setting. Policies and procedures establish authority, responsibility, and accountability. They also serve as operational guidelines and guide development of performance improvement activities. A review of policies and procedures should be included in the orientation and ongoing education of all appropriate staff members in the practice setting.

Glossary

Automated cleaner: A processing unit that uses automated equipment for instrument cleaning and decontamination.

Cavitation: The process whereby sound waves are produced in an ultrasonic cleaner, creating tiny air bubbles on instrument surfaces. When the air bubbles implode, they produce a small amount of suction that pulls debris off of instrument surfaces.

Decontamination: The process by which contaminants are removed, either by hand cleaning or mechanical means, using specific solutions capable of rendering blood and debris harmless and removing them from the surface of an object or instrument.

Ethylene oxide: An alkylating agent that, under the right conditions of time, temperature, concentration, and humidity, can result in microbial death.

Prion: A proteinaceous and infectious agent containing no DNA or RNA.[52]

Ultrasonic cleaner: A processing unit that transmits ultrasonic waves through the cleaning solution in a mechanical process known as cavitation. Ultrasonic cleaning is particularly effective in removing soil deposits from hard-to-reach areas.

Washer/decontaminator: A processing unit that, either by use of single or multiple chambers, automatically decontaminates surgical instruments. It employs a cool water rinse, hot water wash, rinse, and drying. An ultrasonic cleaning feature and lubricant rinse may be added.

Washer/sterilizer: A processing unit that cleans by a spray-force action known as impingement. This machine combines a vigorous agitation bath with jet-stream air to create underwater turbulence. A sterilization cycle follows the washing cycle.

Notes

1. "Recommended practices for sterilization in perioperative practice settings," in *Standards, Recommended Practices, and Guidelines* (Denver: AORN, Inc, 2001) 309-318.

2. N H Fortunato, *Berry & Kohn's Operating Room Technique,* ninth ed (St Louis: Mosby, Inc, 2000) 255, 291, 310; S S Fairchild, *Perioperative Nursing: Principles and Practice,* second ed (Boston: Little, Brown and Co, 1996) 223.

3. J J Perkins, *Principles and Methods of Sterilization in Health Sciences,* second ed (Springfield, Ill: Charles C Thomas Publisher, 1969) 237-238; D Fogg "Infection control," in *Alexander's Care of the Patient in Surgery,* 11th ed, M H Meeker, J C Rothrock, eds (St Louis: Mosby, 1999) 111; Fortunato, *Berry & Kohn's Operating Room Technique,* ninth ed, 310.

4. Fogg, "Infection control," 111; American Society for Healthcare Central Service Professionals of the American Hospital Association, *Training Manual for Central Service Technicians* (Chicago: American Hospital Association, 1997) 98, 101; W A Rutala, "Disinfection, sterilization, and waste disposal," in *Prevention and Control of Nosocomial Infections,* third ed, R P Wenzel, ed (Baltimore: Williams & Wilkins, 1997) 574.

5. "Recommended practices for surgical attire," in *Standards, Recommended Practices, and Guidelines* (Denver: AORN, Inc, 2001) 175-179; "Occupational exposure to bloodborne pathogens; Final rule," *Federal Register* 56 (Dec 6, 1991) 64177; *ANSI/AAMI ST35:1996—Safe Handling and Biological Decontamination of Medical Devices in Health Care Facilities and in Nonclinical Settings* (Arlington, Va: Association for the Advancement of Medical Instrumentation, 1996) 2, 6-7; Fogg, "Infection control," 111; American Society for Healthcare Central Service Professionals of the American Hospital Association, *Training Manual for Central Service Technicians,* 74-75, 80.

6. Fogg, "Infection control," 111.

7. Perkins, *Principles and Methods of Sterilization in Health Sciences,* second ed, 244; American Society for Healthcare Central Service Professionals of the American Hospital Association, *Training Manual for Central Service Technicians,* 82-83; Rutala, "Disinfection, sterilization, and waste disposal," 574; Fortunato, *Berry & Kohn's Operating Room Technique,* ninth ed, 283; Fogg, "Infection control," 111.

8. Perkins, *Principles and Methods of Sterilization in Health Sciences,* second ed, 237-238; Fortunato, *Berry & Kohn's Operating Room Technique,* ninth ed, 310; American Society for Healthcare Central Service Professionals of the American Hospital Association, *Training Manual for Central Service Technicians,* 119.

9. Fogg, "Infection control," 111; American Society for Healthcare Central Service Professionals of the American Hospital Association, *Training Manual for Central Service*

Technicians, 99; Rutala, "Disinfection, sterilization, and waste disposal," 574.

10. *ANSI/AAMI ST35:1996—Safe Handling and Biological Decontamination of Medical Devices in Health Care Facilities and in Nonclinical Settings,* 10-11; American Society for Healthcare Central Service Professionals of the American Hospital Association, *Training Manual for Central Service Technicians,* 88-93; J K Schultz, "Decontamination: Recommended practices," in *Sterilization Technology for the Health Care Facility,* second ed, M Reichert, J H Young, ed (Gaithersburg, Md: Aspen Publishers, Inc, 1997) 14-15.

11. American Society for Healthcare Central Service Professionals of the American Hospital Association, *Training Manual for Central Service Technicians,* 92-93; Fortunato, *Berry & Kohn's Operating Room Technique,* ninth ed, 306-307; Fogg, "Infection control," 113.

12. Fortunato, *Berry & Kohn's Operating Room Technique,* ninth ed, 307.

13. *Ibid,* 306; American Society for Healthcare Central Service Professionals of the American Hospital Association, *Training Manual for Central Service Technicians,* 90-92; B J Gruendemann, B Fernsebner, *Comprehensive Perioperative Nursing, Volume 1: Principles* (Boston: Jones and Bartlett Publishers, 1995) 229-230.

14. "Recommended practices for surgical attire," 175-179.

15. *ANSI/AAMI ST35:1996—Safe Handling and Biological Decontamination of Medical Devices in Health Care Facilities and in Nonclinical Settings,* 10, 11; American Society for Healthcare Central Service Professionals of the American Hospital Association, *Training Manual for Central Service Technicians,* 74-75, 80, 98-99.

16. "Recommended practices for product selection in perioperative practice settings," in *Standards, Recommended Practices, and Guidelines* (Denver: AORN, Inc, 2004) 347-350.

17. Fogg, "Infection control," 111.

18. *Ibid,* 114.

19. M S Favero, W W Bond, "Chemical disinfection of medical and surgical materials," in *Disinfection, Sterilization, and Preservation,* fifth ed, S S Block, ed (Philadelphia: Lippincott Williams & Wilkins, 2001) 910-911.

20. *Ibid,* 911.

21. *Ibid;* W A Rutala, D J Weber, "Creutzfeldt-Jakob disease: Recommendations for disinfection and sterilization," *Healthcare Epidemiology* 32 (May 1, 2001) 1348-1356.

22. Favero, Bond, "Chemical disinfection of medical and surgical materials," 910-913; Rutala, Weber, "Creutzfeldt-Jakob disease: Recommendations for disinfection and sterilization," 1353-1355.

23. World Health Organization, Department of Communicable Disease Surveillance and Response, *WHO Infection Control Guidelines for Transmissible Spongiform Encephalopathies* (Geneva: World Health Organization, 1999) 15.

24. *Ibid;* Rutala, Weber, "Creutzfeldt-Jakob disease: Recommendations for disinfection and sterilization," 1355.

25. World Health Organization, Department of Communicable Disease Surveillance and Response, *WHO Infection Control Guidelines for Transmissible Spongiform Encephalopathies,* 31.

26. *Ibid*, 29-31; "Questions and answers regarding Creutzfeldt-Jakob disease infection-control practices," Centers for Disease Control and Prevention, http://www.cdc.gov/ncidod/diseases/cjd/cjd_inf_ctrl_qa.htm (accessed 6 Nov 2001); Rutala, Weber, "Creutzfeldt-Jakob disease: Recommendations for disinfection and sterilization," 1354-1355; Favero, Bond, "Chemical disinfection of medical and surgical materials," 910-917.

27. World Health Organization, Department of Communicable Disease Surveillance and Response, *WHO Infection Control Guidelines for Transmissible Spongiform Encephalopathies,* 29.

28. Rutala, Weber, "Creutzfeldt-Jakob disease: Recommendations for disinfection and sterilization," 1354-1355.

29. Rutala, Weber, "Creutzfeldt-Jakob disease: Recommendations for disinfection and sterilization," 1354-1355; Favero, Bond, "Chemical disinfection of medical and surgical materials," 913.

30. *Ibid.*

31. *Ibid.*

32. Rutala, Weber, "Creutzfeldt-Jakob disease: Recommendations for disinfection and sterilization," 1355.

33. *Ibid.*

34. *Ibid;* Favero, Bond, "Chemical disinfection of medical and surgical materials," 913.

35. Favero, Bond, "Chemical disinfection of medical and surgical materials," 913.

36. American Society for Healthcare Central Service Professionals of the American Hospital Association, *Training Manual for Central Service Technicians,* 116-119; Fogg, "Infection control," 114.

37. Perkins, *Principles and Methods of Sterilization in Health Sciences,* second ed, 266; Fortunato, *Berry & Kohn's Operating Room Technique,* ninth ed, 307, 308.

38. Fortunato, *Berry & Kohn's Operating Room Technique,* ninth ed, 308.

39. Perkins, *Principles and Methods of Sterilization in Health Sciences,* second ed, 266.

40. American Society for Healthcare Central Service Professionals of the American Hospital Association, *Training Manual for Central Service Technicians,* 102; Fogg, "Infection control," 111.

41. *ANSI/AAMI ST33: 1996—Guidelines for the Selection and Use of Reusable Rigid Container Systems for Ethylene Oxide Sterilization and Steam Sterilization in Health Care Facilities* (Arlington, Va: Association for the Advancement of Medical Instrumentation, 1996) 183.

42. Fortunato, *Berry & Kohn's Operating Room Technique,* ninth ed, 312; American Society for Healthcare Central Service Professionals of the American Hospital Association, *Training Manual for Central Service Technicians,* 102-103.

43. *Ibid.*

44. *Ibid;* Rutala, Weber, "Creutzfeldt-Jakob disease: Recommendations for disinfection and sterilization," 541-542, 552.

45. American Society for Healthcare Central Service Professionals of the American Hospital Association, *Training Manual for Central Service Technicians,* 121-122; Fortunato, *Berry & Kohn's Operating Room Technique,* ninth ed, 312.

46. Fortunato, *Berry & Kohn's Operating Room Technique,* ninth ed, 312.

47. Perkins, *Principles and Methods of Sterilization in Health Sciences,* second ed, 258; American Society for Healthcare Central Service Professionals of the American Hospital Association, *Training Manual for Central Service Technicians,* 161; Rutala, Weber, "Creutzfeldt-Jakob disease: Recommendations for disinfection and sterilization," 568.

48. American Society for Healthcare Central Service Professionals of the American Hospital Association, *Training Manual for Central Service Technicians,* 122.

49. Fortunato, *Berry & Kohn's Operating Room Technique,* ninth ed, 312; American Society for Healthcare Central Service Professionals of the American Hospital Association, *Training Manual for Central Service Technicians,* 172-173; C O Hancock, "Steam sterilization: Sterilizer operation," in *Sterilization Technology for the Health Care Facility,* second ed, M Reichert, J H Young, eds (Gaithersburg, Md: Aspen Publishers, Inc, 1997) 139; J K Schultz, "Steam sterilization: Recommended practices," in *Sterilization Technology for the Health Care Facility,* second ed, M Reichert, J H Young, eds (Gaithersburg, Md: Aspen Publishers, Inc, 1997) 148-149.

50. L K Groah, *Perioperative Nursing,* third ed (Stamford, Conn: Appleton & Lange, 1996) 284-285; Fortunato, *Berry & Kohn's Operating Room Technique,* ninth ed, 311.

51. *Ibid.*

52. Favero, Bond, "Chemical disinfection of medical and surgical materials," 910-911.

Originally published February 1988, *AORN Journal.*

Revised March 1992.

Revised November 1996; published January 1997, *AORN Journal.*

Reformatted July 2000.

Revised November 2001; published March 2002, *AORN Journal.*

Recommended Practices for Laser Safety in Practice Settings

The following recommended practices were developed by the AORN Recommended Practices Committee and have been approved by the AORN Board of Directors. They were presented as proposed recommended practices for comment by members and others. They are effective January 1, 2004.

These recommended practices are intended as achievable recommendations representing what is believed to be an optimal level of practice. Policies and procedures will reflect variations in practice settings and/or clinical situations that determine the degree to which the recommended practices can be implemented.

AORN recognizes the numerous types of settings in which perioperative nurses practice. These recommended practices are intended as guidelines adaptable to various practice settings. These practice settings include traditional ORs, ambulatory surgery units, physicians' offices, cardiac catheterization suites, endoscopy suites, radiology departments, and all other areas where operative and other invasive procedures may be performed.

Purpose

These recommended practices provide guidance to assist practitioners in providing a safe environment for patients and health care workers exposed to a laser environment. This document incorporates activities described in the American National Standards Institute's (ANSI's) *American National Standard for the Safe Use of Lasers in Health Care Facilities,* which specifies standards for the use of class 3 and class 4 laser devices in the health care environment. Health care facilities are encouraged to obtain a copy of the ANSI document and have it readily available for reference in the practice environment.

Recommended Practice I

A laser safety program should be established for private practitioners and/or health care facilities.

1. According to ANSI, facilities in which laser procedures are performed must develop a laser safety program to include, but not be limited to,
   - delegation of authority and responsibility for supervising laser safety to a laser safety officer;
   - establishment of use criteria and authorized procedures for all health care personnel working in laser nominal hazard zones;
   - identification of laser hazards and appropriate control measures;

   - education of personnel (ie, operators and others) regarding assessment and control of hazards; and
   - management and reporting of accidents or incidents related to laser procedures, including action plans to prevent recurrences.

2. Incidents of safety regulation violation should be reported to the laser safety officer and reviewed by the safety committee.[1]

3. People working in a laser environment should have knowledge of the established laser safety program.

Recommended Practice II

Personnel working in laser environments should demonstrate competency commensurate with their responsibilities. Education programs should be specific to laser systems used and procedures performed in the facility.

1. Program criteria and content should be in accordance with applicable standards; the facility's policies and procedures; and federal, state, and local regulations.

2. Personnel should be required to demonstrate laser competency periodically and when new laser equipment, accessories, or safety equipment is purchased or brought into the practice environment.

3. The laser safety program should provide participants with a thorough understanding of laser procedures and the technology required for establishing and maintaining a safe environment during laser procedures.

4. Educational activities should be documented and maintained on file in the facility.[1]

Recommended Practice III

All people should know where lasers are being used, and access to these areas should be controlled.

1. A nominal hazard zone (ie, the space in which the level of direct, reflected, or scattered radiation used during normal laser operation exceeds the applicable maximum permissible exposure) should be identified to prevent unintentional exposure to the laser beam.

♦ The laser safety officer can determine the nominal hazard zone with reference from ANSI Z136.1 and ANSI Z136.3, as well as the safety information supplied by the laser manufacturer.[1]

♦ The nominal hazard zone usually is contained within the room but may extend through open doors and/or transparent windows, depending on the type of laser used.

♦ Personnel in the nominal hazard zone should be aware of all laser safety precautions that are implemented to avoid inadvertent exposure to laser hazards.[1]

2. Regulation laser signs should be placed at all entrances to laser treatment areas when these areas are in service.

♦ Recognizable warning signs specific to the type of laser being used should be designed according to the information described in *American National Standard for Safe Use of Lasers in Health Care Facilities.*[1]

♦ Warning signs should be placed conspicuously to alert bystanders of potential hazards.

♦ Signs should be removed when the laser procedure is completed.[2]

3. Doors in the nominal hazard zone should remain closed, and windows, including door windows, should be covered with a barrier that blocks transmission of a beam as appropriate to the type of laser being used.[2]

Recommended Practice IV

All people in the laser treatment area should be protected from unintentional laser beam exposure.

1. Procedures should be implemented to prevent accidental activation or misdirection of laser beams.

♦ Access to laser keys should be restricted to authorized personnel skilled in laser operation.[3]

♦ Lasers should be placed in standby mode when not in active use.[3]

♦ The laser foot switch should be placed in a position convenient to the operator, and the activation mechanism should be identified. Attention to proper placement of the foot switch and use of the standby switch can reduce unintended activation of the laser beam and potential injury to the patient, operator,

and/or bystander(s). Removing unneeded foot switches prevents confusion and accidents related to inadvertent activation.[2]

♦ The laser operator managing the laser equipment should have no competing responsibilities that would require leaving the laser unattended during active use. Note that continual circulating responsibilities may preclude ability to assume the responsibility of laser operation.

2. Anodized, dull, nonreflective, or matte-finished instruments should be used near the laser site. Such instruments decrease the reflectivity of laser beams. Instruments that have been coated (ie, ebonized) should be inspected regularly to ensure the integrity of the coating.[2]

3. Exposed tissues around the surgical site should be protected with saline-saturated or water-saturated materials (eg, towels, sponges) when thermally intensive lasers are being used. These materials should be remoistened periodically to ensure that they do not dry out and become a source for ignition. The solution (eg, saline, water) absorbs or disperses the energy of the laser beam in areas not intended for laser application.[4]

4. Appropriate backstops (eg, titanium rods, quartz rods) or guards should be used during laser surgery to prevent the laser beam from striking normal tissue. Mirrors made of rhodium or stainless steel may be used in hard-to-reach areas. Mirrors made of glass are not used because they will absorb heat from the laser energy and may shatter.[2] Glass rods should not be used because thermal stress from laser beams may cause breakage.[3]

5. When a fiber is used to deliver laser energy through an endoscope, the end of the fiber should extend at least 1 cm past the end of the endoscope and be in view at all times during active use.[2]

When using lasers with flexible endoscopic delivery systems, care should be taken to avoid laser beam exposure within the sheath. Most flexible fiber-optic endoscopic sheaths are damaged easily by heat.[3] Most flexible fiber-optic endoscope sheaths are flammable.[1]

♦ Backscatter from the laser beam can cause thermal damage, resulting in lens pitting if the fiber is too close to the end of the endoscope.[2]

◆ For rigid endoscopic delivery systems (eg, laryngoscopes, bronchoscopes, laparoscopes), care should be taken to avoid beam heating of the sheath wall. If the metallic tubular system is used improperly, the heat inside the endoscope will cause thermal damage to adjoining tissues.[1]

Recommended Practice V

All people in the nominal hazard zone should wear appropriate eyewear approved by the laser safety officer.

1. People in the nominal hazard zone should wear protective eyewear of specific wavelength and density. Scattered, diffused, and reflected laser beams, in addition to direct exposure from misdirected and damaged fibers, can cause eye injuries.[1] Appropriate laser safety eyewear filters out the hazardous wavelength of laser radiation to prevent thermal eye injuries.

   ◆ Eyewear must be labeled with the appropriate optical density and wavelength for the laser in use. Laser eyewear is not interchangeable for a variety of lasers.[1]

   ◆ A lens filter of appropriate laser wavelength may be used over the top of an endoscope viewing port to protect the eye from laser backscatter. The other eye, however, would be left unprotected should a break in a light fiber occur. Using an eye lens filter does not reduce or cancel out the need for protective eyewear for other people in the nominal hazard zone.[2]

2. Patients' eyes and eyelids should be protected from the laser beam by a method approved by the laser safety officer.[1]

   ◆ Patients who remain awake during laser procedures should wear goggles or glasses designated for the type of laser being used.

   ◆ Patients undergoing general anesthesia should be provided other appropriate protection, such as wet eye pads or laser-specific eye shields.[2]

   ◆ Patients undergoing laser treatments on or around the eyelids should have their eyes protected by corneal eye shields.[1]

Recommended Practice VI

Personnel working in the laser environment should avoid exposure to smoke plume generated during laser surgery.

1. To reduce smoke plume inhalation, local exhaust ventilation controls should be implemented. These controls include, but may not be limited to,

   ◆ wall suction units with in-line filters, and
   ◆ smoke evacuator units.

   Laser smoke plume should be removed by use of local exhaust ventilation. The collection device should be placed as near as possible to the point where plume is produced.[1]

2. Personnel should wear high-filtration surgical masks designed for use during laser procedures that generate smoke plume. These specially designed masks help filter particulate matter and may reduce noxious odors.[5] These masks should not be viewed as absolute protection from chemical contaminants.[1]

3. In situations in which minimal plume is generated, a central wall suction system with an in-line filter can be used to evacuate the plume. Central wall suction units are designed to capture liquids, making the use of in-line filters necessary. Low suction rates associated with wall suction units limit their efficacy in evacuating plume, making them suitable for minimal plume only.[6]

4. In circumstances in which large amounts of plume are generated, a mechanical smoke evacuation system with a high-efficiency filter should be used to remove laser smoke plume according to manufacturers' instructions. The evacuator collection apparatus should be placed as close as possible to the laser site. Detectable odor during the use of a laser and smoke evacuation system is a signal that either smoke is not being captured at the site, the airflow through the system is too fast for absorption to occur, or the filter has exceeded its usefulness and should be replaced.[6]

5. Standard precautions should be used when working in the laser environment.[1] Laser gas airborne contaminants produced during laser procedures

have been analyzed and are shown to contain gaseous toxic compounds, bioaerosols, and dead and living cell material. At some level these have been shown to have an unpleasant odor, cause visual problems for physicians, cause ocular and upper respiratory tract irritation, and have demonstrated mutagenic and carcinogenic potential.[1] The potential for bacterial and/or viral contamination of smoke plume remains controversial.

Recommended Practice VII

All people in the laser treatment area should be protected from electrical hazards associated with laser use.

1. The laser safety officer should approve laser systems and equipment before they are placed in service and after they are evaluated for electrical hazards.[1]

2. Laser service and preventive maintenance should be performed on a regular basis by people who have knowledge of laser systems. Service and maintenance activities should be documented. The laser safety officer should review maintenance documents before allowing any laser to be reentered into service. Documentation of actions taken to ensure the reliability and safe operation of lasers assists the laser safety officer in maintaining a safe laser environment. Recurring problems can be detected and solved with appropriate follow-up.[1]

3. Solutions should not be placed on laser units. Lasers are high-voltage equipment that should be protected against short circuiting associated with spillage or splatter.[3]

Recommended Practice VIII

All people in the laser treatment area should be protected from flammability hazards associated with laser use.

1. Personnel using lasers should be knowledgeable of the fire hazards associated with laser use. Fire is one of the most significant hazards of laser use. The intense heat of laser beams can ignite combustible/flammable solids, liquids, and gases. Flammable and combustible items in the laser environment include, but may not be limited to,

- flammable liquids or combustible ointments (eg, skin prep solutions, oil-based lubricants);
- gases (eg, oxygen, methane, anesthetic agents, alcohol vapor);
- plastics;
- paper or gauze materials;
- surgical drapes;
- adhesive or plastic tapes; and
- endotracheal tubes.

The presence of increased oxygen concentrations enhances combustion of these products and leads to the rapid spread of flames.[1] Pooled skin prep solutions also can retain laser heat, resulting in patient tissue burns. Pooled solutions should be removed and/or patted dry. Prep solutions can be absorbed into linens and body fibers (eg, hair). These solutions should be allowed enough time to evaporate before drapes are applied. Alcohol-based skin prep vapors can become trapped under drapes and coverings, and the volatility of vapors can increase the risk of surgical drape fires.[2]

2. Laser-appropriate fire extinguishers and water should be immediately available where lasers are used. Immediate action can reduce the magnitude of injury.[1]

3. Special ignition-resistant drapes and/or moistened, reusable fabrics should be used to drape around areas that are close to the laser treatment site to decrease the potential for fire.[7]

4. Protected or specially designed endotracheal tubes should be used to minimize the potential for fire during laser procedures in the patient's airway or aerodigestive tract. Standard endotracheal tubes are combustible and should not be used. Other flammable items associated with endotracheal tube use during laser procedures include

- plastic,
- plastic tape,
- ointment/lubricant, and
- surgical prep solution.

Endotracheal tube cuffs should be inflated with dyed saline so that punctures can be recognized and action taken immediately. Moistened packs around the tube may provide additional protection.[1]

Recommended Practice IX

Policies and procedures for laser safety should be developed with regard to individual practice settings, applicable standards, and federal and state regulations. Administrative and procedural controls are required according to ANSI Z136.3, section 4, "Control measures." Policies should be reviewed periodically, revised as necessary, and readily available to all personnel.

1. Administrative controls (eg, job description of the laser safety officer, laser committee structure/function, documentation, education and training, medical surveillance [eg, eye examination], laser service, maintenance) describe instructions or methods that regulate work practices and specify criteria for personnel protection.[1]

2. Procedural controls (eg, assignment of a laser operator, requiring special storage of laser keys to prevent unauthorized use, assuring standby function if the laser is activated during standby periods) are determined by the laser safety officer and used to avoid potential hazards in the use of lasers.[1]

3. Documentation should be consistent with AORN's "Recommended practices for documentation of perioperative nursing care."[8]
   ♦ The Perioperative Nursing Data Set nomenclature should be used when documenting on the patient's record.[9]
   ♦ Documentation regarding the laser procedure should include the type of laser used and safety measures implemented during laser use.[3]

4. A medical surveillance program should be established for health care personnel participating in laser use.
   ♦ Medical surveillance is required for laser users or health care personnel within the nominal hazard zone.
   ♦ All laser accidents require reporting and follow-up.[1]

Glossary

American National Standards Institute (ANSI): Organization that provides guidance for the safe use of lasers for diagnostic and therapeutic uses in health care facilities.

Authorized laser operator: A person educated and trained in laser safety and approved by the facility to operate the laser.

Class 3 laser: Those lasers potentially hazardous for direct exposure to specular (ie, mirror-like) reflection.

Class 4 laser: Those lasers that present significant skin and fire hazards. Most surgical lasers are class 4 lasers.

Combustible: A substance that is capable of catching fire and burning.

Corneal eye shield: A device placed over the eye to protect the cornea from self-induced trauma, such as rubbing, pressure, or excessive use.

Controlled access area: The area where the laser is to be used. Access to this area is restricted to laser team members and/or those given permission to enter the area. Access is granted only to those who have been approved by the laser safety officer.

Fire/flame retardant: A substance that by chemical or physical action reduces flammability of combustibles.

Health care laser system: A system used in health care applications that includes a delivery apparatus to direct the output of the laser, a power supply with control and calibration functions, a mechanical house with interlocks, and associated fluids and gases required for the operation of the laser.

High-efficiency filter or high-efficiency particulate air filter: Filters having a filtration rating of 0.3 microns at 99.7% efficiency.

High filtration masks: Masks having a filtering capacity of particulate matter at 0.3 microns to 0.1 microns in size.

Laser: A device that produces an intense, coherent, directional beam of light by stimulating electronic or molecular transitions to lower energy levels. An acronym for "light amplification by stimulated emission of radiation."

Laser-generated airborne contaminants: Particles, toxins, and steam produced by vaporization of target tissues.

Laser safety officer: Person responsible for effecting the knowledgeable evaluation of laser hazards and authorized and responsible for monitoring and overseeing the control of such laser hazards.

Laser treatment area: Area in which the laser is being operated.

Limiting-exposure duration: The length of time for which tissue can be exposed to the laser beam. This duration is determined by the design and/or intended use of the laser.

Maximum permissible exposure: The level of laser radiation to which a person may be exposed without hazardous effects of adverse biologic changes in his or her eyes or skin.

Nominal hazard zone: The space in which the level of direct, reflected, or scattered radiation used during normal laser operation exceeds the applicable maximum permissible exposure. Exposure levels beyond the boundary of the nominal hazard zone should be below the appropriate maximum permissible exposure level of the laser. Special eye and skin precautions must be enforced in the nominal hazard zone.

Optical density: Ability to absorb a specific laser wavelength.

NOTES

1. American National Standards Institute, Laser Institute of America, *American National Standard for Safe Use of Lasers in Health Care Facilities* (Orlando, Fla: The Laser Institute of America, 1996).

2. K A Ball, *Lasers: The Perioperative Challenge,* second ed (St Louis: Mosby, 1995).

3. K A Ball, "Surgical modalities" in *Alexander's Care of the Patient in Surgery,* 12th ed, J C Rothrock, ed (St Louis: Mosby, 2003) 41-96.

4. J A Kneedler, G H Dodge, *Perioperative Patient Care: The Nursing Perspective,* third ed (Boston: Jones and Bartlett Publishers, 1994).

5. C L Romig, P J Smalley, "Regulation of surgical smoke plume," (Health Policy Issues) *AORN Journal* 65 (April 1997) 824-828.

6. "Smoke evacuation systems, surgical," *Healthcare Product Comparison System* (March 2002).

7. *NFPA 115: Recommended Practice on Laser Fire Protection* (Quincy, Mass: National Fire Protection Association, 1999).

8. "Recommended practices for documentation of perioperative nursing care," in *Standards, Recommended Practices, and Guidelines* (Denver: AORN, Inc, 2003) 233-235.

9. S Beyea, ed, *Perioperative Nursing Data Set,* second ed (Denver: AORN,Inc, 2002).

Originally published November 1989, *AORN Journal.* Revised November 1993.

Revised November 1997; published January 1998, *AORN Journal.* Reformatted July 2000.

Revised November 2003; published April 2004, *AORN Journal.*

Recommended Practices for Managing the Patient Receiving Local Anesthesia

The following recommended practices were developed by the AORN Recommended Practices Committee and have been approved by the AORN Board of Directors. They were presented as proposed recommended practices for comments by members and others. They are effective January 1, 2002.

These recommended practices are intended as achievable recommendations representing what is believed to be an optimal level of practice. Policies and procedures will reflect variations in practice settings and/or clinical situations that determine the degree to which the recommended practices can be implemented.

AORN recognizes the various settings in which perioperative nurses practice. These recommended practices are intended as guidelines adaptable to various practice settings. These practice settings include traditional ORs, ambulatory surgery units, physicians' offices, cardiac catheterization laboratories, endoscopy suites, radiology departments, and all other areas where operative and other invasive procedures may be performed.

Purpose

These recommended practices provide guidelines for RNs managing patients receiving local infiltration anesthesia only. If any sedation is used, AORN's "Recommended practices for managing the patient receiving moderate sedation/analgesia" should be followed. It is not the intent of these recommended practices to address situations that require the services of anesthesia care providers or to substitute RN services in those situations that require the services of anesthesia care providers, regardless of the complexity of the surgical procedure.

Recommended Practice I

Patients receiving local anesthesia during a surgical procedure should be assessed throughout the perioperative experience by an RN.

1. The selection of patients who are to receive local anesthesia should be determined by established criteria developed through an interdisciplinary collaboration of health care professionals.

2. Many healthy patients undergo simple surgical procedures that require only small doses of local anesthetic medications. These patients are at low risk for anesthetic complications and require minimal observation and intervention.

3. The decision to monitor, the parameters monitored, and the frequency of observation should be tailored to the patient and the surgical procedure.[1] If/when administering medications, the perioperative nurse must work within his or her scope of practice.

4. Local anesthesia is not practical for all patients or all types of surgical procedures.[2] Highly nervous, apprehensive, or excitable patients or those who are unable to cooperate because of their mental state or age may not be good candidates for local anesthesia.[3] Each patient has a variety of unique physical characteristics that can influence his or her response to medications. Considerations include, but are not limited to, the patient's weight, age, and medication tolerance and the presence of disease.[4]

5. In the preoperative phase, the RN should review the patient's history, physical examination findings, laboratory results, and other diagnostic test results if indicated. During this preoperative assessment, the perioperative nurse should determine, at a minimum,
   ◆ the patient's allergies and sensitivities (eg, medications, tape, latex, prep solutions);
   ◆ the patient's age, current medications, alternative/complementary therapies, and emotional status;
   ◆ when the patient last consumed solids and/or liquids by mouth (ie, NPO status);
   ◆ whether the surgical site can be anesthetized completely with a local injection; and
   ◆ pulse, blood pressure, arterial oxygen percent saturation, skin status, mental status, and pain management status.[5]

   The need for IV access and/or fluids should be based on patient assessment data and facility policy.

6. The RN should develop a plan of care to include potential problems and stress responses to local anesthesia. Surgery may elicit physiological (eg, autonomic disturbances that may cause fainting) and psychological (eg, fear of the

unknown that may cause anxiety) responses in the patient. The degree of combined stressful stimuli directly determines the response of the patient.[6]

7. The RN should ensure the availability of emergency equipment and be prepared to intervene should an adverse reaction occur. Serious cardiac or respiratory complications can occur abruptly after the administration of local anesthetic medications. If the medication enters the bloodstream directly, convulsions, circulatory and respiratory distress, cardiovascular collapse, or even death can result.[7] Emergency medications, suction apparatus, resuscitative equipment, and qualified personnel should be readily available.[8] At a minimum, personnel should be competent in cardiopulmonary resuscitation.

Recommended Practice II

The RN managing the nursing care of the patient receiving local anesthesia should monitor the patient's physiological and psychosocial status throughout the procedure.

1. At a minimum, the perioperative RN should monitor the patient's heart rate and regularity, respiratory rate, and mental status throughout the procedure. Other monitoring parameters include, but are not limited to,[9]
   ♦ blood pressure,
   ♦ oxygen saturation by pulse oximetry,
   ♦ body temperature,
   ♦ skin temperature and color, and
   ♦ mental status and level of consciousness.

2. The perioperative RN should monitor the patient for physiological reactions to medications and for behavioral changes that may occur due to medications and/or other factors related to the surgical encounter.[10] Continuously monitoring the patient's physiological and psychosocial status facilitates early detection of potential complications.

3. The perioperative RN should monitor the dose, route, and time of administration for all local anesthetic medications given to the patient during the surgical procedure.[11]

4. The perioperative RN should be knowledgeable about medication administration and be able to recognize both desired responses and adverse reactions to anesthetic medications. Local anesthetic agents may cause cardiovascular, respiratory, or central nervous system depression. Adverse reactions may stem from hypersensitivity to the anesthetic agent and/or toxicity due to excessive levels of the medication.[12]

Symptoms of hypersensitivity include, but are not limited to,
♦ urticaria,
♦ tachycardia,
♦ laryngeal edema leading to breathing difficulties,
♦ nausea,
♦ vomiting,
♦ elevated temperature,
♦ severe hypotension, and
♦ anaphylactic shock.

Symptoms of toxicity include, but are not limited to,
♦ restlessness,
♦ unexplained anxiety or fearfulness,
♦ diaphoresis,
♦ nausea,
♦ palpitations,
♦ disturbed respiration,
♦ pallor or flushing,
♦ syncope, and
♦ convulsive movements.

A hypotensive reaction also may occur as a toxic response to local anesthetic medications. A patient's blood pressure may fall gradually or abruptly, and the heart rate may change from normal to tachycardiac to bradycardiac with faintness and/or dizziness. Cardiac arrest may follow.[13] Injury to the anesthetized surgical site can occur because a patient's sensation is absent.[14] A patient undergoing a surgical procedure with local anesthesia may experience significant intraoperative bleeding.[15] He or she may be at risk for hypothermia from cool ambient temperatures, the use of unwarmed IV and irrigation fluids, or prolonged surgical time.[16] Knowledge of undesirable medication reactions and implementation of appropriate interventions help protect the patient from undue harm.[17]

5. The perioperative RN should recognize and report to the physician significant changes in the patient's status and should be prepared to initiate appropriate interventions.[18]

Recommended Practice III

The RN monitoring the patient's care should be clinically competent in the function and use of monitoring equipment, resuscitation equipment, and emergency medications. The monitoring RN should be able to interpret data obtained from the patient.

1. Serious cardiac or respiratory complications can occur abruptly after administration of local anesthetic medication. Knowledge of the function and proper use of monitoring equipment and emergency medications is essential to provide safe patient care.[19]

Recommended Practice IV

Documentation should be consistent with AORN's "Recommended practices for documentation of perioperative nursing care."[20] The Perioperative Nursing Data Set (PNDS) nomenclature should be used when documenting nursing activities on the patient record.[21]

1. Documentation should reflect use of the nursing process. When the nursing process is used, it demonstrates the critical thinking skills practiced by perioperative RNs caring for the surgical patient.[22]

2. The PNDS nomenclature should be used to document desired patient outcomes, nursing diagnoses, and nursing interventions and activities. Use of a standardized language ensures meaningful data collection and analysis within and across practice settings.

3. Documentation of patient care provides a record of the patient's response to local anesthetic medications.

4. Documentation of all nursing interventions and activities performed is legally and professionally important for clear communication, collaboration among health care providers, and continuity of patient care.[23]

Recommended Practice V

Policies and procedures for managing the patient receiving local anesthesia should be developed, reviewed and revised at regularly scheduled intervals, and readily available in the practice setting.

1. Policies and procedures for managing patients receiving local anesthesia should include, but are not limited to,
   ◆ patient selection criteria,
   ◆ type and frequency of monitoring,
   ◆ method and frequency of documentation,
   ◆ medications that may be administered by the perioperative nurse and the level of monitoring skills required,
   ◆ interventions that may be implemented based on preapproved protocol and that are within the scope of nursing practice, and
   ◆ discharge criteria.[24]

2. These recommended practices should be used as guidelines for developing policies and procedures in the practice setting. Policies and procedures establish authority, responsibility, and accountability. They also serve as operational guidelines and assist in the development of performance improvement activities. A review of policies and procedures should be included in orientation and ongoing staff member education.

NOTES
1. J L Hoffer, "Anesthesia," in *Alexander's Care of the Patient in Surgery*, 11th ed, M H Meeker, J C Rothrock, eds (St Louis: Mosby, Inc, 1999) 209, 231-232.
2. *Ibid*, 231; N H Fortunato, *Berry & Kohn's Operating Room Technique*, ninth ed (St Louis: Mosby, 2000) 427; M Kost, "Local and regional anesthesia," in *Ambulatory Surgical Nursing*, second ed, N Burden et al, eds (Philadelphia: W B Saunders Co, 2000) 286-287.
3. Fortunato, *Berry & Kohn's Operating Room Technique*, ninth ed, 427.
4. A M Martinelli, "Administering drugs and solutions," in *Patient Care During Operative and Invasive Procedures*, second ed, M L Phippen, M P Wells, eds (Philadelphia: W B Saunders Co, 2000) 114, 117.
5. Hoffer, "Anesthesia," 232; Fortunato, *Berry & Kohn's Operating Room Technique*, ninth ed, 424-425; Kost, "Local and regional anesthesia," 293.
6. R P Shumaker, "Perioperative nursing," in *Medical-Surgical Nursing: Clinical Management for Continuity of Care*, fifth ed, J M Black, E Matassarin-Jacobs, eds (Philadelphia: W B Saunders Co, 1997) 451; J Luckmann,

K C Sorensen, *Medical-Surgical Nursing: A Psychophysiologic Approach,* third ed (Philadelphia: W B Saunders Co, 1987) 265; K Blais, "Perioperative nursing process," in *Perioperative Nursing: Principles and Practice,* second ed, S S Fairchild, ed (Boston: Little, Brown and Co, 1996) 274.

7. Kost, "Local and regional anesthesia," 290; Fortunato, *Berry & Kohn's Operating Room Technique,* ninth ed, 427; Hoffer, "Anesthesia," 232.

8. Hoffer, "Anesthesia," 232.

9. *Ibid;* Fortunato, *Berry & Kohn's Operating Room Technique,* ninth ed, 426-427.

10. Fortunato, *Berry & Kohn's Operating Room Technique,* ninth ed, 425-427.

11. Hoffer, "Anesthesia," 232.

12. *Ibid;* Kost, "Local and regional anesthesia," 290-291.

13. A M Martinelli, "Physiologically monitoring the patient," in *Patient Care During Operative and Invasive Procedures,* second ed, M L Phippen, M P Wells, eds (Philadelphia: W B Saunders Co, 2000) 146.

14. D Rivellini, "Local and regional anesthesia: Nursing implications," *The Nursing Clinics of North America* 28 (September 1993) 560.

15. Martinelli, "Physiologically monitoring the patient," 142.

16. *Ibid,* 139-140, 143.

17. C J Smith, "Preparing nurses to monitor patients receiving local anesthesia," *AORN Journal* 59 (May 1994) 1036; Martinelli, "Physiologically monitoring the patient," 146.

18. Hoffer, "Anesthesia," 232; Fortunato, *Berry & Kohn's Operating Room Technique,* ninth ed, 426-427; Kost, "Local and regional anesthesia," 291.

19. *Ibid.*

20. "Recommended practices for documentation of perioperative nursing care," in *Standards, Recommended Practices, and Guidelines* (Denver: AORN, Inc, 2001) 199-201.

21. S Beyea, ed, *Perioperative Nursing Data Set: The Perioperative Nursing Vocabulary,* second ed (Denver: AORN, Inc, 2002).

22. C S Ladden, "Concepts basic to perioperative nursing," in *Alexander's Care of the Patient in Surgery,* 11th ed, M H Meeker, J C Rothrock, eds (St Louis: Mosby, Inc, 1999) 6-13; J Gill et al, "Incorporating nursing diagnosis and King's theory in the OR documentation," *Canadian Operating Room Nursing Journal* (March/April 1995) 10-11; Blais, "Perioperative nursing process," 271-272, 280, 284, 286-288; Fortunato, *Berry & Kohn's Operating Room Technique,* ninth ed, 19-24.

23. L C A Simunek, "Legal and ethical dimensions of perioperative nursing practice," in *Perioperative Nursing: Principles and Practice,* second ed, S S Fairchild, ed (Boston: Little, Brown and Co, 1996) 390-394; Blais, "Perioperative nursing process," 286-290; B J Gruendemann, B Fernsebner, *Comprehensive Perioperative Nursing, Volume I: Principles* (Boston: Jones and Bartlett Publishers, 1995) 95.

24. L K Groah, "Anesthesia," in *Perioperative Nursing,* third ed, L K Groah, ed (Stamford, Conn: Appleton & Lange, 1996) 245, 248; A Ferrari, "Anesthesia and perioperative nursing implications," in *Perioperative Nursing: Principles and Practice,* second ed, S S Fairchild, ed (Boston: Little, Brown and Co, 1996) 105.

RESOURCES

Burden, N. "Ambulatory approach: A case study: Identification and treatment of narcotic depression in the ambulatory surgical patient," *Journal of Post Anesthesia Nursing* 10 (April 1995) 94-99.

Burden, N; Iyer, J. "Ambulatory approach: Local anesthesia: Not always benign," *Journal of Post Anesthesia Nursing* 2 (February 1987) 45-50.

Chang, W K; Mulford, G J. "Iatrogenic trigeminal sensorimotor neuropathy resulting from local anesthesia: A case report," *Archives of Physical Medicine and Rehabilitation* 81 (December 2000) 1591-1593.

Kern, K; Langevin, P B; Dunn, B M. "Methemoglobinemia after topical anesthesia with lidocaine and benzocaine for a difficult intubation," *Journal of Clinical Anesthesia* 12 (March 2000) 167-172.

Schecter, W P; Swisher, J L. "Local anesthesia in surgical practice," *Current Problems in Surgery* (January 2000) 10-66.

Originally published May 1984, *AORN Journal.*

Revised September 1989.

Revised August 1993.

Revised November 1997; published February 1998.

Reformatted July 2000.

Revised November 2001; published April 2002, *AORN Journal.*

Recommended Practices for Selection and Use of Packaging Systems

The following recommended practices were developed by the AORN Recommended Practices Committee and have been approved by the AORN Board of Directors. They were presented as proposed recommended practices for comments by members and others. They are effective January 1, 2001.

These recommended practices are intended as achievable recommendations representing what is believed to be an optimal level of practice. Policies and procedures will reflect variations in practice settings and/or clinical situations that determine the degree to which the recommended practices can be implemented.

AORN recognizes the numerous types of settings in which perioperative nurses practice. These recommended practices are intended as guidelines adaptable to various practice settings. These practice settings include traditional ORs, ambulatory surgery units, physicians' offices, cardiac catheterization suites, endoscopy suites, radiology departments, and all other areas where operative and other invasive procedures may be performed.

Purpose

These recommended practices provide guidelines for evaluation, selection, and use of packaging systems for items to be sterilized. These packaging systems include woven fabrics, nonwoven materials, peel pouches of plastic and/or paper, and container systems. Packaging systems should ensure sterility of package contents until opened for use and should permit removal of contents without contamination.

Recommended Practice I

Packaging systems should be evaluated according to the AORN "Recommended practices for product selection in perioperative practice settings."[1]

1. Packaging systems should
   - be appropriate to item(s) being sterilized (ie, permit identification of contents; permit complete and secured enclosure of item(s); protect package contents from physical damage; resist tears, punctures, and abrasions; be free of holes; be free of toxic ingredients; be low-linting; permit delivery of contents without contamination; maintain sterility of package contents until opened);

   - be appropriate to the method of sterilization (ie, provide adequate seal integrity; be tamperproof and able to seal only once; provide an adequate barrier to particulate matter and fluids; be compatible with and able to withstand physical conditions of the sterilization process; permit adequate air removal; allow penetration and removal of sterilant);
   - have a favorable cost/benefit ratio; and
   - be used according to manufacturers' instructions.[2]

2. Each facility should evaluate and test the performance of each packaging system before selection and implementation to ensure conditions for sterilization, storage, and handling can be met.

Recommended Practice II

Packaging systems should be compatible with the sterilization process.

1. Packaging systems for steam sterilization should
   - provide adequate air removal,
   - permit steam penetration and direct contact with item(s) surfaces,
   - permit adequate drying,
   - permit use of material compatible (ie, nondegradable) with the sterilization process, and
   - maintain the integrity of the system.

   The purpose of packaging systems is to permit sterilization of the package contents, maintain sterility of the contents until the package is opened, and permit delivery of contents without contamination.[3]

   Steam sterilization parameters can vary according to humidity, altitude, packaging material, package contents, load, position of item within each sterilizer, size of pack, weight of pack, density of pack, and efficacy of the sterilization cycle.

2. Manufacturers of packaging systems should provide materials data relevant to sterilization. Practice settings should follow manufacturers' instructions for each packaging system for steam sterilization.[4]

3. Packaging systems for ethylene oxide (EO) should
   - be permeable to EO, moisture, and air;
   - permit aeration;

♦ maintain material compatibility (ie, non-degradable) with the sterilization process; and

♦ maintain the integrity of the system.

The purpose of packaging systems for EO sterilization is to permit sterilization and aeration of package contents and packaging material, maintain sterility of package contents until opened, and permit delivery of contents without contamination.[5] Woven, nonwoven, peel pouch package, and some rigid container materials are permeable to EO and do not impede rapid aeration of contents. Woven materials, however, absorb a large amount of the relative humidity needed for EO sterilization, which may prevent adequate penetration of EO to all surfaces of the package contents.[6]

4. Packaging systems for hydrogen peroxide plasma sterilization should

♦ be permeable to the process,

♦ maintain compatibility (ie, nondegradable, nonabsorptive) with the sterilization process,

♦ be made of a material recommended by manufacturers and used according to the manufacturers' instructions, and

♦ maintain the integrity of the system.

The purpose of packaging systems is to permit sterilization of the package contents, maintain sterility of the contents until the package is opened, and permit delivery of contents without contamination.[7] The low temperature plasma sterilization process is affected by altitude and peel pouch packaging material.

5. Manufacturers of low-temperature plasma sterilizers should provide materials data relevant to peel pouch material. Because the absorption of the plasma sterilant (ie, hydrogen peroxide) could have an adverse affect on the effectiveness of the sterilization process and be absorbed by paper peel pouches, it is recommended that peel pouch material be made with polyester/nonwoven polyoletin laminate.[8]

Recommended Practice III

Packaging materials should be processed to maintain the properties required for sterilization.

1. Packaging materials should be maintained at room temperature (ie, 18° C to 22° C [64° F to 72° F]) and at a relative humidity of 35% to 70%. Maintaining room temperature and moisture content of packaging material facilitates steam penetration and prevents superheating during the sterilization process.[9]

2. Woven materials should be laundered between every use for rehydration. Resterilization without laundering may lead to superheating and could be a deterrent to achieving sterilization.[10] Overdrying and/or pressing and storage in areas of low humidity may lead to overheating and sterilization failure. Woven packaging that is adequately hydrated should withstand multiple sterilization processes. For barrier quality wrappers, manufacturers' instructions should be followed for the suggested number of processings.[11]

3. Reusable textiles should maintain a protective barrier throughout the life of the product. Multiple processings eventually will diminish the protective barrier of the material. A method should be established to monitor, control, and determine useful life when reprocessing woven materials. This should include, but not be limited to, the number of sterilization processes and washing cycles that may occur while maintaining the acceptable barrier of the material.[12]

Recommended Practice IV

Package contents should be assembled, handled, and wrapped in a manner that provides for an aseptic presentation of package contents.

1. The appropriate size wrapping material should be selected to achieve adequate coverage of the item being packaged. It is essential to wrap the item securely to prevent gapping, billowing, and air pockets from forming, which could compromise sterility.

Sequential wrapping using two barrier-type wrappers provides a tortuous pathway to impede microbial migration and permits ease of presentation to the sterile field without compromising sterility. A fused or bonded, double-layer, disposable, nonwoven wrapper used according to manufacturers' recommendations may provide a bacterial barrier comparable to the sequential double wrap, allowing safe and easy presentation to the sterile field. Correct use of a single, disposable, nonwoven wrapper may eliminate the need to double wrap sequentially.[13]

2. The technology of woven and nonwoven packaging material is rapidly evolving.[14] Individuals involved in product selection should evaluate each specific product's capability to meet the defined criteria for a packaging system.

Recommended Practice V

Peel packages should be used according to manufacturers' instructions.

1. Peel packages should have as much air removed as possible before sealing. Air acts as a barrier to heat and moisture. Expansion of air may cause rupturing of packages during the sterilization process.[15]

2. Peel packages should provide a seal of proven integrity and not allow resealing. A break in the seal may allow microorganisms to enter and contaminate package contents.[16]

3. Peel pouches should be hermetically sealed. Heat is applied to the open end of the peel pouch. Pressure is applied to the mating surfaces of 'self-sealing' pouches. During the sterilization process, the seal adhesive 'cures' to become a permanent seal.[17] Packages should be inspected for intact seals before and after sterilization and before use.

4. Double-peel packaging is not routinely required for sterilization; however, double packaging may facilitate containment of multiple small items to be sterilized and facilitate aseptic presentation to the sterile field.[18]

5. Double-peel packages should be used in such a manner as to avoid folding the inner package to fit into the outer package. Folding edges of inner peel packages may entrap air and inhibit the sterilization process.[19]

6. Peel packages made of plastic and paper combinations should be used according to manufacturers' instructions. When using double-peel packages, the paper portions should be placed together to ensure penetration and removal of the sterilant, air, and moisture. Sterilizing agents penetrate paper portions of peel packages, and plastic portions allow items to be viewed.[20] When loading peel packages into the sterilizer, place the packages on the rack or in the sterilizing pan in the same direction (ie, paper/plastic, paper/ plastic, paper/plastic). Do not place packages randomly in the sterilizer or with plastic surfaces facing one another. Plastic impedes the movement of the sterilizing agent into and out of the package.

7. Peel packages should open without tearing, linting, shredding, or delaminating. Contamination of sterile contents can occur due to functional failure of peel packages.[21]

8. The peel packaging should be compatible with the sterilization process, permit sterilization of the contents, and maintain package sterility until opened.[22]

Recommended Practice VI

Rigid container systems should be used according to manufacturers' instructions.

1. The approved sterilization method and cycle exposure times for each rigid container system should be provided in the manufacturers' data and instructions. Construction materials and container design may affect compatibility with the sterilization process (eg, penetration of sterilant [gas plasma], release of moisture or sterilant [EO]). Recommendations related to the type of sterilization method vary by the manufacturer. Prevacuum sterilizers may be preferred, as air removal is difficult in gravity displacement sterilizers.[23]

2. Rigid containers have filter and/or valve systems that should be secure and in proper working order before sterilization. The filter plate should be examined for integrity both before installation and after the sterilization process. If the filter is damp or dislodged or has holes, tears, or punctures, the contents should be considered contaminated. It is recommended that only components of the rigid container system specified by the manufacturer and compatible with the system be used in the practice setting.[24]

3. The integrity of the rigid container system should be evaluated periodically.

4. The purpose of packaging systems is to permit sterilization of the package contents, maintain sterility of contents until the package is opened, and permit delivery of contents without contamination.[25]

Loosened rivets, improperly maintained valves, worn gaskets, dents, or other compromises to the integrity of the container system will compromise the sterilization process and may not permit the contents to remain sterile or be delivered aseptically.[26]

Recommended Practice VII

Packages to be sterilized should be labeled according to the policies and procedures of the practice setting and according to manufacturers' instructions.

1. Packaging systems should be labeled before sterilization. The label information should include, but not be limited to,
   ◆ a description of package contents,
   ◆ initials of the package assembler, and
   ◆ a lot control number.

2. Label information should be documented on pressure-sensitive tape and not on the packing material. Peel packages may be labeled on the plastic portion or on the self-sealing tab. Markers used to label packaging systems should be indelible, nonbleeding, and nontoxic. Felt-tip ink pens or a very soft lead pencil may be used.[27]

Recommended Practice VIII

According to the AORN "Recommended practices for sterilization in perioperative practice settings," shelf life of a packaged sterile item is event related.[28]

1. The length of time an item is considered sterile depends on the
   ◆ type and configuration of packaging materials used,
   ◆ number of times a package is handled before use,
   ◆ number of personnel who may have handled the package,
   ◆ storage on open or closed shelves,
   ◆ environmental conditions of the storage area (eg, cleanliness, temperature, humidity), and
   ◆ use of dust covers and method of sealing.[29]

Recommended Practice IX

Policies and procedures for the selection and use of packaging systems should be written, reviewed periodically, and readily available within the practice setting.

1. These recommended practices should be used as guidelines for the development of policies and procedures for packaging. The AORN recommended practices that deal with sterilization and protective barrier materials also should be consulted when developing policies and procedures. Policies and procedures establish authority, responsibility, and accountability for the selection and use of packaging systems within the practice setting. Policies and procedures also establish guidelines for performance improvement activities to be used in monitoring packaging system efficacy.

2. An introduction to related policies and procedures should be included in the orientation and ongoing education of personnel to assist in the development of knowledge, skills, and behaviors that affect patient outcomes.

Glossary

Hydrogen peroxide plasma sterilization: An ionizing hydrogen peroxide gas or cloud or low-temperature plasma produced by exciting a strong electrical field over a contained precursor vapor that serves as a sterilizing agent in this type of sterilization process.

Nonwoven materials: A sheet, web, or batt of natural and/or synthetic fibers of filaments, excluding paper, that have not been converted into yarns and that are not bonded to each other by several means.

Packaging systems: A generic term meant to include all types of packaging, such as wrapping materials, pouches, and rigid container systems.

Rigid sterilization container system: Specifically designed heat-resistant, metal, plastic, or anodized aluminum receptacles used to package items, usually surgical instruments, for sterilization. The lids and/or bottom surfaces contain steam- or gas-permeable, high-efficiency microbial filters.

Sequential wrapping: A double-wrapping procedure that creates a package within a package.

Superheating: A condition in which dehydrated textiles are subjected to steam sterilization. The package or product becomes too dry and causes destructive effects on the strength of the cloth fibers.

Useful life: Length of time, as determined by the manufacturer, for which a product maintains acceptable safety and performance characteristics. The manufacturer should provide materials data to support useful life.

Woven textile: A reusable fabric constructed from yarns made of natural and/or synthetic fibers or filaments that are woven or knitted together to form a web in a repeated interlocking pattern.

NOTES

1. "Recommended practices for product selection in perioperative practice settings," in *Standards, Recommended Practices, and Guidelines* (Denver: AORN, Inc, 2004) 347-350.

2. Association for the Advancement of Medical Instrumentation, "Good hospital practice: Steam sterilization and sterility assurance. ANSI/AAMI ST46-1993," in *AAMI Standards and Recommended Practices vol 1.1: Sterilization, part 1: Sterilization in Health Care Facilities* (Arlington, Va: Association for the Advancement of Medical Instrumentation, 1998) 19-20; A J Eagleton, "Packaging: Selection and use," in *Sterilization Technology for the Health Care Facility,* second ed, M Reichert, J H Young, eds (Gaithersburg, Md: Aspen Publishers, Inc, 1997) 85.

3. *Ibid;* L H Nicolette, "Sterilization and disinfection," in *Perioperative Nursing,* third ed, L K Groah, ed (Stamford, Conn: Appleton & Lange, 1996) 169.

4. Eagleton, "Packaging: Selection and use," 87.

5. *Ibid,* 85; Association for the Advancement of Medical Instrumentation, "Good hospital practice: Steam sterilization and sterility assurance. ANSI/AAMI ST46-1993," 19-20.

6. M L Young, "Ethylene oxide sterilization: Recommended practices," in *Sterilization Technology for the Health Care Facility,* second ed, M Reichert, J H Young, eds (Gaithersburg, Md: Aspen Publishers, Inc, 1997) 209-210; Association for the Advancement of Medical Instrumentation, *Ethylene Oxide Sterilization in Health Care Facilities: Safety and Effectiveness ANSI/AAMI ST41-1999* (Arlington, Va: Association for the Advancement of Medical Instrumentation, 2000) 27.

7. Eagleton, "Packaging: Selection and use," 85; Nicolette, "Sterilization and disinfection," 167.

8. D Alexander, "Packaging: Pouches," in *Sterilization Technology for the Health Care Facility,* second ed, M Reichert, J H Young, eds (Gaithersburg, Md: Aspen Publishers, Inc, 1997) 69; Eagleton, "Packaging: Selection and use," 90.

9. Nicolette, "Sterilization and disinfection," 169; Association for the Advancement of Medical Instrumentation, "Good hospital practice: Steam sterilization and sterility assurance. ANSI/AAMI ST46-1993," 19.

10. Association for the Advancement of Medical Instrumentation, "Good hospital practice: Steam sterilization and sterility assurance. ANSI/AAMI ST46-1993," 20; N Fortunato, *Berry & Kohn's Operating Room Technique,* ninth ed (St Louis: Mosby, Inc, 2000) 259; American Society for Healthcare Central Service Professionals, *Training Manual for Central Service Technicians* (Chicago: American Hospital Association, 1997) 141.

11. Association for the Advancement of Medical Instrumentation, *Processing of Reusable Surgical Textiles for Use in Health Care Facilities ANSI/AAMI ST65-2000* (Arlington, Va: Association for the Advancement of Medical Instrumentation, 2000) 22-26; Eagleton, "Packaging: Selection and use," 87; B Stanewick, W Kogut, "Packaging: Textiles," in *Sterilization Technology for the Health Care Facility,* second ed, M Reichert, J H Young, eds (Gaithersburg, Md: Aspen Publishers, Inc, 1997) 82-83.

12. Eagleton, "Packaging: Selection and use," 85, 87; Stanewick, Kogut, "Packaging: Textiles," 82, 83; "Recommended practices for use and selection of barrier materials for surgical gowns and drapes," in *Standards, Recommended Practices, and Guidelines* (Denver: AORN, Inc, 2000) 267-270; Association for the Advancement of Medical Instrumentation, *Processing of Reusable Surgical Textiles for Use in Health Care Facilities ANSI/AAMI ST65-2000,* 25.

13. N Gorman-Annis, "Nonwovens," in *Sterilization Technology for the Health Care Facility,* second ed, M Reichert, J H Young, eds (Gaithersburg, Md: Aspen Publishers, Inc, 1997) 60; Eagleton, "Packaging: Selection and use," 85-87.

14. Gorman-Annis, "Nonwovens," 61.

15. Fortunato, *Berry & Kohn's Operating Room Technique,* ninth ed, 259; Eagleton, "Packaging: Selection and use," 90; Alexander, "Packaging: Pouches," 65-66.

16. Alexander, "Packaging: Pouches," 62, 65-66; Nicolette, "Sterilization and disinfection," 169-170; Fortunato, *Berry & Kohn's Operating Room Technique,* ninth ed, 258-259.

17. Alexander, "Packaging: Pouches," 65-66; American Society for Healthcare Central Service Professionals, *Training Manual for Central Service Technicians,* 149-150.

18. Eagleton, "Packaging: Selection and use," 90; Nicolette, "Sterilization and disinfection," 169-170.

19. Eagleton, "Packaging: Selection and use," 90.

20. American Society for Healthcare Central Service Professionals, *Training Manual for Central Service Technicians,* 149-150; Nicolette, "Sterilization and disinfection," 169.

21. Nicolette, "Sterilization and disinfection," 169; Alexander, "Packaging: Selection and use," 67.

22. Alexander, "Packaging: Selection and use," 62-67; American Society for Healthcare Central Service Professionals, *Training Manual for Central Service Technicians,* 131; Fortunato, *Berry & Kohn's Operating Room Technique,* ninth ed, 258-259.

23. ECRI, "Sterilization containers," in *Healthcare Product Comparison System* (Plymouth Meeting, Pa: ECRI, August 1997) 2; J Whitbourne, "Packaging: Rigid containers," in *Sterilization Technology for the Health Care Facility,* second ed, M Reichert, J H Young, eds (Gaithersburg, Md: Aspen Publishers, Inc, 1997) 70-75; Association for the Advancement of Medical Instrumentation, "Guidelines for the selection and use of reusable rigid sterilization container systems for ethylene oxide sterilization and steam sterilization in health care facilities. ANSI/AAMI ST33-1996," in *AAMI Standards and Recommended Practices vol 1.1: Sterilization, part 1: Sterilization in Health Care Facilities* (Arlington, Va: Association for the Advancement of Medical Instrumentation, 1998) 185-186; Nicolette, "Sterilization and disinfection," 170; American Society for

Healthcare Central Service Professionals, *Training Manual for Central Service Technicians*, 152.

24. Association for the Advancement of Medical Instrumentation, "Guidelines for the selection and use of reusable rigid sterilization container systems for ethylene oxide sterilization and steam sterilization in health care facilities. ANSI/AAMI ST33-1996," 181-183; Eagleton, "Packaging: Selection and use," 88; American Society for Healthcare Central Service Professionals, *Training Manual for Central Service Technicians*, 151.

25. Eagleton, "Packaging: Selection and use," 85.

26. ECRI, "Sterilization containers," 2; American Society for Healthcare Central Service Professionals, *Training Manual for Central Service Technicians*, 151; Association for the Advancement of Medical Instrumentation, "Guidelines for the selection and use of reusable rigid sterilization container systems for ethylene oxide sterilization and steam sterilization in health care facilities. ANSI/AAMI ST33-1996," 181.

27. Association for the Advancement of Medical Instrumentation, "Guidelines for the selection and use of reusable rigid sterilization container systems for ethylene oxide sterilization and steam sterilization in health care facilities. ANSI/AAMI ST33-1996," 182; American Society for Healthcare Central Service Professionals, *Training Manual for Central Service Technicians*, 154.

28. "Recommended practices for sterilization in perioperative practice settings," in *Standards, Recommended Practices, and Guidelines* (Denver: AORN, Inc, 2000) 347-358.

29. *Ibid*; Association for the Advancement of Medical Instrumentation, *Ethylene Oxide Sterilization in Health Care Facilities: Safety and Effectiveness ANSI/AAMI ST41-1999*, 33; N F Japp, "Packaging: Shelf life," in *Sterilization Technology for the Health Care Facility*, second ed, M Reichert, J H Young, eds (Gaithersburg Md: Aspen Publishers, Inc, 1997) 99.

Originally published February 1983, *AORN Journal*.
Revised November 1988, February 1992.
Revised November 1995; published May 1996, *AORN Journal*.
Revised and reformatted; published December 2000, *AORN Journal*.

Recommended Practices for Use of the Pneumatic Tourniquet

The following recommended practices were developed by the AORN Recommended Practices Committee and have been approved by the AORN Board of Directors. They were presented as proposed recommended practices for comments by members and others. They are effective January 1, 2002.

These recommended practices are intended as achievable recommendations representing what is believed to be an optimal level of practice. Policies and procedures will reflect variations in practice settings and/or clinical situations that determine the degree to which the recommended practices can be implemented.

AORN recognizes the numerous types of settings in which perioperative nurses practice. These recommended practices are intended as guidelines adaptable to various practice settings. These practice settings include traditional ORs, ambulatory surgery units, physicians' offices, cardiac catheterization suites, endoscopy suites, radiology departments, and all other areas where operative and other invasive procedures may be performed.

Purpose

These recommended practices provide guidelines for use of pneumatic tourniquets, which primarily are used to occlude blood flow and obtain a near bloodless field for extremity surgery. Pneumatic tourniquets also are used to confine a bolus of local anesthetic in an extremity during IV regional anesthesia (IVRA [ie, Bier's block]). These recommended practices provide information for testing, applying, cleaning, and documenting the use of pneumatic tourniquet equipment. Pneumatic tourniquets consist of an inflatable cuff, pressure source, pressure regulator, connective tubing, and pressure display. These recommended practices provide general guidelines for developing policies and procedures for tourniquet use in the practice setting. Due to the variety and complexity of current tourniquet equipment, policies and procedures will reflect considerations for the specific tourniquet system being used.

Recommended Practice I

Personnel should demonstrate competency in use of pneumatic tourniquets in the practice setting.

1. Perioperative personnel should be instructed in the proper operation of pneumatic tourniquets before use. Instruction and return demonstration of proper use of a pneumatic tourniquet reduces the risk of patient injury and extends the life of the pneumatic tourniquet.

2. Personnel should participate in ongoing competency assessment and educational activities that will facilitate acquisition of knowledge and skills that affect patient outcomes.[1]

Recommended Practice II

Pneumatic tourniquets should be cleaned, inspected, tested, and maintained before and after use according to manufacturers' written instructions.

1. Preoperatively, the entire tourniquet system should be checked. Before each use, pneumatic tourniquets should be inspected for cleanliness and tested for integrity and function. Most electric tourniquets automatically self-test and calibrate upon activation. The cuff, tubing, connectors, gauges, and pressure source should be clean and kept in working order. The cuff and tubing should be inspected for cracks and leaks. Patient safety demands that all tourniquet parts function properly before a procedure. Connectors should be fastened securely to the tourniquet pressure source to prevent accidental deflation of the cuff during use. Unintentional pressure loss can result from loose tubing connectors, deteriorated tubing, stopcock leaks, cuff bladder leaks, or worn cuff closures.[2]

2. Reusable cuffs and bladders should be cleaned, rinsed, and dried between patient use according to the manufacturers' instructions and AORN's "Recommended practices for high-level disinfection."[3] The cuff and bladder should be rinsed thoroughly because cleaning solution residue may increase the chance of allergic reactions and decrease the life of the cuff and bladder. All tubing should be wiped with a US Environmental Protection Agency (EPA) high- or intermediate-level tuberculocidal disinfectant and dried before storage. Care must be taken to prevent introduction of solutions into the ports. Water in the ports contributes to microbial

growth. Subsequent deflation of wet bladders may cause minute droplets of solution to be forced into the tourniquet regulating mechanism, causing damage.[4]

3. If blood or other body fluids come in contact with tourniquet components, more extensive cleaning with an enzymatic solution and an EPA high- or intermediate-level tuberculocidal disinfectant capable of inactivating bloodborne pathogens is necessary.

4. The frequency, method, and criteria for pneumatic tourniquet testing should be established according to manufacturers' written instructions. A pneumatic tourniquet management program assists in identifying equipment problems that may have adverse effects on patient safety.[5]

5. Documentation should reflect the biomedical equipment and/or serial number, date of inspection, preventive maintenance, and status of all equipment. Records of equipment failure and preventive maintenance assist in identifying equipment performance problems or hazards and minimize clinical and physical risks.[6]

6. If a pneumatic tourniquet has malfunctioned, causing serious injury or contributing to the death of a patient or other individual, the health care facility must report this information to the manufacturer and the US Food and Drug Administration as required by the Safe Medical Devices Act of 1990.[7] Device identification, service, maintenance, and event information should be included in the report.

Recommended Practice III

The pneumatic tourniquet should be used as designed and in a manner that reduces risk of patient injury. Perioperative personnel should be aware of the most common tourniquet-related complications and implement prevention strategies to minimize complication occurrence.

1. Tourniquet systems use compressed gas to apply a carefully controlled amount of tourniquet pressure. The appropriate gas source must be selected according to manufacturers' written instructions. The specific tourniquet system determines whether this gas is nitrogen or air. Gas may be delivered from a portable canister, tank, or built-in system. Tourniquets should never be inflated with nitrous oxide or oxygen because of fire risk.[8] Gases used incorrectly for inflation are potentially hazardous.[9] Some systems offer an automated microprocessor that performs self-calibration, displays elapsed inflation time, and sounds alarms when parameters are not met.

2. Tourniquet cuff length and width should be individualized, taking into consideration the size and shape of the patient's limb and specific demands of the procedure. The widest cuff possible, based on appropriate tourniquet length, should be selected. A wider bladder occludes blood flow at a lower pressure.[10] The cuff should overlap at least 3 inches but not more than 6 inches.[11] Too much overlap causes increased pressure and potential rolling or wrinkling of underlying soft tissue, which increases pressure on the area of overlap.

3. Contour tourniquet cuffs specifically designed to fit conical extremities occlude arterial flow at lower pressures than straight tourniquet cuffs of equal width.[12] A contour cuff may be more appropriate than a straight cuff on an extremity that is highly muscular or on the extremity of a patient who is obese because use of contour cuffs enhances comfort and reduces risk of shearing.[13]

4. Manufacturers' instructions may suggest that a soft, wrinkle-free padding (eg, cast padding, stockinette) be placed around the limb as proximal to the incision as possible, being careful not to pinch the skin folds where the tourniquet is applied. To improve tourniquet positioning on an obese extremity, an assistant can manually grasp the tissue of the extremity and gently apply and hold traction distal to the tourniquet site until the padding and cuff are placed. Traction should be maintained until the cuff is secured.[14]

5. Upper arm, thigh, and calf/supramalleolar tourniquet cuffs should be positioned on the limb at the point of maximum circumference proximal to the incision.[15] Calf tourniquets should be of the widest contour cuff possible and should be placed with the proximal edge near the largest calf circumference and at least 2 cm distal to the head of the fibula and 2 cm

proximal to the malleoli.[16] There is a potential risk to superficial nerves in unprotected areas during cuff placement. When the tourniquet cuff is inflated, nerves and blood vessels are compressed.

6. The tourniquet cuff should be protected to keep fluids (eg, skin prep solutions) from collecting under the cuff and causing chemical burns.[17] The tourniquet cuff also should be protected from contamination during surgery. Tourniquet protectors (eg, U-shaped drapes, adhesive drapes, plastic bags, tourniquet covers) should be used to minimize soiling.

7. Skin integrity under the tourniquet should be maintained. The cuff should be applied to the extremity so that underlying skin and tissue are not traumatized unduly. Some tourniquets are manufactured with gel padding for conforming pressures. If at any time cuff adjustment is necessary, the cuff should be removed and reapplied to the desired position to avoid shearing forces.[18]

8. An elastic wrap (eg, Esmarch's bandage) should be available for exsanguination. After the extremity is elevated, an elastic wrap often is used to compress superficial vessels to force blood out of the extremity. Adequate exsanguination helps reduce the pain associated with tourniquet use. Exsanguination with an elastic wrap may not be appropriate following traumatic injury or if the extremity has been in a cast. Thrombi in vessels could become dislodged, resulting in emboli.[19] In the presence of infection, painful fractures, or malignant tumors, exsanguination is accomplished by extremity elevation only.[20]

9. The use of a pneumatic tourniquet is contraindicated for patients with vascular disease or poor peripheral circulation.[21]

10. Tourniquets should be inflated rapidly. Rapid cuff inflation occludes arteries and veins almost simultaneously, preventing filling of superficial veins before occlusion of arterial blood flow.[22]

11. Tourniquet inflation pressure should be kept to a minimum. Nerve damage may result from excessive tourniquet pressure or uneven padding.[23] While the cuff is inflated, the pressure gauge or digital display should be clearly visible and monitored for excessive fluctuation. Catastrophic neurological complications (eg, permanent nerve palsy) can occur with excessive tourniquet inflation pressures.[24] The physician considers the patient's age and systolic blood pressure, circumference of the extremity, tourniquet width, and other clinical factors when determining tourniquet inflation pressure. The ideal pressure to which a tourniquet should be inflated has not been determined. The minimum pressure that will produce a bloodless field should be used as a guideline for inflation pressure. The basic guidelines are to add

♦ 50 to 75 mm Hg to the patient's systolic blood pressure for the upper extremities of adult patients,

♦ 100 to 150 mm Hg to the patient's systolic blood pressure for the lower extremities of adult patients,[25] and

♦ 100 mm Hg to the patient's systolic blood pressure for pediatric patients.[26]

12. Tourniquet technology continues to evolve. Emerging technology includes a modified tourniquet control unit that automatically measures the limb occlusion pressure (LOP) (ie, the minimum cuff pressure necessary to stop arterial blood flow distal to the cuff). This feature maintains the cuff at the lowest pressure necessary to maintain a bloodless surgical field. Clinical trials in 2001 established suggested pressures for adult and pediatric limb occlusion using this technology. Over time, technology may change the way tourniquets are used. It is the responsibility of the health care practitioner and facility to stay abreast of new technology and its impact on patient care and safety, as well as its cost.

13. Tourniquet inflation time should be kept to a minimum. The surgeon should be informed of the duration of the tourniquet time at regular, established intervals. Paralysis may result from prolonged use of the tourniquet. It has not been determined exactly how long a tourniquet may be inflated safely. The time varies with the patient's age and physical status and the vascular supply to the extremity. One hour is the recommended inflation time limit for an upper extremity and one and one-half to two

hours for a lower extremity. In addition, after a period of reperfusion (ie, 10 minutes or more), the tourniquet may be reinflated for another full period as above.[27]

14. Use of bilateral extremity tourniquets has become more common and presents a unique set of potential complications. Tourniquet use causes anaerobic metabolism, which produces lactic acid and other metabolites. Lactic acidosis causes a decrease in vascular resistance and allows an increased blood flow when the tourniquet is deflated. The larger the muscle mass, the greater the production of these by-products. To reduce the rapid release of large amounts of these metabolic by-products, tourniquets should be deflated individually 30 to 45 minutes apart when bilateral tourniquets are used (eg, during simultaneous bilateral total knee arthroplasty). Sequential deflation lessens the potential for adverse patient reactions (eg, fat embolism) to these by-products.[28]

15. Tourniquets should be deflated as recommended by the manufacturer. Upon deflation of the tourniquet, the cuff and sleeve/padding should be removed from the extremity. Even slight impedance of venous return by the padding or deflated cuff may lead to congestion and pooling of blood at the surgical site.[29]

16. A number of adverse reactions have been identified in relation to tourniquet use. Over-pressurization may cause pain at the cuff site; muscle weakness; compression injuries to blood vessels, nerves, muscle, or skin; or extremity paralysis. Underpressurization may result in blood in the surgical field, passive congestion of the limb, shock, and hemorrhagic infiltration of a nerve. Excessive inflation time may result in excessive hyperemia, muscle weakness, ischemic injury, or extremity paralysis. Improper cuff application may lead to venous congestion, bruising, blistering, pinching, ecchymosis, or necrosis of the skin.

17. Safety measures should be implemented to prevent injury. These measures include, but are not limited to,
    ♦ following manufacturers' written instructions,
    ♦ performing a complete patient assessment preoperatively,

♦ applying the cuff to the extremity with care and attention,
♦ ensuring proper fit of the cuff on the extremity,
♦ avoiding fluid retention under the cuff,
♦ using the minimal effective pressure required to suppress arterial circulation in an extremity,
♦ monitoring the pressure display to ensure that it accurately reflects the pressure in the cuff bladder, and
♦ monitoring tourniquet inflation time.

Monitoring safety parameters during use of a pneumatic tourniquet reduces the risk for complications and patient injury.

Recommended Practice IV

Potential patient injuries and complications associated with intravenous regional anesthesia (IVRA [ie, Bier's block]) should be identified, and safe practices should be established.

1. Although anesthesia care providers monitor the patient for complications, perioperative personnel should be aware of the patient's physiological status. Adverse reactions to local anesthetic agents are potential complications of IVRA. The major danger is of an inadvertent bolus of local anesthetic entering the general circulation. This can occur when there is accidental or sudden deflation of the tourniquet, from deflation soon after injection of local anesthetic, or if the bolus is released too rapidly at the end of the procedure. The sudden rush of anesthetic and metabolic waste into the circulatory system affects the central nervous system (eg, ringing in the ears, tingling, numbness, loss of consciousness, convulsions) and the heart.[30] To minimize the potential for an adverse reaction, the tourniquet should be deflated gradually as determined by the physician.

Recommended Practice V

Documentation should be consistent with AORN's "Recommended practices for documentation of perioperative nursing care."[31] The Perioperative Nursing Data Set nomenclature should be used when documenting on the patient record.[32]

1. Documentation during the use of pneumatic tourniquets should include, but not be limited to,

♦ cuff location,

♦ skin protection (eg, padding, stockinette, gel lining),

♦ cuff pressure,

♦ time of inflation and deflation,

♦ skin and tissue integrity under the cuff before and after use of the pneumatic tourniquet,

♦ assessment and evaluation of the entire extremity,

♦ identification/serial number and model of the specific tourniquet, and

♦ identification of the person who applied the cuff.

Facility policy should differentiate between documentation required for the perioperative record and the anesthesia record.

2. Documentation provides information for continuity of care and retrospective review of the patient's progress. Documented events may provide data for research studies. Personnel should be familiar with facility documentation policies and procedures.

Recommended Practice VI

Policies and procedures for the use of a pneumatic tourniquet should be developed, reviewed at regular intervals, and readily available in the practice setting.

1. Policies and procedures for pneumatic tourniquet use should include, but not be limited to,

♦ responsibility for cuff application;

♦ responsibility for monitoring the tourniquet while in use;

♦ patient care documentation;

♦ potential adverse reactions;

♦ documentation of maintenance, testing, inspection, and cleaning; and

♦ care of the tourniquet after use.

2. These recommended practices should be used as guidelines for developing policies and procedures in the practice setting. Policies and procedures establish authority, responsibility, and accountability. They also serve as operational guidelines and guide development of performance improvement activities. A review of policies and procedures should be included in the orientation and ongoing education of all appropriate staff members in the practice setting.

Glossary

Adverse reaction: A response that produces a detrimental effect.

Exsanguination: The process of forcible expulsion of blood from an extremity. The state of being deprived of blood.

Pneumatic: Pertaining to gas or air; filled with compressed gas or air.

NOTES

1. "Competency statements in perioperative nursing," in *Standards, Recommended Practices, and Guidelines* (Denver: AORN, Inc, 2001) 19-21.

2. ECRI, "Tourniquets, pneumatic," in *Healthcare Product Comparison System* (Plymouth Meeting, Pa: ECRI, June 1997) 2.

3. "Recommended practices for high-level disinfection," in *Standards, Recommended Practices, and Guidelines* (Denver: AORN, Inc, 2001) 196.

4. L K Groah, *Perioperative Nursing,* third ed (Stamford, Conn: Appleton & Lange, 1996) 304.

5. Joint Commission on Accreditation of Healthcare Organizations, "Management of the environment of care (EC)," *Comprehensive Accreditation Manual for Hospitals* (Oakbrook Terrace, Ill: Joint Commission on Accreditation of Healthcare Organizations, 2000) EC12.

6. *Ibid.*

7. M A Heller, *Guide to Medical Device Regulation,* vol 2 (Washington, DC: Thompson Publishing Group, 1998) 359; A V Harris, S E Ziel, "Reporting requirements under the Safe Medical Devices Act," *AORN Journal* 64 (September 1996) 461.

8. ECRI, "Tourniquets, pneumatic," 2.

9. *Ibid.*

10. R S Pauers, M A Carocci, "Low pressure pneumatic tourniquets: Effectiveness at minimum recommended inflation pressures," *The Journal of Foot and Ankle Surgery* 33 no 6 (1994) 605; J P Estebe et al, "Tourniquet pain in a volunteer study: Effect of changes in cuff width and pressure," *Anaesthesia* 55 (January 2000) 21.

11. Groah, *Perioperative Nursing,* third ed, 303.

12. Zimmer, *Tourniquet Safety* (Warsaw, Ind: Zimmer, Inc, 1997) 8; Pauers, Carocci, "Low pressure pneumatic tourniquets: Effectiveness at minimum recommended inflation pressures," 605.

13. *Ibid.*

14. K A Krackow, "A maneuver for improved positioning of a tourniquet in the obese patient," *Clinical Orthopedics and Related Research* 168 (August 1982) 80.

15. N H Fortunato, *Berry & Kohn's Operating Room Technique,* ninth ed (St Louis: Mosby, Inc, 2000) 528.

16. N S Lichtenfeld, "The pneumatic ankle tourniquet with ankle block anesthesia for foot surgery," *Foot and Ankle* 13 (July/August 1992) 344-349.

17. Groah, *Perioperative Nursing,* third ed, 304.

18. R Waldo, A Kamino, M L Phippen, "Providing instruments, equipment, and supplies," in *Patient Care During*

Operative and Invasive Procedures, ed M L Phippen, M P Wells (Philadelphia: W B Saunders, Co, 2000) 102.

19. Y Ogino et al, "Cerebral infarction after deflation of a pneumatic tourniquet during total knee replacement," *Anesthesiology* 90 (January 1999) 297; Groah, *Perioperative Nursing,* third ed, 304.

20. Zimmer, *Tourniquet Safety,* 15; Groah, *Perioperative Nursing,* third ed, 304.

21. Groah, *Perioperative Nursing,* third ed, 304.

22. *Ibid.*

23. A J Hodgson, "A proposed etiology for tourniquet-induced neuropathies," *Journal of Biomedical Engineering* 116 (May 1994) 224.

24. Zimmer, *Tourniquet Safety,* 31; M D Jacobson et al, "Muscle functional deficits after tourniquet ischemia," *The American Journal of Sports Medicine* 22 no 3 (1994) 372.

25. Waldo, Kamino, Phippen, "Providing instruments, equipment, and supplies," 102; C L Henderson et al, "A North American survey of intravenous regional anesthesia," *Anesthesia Analgesia* 85 (1997) 858-863.

26. J R Lieberman, L T Staheli, M C Dales, "Tourniquet pressures on pediatric patients: A clinical study," *Orthopedics* 20 (December 1997) 1146.

27. Groah, *Perioperative Nursing,* third ed, 304.

28. J J Branson, W M Goldstein, "Sequential bilateral total knee arthroplasty," *AORN Journal* 73 (March 2001) 615-616.

29. S J Tredwell et al, "Pediatric tourniquets: Analysis of cuff and limb interface, current practice, and guidelines for use," *Journal of Pediatric Orthopedics* 21 (September/October 2001) 671-676; Zimmer, *Tourniquet Safety,* 23.

30. Zimmer, *Tourniquet Safety,* 34.

31. "Recommended practices for documentation of perioperative nursing care," in *Standards, Recommended Practices, and Guidelines* (Denver: AORN, Inc, 2001) 199-201.

32. S Beyea, ed, *Perioperative Nursing Data Set,* second ed (Denver: AORN, Inc, 2001).

Originally published April 1984, *AORN Journal.*
Revised November 1990.

Published as proposed recommended practices March 1994.

Revised November 1998; published December 1998.
Reformatted July 2000.

Revised November 2001; published February 2002, *AORN Journal.*

Recommended Practices for Positioning the Patient in the Perioperative Practice Setting

The following recommended practices have been developed by the AORN Recommended Practices Committee and have been approved by the AORN Board of Directors. They were presented as proposed recommended practices for comment by members and others. They are effective January 1, 2001.

These recommended practices are intended as achievable recommendations representing what is believed to be an optimal level of practice. Policies and procedures will reflect variations in practice settings and/or clinical situations that determine the degree to which the recommended practices can be implemented.

AORN recognizes the numerous types of settings in which perioperative nurses practice. These recommended practices are intended as guidelines adaptable to various practice settings. These practice settings include traditional ORs, ambulatory surgery units, physicians' offices, cardiac catheterization suites, endoscopy suites, radiology departments, and all other areas where operative or other invasive procedures may be performed.

Purpose

These recommended practices provide guidelines for positioning the patient in the perioperative setting. They are not intended to cover aspects of perioperative patient care addressed in other recommended practices. The patient's position should provide optimum exposure for the procedure and access to IV lines and monitoring devices. Attention must be given to patient comfort and safety, as well as circulatory, respiratory, musculoskeletal, and neurologic structure. The procedure, surgeon preference, and patient condition determine equipment used for positioning. Working as a member of the team, the perioperative nurse can minimize the risk of perioperative complications related to positioning.

Recommended Practice I

Preoperative assessment for positioning needs should be made before transferring the patient to the procedure bed.

1. The preoperative interview should include questions to determine patient tolerance to the planned position. Assessment includes both patient and intraoperative factors. Patient factors include, but are not limited to,
   - age,

   - height and weight,
   - skin condition,
   - nutritional status,
   - preexisting conditions (eg, vascular, respiratory, circulatory, neurologic, immunocompromise), and
   - physical/mobility limits (eg, prostheses, implants, range of motion).

   Intraoperative factors include, but are not limited to,
   - anesthesia,
   - length of surgery, and
   - position required.

   Preplanning is necessary to ensure that the appropriate positioning devices and an adequate number of personnel are available to position the patient on the procedure bed. Positioning requires knowledge and understanding of the physiologic effects and implications of the position in relation to the patient's assessed status and limitations.[1] Patient injury (eg, burns, nerve damage, pressure ulcers, alopecia) can occur as normal defense mechanisms are altered due to anesthetic agents and medications, as well as forced prolonged immobility during the procedure.[2]

2. The perioperative nurse should actively participate in safely positioning the patient. Safe and appropriate positioning requires teamwork. Communicating specific patient needs to surgical team members contributes to safe positioning. Safely positioning the patient is a priority of perioperative nurses. Outcomes of safe and appropriate positioning may include
   - optimal exposure of the surgical site;
   - airway management, ventilation, and monitoring access for the anesthesia care provider;
   - physiologic safety for the patient; and
   - maintenance of patient dignity by controlling unnecessary exposure.[3]

Recommended Practice II

Positioning devices should be readily available, clean, and in proper working order before placing the patient on the procedure bed.

1. Equipment should be maintained and used according to manufacturers' written instructions. Equipment function should be verified

before use. Properly functioning equipment and devices contribute to patient safety and assist in providing adequate exposure of the surgical site.[4]

2. Positioning devices should be provided for each surgical position and its variations. These devices include padding and pressure relief devices. Firm and stable devices help distribute pressure evenly and decrease the potential for injury. Anatomic and physical limitations will dictate the types of positioning devices that can be used for any individual patient.[5]

3. Personnel should be familiar with the proper function and use of positioning equipment and devices. The appropriate device(s) should be selected to achieve the desired effect. Excessive stretching of neuromuscular and vascular structures should be avoided. Selection criteria for positioning equipment and devices include, but are not limited to,
   ♦ availability in a variety of appropriate sizes and shapes;
   ♦ durable material and design;
   ♦ ability to maintain normal capillary interface pressure;
   ♦ resistance to moisture and microorganisms;
   ♦ radiolucency;
   ♦ fire resistance;
   ♦ nonallergenic to the patient;
   ♦ ease of use;
   ♦ easily cleaned/disinfected if not disposable;
   ♦ easily stored, handled, and retrieved; and
   ♦ cost effectiveness.[6]

Studies suggest that positioning devices should maintain normal capillary interface pressure of 32 mm Hg or less.

Procedure beds and accessory parts often are covered with vinyl or nylon fabrics. Foam pads are not effective in reducing capillary interface pressure because they quickly compress under heavy body areas. Use of gel pads or similar devices over the OR bed decreases pressure at any given point by redistributing overall pressures across a larger surface area. Convoluted foam mattress overlays are effective in reducing pressure only if they are made of a thick and dense foam that resists compression. Pillows, blankets, and molded foam devices may produce only a minimum of pressure reduction.

Towels and sheet rolls do not reduce pressure and may contribute to friction injuries.[7]

Recommended Practice III

The perioperative nurse should actively participate in monitoring patient body alignment and tissue integrity based on sound physiologic principles.

1. The number of personnel and/or devices should be adequate to safely transfer and/or position the patient. An inadequate number of personnel and/or insufficient equipment can result in patient injury.[8] Indwelling catheters, tubes, or cannulas may be dislodged without proper support. Sliding or pulling the patient can result in shearing force and/or friction. Shearing refers to the patient's skin remaining stationary while underlying tissues shift or move, as might occur when the patient is pulled or dragged without support to the skeletal system or when a draw sheet is used. Friction occurs when skin rubs over a rough stationary surface. Maintaining the patient's correct body alignment and supporting extremities and joints decreases the potential for injury during transfer and positioning.[9] Refer to Table 1 for injury risks and safety considerations to be followed when positioning the patient. The table is not all-inclusive but is presented to provide general guidance for personnel who position the patient.[10]

Recommended Practice IV

After positioning, the perioperative nurse should evaluate the patient's body alignment and tissue integrity.

1. After the desired position is attained, the perioperative nurse should evaluate the patient again. This evaluation should include, but not be limited to, the following systems:
   ♦ respiratory,
   ♦ circulatory,
   ♦ neurologic,
   ♦ musculoskeletal, and
   ♦ integumentary.

   Respiratory function can be decreased by mechanical restriction of the rib cage, which can occur with certain positions (eg, prone, lateral, lithotomy). Circulatory function is influenced by anesthetic agents and surgical techniques that

Table 1

INJURY RISKS AND SAFETY CONSIDERATIONS WHEN POSITIONING PATIENTS		
Position	**Risks**	**Safety considerations**
Supine	Pressure points, including occiput, scapulae, thoracic vertebrae, olecranon process, sacrum/coccyx, calcaneae, and knees.	♦ Padding to heels, elbows, knees, spinal column, and occiput alignment with hips, legs parallel and uncrossed ankles.
	Neural injuries of extremities, including brachial plexus and ulna, and pudendal nerves.	♦ Arm boards at less than 90-degree angle and level with floor. ♦ Head in neutral position. ♦ Arm board pads level with table pads.
Prone	Head Eyes Nose	♦ Maintain cervical neck alignment. ♦ Protection for forehead, eyes, and chin. ♦ Padded headrest to provide airway access.
	Chest compression, iliac crests	♦ Chest rolls (ie, clavicle to iliac crest) to allow chest movement and decrease abdominal pressure.
	Breasts, male genitalia	♦ Breasts and male genitalia free from torsion.
	Knees Feet	♦ Knees padded with pillow to feet. ♦ Padded footboard.
Lateral	Bony prominence and pressure points on dependent side	♦ Axillary role for dependent axilla. ♦ Lower leg flexed at hip. ♦ Upper leg straight with pillow between legs. ♦ Padding between knees, ankles, and feet.
	Spinal alignment	♦ Maintain spinal alignment during turning. ♦ Padded support to prevent lateral neck flexion.
Lithotomy	Hip and knee joint injury Lumbar and sacral pressure Vascular congestion	♦ Place stirrups at even height. ♦ Elevate and lower legs slowly and simultaneously from stirrups.
	Neuropathy of obturator nerves, saphenous nerves, femoral nerves, common peroneal nerves, and ulnar nerves.	♦ Maintain minimal external rotation of hips. ♦ Pad lateral or posterior knees and ankles to prevent pressure and contact with metal surface.
	Restricted diaphragmatic movement Pulmonary region	♦ Keep arms away from chest to facilitate respiration. ♦ Arms on arm boards at less than 90-degree angle or over abdomen.

may result in vasodilatation, hypertension, decreased cardiac output, and inhibition of normal compensatory mechanisms. Positions such as lithotomy and Trendelenburg's can cause redistribution and congestion of the blood supply. Circulatory responses to certain positions or position changes can be rapid and dramatic. Nerve and muscle trauma result from stretching or compression when upper extremities are abducted at greater than 90 degrees to the body, hips are placed in excessive external rotation, and/or the head and neck is hyperflexed or hyperextended.[11]

Intraoperative skin injury is a function of unrelieved pressure, duration of the pressure, and the location of the pressure on the body surface. Several studies indicate that procedures longer than two and one-half to three hours significantly increase the patient's risk for pressure ulcer formation. External pressure exceeding normal capillary interface pressure (ie, 23 to 32 mm Hg) can cause occlusion that will restrict or block blood flow. The resulting tissue ischemia will lead to tissue breakdown. Both high pressure for a short duration and low pressure for extended duration are risk factors. As noted, other extrinsic factors for skin injury are shear forces and friction.

The incidence of pressure ulcers occurring as a result of surgery may be as high as 66%, with most being stage I, and fewer than 10% being stage II or higher. Pressure ulcers are staged according to the degree of tissue damage.

- Stage I: Intact, reddened skin does not blanch to fingertip pressure.
- Stage II: Partial skin loss involving the epidermis and dermis. Skin is abraded or blistered or has shallow craters.
- Stage III: Full thickness skin loss possibly down to, but not through, the fascial layer. Deep craters with or without sinus tracts in tissues.
- Stage IV: Muscle, bone, and supporting structures show extensive damage.[12]

2. After repositioning or any movement of the patient, procedure bed, or devices that attach to the procedure bed, the patient should be reassessed for body alignment. Changing position may expose or damage otherwise protected body tissue. This position change may be perceptible or imperceptible and may result from adding or deleting positioning devices, adjusting the procedure bed in some manner, or moving the patient on the procedure bed.[13]

Recommended Practice V

Documentation of surgical positioning should be consistent with AORN's "Recommended practices for documentation of perioperative nursing care."[14]

1. Documentation should include, but not be limited to,
   - preoperative assessment,
   - type and location of positioning and/or padding devices,
   - names and titles of persons positioning the patient, and
   - postoperative outcome evaluation.

   Documentation of the perioperative care plan includes the nursing assessments and interventions, as well as an appraisal of the quality of care delivered. Documenting nursing activities provides an accurate picture of the perioperative nursing care administered and the outcomes of the care delivered.[15]

Recommended Practice VI

Policies and procedures related to positioning should be developed and reviewed annually, revised as necessary, and be available in the practice setting.

1. These policies and procedures should include, but not be limited to,
   - assessment and evaluation criteria and documentation;
   - anatomic and physiologic considerations;
   - safety interventions;
   - documentation of patient position and/or repositioning, positioning devices, and personnel positioning the patient; and
   - positioning device care and maintenance.

2. These recommended practices should be used as guidelines for developing policies and procedures in the practice setting. Policies and procedures establish authority, responsibility, and accountability. They also serve as operational guidelines. An introduction and review of policies and procedures should be included in the orientation and ongoing education of personnel to assist them in obtaining knowledge and developing skills and attitudes that will affect patient outcomes. Policies also assist in the development of performance improvement activities.

Glossary

Positioning device: Any device or piece of equipment used for positioning the patient and/or providing maximum anatomic exposure. Devices include, but are not limited to,

- support devices for head, arms, chest, iliac crests, and lumbar areas;
- pads in a variety of sizes and shapes for pressure points (eg, head, elbows, knees, ankles, heels, sacral areas);
- securing devices (eg, safety belts, tapes, kidney rests, vacuum pack positioning devices);
- procedure bed equipment (eg, headrest/holders, overhead arm supports, stirrups, foot boards); and
- specialty surgical beds (eg, fracture tables, ophthalmology carts/stretcher chairs).

NOTES

1. ECRI, "Patient positioning," in *Operating Room Risk Management* (Plymouth Meeting, Pa: ECRI, July 1992) 1-12; D McEwen, "Intraoperative positioning of surgical patients," *AORN Journal* 63 (June 1996) 1059-1079; J Ramsay, "Pressure ulcer risk factors in the operating room," *Advances in Wound Care* 11 no 3 suppl (May/June 1998) 5-6.

2. V M Hoshowsky, C A Schramm, "Intraoperative pressure sore prevention: An analysis of bedding materials," *Research in Nursing and Health* 17 (October 1994) 333-339; B J Gruendemann, B Fernsebner, *Comprehensive Perioperative Nursing, Volume 1: Principles* (Boston: Jones and Bartlett Publishers, 1995) 389-410; C Biddle, M J Cannady, "Surgical positions: Their effects on cardiovascular, respiratory systems," *AORN Journal* 52 (August 1990) 359; D Ben-Amitai, B Z Garty, "Alopecia in children after cardiac surgery," *Pediatric Dermatology* 10 (March 1993) 32-33; M K Gillette, C C Caruso, "Intraoperative tissue injury: Major causes and preventative measures," *AORN Journal* 50 (July 1989) 72; T P Beach, "Unusual patients: Pediatrics," in *Positioning in Anesthesia and Surgery*, second ed (Philadelphia: W B Saunders Co, 1987) 255-264: P R Graling, D B Colvin, "The lithotomy position in colon surgery: Postoperative complications," *AORN Journal* 55 (April 1992) 1039.

3. Gruendemann, Fernsebner, *Comprehensive Perioperative Nursing, Volume 1: Principles*, 390; B Tettenborn et al, "Postoperative brainstem and cerebellar infarcts," *Neurology* 43 (March 1993) 476; E A Lachmann et al, "Complications associated with intermittent pneumatic compression," *Archives of Physical Medicine and Rehabilitation* 73 (May 1992) 483; Gillette, Caruso, "Intraoperative tissue injury: Major causes and preventative measures," 70, 76; J M Head, "Multilevel spine fractures: Intraoperative nursing management," *Journal of Neuroscience Nursing* 22 (December 1990) 373; E K Murphy, "Liability for injury resulting from poor patient positioning," (OR Nursing Law) *AORN Journal* 53 (June 1991) 1361-1365; J T Martin, "Introduction to positioning," in *Positioning in Anesthesia and Surgery*, second ed (Philadelphia: W B Saunders Co, 1987) 1-2; J T Martin, "General aspects of safe positioning for the surgical patient," in *Positioning in Anesthesia and Surgery*, second ed (Philadelphia: W B Saunders Co, 1987) 5-9; D Jacobs et al, "Unusual complication after pelvic surgery: Unilateral lower limb crush syndrome and bilateral common peroneal nerve paralysis," *Acta Anaesthesiologica Belgica* 43 no 2 (1992) 139-143.

4. ECRI, "Patient positioning," 5; Martin, "General aspects of safe positioning for the surgical patient," 5-8; C R Paschal, L R Strzelecki, "Lithotomy positioning devices: Factors that contribute to patient injury," *AORN Journal* 55 (April 1992) 1022; Gillette, Caruso, "Intraoperative tissue injury: Major causes and preventative measures," 76, 77.

5. Hoshowsky, Schramm, "Intraoperative pressure sore prevention: An analysis of bedding materials," 334; McEwen, "Intraoperative positioning of surgical patients," 1063; Gruendemann, Fernsebner, *Comprehensive Perioperative Nursing, Volume 1: Principles*, 408; Martin, "General aspects of safe positioning for the surgical patient," 6; S G Welborn, "The lithotomy position: Anesthesiologic considerations," in *Positioning in Anesthesia and Surgery*, second ed (Philadelphia: W B Saunders Co, 1987) 62; L B Schwartz, R S Stahl, A H DeCherney, "Unilateral compartment syndrome after prolonged gynecologic surgery in the dorsal lithotomy position: A case report," *Journal of Reproductive Medicine* 38 (June 1993) 471; Paschal, Strzelecki, "Lithotomy positioning devices: Factors that contribute to patient injury," 1011-1022; S W Wolfe, M F Lospinuso, S W Burke, "Unilateral blindness as a complication of patient positioning from spinal surgery: A case report," *Spine* 17 (May 1992) 604; Lachmann et al, "Complications associated with intermittent pneumatic compression," 482-485; L Romanowski et al, "Brachial plexus neuropathies after advanced laparoscopic surgery," *Fertility and Sterility* 60 (October 1993) 730; Gillette, Caruso, "Intraoperative tissue injury: Major causes and preventative measures," 66-78.

6. McEwen, "Intraoperative positioning of surgical patients," 1060, 1063; Gruendemann, Fernsebner, *Comprehensive Perioperative Nursing, Volume 1: Principles*, 408.

7. E M Landis, "Micro-injection studies of capillary blood pressure in human skin," *Heart* 15 (1930) 209-228; Hoshowsky, Schramm, "Intraoperative pressure sore prevention: An analysis of bedding materials," 333; McEwen, "Intraoperative positioning of surgical patients," 1060; M G Kemp et al, "Factors that contribute to pressure sores in surgical patients," *Research in Nursing & Health* 13 (October 1990) 293, 294; D Doughty, P Fairchild, S Stogis, "Your patient: Which therapy?" *Journal of Enterostomal Therapy* 17 (July/August 1990) 155; Gruendemann, Fernsebner, *Comprehensive Perioperative Nursing, Volume 1: Principles*, 391-394.

8. N H Fortunato, "Positioning the patient," in *Berry & Kohn's Operating Room Technique*, ninth ed (St Louis: Mosby, 2000) 487-500; J T Martin, "The prone position: Anesthesiologic considerations," in *Positioning in Anesthesia and Surgery*, second ed (Philadelphia: W B Saunders Co, 1987) 198; Gruendemann, Fernsebner, *Comprehensive Perioperative Nursing, Volume 1: Principles*, 400.

9. McEwen, "Intraoperative positioning of surgical patients," 1069-1073; Gruendemann, Fernsebner, *Comprehensive Perioperative Nursing, Volume 1: Principles*, 391-392, 396-404; Martin, "The prone position: Anesthesiologic considerations," 210-211; Biddle, Cannady, "Surgical positions: Their effects on cardiovascular, respiratory systems," 350-359; B L Smith, "Physiologic changes in the normal conscious human subject on changing from the erect to the supine position," in *Positioning in Anesthesia and Surgery*, second ed (Philadelphia: W B Saunders Co, 1987) 13-32; J Walsh, "AANA journal course: Update for nurse anesthetists—Patient positioning," *Journal of the American Association of Nurse Anesthetists* 62 (June 1994) 289-298.

10. *Ibid*; A N Thomas, "The lateral decubitus position: Surgical aspects," in *Positioning in Anesthesia and Surgery*, second ed (Philadelphia: W B Saunders Co, 1987) 148-49; Romanowski, "Brachial plexus neuropathies after advanced laparoscopic surgery," 730; Paschal, Strzelecki, "Lithotomy positioning devices: Factors that contribute to patient injury," 1011-1022; Welborn, "The lithotomy position: Anesthesiologic considerations," 60-61; K K Gombar et al, "Femoral neuropathy: A complication of the lithotomy position," *Regional Anesthesia* 17 (September/October 1992) 306-308; J T Martin, "The trendelenburg's position: A review of current slants about head down tilt," *Journal of the American Association of Nurse Anesthetists* (February 1995) 29-36.

11. McEwen, "Intraoperative positioning of surgical patients," 1069-1073; Gruendemann, Fernsebner, *Comprehensive Perioperative Nursing Volume 1: Principles,* 396-404; Biddle, Cannady, "Surgical positions: Their effects on cardiovascular, respiratory systems," 350-359; Smith, "Physiologic changes in the normal conscious human subject on changing from the erect to the supine position," 13-32; Gillette, Caruso, "Intraoperative tissue injury: Major causes and preventative measures," 72; Gombar et al, "Femoral neuropathy: A complication of the lithotomy position," 307.

12. Landis, "Micro-injection of capillary blood pressure in human skin," 209-228; Hoshowsky, Schramm, "Intraoperative pressure sore prevention: An analysis of bedding materials," 333-334; McEwen, "Intraoperative positioning of surgical patients," 1059-1062; Gruendemann, Fernsebner, *Comprehensive Perioperative Nursing, Volume 1: Principles,* 391-395; Ramsay, "Pressure ulcer risk factors in the operating room," 5-6.

13. Martin, "General aspects of safe positioning for the surgical patient," 8-11.

14. "Recommended practices for documentation of perioperative nursing care," in *Standards, Recommended Practices, and Guidelines* (Denver: AORN, Inc, 2000) 229-231.

15. *Ibid.*

RESOURCES

"OR acquired pressure ulcers," *Advances in Wound Care* 11 suppl no 3 (May/June 1998) 2-16.

Dybec, R B. "Nerve injuries following TRAM flap surgery," *Plastic Surgical Nursing* 17 (Summer 1997) 77-79.

Originally published November 1990, *AORN Journal.*

Revised November 1995; published August 1996, *AORN Journal.*

Revised and reformatted; published January 2001, *AORN Journal.*

Recommended Practices for
Product Selection in Perioperative Practice Settings

The following recommended practices were developed by the AORN Recommended Practices Committee and have been approved by the AORN Board of Directors. They were presented as proposed recommended practices for comment to members and others. These recommended practices are effective January 1, 2004.

These recommended practices are intended as achievable recommendations representing what is believed to be an optimal level of practice. Policies and procedures will reflect variations in practice settings or clinical situations that determine the degree to which the recommended practices can be implemented.

AORN recognizes the numerous types of settings in which perioperative nurses practice. These recommended practices are intended as guidelines adaptable to various practice settings. These practice settings include traditional ORs, ambulatory surgery units, physicians' offices, cardiac catheterization suites, endoscopy suites, radiology departments, and all other areas where surgical and other invasive procedures may be performed.

Purpose

These recommended practices provide guidelines for selecting medical devices and other products used in perioperative settings. AORN recognizes that many facilities belong to purchasing organizations and may be limited to selecting products from contract vendors. As new medical devices and products are introduced, choices continue to exist, and perioperative nurses continue to have an integral role in evaluating and selecting products that may affect the quality and safety of perioperative patient care.

Patient safety is a primary concern of perioperative nurses, and safety concerns must continue to drive perioperative nurses as they participate in evaluating and selecting medical devices and products for use in practice settings. Patient safety is one of the four domains of perioperative nursing (ie, safety, physiologic responses, behavioral responses, structural data elements) as specified in the Perioperative Nursing Data Set.[1] This nursing vocabulary was defined and published by AORN and is a Health Level Seven registered vocabulary. The National Library of Medicine is considering including the data set in the Unified Medical Language System.

Recommended Practice I

A mechanism for product and medical device standardization and evaluation should be implemented.

1. Capital equipment and medical device procurement are collaborative processes requiring clinical, business, financial, and legal acumen. Goals of product standardization and value analysis processes are to select functional and reliable products that are safe, cost-effective, and environmentally conscious and that promote quality care and avoid duplication or rapid obsolescence.[2] All departments involved in the selection, purchase, and use of products and medical devices should be represented on a multidisciplinary product evaluation and selection committee.[3,4] These departments may include, but are not limited to,
   - surgical services;
   - nursing services;
   - administration;
   - infection control;
   - surgeons, surgical staff members, OR committee members;
   - central/sterile processing;
   - pharmacy;
   - education;
   - materiel management and purchasing;
   - anesthesia;
   - biomedical engineering;
   - environmental services;
   - risk management;
   - radiology;
   - laboratory; and
   - institutional review board (IRB).

   Committee members other than perioperative personnel should be consulted to obtain input from departments with similar needs to select the most appropriate products and medical devices.[4,5]

2. Additional subcommittees or task forces may be needed because of the size of the facility or because a specialty product may have a limited user group.

3. The role of a perioperative multidisciplinary team may include initiating, coordinating, and participating in clinical evaluation of products and medical devices. Perioperative nurses frequently are involved in direct surgical patient care and in

the use and evaluation of products and medical devices.[4] Manufacturers' representatives should be contacted to serve as resource people for information about new or existing products and medical devices. These individuals have access to information concerning products currently on the market.[4,6] Manufacturers' representatives should be able to provide both clinical and technical data related to product research, new products and medical devices, packaging, sterilization, and environmental conservation.

4. E-commerce business-to-business applications should be used when applicable. Use of e-commerce applications can help with
   - ◆ collecting product data,
   - ◆ assessing group purchasing organization (GPO) catalogs,
   - ◆ soliciting pricing information,
   - ◆ comparing prices,
   - ◆ exploring online auctions for surplus or refurbished equipment,
   - ◆ enhancing buying power,
   - ◆ consolidating or reducing inventory, and
   - ◆ purchasing items online.[7]

Recommended Practice II

Product and medical device evaluations should be based on objective criteria specific to an item's function and use.

1. Criteria to evaluate medical devices and other products, including implants, may include, but are not limited to,
   - ◆ safety, performance, quality, and improved efficiency;
   - ◆ purpose and use;
   - ◆ ease of use;
   - ◆ compatibility with other products or medical devices;
   - ◆ impact on quality patient care and clinical outcomes;
   - ◆ efficacy;
   - ◆ cost/value analysis;
   - ◆ reimbursement potential;
   - ◆ compliance with GPOs;
   - ◆ sterilization/reprocessing parameters;
   - ◆ liability (eg, for investigational devices);
   - ◆ regulatory control (eg, from the US Food and Drug Administration);

   - ◆ standardization;
   - ◆ new technology competitiveness;
   - ◆ adaptability to future technology;
   - ◆ environmental impact;
   - ◆ availability and quality of service after purchase;
   - ◆ investment in personnel training; and
   - ◆ e-commerce applications (eg, support information, access, operational efficiency, availability).

2. Careful selection of criteria ensures the reliability and validity of trial evaluation results.[3,4,6] Cost considerations should be weighed against patient and personnel safety and user preference. All direct and indirect costs of products and medical devices (eg, waste disposal, processing, training, storage) should be identified and evaluated.[8]

3. Each product or medical device, disposable supply, or capital equipment purchase should be evaluated with criteria pertinent to the item. Specific and unique information may be required. Use a product-specific, written evaluation tool to facilitate objective review and analysis.[3,4,6]

Recommended Practice III

A clinical evaluation should be initiated based on an identified need or opportunity.

1. Appropriate committee members should screen products and medical devices before clinical evaluations are conducted. Unnecessary expenditure of time and money can be avoided if a viable need, issue, or concern is established first. A review of the literature on products and medical devices being evaluated may prevent clinical evaluations of inappropriate items.[2,3,9]

2. All departments and clinical areas affected by a product or medical device should be represented during the clinical evaluation process. Clinical functioning can best be measured in the practice setting by knowledgeable end users. Including all clinical areas in the evaluation process provides direct feedback from staff members whose practices will be affected by the item.[3-6,9,10] Standardization within the practice setting is increased when all clinical areas are involved.

◆ 594 ◆

3. Limits should be placed on the scope and time of the clinical evaluation. These limits should include, but are not limited to,
   - number of users,
   - cost,
   - number of products or medical devices to be evaluated,
   - time span,
   - number of departments and clinical areas involved,
   - desired patient outcomes, and
   - follow-up patient data, if indicated.

   Limits for evaluating products or medical devices increase the usefulness of user feedback. Unlimited time to evaluate products or medical devices may result in decreased evaluator input and enthusiasm.[6]

4. Demonstration of and instruction on use of the product or medical device being evaluated should be conducted before the clinical evaluation begins. Instructing all individuals involved in the clinical evaluation facilitates safe clinical practice and helps establish validity of the product or medical device evaluation.[4-6]

Recommended Practice IV

Evaluation data should be analyzed to determine product recommendations.

1. When evaluating data, actual clinical performance should be compared to predetermined standards.[4,6] Individuals participating in the clinical evaluation should provide data about the product or medical device to complete the evaluation tool.

2. Data should be analyzed and a summary of findings, conclusions, and recommendations presented. This information facilitates efficient and consistent decisions based on preestablished criteria and an evidence-based product assessment.[2,3]

3. A value analysis may be performed as part of the evaluation and selection process.[2,10] Whenever possible, selected products should have a positive cost-benefit ratio. Products that do not have a positive cost-benefit ratio should have other, more critical redeeming factors that make them an appropriate selection for purchase.

4. Upon completion of the evaluation process, a list of products or medical devices can be compiled as a basis for obtaining competitive bids and making alternative product or medical device purchases.[2-4,6]

5. After a product or medical device has been selected, a comprehensive plan for introduction, use, and further evaluation of the item should be developed and implemented in the facility.[2,4] New product performance and user satisfaction should be evaluated at planned intervals. This evaluation helps ensure that new products are meeting expected performance criteria—including cost-effectiveness performance criteria—and that the preselection evaluation process has met its objectives.

Recommended Practice V

Policies and procedures for evaluating and selecting products and medical devices should be written, reviewed periodically, and readily available in perioperative practice settings.

1. Policies and procedures establish authority, responsibility, and accountability for product evaluation and selection. They serve as operational guidelines and provide a framework for continuous quality improvement activities related to product evaluation and selection.

2. Written guidelines should be available for all health care personnel involved in the selection and evaluation of commonly used products and medical devices. Orientation and ongoing education activities for personnel should include an introduction to and review of policies and procedures to be applied in the practice setting. Compliance with policies and procedures helps develop and reinforce knowledge, skills, and attitudes that affect patient outcomes.

NOTES

1. S Beyea, ed, *Perioperative Nursing Data Set,* second ed (Denver: AORN, Inc, 2002).

2. A M Fernandez et al, "Technology assessment in healthcare: A review and description of a 'best practice' technology assessment process," *Best Practices and Benchmarking in Healthcare* 2 (November/December 1997) 241.

3. R Podabinski, D Monckton, J Thompson, "A new product selection model," (Material Management) *OR Manager* 15 (September 1999) 34-40.

4. M Dickerson, "Product evaluation: A key to controlling costs," *Nursing Economic$* 5 (March/April 1987) 60-64.

5. C Rupert, S Kitzman, "The clinical voice in product selection and implementation," *SSM* 8 (August 2002) 24-26.

6. P Barone-Ameduri, "Equipment trials make sense," *Nursing Management* 17 (June 1986) 43-44.

7. F Doyle C Weisbrod, "Endless possibilities: Using the Internet in the supply chain process," *SSM* 8 (February 2002) 24-28.

8. P S Hunt, "Speaking the language of finance," *AORN Journal* 73 (April 2001) 774-787.

9. E Beaumont, "Technology scorecard: Are you up to date?" *American Journal of Nursing* 96 (December 1996) 23-28.

10. S B Wilen, B M Stone, "Cost versus cost effectiveness: The Achilles' heel for healthcare delivery," (Editorial) *Best Practices and Benchmarking in Healthcare* 2 (May/June 1997) 142-144.

RESOURCES

Baird, M V G. "Product selection in the OR: A decision-making model," *AORN Journal* 48 (September 1988) 512-517.

Weatherly, K S, et al. "Product evaluation process: A systems approach to controlling health care costs," *AORN Journal* 59 (February 1994) 489-494, 496-498.

Wilhelm-Hass, E. "Breaking the time barrier: Learning from a new product evaluation," *AORN Journal* 56 (December 1992) 1074-1081.

Originally published April 1989, *AORN Journal.*

Revised August 1993.

Revised November 1997; published January 1998, *AORN Journal.* Reformatted July 2000.

Revised November 2003; published March 2004, *AORN Journal.*

Recommended Practices for Reducing Radiological Exposure in the Practice Setting

T
he following recommended practices have been developed by the AORN Recommended Practices Committee and have been approved by the AORN Board of Directors. They were presented as proposed recommended practices for comments by members and others. They are effective January 1, 2001.

These recommended practices are intended as achievable recommendations representing what is believed to be an optimal level of practice. Policies and procedures will reflect variations in practice settings and/or clinical situations that determine the degree to which the recommended practices can be implemented.

AORN recognizes the various settings in which perioperative nurses practice. These recommended practices are intended as guidelines adaptable to various practice settings. These practice settings include traditional ORs, ambulatory surgery units, physicians' offices, cardiac catheterization suites, endoscopy suites, radiology departments, and all other areas where operative and other invasive procedures may be performed.

Purpose

These recommended practices will assist the perioperative nurse in reducing radiation exposure in the practice setting. These recommended practices do not refer to therapeutic intraoperative radiation therapy or to lasers, which are recognized as non-ionizing radiation and, therefore, are not within the scope of these recommended practices.

Ionizing radiation can damage living tissues and may produce long-term effects. Patients and personnel should be protected from unsafe levels of radiation that are not medically indicated because of the effects of ionizing radiation exposure on tissue. Radiation safety in the practice setting is a responsibility shared by the department of radiology, the department of surgical services, the radiation safety officer for the facility, and perioperative personnel.

Recommended Practice I

The patient should be exposed to radiation only if medically indicated.

1. All reasonable means of reconciling an incorrect sponge, sharp, or instrument count should be implemented before using a radiological examination to locate a sponge, sharp, or

instrument not located during the intraoperative count. Exposure to radiation may have some finite risk; therefore, radiation exposure to patients and personnel should be kept as low as reasonably achievable (ALARA).[1]

Recommended Practice II

During medically indicated radiological procedures, the patient should be protected from unnecessary radiation exposure.

1. X-rays to the abdomen and pelvis of women who are pregnant or may be pregnant should be avoided if possible. Exposing the fetus to radiation during the first trimester may result in abnormalities in rapidly dividing embryonic cells.[2]

2. A leaded shield should be used to protect the fetus when other areas of a pregnant woman's body are x-rayed. The fetus is highly sensitive to ionizing radiation. Scattered radiation may expose the fetus to low-level radiation.[3]

3. Leaded shields should be used, when possible, to protect the patient's ovaries or testes (ie, gonads) during x-ray studies of the hips and upper legs. Protective shielding should be placed between the patient and the source of radiation. Radiation may cause damage to gonadal cells.[4]

4. Leaded shields should be used, when possible, to protect the thyroid during x-ray studies of the upper extremities, trunk, and head. Thyroid and lymphoid tissues appear to be sensitive to radiation exposure.[5]

Recommended Practice III

Occupational exposure to radiation should be minimized in the practice setting.

1. During radiation exposure, all personnel should stand at least 6 ft (ie, 2 m) from the x-ray tube and behind leaded shielding. Distance from the radiation beam and attenuation by leaded shielding and wall materials will decrease radiation exposure.[6]

2. Leaded shielding should be provided to personnel who cannot leave the room or cannot stand approximately 6 ft (ie, 2m) away from

the x-ray tube and the patient. Leaded screens and/or leaded aprons and thyroid shields minimize exposure to scattered radiation.[7]

3. Personnel should be positioned out of the direct line of the primary projection beam.[8] Personnel, even when protected by leaded aprons, leaded shields, and thyroid shields, should position themselves behind or to the side of and as far away as possible from the radiation beam. Leaded aprons do not attenuate 100% of the radiation beam.

4. Personnel wearing leaded aprons should face the unit that is emitting radiation. To provide protection, the leaded apron must be between the source of radiation and the body.[9]

5. Slings, traction devices, and sandbags should be used to maintain patient position during radiation exposure. Cassette holders should be used to position films. Personnel should not hold the patient unless absolutely necessary and should avoid exposure to the direct beam. Protective gloves and leaded aprons should be worn if the patient must be held. Holding devices allow personnel to reduce their exposure by distancing themselves from direct and scattered radiation.[10]

6. During fluoroscopy, personnel should wear
   ♦ leaded aprons,
   ♦ thyroid shields if they are in proximity to the patient,
   ♦ eye protection (eg, lead-glass lenses, face masks with lead-acrylic windows) if they are next to the patient during frequent or long periods of fluoroscopy, and
   ♦ radioprotective gloves if their hands are exposed to the direct beam.

The potential for exposure to radiation is greater during fluoroscopy than during conventional radiographic studies due to increased radiation scatter and exposure time. The areas at greatest risk of radiation exposure for personnel within a 6-ft (ie, 2-m) range of the radiation source are the head, neck, and hands. In practice, perioperative personnel may receive the same exposure to their unprotected thyroid as the surgeon. Moving and holding the C-arm unit during fluoroscopy exposes the surgeon's fingers to high dosages of radiation. Radiation-attenuating

surgical gloves block 50% of the dosage.[11] The lens structure of the eye is sensitive to radiation.[12] Lead-glass lenses and face masks with lead-acrylic windows afford a high degree of protection. There is a significant degree of lens and brain dose reduction afforded by the use of glass or photochromic lenses.[13]

7. During lateral/oblique radiation, including fluoroscopy, personnel remaining in the OR should wear leaded aprons and thyroid shields and stand at least 6 ft away from the projected beam. Levels of scattered radiation can increase up to four times when the radiation is directed at an oblique angle. This results in greater exposure to the head and neck areas of personnel in proximity.[14]

8. Guidelines for radiation safety are based on the principles of time, distance, and shielding. When exposed to radiation at a constant rate, the total dose equivalent received depends on the length of time exposed. If the distance from the point source of radiation is doubled, the exposure is quartered. Radiation that scatters as the x-ray beam passes through the patient also can be a source of radiation exposure. Passage through materials reduces the amount of radiation. Government regulations stipulate the dose limits for occupational exposure and are described in the glossary.

At the time of the publishing of this document, there was no industry consensus regarding the management of the patient undergoing sentinel node biopsy.

Recommended Practice IV

Shielding devices should be handled carefully and examined periodically to prevent and detect damage that could diminish their effectiveness.

1. When leaded aprons and thyroid shields are stored, they should be laid flat or hung vertically and should not be folded. Leaded aprons and shields are very susceptible to cracking, which can reduce the apron's effectiveness as a shielding barrier.[15]

2. Leaded protective devices should be tested for effectiveness at defined intervals by radiology department staff members or radiation safety

experts. Visual inspection is not always adequate to detect cracks. A radiographic test performed at least every 12 months, or whenever damage is suspected, will ascertain integrity of the apron or shield.[16]

Recommended Practice V

Individuals should be protected from exposure to patients who have received diagnostic or therapeutic radionuclides that may pose a radiation risk.

1. Facilities that use therapeutic radionuclides should employ a radiation safety officer (RSO). This individual should determine specific site regulations. The primary function of the RSO is supervision of the daily operation of the radiation safety program to ensure that individuals are protected from radiation. The RSO should determine which people are in frequent proximity to radiation, which should receive monitoring devices, and how occupational exposure is recorded.

2. Radionuclide materials are absorbed by the body, and safety precautions are required depending on the absorption and excretion of the radionuclide.[17] Patients who have received radionuclides may emit radiation.[18] If patients require surgery before the material has decayed to background levels, patients may expose surgical personnel to radiation.[19] Body fluids and tissue removed from patients who have undergone recent diagnostic nuclear medicine studies should be handled according to radiation safety procedures and standard precautions. These standards should be based on government regulations and recommendations. Personnel should use the principles of time, distance, and shielding when caring for patients who have received therapeutic radionuclides.

3. In addition to time, distance, and shielding, contamination-control measures also should apply to the use of radioactive materials.[20] When transferring patients who received therapeutic radionuclides in the OR, perioperative personnel should notify personnel receiving the patients of the radiation source and anatomical location before patient transfer. All radiation precautions should be observed during transport. The RSO should establish precautions.

Advance communication allows personnel to protect themselves and other patients from unnecessary exposure to radiation.[21]

Recommended Practice VI

Radiation monitoring devices should be worn by personnel who are in frequent proximity to radiation, as determined by the RSO.

1. When single monitoring devices are used, they should be worn on the same area of the body by all health care personnel. Radiation monitoring devices are the principal mechanism for monitoring radiation exposure of personnel on a day-to-day basis and, therefore, should be used consistently by health care personnel working with radiation.[22]

2. When two monitoring devices are used, one should be worn at the neckline outside the leaded apron, and the other should be worn inside the leaded apron. The monitor worn under the apron measures whole-body and gonad exposure, and the one at the neckline measures head and neck exposure.[23] Personnel monitoring is required for individuals who have a reasonable probability of exceeding 25% of the occupational dose equivalent limit of five rem (ie, a special unit of dose equivalent) per year in the course of their work.[24]

Recommended Practice VII

Appropriate handling of therapeutic radiation sources in the practice setting should minimize exposure.

1. Radioactive materials should be kept in a protective, lead-lined container. The container effectively shields personnel from exposure to radiation.[25]

2. Radioactive capsules and/or needles must be handled with forceps. Forceps are used to increase the distance between the health care worker and the radiation source. Gloves do not provide shielding for therapeutic radionuclides. They may serve to control contamination if the radionuclide is liquid.[26]

3. Standardized radiation warning signs should be posted at doors to alert persons entering a

room that radioactive material is present. Signs warn persons of the potential for radiation exposure.[27]

Recommended Practice VIII

Measures taken to protect patients from direct and indirect radiation exposure should be documented on the perioperative nursing record.

1. Perioperative nursing documentation should include the type of patient protection and the area(s) protected. Documentation of nursing interventions promotes continuity of patient care, improves communication among health care team members, and serves as a medical legal record of patient care.[28]

Recommended Practice IX

Policies and procedures regarding radiation exposure should be written, reviewed periodically, and readily available within the practice setting.

1. Policies and procedures should be developed collaboratively and approved by perioperative personnel, the RSO, or the director of the radiology department in cooperation with safety committee members or the radiation safety expert in accordance with government regulation. Policies and procedures should be reviewed by a medical radiation physicist. Collaboration should ensure compliance with current radiation safety policies and contribute to quality patient care.[29]

2. Policies and procedures should include, but not be limited to,
   ♦ identifying measures for protecting patients and personnel from unnecessary exposure to ionizing radiation;
   ♦ establishing authority, responsibility, and accountability for radiation safety;
   ♦ developing procedures for handling and disposing of body fluids and tissue that may be radioactive;
   ♦ ensuring that appropriate personnel wear radiation monitoring devices; and
   ♦ scheduling of radiographic testing of the leaded protective devices.

   Policies and procedures establish guidelines for performance improvement activities to be used in

monitoring radiation safety.[30] Radiation safety policies and procedures should be included in the orientation and ongoing education of all perioperative personnel in the practice setting. Education programs should be developed to enhance knowledge that minimizes patient, personnel, and public risk of unnecessary exposure. Personnel should be educated to the risks of radiation exposure and the precautions to minimize it.[31]

Glossary

Absorbed dose: The energy imparted to matter by ionizing radiation per unit mass of irradiated material at the place of interest. The special unit of absorbed dose is the rad.

ALARA: As low as reasonably achievable.

Attenuation: The process by which a beam of radiation is reduced in intensity when passing through some material.

Beam: A unidirectional flow of particle or electromagnetic radiation.

Deep dose equivalent: The dose equivalent at a tissue depth of 1 cm; applies to the external whole body exposure.

Distance: The greater the distance from the source of radiation, the less the exposure. The inverse-square law applies—at a 4-ft distance from the source, the exposure received is one quarter of that received at a 2-ft distance.

Exposure: A measure of the total quantity of radiation reaching a specific point measured in the air. The unit of measure is based on the amount of ionization produced in air by a specified amount of x-ray or gamma-ray energy. Radiation exposure is controlled in three ways—shielding, distance, and time.

External dose: That portion of the dose equivalent received from radiation sources outside the body.

Film badge: A personnel monitoring device that uses film as a sensing medium to determine a worker's occupational exposure to ionizing radiation.

Fluoroscopy: The observation of the internal features of an object by means of the fluorescence produced on a screen by x-rays transmitted through the object.

Gamma radiation: The emission of electromagnetic energy from the nucleus of an atom.

Gonad: Ovary or testis.

Gonad shield: A leaded device used to reduce x-ray exposure to the reproductive organs.

High radiation area: An area in which radiation levels could result in an individual receiving a dose equivalent in excess of 0.1 rem per hour.

Internal dose: That portion of the dose equivalent received from radioactive material taken into the body.

Ionizing radiation: Electromagnetic radiation (eg, x-rays, gamma rays) that yields ions as it passes through tissue.

Leaded apron: A leaded-rubber material worn to protect personnel from scattered radiation.

Occupational dose: Annual exposure limits that took effect in 1994 are

- ♦ total-dose equivalent (internal and external combined)—50 mSv;
- ♦ lenses of eyes—150 mSv; and
- ♦ skin, extremities, and individual organs—500 mSv.[32]

Quantify amount: A millirem is one one-thousandth of a rem.

Rad: Radiation absorbed dose.

Radioactivity: The property, possessed by certain nuclides, of spontaneously emitting particles of gamma radiation or of emitting radiation following orbital electron capture or spontaneous fission.

Radionuclide: A radioactive atom used in nuclear medicine that shows radioactive disintegration and emits alpha and beta particles or gamma rays. Some radionuclides are used for diagnostic studies to trace the function and structure of most organs. Those emitting alpha and beta particles are used primarily for treating malignant tumors.

Rem: A special unit of dose equivalent. The dose equivalent in rems is numerically equal to the absorbed dose in rads multiplied by the quality factor, which, for most medical radiation, is one.

Scatter radiation: Radiation is scattered when an x-ray beam strikes a patient's body, as it passes through the patient's body, and as it strikes surrounding structures (eg, walls, OR furniture).

Shallow dose equivalent: The dose equivalent at a tissue depth of 0.007 cm averaged over an area of 1 cm[2].

Shielding: Radiation interacts with any type of material, and the amount of radiation is reduced during passage through materials. A thin layer of lead can absorb most scattered x-rays. Gamma radiation from medically useful radionuclides is substantially attenuated by 1 to 2 inches of lead.

Thermoluminescent dosimeter: A monitoring device that uses a special crystalline material as a sensing medium in place of film.

Time factor: The less time one is exposed to radiation, the less radiation one absorbs. Remaining close to a source of radiation for 15 minutes, an individual receives one-half the radiation dose received if the exposure time was 30 minutes.

Total effective dose equivalent: The sum of deep dose equivalent (for external exposures) and the committed effective dose equivalent (for internal exposures).

NOTES

1. W K Sinclair, "Radiation protection recommendations on dose limits: The role of the NCRP and the ICRP and future developments," *International Journal of Radiation Oncology, Biology, Physics* 31 (Jan 15, 1995) 388-389; N L Frederiksen, "X-rays: What is the risk?" *Texas Dental Journal* 112 (February 1995) 68-72.

2. M H Barnett, *The Biological Effects of Ionizing Radiation: An Overview*, US Department of Health, Education, and Welfare, publ no 77-8004 (Washington, DC: US Government Printing Office, 1976) 11; H M Cullings, W R Hendee, "Radiation risks in the orthopedic operating room," *Contemporary Orthopaedics* 8 (April 1984) 48; L U Krebs, "Sexual and reproductive dysfunction," in *Cancer Nursing Principles and Practice,* fourth ed, S L Groenwald et al, eds (Boston: Jones and Bartlett Publishers, 1997) 760; National Council on Radiation Protection and Measurements, *Radiation Protection for Medical and Allied Health Personnel* (Bethesda, Md: National Council on Radiation Protection and Measurements, 1989) 12; National Council on Radiation Protection and Measurements, *Limitation of Exposure to Ionizing Radiation* (Bethesda, Md: National Council on Radiation Protection and Measurements, 1993) 38; Committee on the Biological Effects of Ionizing Radiations et al, *Health Effects of Exposure to Low Levels of Ionizing Radiation, Beir V* (Washington, DC: National Academy Press, 1990) 352-354.

3. N H Fortunato, *Berry & Kohn's Operating Room Technique,* ninth ed (New York: Mosby, 2000) 189.

4. B J Gruendemann, B Fernsebner, *Comprehensive Perioperative Nursing, Volume 1: Principles* (Boston: Jones and Bartlett Publishers, 1995) 326; Committee on the Biological Effects of Ionizing Radiations et al, *Health Effects of Exposure to Low Levels of Ionizing Radiation, Beir V,* 365.

5. N H Fortunato, *Berry & Kohn's Operating Room Technique,* ninth ed, 190; Committee on the Biological Effects of Ionizing Radiations et al, *Health Effects of Exposure to Low Levels of Ionizing Radiation, Beir V,* 281

6. National Council on Radiation Protection and Measurements, *Radiation Protection for Medical and Allied Health Personnel,* 27-29; J A Kneedler, G H Dodge, *Perioperative Patient Care: The Nursing Perspective,* third ed (Boston: Jones and Bartlett Publishers, 1994) 131; L Strangio, "Interventional uroradiologic procedures," *AORN Journal* 66 (August 1997) 288.

7. L W Johnson, R J Moore, S Balter, "Review of radiation safety in the cardiac catheterization laboratory," *Catheterization and Cardiovascular Diagnosis* 25 (March 1992) 186-194; M L Phippen, M P Wells, *Patient Care During Operative and Invasive Procedures* (Philadelphia: W. B. Saunders Co, 2000) 156; National Council on Radiation Protection and Measurements, *Radiation Protection for Medical and Allied Health Personnel,* 28.

8. L K Groah, *Perioperative Nursing,* third ed (Stamford, Conn: Appleton & Lange, 1996) 37.

9. *Ibid.*

10. *Ibid.*

11. D H Bagley, A Cubler-Goodman, "Radiation exposure during ureteroscopy," *The Journal of Urology* 144 (December 1990) 1356-1358.

12. *Ibid.*

13. N W Marshall, K Faulkner, P Clarke, "An investigation into the effect of protective devices on the dose to radiosensitive organs in the head and neck," *The British Journal of Radiology* 65 (September 1992) 799-802.

14. Cullings, Hendee, "Radiation risks in the orthopedic operating room," 48-57; Fortunato, *Berry & Kohn's Operating Room Technique,* ninth ed, 190.

15. Gruendemann, Fernsebner, *Comprehensive Perioperative Nursing, Volume 1: Principles,* 330.

16. Groah, *Perioperative Nursing,* third ed, 38.

17. Kneedler, Dodge, *Perioperative Patient Care: The Nursing Perspective,* third ed, 132.

18. Fortunato, *Berry & Kohn's Operating Room Technique,* ninth ed, 189.

19. *Ibid.*

20. Kneedler, Dodge, *Perioperative Patient Care: The Nursing Perspective,* third ed, 132.

21. Groah, *Perioperative Nursing,* third ed, 38.

22. Gruendemann, Fernsebner, *Comprehensive Perioperative Nursing, Volume 1: Principles,* 328-329.

23. Kneedler, Dodge, *Perioperative Patient Care: The Nursing Perspective,* third ed, 131.

24. National Council on Radiation Protection and Measurements, *Radiation Protection for Medical and Allied Health Personnel,* 19; Gruendemann, Fernsebner, *Comprehensive Perioperative Nursing, Volume 1: Principles,* 328.

25. National Council on Radiation Protection and Measurements, *Radiation Protection for Medical and Allied Health Personnel,* 31; Groah, *Perioperative Nursing,* third ed, 38.

26. Groah, *Perioperative Nursing,* third ed, 38; Kneedler, Dodge, *Perioperative Patient Care: The Nursing Perspective,* third ed, 132.

27. National Council on Radiation Protection and Measurements, *Radiation Protection for Medical and Allied Health Personnel,* 30-31.

28. "Recommended practices for documentation of perioperative nursing care," in *Standards, Recommended Practices, and Guidelines* (Denver: AORN, Inc, 2000) 229-231.

29. National Council on Radiation Protection and Measurements, *Radiation Protection for Medical and Allied Health Personnel,* 18-19.

30. "Patient outcomes: Standards of perioperative care," *Standards, Recommended Practices, and Guidelines* (Denver: AORN, Inc, 2000) 181-189.

31. J G Giblin et al, "Radiation risk to the urologist during endourologic procedures and a new shield that reduces exposure," *Urology* 48 (October 1996) 627; Johnson et al, "Review of radiation safety in the cardiac catheterization laboratory," 193.

32. National Council on Radiation Protection and Measurements, *Limitation of Exposure to Ionizing Radiation,* 56.

Originally published October 1989, *AORN Journal.*

Published as proposed recommended practices September 1993.

Revised and reformatted; published January 2001, *AORN Journal.*

Recommended Practices for Skin Preparation of Patients

The following recommended practices were developed by the AORN Recommended Practices Committee and have been approved by the AORN Board of Directors. They were presented as proposed recommended practices for comments by members and others. They are effective January 1, 2002.

These recommended practices are intended as achievable recommendations representing what is believed to be an optimal level of practice. Policies and procedures will reflect variations in practice settings and/or clinical situations that determine the degree to which the recommended practices can be implemented.

AORN recognizes the numerous types of settings in which perioperative nurses practice. These recommended practices are intended as guidelines adaptable to various practice settings. These practice settings include traditional ORs, ambulatory surgery units, physicians' offices, cardiac catheterization suites, endoscopy suites, radiology departments, and all other areas where operative and other invasive procedures may be performed.

Purpose

These recommended practices provide a guideline for achieving skin preparation of the surgical site. The goal of preoperative skin preparation is to reduce the risk of postoperative surgical site infection by removing soil and transient microorganisms from the skin, reducing the resident microbial count to subpathogenic levels in a short period of time and with the least amount of tissue irritation, and inhibiting rapid rebound growth of microorganisms.

Recommended Practice I

The surgical site should be assessed before skin preparation.

1. Skin should be assessed before skin preparation, and the presence of moles, warts, rashes, or other skin conditions at the surgical site should be noted and documented. Inadvertent removal of lesions traumatizes the skin at the surgical site and provides an opportunity for wound colonization by microorganisms.[1]

Recommended Practice II

Whenever possible, hair should be left at the surgical site. If it is determined that hair should be removed, removal should be performed according to physicians' orders and/or according to policies and procedures in the practice setting.[2]

1. An assessment of the amount and degree of hair at the site should be performed. The necessity of hair removal depends on the amount of hair, location of the incision, and type of surgical procedure to be performed. Inappropriate hair removal techniques can traumatize skin and provide an opportunity for colonization of microorganisms at the surgical site.

2. If hair is to be removed at the surgical site, these guidelines should be followed.[3]
   - Personnel skilled in hair removal techniques should perform the removal.
   - Hair removal should be performed as close to the time of surgery as possible, except when a depilatory is to be used (see number four).
   - Hair removal should be performed in an area outside of the room where the procedure will be performed.
   - Hair removal should be performed in a manner that preserves skin integrity.

3. Microscopic exudative rashes and skin abrasions can occur during hair removal. These rashes and skin abrasions can provide a portal of entry for microorganisms.[4] When hair removal is necessary, an electric or battery-powered clipper with a disposable or reusable head that can be disinfected between patients should be used, if possible. This is the simplest and least irritating method of hair removal.[5] If hair is removed, removal should take place away from the sterile field, preferably in an area outside of the room where the procedure will be performed. The dispersal of loose hair has the potential to contaminate the surgical site and sterile field.[6]

4. Depilatories have caused skin reactions in some individuals, causing surgeries to be cancelled.[7] If a depilatory is to be used, manufacturers' written instructions regarding preapplication skin testing should be followed. Depending on the manufacturers' instructions, some depilatories may require use before the patient's arrival in the practice setting.[8]

5. Hair removal with a razor can disrupt skin integrity and is not recommended.

6. All items used in hair removal should be disposed of or disinfected between surgical procedures.

Recommended Practice III

The surgical site and surrounding areas should be clean.

1. The skin around the surgical site should be free of soil and debris. Removal of superficial soil, debris, and transient microbes before applying antiseptic agent(s) reduces the risk of wound contamination by decreasing the organic debris on the skin.[9]

2. Cleansing should be accomplished by any of the following methods before surgical skin preparation:
    ♦ patient showering and/or shampooing before arrival in the practice setting,
    ♦ washing the surgical site before arrival in the practice setting, or
    ♦ washing the surgical site immediately before applying the antiseptic agent in the practice setting.

Recommended Practice IV

When indicated, the surgical site and surrounding area should be prepared with an antiseptic agent.

1. Antiseptic agent(s) should be selected according to AORN's "Recommended practices for product selection in perioperative practice settings"[10] and used in accordance with the manufacturers' written instructions. Antiseptic agent(s) should have a broad range of germicidal action.[11]

2. Data from current research, manufacturers' literature, the Association for Professionals in Infection Control and Epidemiology, and the US Food and Drug Administration should be consulted when selecting an antiseptic agent for skin preparation.

3. Products for skin antisepsis should be chosen carefully according to the patient's condition. Antiseptic agents used on the skin of patients with known hypersensitivity reactions may cause adverse outcomes (eg, blisters, rashes). Some antiseptic agents may be absorbed by the skin or mucous membranes and become neurotoxic or ototoxic.[12] Certain antiseptic agents are believed to be potentially harmful to fetuses or neonates if used on pregnant women and/or nursing mothers.

4. Antiseptic agents used for skin preparation should be applied using sterile supplies. Infection can occur due to a high microbial count at the incision site; therefore, skin preparation should progress from the incision site to the periphery using a sponge/applicator, which should be discarded after the periphery has been reached.[13]

    The use of sterile supplies alone does not reduce microbial counts and rebound microbial activity. Friction during the cleansing process and application of antimicrobial agents are the primary methods for removing soil and transient organisms.[14] Data from one limited study suggest that a clean prep kit may be as effective as a sterile kit for disinfecting skin.[15] Additional research is needed to establish definitive patient outcomes and/or support for a change in practice. Antiseptic products that are marketed with applicators may be applied with clean gloves per the manufacturers' written recommendations; however, there presently are no published data that support the use of clean, as opposed to sterile, gloves.

5. The prepared area of skin and the drape fenestration should be large enough to accommodate extension of the incision, the need for additional incisions, and all potential drain sites.[16] Enlarging the drape fenestration or inadvertent shifting of the drapes can result in contamination, as an unprepared area may be exposed.[17]

Recommended Practice V

Personnel who are knowledgeable about the patient and skilled in skin preparation techniques should prepare the surgical site in a manner that preserves skin integrity and prevents injury to the skin.

1. When preparing the skin for a surgical procedure, special considerations should include
    ♦ preparing areas of high microbial counts (eg, umbilicus, pubis, open wounds) within the prepared areas last;[18]

◆ isolating the colostomy site(s) from the prepared area, covering the site(s) with an antiseptic-soaked sponge, and preparing the colostomy site(s) last;[19]

◆ using normal saline to prepare burned, denuded, or traumatized skin;[20]

◆ avoiding the use of chlorhexidine gluconate and/or alcohol or alcohol-based products on mucous membranes;[21]

◆ using gentle preparation techniques when preparing skin of patients with certain medical conditions (eg, diabetes, skin ulcerations);[22]

◆ allowing sufficient contact time of antiseptic agents before applying sterile drapes to achieve maximum effectiveness of the agent;[23]

◆ allowing sufficient time for complete evaporation of any flammable antiseptic agent (eg, alcohol, alcohol-based preparations) to reduce the possibility of fire;[24] and

◆ preventing antiseptic agent pooling beneath patients, pneumatic tourniquet cuffs, electrodes, or electrosurgical unit dispersive pads to reduce the risk of chemical burns.

Recommended Practice VI

Patient skin preparation should be documented in the patient record according to AORN's "Recommended practices for documentation of perioperative nursing care."[25]

1. Documentation should include, but not be limited to,
   ◆ the condition of the skin at the surgical site (eg, presence of rashes, skin eruptions, abrasions);
   ◆ hair removal, if performed, including method, time of removal, and area;
   ◆ type of skin preparation used (eg, cleansing agent, solvent, antiseptic agent);
   ◆ name(s) of person(s) performing skin preparation; and
   ◆ development of any patient hypersensitivity reactions.

   Documentation of surgical skin preparation may assist in performance improvement and infection control follow-up. Accountability and source of information are established by recording names of personnel who perform procedures. Documentation provides communication for all care providers in developing an ongoing plan of care.[26]

Recommended Practice VII

Policies and procedures on the skin preparation of patients should be written, reviewed annually, and readily available within the practice setting.

1. These recommended practices should be used as guidelines for developing policies and procedures in the practice setting. An introduction and review of policies and procedures should be included in the orientation and ongoing education of staff members to assist in the development of knowledge, skills, and attitudes that affect patient outcomes. Policies and procedures establish authority, responsibility, and accountability and serve as operational guidelines. Policies and procedures also assist in the development of performance improvement activities.

Glossary

Antisepsis: The prevention of sepsis by preventing or inhibiting the growth of resident and transient microbes.

Antiseptic: A product with antimicrobial activity that formerly may have been referred to as an "antimicrobial agent."

Antiseptic agent: An agent capable of producing antisepsis.

NOTES

1. O B Jepsen, K A Bruttomesso, "The effectiveness of preoperative skin preparations: An integrative review of the literature," *AORN Journal* 58 (September 1993) 483; P A Mews, "Establishing and maintaining a sterile field," in *Patient Care During Operative and Invasive Procedures,* ed M L Phippen, M P Wells (Philadelphia: W B Saunders Co, 2000) 78-79; D Fogg, "Infection control," in *Alexander's Care of the Patient in Surgery,* 11th ed, M H Meeker, J C Rothrock, eds (St Louis: Mosby, 1999) 145; A J Mangram et al, "Guideline for prevention of surgical site infection, 1999," *Infection Control and Hospital Epidemiology* 20 (April 1999) 257.

2. Mews, "Establishing and maintaining a sterile field," 78; Fogg, "Infection control," 144; Mangram, "Guideline for prevention of surgical site infection, 1999," 257, 266.

3. M Briggs, "Principles of closed surgical wound care: A review of the factors before, during and after surgical procedures that may predispose patients to post-operative wound infection," *Journal of Wound Care* 6 (June 1997) 290; D J Little, "Preoperative phase," in *Perioperative Nursing: Principles and Practice,* second ed, S S Fairchild, ed (Boston: Little, Brown and Co, 1996) 311; M Simmons, "Preoperative skin preparation," *Professional Nurse* 13 (April 1998) 447; Jepsen, Bruttomesso, "The effectiveness of preoperative skin preparations: An integra-

tive review of the literature," 483; Fogg, "Infection control," 145; Mangram, "Guideline for prevention of surgical site infection, 1999," 257, 266.

4. Briggs, "Principles of closed surgical wound care," 289; Mangram et al, "Guideline for prevention of surgical site infection, 1999," 257, 266.

5. *Ibid*; Fogg, "Infection control," 145.

6. Mews, "Establishing and maintaining a sterile field," 78.

7. M M Olson, J MacCallum, D G McQuarrie, "Preoperative hair removal with clippers does not increase infection rate in clean surgical wounds," *Surgery, Gynecology, & Obstetrics* 62 (February 1986) 181; Jepsen, Bruttomesso, "The effectiveness of preoperative skin preparations: An integrative review of the literature," 483; Mangram et al, "Guideline for prevention of surgical site infection, 1999," 257.

8. Mews, "Establishing and maintaining a sterile field," 78; D S Wendelin, G B Mallory, S B Mallory, "Depilation in a 6-month-old with hypertrichosis: A case report," *Pediatric Dermatology* 16 (July/August 1999) 311; E A Olsen, "Methods of hair removal," *Journal of the American Academy of Dermatology* 40 (February 1999) 147.

9. Mangram et al, "Guideline for prevention of surgical site infection, 1999," 258; Mews, "Establishing and maintaining a sterile field," 79.

10. "Recommended practices for product selection in perioperative practice settings," in *Standards, Recommended Practices, and Guidelines* (Denver: AORN, Inc, 2004) 347-350.

11. K S Hagen, J Treston-Aurand, "A comparison of two skin preps used in cardiac surgical procedures," *AORN Journal* 62 (September 1995) 395; Mews, "Establishing and maintaining a sterile field," 79; Mangram et al, "Guideline for prevention of surgical site infection, 1999," 257.

12. Mews, "Establishing and maintaining a sterile field," 79.

13. *Ibid*; Mangram et al, "Guideline for prevention of surgical site infection, 1999," 258; A Earl, "Operating room," in *APIC Infection Control and Applied Epidemiology: Principles and Practice* (St Louis: Mosby, 1996) 95-1.

14. Mews, "Establishing and maintaining a sterile field," 77, 79; Mangram et al, "Guideline for prevention of surgical site infection, 1999," 258; D K Gauthier, P T O'Fallon, D Coppage, "Clean vs sterile surgical skin preparation kits," *AORN Journal* 58 (September 1993) 486-495.

15. Gauthier, O'Fallon, Coppage, "Clean vs sterile surgical skin preparation kits," 494.

16. Mangram "Guideline for prevention of surgical site infection, 1999," 258.

17. *Ibid*, 267; S S Fairchild, "Foundations of surgery" in *Perioperative Nursing: Principles and Practice,* second ed, S S Fairchild, ed (Boston: Little, Brown and Co, 1996) 255; Fogg, "Infection control," 148.

18. Earl, "Operating room," 95-1; N H Fortunato, *Berry & Kohn's Operating Room Technique,* ninth ed (St Louis: Mosby, 2000) 507; S S Fairchild, "Patient care management," in *Perioperative Nursing: Principles and Practice,*

second ed, S S Fairchild ed (Boston: Little, Brown and Co, 1996) 333; Fogg, "Infection control," 145.

19. Fortunato, *Berry & Kohn's Operating Room Technique,* 507; Fairchild, "Patient care management," 333.

20. Fortunato, *Berry & Kohn's Operating Room Technique,* 507.

21. Briggs, "Principles of closed surgical wound care," 290; Mews, "Establishing and maintaining a sterile field," 79-80.

22. Mews, "Establishing and maintaining a sterile field," 79.

23. E Larson, "APIC guideline for infection control practice: Guideline for use of topical antimicrobial agents," *American Journal of Infection Control* 16 (December 1988) 259; W Rutala, "APIC guidelines for infection control practice: APIC guideline for selection and use of disinfectants," *American Journal of Infection Control* 24 (August 1996) 330, 334; Groah, "Preparation of the patient and surgical team members," 207-208; Mangram et al, "Guideline for prevention of surgical site infection, 1999," 258.

24. Mews, "Establishing and maintaining a sterile field," 79; Mangram et al, "Guideline for prevention of surgical site infection, 1999," 257.

25. Fogg, "Infection control," 145; K J Donahoe, "Plastic and reconstructive surgery," in *Alexander's Care of the Patient in Surgery,* 11th ed, M H Meeker, J C Rothrock, eds (St Louis: Mosby, 1999) 1032; Fortunato, *Berry & Kohn's Operating Room Technique,* 317, 506; "Recommended practices for documentation of perioperative nursing care," in *Standards, Recommended Practices, and Guidelines* (Denver: AORN, Inc, 2001) 199-201.

26. "Recommended practices for documentation of perioperative nursing care," 199-201.

RESOURCES

Association for Professionals in Infection Control and Epidemiology, http://www.apic.org (accessed 11 Oct 2001).

Bryne, D, et al. "Wound infection rates: The importance of definition and post-discharge wound surveillance," *Journal of Hospital Infection* 26 (January 1994) 37-43.

Centers for Disease Control and Prevention, http://www.cdc.gov (accessed 11 Oct 2001).

Hallstrom R; Beck S L. "Implementation of the AORN skin shaving standard. Evaluation of a planned change," *AORN Journal* 58 (September 1993) 498-506.

US Food and Drug Administration, http://www.fda.gov (accessed 11 Oct 2001).

Originally published May 1976, *AORN Journal,* as "Standards for preoperative skin preparation of patients." Format revision March 1978, July 1982.

Revised February 1983, November 1988, November 1992; June 1996. Published November 1996, *AORN Journal;* reformatted July 2000.

Revised November 2001; published January 2002, *AORN Journal.*

Recommended Practices for the Care and Handling of Specimens in the Perioperative Environment

The following recommended practices were developed by the AORN Recommended Practices Committee and have been approved by the AORN Board of Directors. They were presented as proposed recommended practices for comments by members and others. They are effective January 1, 2006.

These recommended practices are intended as achievable recommendations representing what is believed to be an optimal level of practice. Policies and procedures will reflect variations in practice settings and/or clinical situations that determine the degree to which the recommended practices can be implemented.

AORN recognizes the numerous types of settings in which perioperative nurses practice. These recommended practices are intended as guidelines adaptable to various practice settings. These practice settings include traditional ORs, ambulatory surgery centers, physicians' offices, cardiac catheterization suites, endoscopy suites, radiology departments, and all other areas where operative and other invasive procedures may be performed.

Purpose

These recommended practices provide guidance for the implementation of containment, identification, labeling, preservation, transfer, transport, and disposition of surgical specimens. *Specimens* in this document include tissue, blood, body fluids, or foreign bodies (eg, plates, screws) removed from a patient for pathological, microbiological, or gross examination. Specimen identification, collection, and handling are multidisciplinary tasks that require vigilant attention to detail so that each person in the chain of custody understands the patient's needs and is aware of information about the specimen. Mishandling or misidentification of specimens can lead to inaccurate or incomplete diagnosis or the need for additional procedures.[1,2] These recommended practices are not intended to address aspects of perioperative patient care addressed in other recommended practices.

Recommended Practice I

Assessment of specimen collection and special handling needs should begin when the procedure is scheduled.

1. Specimen handling should be assessed and planned before the procedure. This assessment includes persons and departments to be notified (eg, pathology for frozen section), supplies needed for transfer or transport, availability of personnel, or specific requirements necessary for collection or handling of the specimen (eg, timing of transfer, solution, container). Early patient assessment and preplanning minimizes the time required during the surgical procedure and reduces the potential for mishandling specimens.

2. Containers and collection devices of appropriate size and type with correct preservatives should be determined and obtained before the procedure. Containers should be large enough to safely secure the specimen and fluids, if used, to prevent leakage and unnecessary exposure of personnel or others handling the container or its contents. The container and collection device also should be of a size appropriate to allow the preservatives or solutions, if used, to contact all surfaces of the specimen. Collection containers may be sterile or clean, depending on collection requirements.

3. The patient's cultural considerations should be assessed to determine appropriate handling and disposal of specimens. Circumstances may require that specimens be handled or disposed of differently than routine requirements. The patient's written permission may be needed in advance for special requests.

Recommended Practice II

Procedures for correct patient and specimen identification should be implemented, including confirmation of consistent and accurate patient information on labels and forms.

1. Patient identification should be confirmed using two unique identifiers according to health care organization policy at the time the specimen is removed from the patient and when it is placed in the container for transfer and transport. Two unique patient identifiers should be used to minimize the risk of misidentification. Misidentification of a specimen, margins, or other information about a specimen can result in adverse outcomes, delay, error in diagnosis or treatment, or the need for an additional procedure.[2]

2. Specimen identification should begin at the time the specimen is removed from the patient with both verbal and written communication

to confirm information. Communication should include a "read back" verification of the information. Using a "write down, read back" process to confirm the communication minimizes the risk of miscommunication.

3. Identification of the specimen should be confirmed verbally between the surgeon and registered nurse circulator and documented completely on the appropriate form(s). Identification should include, but is not limited to,
   ♦ originating source of specimen (eg, site or side),
   ♦ type of tissue,
   ♦ clinical diagnosis, and
   ♦ pertinent clinical information.

   Specific types of specimens may require additional information (eg, breast masses, which may include tissue markers of various types and suture tags for orientation.)

4. Each specimen removed for examination should be clearly documented on the specimen container, operative record, and pathology documents.

5. Specimens should be protected and secured on the sterile field to maintain the integrity of the specimen. Specimens should be passed off the sterile field as soon as possible. Specimens that must be kept on the surgical field before transfer should be maintained and labeled appropriately to prevent loss, damage, or mishandling.

6. Specimens transferred from the sterile field should be visibly labeled by the scrub person to prevent errors and misidentification, following verbal communication and verification (ie, "write down, read back") of the information. Written communication about the specimen at the time of removal, confirmed with the surgeon, minimizes opportunities for errors during the transfer/transport process.

Recommended Practice III

Collection and handling of a specimen should be completed in a manner that protects and secures the specimen and prevents contamination of personnel handling the specimen.

1. Specimens secured on the sterile field before transfer should be maintained in a manner to prevent misidentification or mishandling. The method of maintaining the tissue should be consistent with the specimen type; this often requires that tissue remain moistened with sterile saline to prevent drying.

2. The specimen should be contained and labeled immediately to prevent mishandling and errors. Securing specimens at the point of removal (eg, specimen cup) prevents damage and minimizes the risk of mishandling.

   Specimens and containers removed from the surgical field should be handled using standard precautions. The sterility (if indicated) and integrity of the specimen should be maintained during transfer from the sterile field to the container. Clean secondary packaging should be used to prevent contamination of personnel and the environment during transport of specimens.

3. Specimen containers containing a preservative or anticoagulant should be mixed thoroughly before the specimen is placed in the container. The use of preservatives or chemical additives for tissue preservation should be confirmed with the physician. Personnel should practice safety and protective precautions when working with chemical agents.[3]

4. Specimens removed from the procedural area should be secured in an impervious container. The size or type of container is dependent on size of the specimen, timing of the specimen review, preservatives, and containment for transport of the specimen. Containers and collection devices should allow for transfer and transport of biohazardous material without leaking or spilling. Containers should be rigid, leak-proof, sturdy, and nonreactive to fixative solutions such as formalin and alcohol. Lids should fit tightly to prevent spillage.[4]

5. Syringes used for specimen collection and containment should be capped without needles. Needles should not be left on syringes that will be transported. Needles create an unnecessary hazard to those transporting and receiving specimens and may invalidate results due to exposure to air.

6. Caution should be used when handling or dispensing formalin. It can be absorbed through the skin and nasal passages, splashed in the

eyes, and ingested. Exposure can result in irritation, burns, and allergic reactions.[5]

♦ All formalin in the OR should be stored in one location, along with a material safety data sheet. Storage and use of formalin is regulated by the Occupational Safety and Health Administration and other federal and state health regulatory agencies.[6]

♦ Personnel handling formalin should wear appropriate personal protective equipment, which includes face and eye shields, gloves, and other protective garments.[5-7]

♦ Formalin should be dispensed and stored in an area other than the OR. The room should have a ventilation system incorporating negative pressure and an exhaust hood.[7]

♦ Policies and procedures should be established for safe storage and dispensing of formalin in the surgical environment.

♦ Personnel should be educated about the safe handling of formalin, including containment and cleanup of spills, and other measures to minimize risk of exposure.

♦ Formalin should be disposed of according to state and local regulations. Formalin is a U-listed chemical, hazardous upon disposal, and regulated by the US Environmental Protection Agency.[8]

Recommended Practice IV

Specimen containers should be labeled to communicate patient, specimen, preservative, and biohazard information.

1. Two unique identifiers should be used to identify the patient reference. Information on the label should include, but not be limited to,
   ♦ specimen type and site,
   ♦ health care organization-defined unique identifiers (eg, patient name and hospital number), and
   ♦ current date and time.

   Dark, indelible ink should be used. The label or tag should be secured on the specimen container.

2. Containers should be labeled to indicate that a biohazardous material is being transported to prevent contamination of personnel transporting or receiving the specimen.[4]

3. If chemical preservatives are used, the label should clearly identify these additives.

4. The label should be placed on the container, not the lid. This prevents the loss of appropriate identification after the container is opened for processing.

Recommended Practice V

Tissue specimens should be designated for routine pathological exam, gross identification only, or disposal according to health care organizational policies.

1. All tissue must be disposed of in a manner consistent with state and federal guidelines, whether or not needing pathological examination.[2]

2. Health care organizations should develop policies and procedures regarding which tissues require only gross identification or disposal.[9-11]

3. The pathologist has the ultimate responsibility for making decisions about the extent of the examination of the tissue.

Recommended Practices VI

Health care organizations should establish communication and documentation methods regarding specimen accountability and accurate documentation.

1. Documentation should include, but not be limited to,
   ♦ type of specimen;
   ♦ patient name, age, gender, health care organization, history, and diagnosis;
   ♦ studies required;
   ♦ date and time of collection;
   ♦ information pertinent to the specimen or source;
   ♦ surgeon's name and contact number; and
   ♦ the registered nurse doing the preparation and documentation of the specimen for transport.

2. Documentation via printed tools should be used to minimize errors related to handwriting and inaccuracies. When handwritten documentation is required, it should be accurate and legible. Common reasons for pathology errors are unlabeled containers, insufficient patient

identification, and incomplete or illegible information. Technology applications, such as bar coding, may be used to minimize errors.[12]

3. Specimen identification and requisition forms should accompany the specimen in a manner that protects the form and keeps it secured with the specimen.

4. Documentation should establish the chain of custody from the point of removal until pathological examination. Chain of custody is required for tissue specimens as well as material removed for forensic examination (see Recommended Practice IX).

5. Methods should be implemented to accurately record critical information such as tissue margins or orientation of the tissue as it relates to the anatomy, special tests requested, or disposition of the specimen. Requests for other than routine handling should be noted (eg, decalcification, x-ray, freezing). Delays or misdiagnosis can occur when the information is not accurately or completely communicated for the examination.[1]

6. Criteria for verbal and written specimen identification should be established to prevent misinformation. Commonly used methods include "write down, read back" verification of verbal communication. Communication should include, but not be limited to,
   ♦ physician to physician,
   ♦ physician to scrub person,
   ♦ scrub person to registered nurse circulator, and
   ♦ physician to registered nurse circulator.

7. Any communication between physicians, such as pathologist and surgeon, should be direct (ie, not through an intermediary) when it relates to diagnosis or specific diagnostic information about the specimen. A record of communication should be documented in the patient's record, such as the direct report of frozen section results to the surgeon. If communication directly between physicians is not possible, it should be written, marked with the date and time, and included in the patient's record.

8. If the patient requests to keep a removed item (eg, implanted medical device), the nurse should follow procedures for identification and standard precaution guidelines per health care organization policy.

9. Requests for specimens to be returned to the patient should follow health care organization policy after the pathology examination is complete.

10. Disposition of all removed tissue, devices, and implants should be documented on the operative record according to health care organization policy or state guidelines.

Recommended Practice VII

Explanted defective medical devices must be reported to the manufacturer.[13]

1. Medical devices removed due to apparent failure of the device must be retained by the facility. All portions of the device should be retained together, as well as the packaging, if available.

2. Defective explanted medical devices should be sent for pathology examination for identification purposes.

3. The removed medical device should not be decontaminated or sterilized before it is transported from the surgical suite.

4. A risk management report should be completed regarding the defective device, per health care organization policy, and reported to the manufacturer.

5. Documentation should include the reason for removal, if known.

Recommended Practice VIII

Transfer and transport methods and processes should be established by the health care organization according to the specimen type and diagnostic requirements.

1. Procedures should be established to prevent mishandling of specimens by verifying patient and specimen information before transfer, and by transport personnel at each point of exchange. Proper documentation allows tracking of the specimen from its source to its final

disposition. A logbook should be used to record specimen, date, time, and the name of each person involved in each transfer process.

2. All specimens must be identified as biohazardous and transported in a manner that prevents contamination by chemical, blood, and other potentially infectious material to personnel and the environment.[3]

3. Containers with chemicals must have proper identifiers and labeling.[3]

4. Accompanying documents should be protected from contamination.

5. Specimens should be transferred and transported in a manner that protects their viability. This may include, but is not limited to, protective packaging, temperature control, adequate fluids, or culture media.

6. Specimens that will not be transported immediately to the laboratory should be temporarily stored to maintain integrity for examination. Appropriate equipment with a biohazard sign should be available for holding specimens at the correct temperature until transport can take place according to the guidelines of the Clinical Laboratory Improvement Act.[14]

7. Specimens should be transported in a manner that ensures confidentiality of personal health information and minimizes visibility of the specimen.[15]

8. Documentation should be completed to establish the chain of custody from the point of removal until examination. Chain of custody is required for tissue specimens as well as materials removed for forensic examination.

Recommended Practice IX

Forensic specimens should be handled in a manner that preserves the condition of the evidence and verifies that the evidence has been in secure possession at all times.

1. The surgeon should place the evidence directly into a designated envelope or bag. The contents should be listed and described on the appropriate form (eg, "Release of Evidence" or similar form) and attached to the envelope or bag. The evidence envelope or bag should be labeled with the patient's identification, collection date, time, and name of collector.

2. The sealed evidence envelope should be given to the responsible law enforcement officer. If the law enforcement officer is not immediately available, the health care organization's policy for disposition of a sealed evidence envelope and attached documentation should be followed. Documentation in the operative record should include, but not be limited to,
   ◆ description of the removed item,
   ◆ area of the anatomy from which it was removed, and
   ◆ disposition.

3. Bullets should not be handled with metal instruments, if possible, because these may scratch the bullet surface.[16] After the bullet is removed, it should be placed into a nonmetal container and sealed evidence envelope. Bullets should be submitted per local and state law enforcement requirements.

4. In cases involving an ongoing criminal investigation, all of the patient's clothes and belongings should be secured as evidence, regardless of condition. Clothing removed from the patient should be cut along the seams or around bullet or stab wound holes. Items should be placed in a paper bag with the patient's identification, then into a personal belongings bag with the patient's identification. Plastic bags trap moisture and may facilitate growth of mold, which could destroy evidence. After collecting objects in appropriate paper containers, place heavily saturated objects in plastic to avoid leakage of fluids and contamination to evidence collectors.[17] Disposition must be completed per local and state law enforcement requirements.

5. Informational evidence (eg, patient statements, appearance, behavior, bodily marks) should be documented in detail.

6. Documentation should be completed to establish the chain of custody from the point of removal until examination.[18] Chain of custody is required for tissue specimens as well as clothing and other personal items removed for forensic examination.

Recommended Practice X

Each health care organization should develop written procedures for handling radioactive pathology specimens. These procedures should include, but are not limited to, specimen handling, labeling, transportation, storage, and disposal. The procedures should keep radiation exposure to hospital workers as low as reasonably achievable.[19,20]

1. Procedures should be developed in conjunction with the health care organization's radiation safety officer.

2. Policies should describe how specimen containers are labeled.[21]

3. Specimens containing radioactive materials should be promptly transported from the OR to the pathology department in properly labeled and sealed containers.

4. The health care organization should validate competencies of all personnel handling radioactive specimens.

Recommended Practice XI

Policies and procedures related to the collection and handling of specimens and establishment of safe practices should be developed, reviewed periodically, revised as necessary, and readily available in the practice setting.

1. Policies and procedures for the collection and handling of specimens should be written and approved by the disciplines responsible for collecting, handling, examining, storing, and transporting specimens and other related activities. Policies and procedures establish authority, responsibility, and accountability and serve as operational guidelines. Policies and procedures also assist in the development of patient and health care worker safety, quality assessment, and improvement activities. Nurses should collaborate with all members of the health care team and related law enforcement agencies to develop policies that address collection and handling of surgical or forensic specimens. Multidisciplinary review of policies and procedures ensures that specimen collection and handling policies are based on current knowledge and

legal requirements. Applicable state and federal regulations must be followed.

2. Elements for safe specimen handling should include, but are not limited to,
   ♦ containers, collection devices, and preservatives for each specimen type;
   ♦ specimen, tissue, and patient identification;
   ♦ labeling;
   ♦ transfer and transport;
   ♦ maintenance of the specimen;
   ♦ documentation and communication of test ordered;
   ♦ chain of custody;
   ♦ patient requests or needs;
   ♦ specimen disposition; and
   ♦ communication of test results.

3. Education, competency assessment, and validation should be conducted at the time of employment. This includes, but is not limited to,
   ♦ roles, responsibilities, and methods of communication required when specimens are removed;
   ♦ methods and materials used for various types of specimen collection and handling;
   ♦ regulatory guidelines related to specimen collection and handling; and
   ♦ safety practices that ensure proper collection and handling.

4. Policies and procedures establish authority, responsibility, and accountability and serve as operational guidelines. Introduction and review of policies and procedures should be included in orientation and ongoing education of personnel to assist in the development of knowledge, skills, and attitudes that affect patient care. Policies and procedures also assist in development of performance improvement activities.

5. The uniform perioperative nursing vocabulary should be used to document specimens on the intraoperative patient record. The perioperative nursing vocabulary is a clinically relevant, empirically validated, standardized language describing perioperative nursing care. This standardized language consists of a collection of data elements, the Perioperative Nursing Data Set (PNDS), and includes perioperative nursing diagnoses, interventions, and outcomes.

Table 1

SAMPLE POLICIES AND PROCEDURES FOR PACKAGING AND HANDLING SPECIMENS[1]	
Aerobic culture	Minimize swab exposure to air.
Anaerobic culture	Should be collected via a closed system from deep sites, bypassing normal flora. The best method is an anaerobic tube or sterile container. Do not add fluid. Swabs are the least effective. Tissue or fluid specimens are the best; fluid must be in a capped syringe without air. Tube contains transport medium, and tissue/swab should be imbedded in transport medium. Send to laboratory within 30 minutes. Large specimens may be collected in a closed, sterile container, as they retain anaerobic conditions within the tissue.
Biopsy	Usually sent fresh, no preservative; taken to pathology immediately.
Cultures	Maintain sterility of container when placing specimen.
Cytology	For sputum, bronchial, or peritoneal washings. Saline or heparin may be added to some types.
Frozen section	No fixative, kept moist. Intended for immediate transport to pathology department for a special freezing and slicing process for a tentative diagnostic reading.
Fungal	Examination done on a culture specimen.
Gram stain	Sent with a culture specimen. May request anaerobic or aerobic testing.
Pap smear	A type of cytology in a special pap fixative (99% alcohol).
Routine tissue specimen	Kept moist and placed in a container to protect integrity of tissue. Generally placed in refrigerator for pathology pickup within a few hours or overnight.
Stones	Stones may be placed in a dry specimen container. Tissue specimens that contain stones should be placed in buffered formalin (ie, gallbladder with stones).
Swab	Place in an approved swab transport device.
Urine	Place in a sterile container.

1. *"Specimen collection guide," University of Washington Department of Laboratory Medicine,* http://depts .washington.edu/labweb/PatientCare/Clinical/Specimen.htm *(accessed 12 Jan 2006).*

The expected outcomes of primary importance to these recommended practices are outcome 24 (O24), "The patient's care is consistent with the perioperative plan of care," and outcome 28 (O28), "The patient's value system, lifestyle, ethnicity, and culture are considered, respected, and incorporated in the perioperative plan of care as appropriate." The intervention specific to the domain of Safety is intervention 84 (I84), "Manages specimen handling and disposition."[22]

6. Quality monitoring of specimen collection processes, handling, and transport should be established to identify trends or near misses. A focus on error reduction should be developed. Methods of root cause analysis should be used to examine near misses or specimen handling errors to identify opportunities for improvement.

7. Packaging and handling of specimens should follow policies and procedures developed by the health care organization (Table 1).

Glossary

Cytology: The study of cells, including their formation, origin, structure, function, biochemical activities, and pathologic characteristics.

Forensic evidence: Evidence for use in legal or criminal proceedings.

Microbiology: The study of microorganisms, including bacteria, fungus, algae, and protozoa.

Specimen: Tissue or body substance removed for study.

Frozen section: A method used in preparing a selected portion of tissue for pathologic examination. The tissue is moistened and, fixed or unfixed, is rapidly frozen and cut by a microtome in a cryostat. This method is very rapid, allowing the pathologist to examine the specimen during a surgical procedure.[23]

Chain of custody: A legal term that refers to the ability to guarantee the identity and integrity of the specimen from collection through to reporting of the test results. A process used to maintain, secure, and document the chronological history of the evidence.[24]

NOTES

1. R E Nakhleh, G Gephardt, R J Zarbo, "Necessity of clinical information in surgical pathology: A College of American Pathologists Q-probes study of 771,475 surgical pathology cases from 341 institutions," *Archives of Pathology and Laboratory Medicine* 123 (July 1999) 615-619.

2. L Slavin, M A Best, D C Aron, "Gone but not forgotten: The search for the lost surgical specimens; Application of quality improvement techniques in reducing medical error," *Quality Management in Health Care* 10 no 1 (2001) 45-53.

3. "Occupational exposure to hazardous chemicals in laboratories," 29 CFR 1910.1450, Occupational Safety and Health Administration, *http://www.osha.gov/pls/oshaweb/owadisp.show_document?p_table=STANDARDS&p_id=10106* (accessed 13 Oct 2005).

4. "Guidelines for the safe transport of infectious substances and diagnostic specimens," publ WHO/EMC/97.3 (1997), World Health Organization, *http://www.who.int/csr/emc97_3.pdf* (accessed 29 Nov 2005).

5. "Material safety data sheet: Formalin solution 5%," Science Stuff, Inc, *http://www.sciencestuff.com/msds/C1776.html* (accessed 11 Aug 2005).

6. "Substance technical guidelines for formalin," 29 CFR 1910.1048 App A, Occupational Safety and Health Administration, *http://www.osha.gov/pls/oshaweb/owadisp.show_document?p_table=STANDARDS&p_id=10076* (accessed 13 Oct 2005).

7. "Recommended guidelines for controlling noninfectious health hazards in hospitals (continued)," National Institute for Occupational Safety and Health, *http://www.cdc.gov/niosh/hcwold5a.html* (accessed 29 Nov 2005).

8. "Introduction to hazardous waste identification," 40 CFR Parts 261 (September 2003), US Environmental Protection Agency, *http://www.epa.gov/epaoswer/hotline/training/hwid05.pdf* (accessed 29 Nov 2005).

9. R Zarbo, R Nakhleh, "Surgical pathology specimens for gross examination only and exempt from submission," *Archives of Pathology and Laboratory Medicine* 123 (February 1999) 133-139.

10. P Fitzgibbons, K Cleary, "CAP offers recommendations on selecting surgical specimens for examination," *CAP Today* 10 (July 1996) 40.

11. "College of American Pathologists policy on surgical specimens to be submitted to pathology for examination," (1999) College of American Pathologists, *http://www.cap.org/apps/docs/laboratory_accreditation/surgical_specimens.pdf* (accessed 19 Oct 2005).

12. P N Valenstein, R L Sirota, "Identification errors in pathology and laboratory medicine," *Clinical Laboratory Medicine* 24 (December 2004) 979-996.

13. "Medical device tracking requirements," 21 CFR 821 (April 1, 2005), US Food and Drug Administration, *http://www.accessdata.fda.gov/scripts/cdrh/cfdocs/cfcfr/CFRSearch.cfm?CFRPart=821&showFR=1* (accessed 13 Oct 2005).

14. "CLIA Subpart K—Quality systems for nonwaived testing," Centers for Medicare and Medicaid Services, Clinical Laboratory Improvement Amendments, *http://www.phppo.cdc.gov/clia/regs/subpart_k.aspx#493.1240* (accessed 29 Oct 2005).

15. "Summary of the HIPAA privacy rule," US Department of Health and Human Services, *http://www.hhs.gov/ocr/privacysummary.pdf* (accessed 29 Oct 2005).

16. S L Hanshaw, "Bullet retrieval in the operating room," *Seminars in Perioperative Nursing* 3 (October 1994) 232-236.

17. G A Muro, C R Easter, "Clinical forensics for perioperative nurses," *AORN Journal* 60 (October 1994) 585-593.

18. M M Evans, P A Stagner, "Maintaining the chain of custody: Evidence handling in forensic cases," *AORN Journal* 78 (October 2003) 563-569.

19. P Fitzgibbons, V LiVolsi, et al, "Recommendations for handling radioactive specimens obtained by sentinel lymphadenectomy," *American Journal of Surgical Pathology* 24 (November 2000) 1549-1551.

20. M Cibull, "Handling sentinel lymph node biopsy specimens: A work in progress," *Archives of Pathology and Laboratory Medicine* 123 (July 1999) 620-621.

21. "Exemptions to labeling requirements," 10 CFR 20.1905, Nuclear Regulatory Commission, *http://a257.g.akamaitech.net/7/257/2422/14mar20010800/edocket.access.gpo.gov/cfr_2002/janqtr/10cfr20.1905.htm* (accessed 13 Oct 2005).

22. S C Beyea, ed, *Perioperative Nursing Data Set: The Perioperative Nursing Vocabulary,* second ed (Denver: AORN, Inc, 2002).

23. *Mosby's Medical, Nursing, and Allied Health Dictionary,* sixth ed (St Louis: Mosby, 2002) 710.

24. "Glossary: Chain of custody," Peace-Officers.com, *http://peace-officers.com/content/glossary/def-chain.shtml* (accessed 29 Oct 2005).

Originally approved November 2005, AORN Board of Directors. Scheduled for publication in the *AORN Journal* in 2006.

Recommended Practices for Standard and Transmission-Based Precautions in the Perioperative Practice Setting

The following recommended practices were developed by the AORN Recommended Practices Committee and have been approved by the AORN Board of Directors. They were presented as proposed recommended practices for comments by members and others. They are effective January 1, 1999.

These recommended practices are intended as achievable recommendations representing what is believed to be an optimal level of practice. Policies and procedures will reflect variations in practice settings and/or clinical situations that determine the degree to which the recommended practices can be implemented.

AORN recognizes the numerous types of settings in which perioperative nurses practice. These recommended practices are intended as guidelines adaptable to various practice settings. These practice settings include traditional ORs, ambulatory surgery units, physicians' offices, cardiac catheterization suites, endoscopy suites, radiology departments, and all other areas where operative and other invasive procedures may be performed.

Purpose

These guidelines identify practices that can be employed to protect patients and health care workers from exposure to bloodborne and body fluid pathogens, which are primary potential sources for transmission of disease. They are inclusive of all personnel at risk for exposure to bloodborne pathogens. They are based in part on the "Guideline for isolation precautions in hospitals," published by the US Department of Health and Human Services Centers for Disease Control and Prevention (CDC). The rapidly changing health care environment presents health care workers with continuing challenges in the form of newly recognized pathogens and long known microorganisms that have become more difficult to eradicate using today's therapeutic measures. Protecting patients and their health care providers from pathogen transmission continues to become more difficult and thus more imperative. Following these guidelines consistently may well be the most effective method to prevent the spread of medication-resistant and disease-causing microorganisms.

Recommended Practice I

Standard precautions to prevent pathogen transmission should be used during all invasive procedures.

1. Standard precautions should be implemented as the primary strategy for successful control of disease-producing microorganisms. Standard precautions apply to exposure or potential for exposure to blood; all body fluids and excretions except sweat, whether or not blood is visible; non-intact skin; and mucous membranes. Standard precautions are designed to reduce the risk of transmission of pathogenic organisms, whatever the source.[1]

Recommended Practice II

Standard precautions should include use of protective barriers and prompt and frequent handwashing to reduce the risk of exposure to potentially infectious materials.

1. Personal protective equipment (PPE) should be used when exposure to potentially infectious materials is anticipated. PPE reduces the risk of exposure to potentially infectious materials. Any patient may be infected with pathogens. PPE for standard precautions includes intact gloves, gowns, masks, and eye protection (eg, face shields, goggles, glasses with side shields).[2] Leg coverings, shoe covers, and other PPE may be used where indicated.

2. If contaminated with blood or body fluids, hands and other skin surfaces should be washed as soon as patient safety permits. Hands should be washed as soon as gloves are removed.[3] Prompt and frequent handwashing can be the single most important measure to reduce the spread of microorganisms.[4]

Recommended Practice III

Personnel should take precautions to prevent injuries caused by scalpels and other sharp instruments.

1. Surgical team members should use hands-free techniques whenever possible and practical, instead of passing needles and other sharp items hand to hand. Studies show that most sharps injuries occur when suture needles or sharps are passed between perioperative team members. Changes in surgical practice to minimize manual manipulation of sharps (ie, no-touch techniques) can have a major impact on these injuries.[5] Creation of a "neutral" zone (ie,

where instruments are put down and picked up, rather than passed hand to hand) may decrease injuries from sharp instruments.[6]

2. All sharps should be handled, removed, and disposed of properly. Containing contaminated sharps in impervious disposal containers helps prevent injuries to the personnel cleaning the room or equipment after use.[7] Used needles should not be sheared, bent, broken, recapped, or resheathed by hand. If recapping is required, mechanical devices or the one-hand technique should be used.[8] Knife blades should be removed using an instrument or device. Disposable sharps should be placed in a puncture-resistant, labeled container.[9] Reusable sharps should be placed in a puncture-resistant container or otherwise separated from other instruments as soon as possible after use.

Recommended Practice IV

Personnel should handle specimens as potentially infectious material.

1. Specimens of blood or other potentially infectious materials should be placed in containers that prevent leakage during collection, handling, processing, storage, transport, or shipping. The exterior surfaces of specimen containers received from the surgical field should be cleaned with a chemical germicide. Placing items in leak-proof containers is intended to eliminate or minimize the possibility of inadvertent contact with blood or other potentially infectious materials.[10]

Recommended Practice V

Work practices should be designed to minimize risk of occupational exposure to bloodborne and other potentially infectious pathogens.

1. Work practice controls should include prohibition of eating, drinking, smoking, applying cosmetics or lip balm, and handling contact lenses in work areas where there is reasonable likelihood of occupational exposure. Hepatitis B virus (HBV) transmission can occur by indirect means via common environmental surfaces contaminated with infectious material.

Although the probability of disease transmission with a single exposure of this type may be remote, activities involving hand-to-nose, hand-to-mouth, or hand-to-eye action can contribute to indirect transmission.[11]

2. Personnel should report exposure incidents to their employers according to facility policy. Prompt reporting enables employers to provide timely and confidential post-exposure evaluation, intervention, testing, or appropriate prophylaxis.[12]

Recommended Practice VI

Personnel who have exudative lesions or weeping dermatitis should refrain from providing direct patient care or handling medical devices used in performing invasive procedures.

1. Restricting personnel who have exudative lesions or weeping dermatitis reduces the risk of transmission of bloodborne and other pathogens between workers and patients.[13]

Recommended Practice VII

Personnel who participate in invasive procedures are encouraged to voluntarily know their HIV and HBV antibody status and disclose a positive status to the appropriate facility authority.

1. Refer to AORN's position statement, "AORN revised statement on the patient and health care workers with human immunodeficiency virus (HIV) and other bloodborne diseases."[14]

Recommended Practice VIII

Guidelines of the Centers for Disease Control Advisory Committee on Immunization Practices regarding HBV immunization should be followed.

1. Personnel participating in invasive procedures or postoperative cleaning and processing should receive HBV immunizations unless medically contraindicated. Immunization against HBV is effective in preventing the disease and should be given before occupational exposure occurs.[15] Information about HBV infection should be provided to employees within 10 days of hire, and informed consent should be given before employees accept HBV immunizations. Employees

who decline the vaccine should sign a declination statement.[16] Vaccination should remain available after this declaration in the event the employee changes his or her mind.

Recommended Practice IX

Transmission-based precautions should be used in addition to standard precautions for patients who are known or suspected to be infected with epidemiologically important and highly transmissible pathogens. Types of transmission-based precautions include airborne, droplet, and contact precautions.

1. Airborne precautions should be used when caring for patients who are known or suspected to have epidemiologically important pathogens that can be transmitted by the airborne route (eg, rubeola, varicella, tuberculosis [TB]). Airborne transmission occurs by dissemination of airborne droplet nuclei (ie, small particle residue 5 microns or smaller in size). Airborne precautions include
   - special air handling and ventilation,
   - respiratory protection to be worn by susceptible persons (ie, not immune to measles or varicella), and
   - placing surgical masks on patients during transport.

   Microorganisms carried by airborne transmission can be dispersed widely by air currents and may become inhaled by or deposited on a susceptible host within the same room or over a longer distance from the source patient.[17]

2. Additional OR considerations for patients known or suspected to have pulmonary TB include the following. Elective surgical procedures on patients who have TB should be delayed until the patient is no longer infectious. If surgical procedures must be performed, they should be done, if possible, in ORs that have anterooms. If no anteroom is available, strict traffic control should be enforced. Attempts should be made to perform procedures at times when other patients are not present in the surgical suite and when a minimum number of personnel are present (eg, at the end of the day). Placing a bacterial filter on patients endotracheal tubes when operating on patients who have confirmed or suspected

TB may help reduce the risk for contaminating anesthesia equipment or discharging tubercle bacilli into the ambient air. When surgical procedures are performed on patients who may have infectious TB, respiratory protection worn by the personnel must protect the field from the respiratory secretions of the health care worker and protect the health care worker from the infectious droplets generated by patients. For additional precautions to prevent transmission of TB, refer to the CDC's "Guidelines for preventing the transmission of tuberculosis in health-care facilities."[18]

3. Droplet precautions should be used when caring for patients who are known or suspected to be infected with microorganisms (eg, diphtheria, pertussis, influenza, mumps) that can be transmitted by infectious large particle droplets (ie, larger than 5 microns in size). Droplet precautions include
   - wearing a mask when within three feet of patients,
   - positioning patients at a distance of at least three feet from other patients, and
   - placing surgical masks on patients during transport.

   Droplets are generated from the source person primarily during coughing, sneezing, or talking. Transmission via droplet requires close contact between patients and personnel; droplets do not remain suspended in the air and generally travel short distances, three feet or less.[19]

4. Contact precautions should be used when providing care for patients who are known or suspected to be infected with microorganisms that are transmitted by direct or indirect contact with patients or items and surfaces in patients' environments (eg, herpes simplex, impetigo, multimedication-resistant pathogens, infectious diarrhea). Contact precautions include
   - wearing gloves when caring for patients or coming in contact with items that may contain high concentrations of microorganisms (eg, fecal material, blood, wound drainage),
   - wearing gowns when it is anticipated that clothing will have substantial contact with patients or items in the patients' environment, (see "Recommended practices for selection and use of surgical gowns and drapes"),

♦ ensuring that precautions are maintained during transport, and

♦ adequately cleaning and disinfecting patient care equipment and items before use with each patient.

Gloves are worn for three reasons:

♦ to protect health care personnel from gross contamination,

♦ to protect patients from health care personnel, and

♦ to keep personnel from transmitting microorganisms from one patient to another.[20]

Gowns are worn to prevent contamination of clothing and to protect personnel's skin from blood and body fluid.[21] When patient transport is necessary, it is important that appropriate barriers are used to reduce the opportunity for transmission of pertinent microorganisms to other patients, personnel, and visitors, and to reduce contamination of the environment.[22] Noncritical equipment (eg, equipment that touches intact skin) contaminated with blood, body fluids, secretions, or excretions should be cleaned and disinfected after use, according to hospital policy.[23]

5. When additional measures are indicated to prevent the spread of highly transmissible or epidemiologically important infectious organisms, an infection control practitioner should be consulted for guidance. The CDC's "Guideline for isolation precautions in hospitals" also outlines transmission precautions.[24]

Recommended Practice X

Policies and procedures that address occupational exposure to blood and body fluids and epidemiologically important microorganisms should be written, reviewed periodically, and readily available within the practice setting.

1. The Occupational Safety and Health Administration and other federal and state regulatory agencies have rules that govern occupational exposure to pathogens. Facility policies and procedures that address occupational exposure to pathogens should be consistent with federal, state, and local regulations.

2. These recommended practices should be used as guidelines for developing policies and procedures within the practice setting. Policies and procedures establish authority, responsibility, and accountability, and serve as operational guidelines. Introduction and review of policies and procedures must be included in the orientation and continuing education of personnel to assist in the development of knowledge, skills, and attitudes that affect patient care. Policies and procedures also assist in the development of quality assessment and improvement activities.

Glossary

Airborne precautions: Precautions that reduce the risk of an airborne transmission of infectious airborne droplet nuclei (ie, small particle residue 5 microns or smaller).

Anteroom: An outer room that leads to another room and that is often used as a waiting room.

Contact precautions: Precautions designed to reduce the risk of transmission of epidemiologically important microorganisms by direct or indirect contact.

Droplet precautions: Precautions that reduce the risk of large particle droplet (ie, 5 microns or larger) transmission of infectious agents.

Exposure incident to pathogens: Specific eye, mouth, or other mucous membranes; nonintact skin; or parenteral contact with blood or other potentially infectious materials that results from the performance of an employee's duties.[25]

Hands-free or no-touch technique: Instrument transfer between the scrub person and the surgeon that ensures that neither ever touches the same sharp instrument at the same time. Instruments can be placed in a neutral zone between the scrub person and the surgeon.[26]

Invasive procedures: The surgical entry into tissues, cavities, or organs, or repair of major traumatic injuries.[27]

Personal protective equipment: Personal protective equipment for standard precautions includes intact gloves, gowns, masks, and eye protection (eg, face shields, goggles, glasses with side shields).

Personnel: Paid or unpaid health care workers, students, volunteers, physicians, and others who may have direct patient contact or opportunity for exposure to patients or devices, supplies, or equipment used for patients.

Potentially infectious material: Blood; all body fluids, secretions, and excretions except sweat, regardless of whether they contain visible blood; nonintact skin; mucous membranes; and airborne, droplet, and contact-transmitted epidemiologically important pathogens.[28]

Sharps: Sharps include, but are not limited to, suture needles, scalpel blades, hypodermic needles, electrosurgical needles and blades, safety pins, and instruments with sharp edges or points.

Standard precautions: The primary strategy for successful nosocomial infection control and reduction of worker exposure; precautions used for care of all patients regardless of their diagnosis or presumed infectious status.[29]

Transmission-based precautions: Second tier of precautions designed to be used with patients known or suspected to be infected or colonized with highly transmissible or epidemiologically important pathogens for which additional precautions are needed to prevent transmission in the practice setting.[30]

NOTES

1. J S Garner, "Guideline for isolation precautions in hospitals," *Infection Control and Hospital Epidemiology* 17 (January 1996) 55.

2. *Ibid,* 63.

3. "Occupational exposure to bloodborne pathogens; Final rule," *Federal Register* 56 (Dec 6, 1991), 64176.

4. Garner, "Guideline for isolation precautions in hospitals," 61.

5. J L Gerberding, "Procedure-specific infection control for preventing intraoperative blood exposures," *American Journal of Infection Control* 21 (December 1993) 365-366.

6. *Ibid,* 366.

7. *Ibid.*

8. "Occupational exposure to bloodborne pathogens; Final rule," 64118.

9. *Ibid.*

10. *Ibid,* 64122.

11. *Ibid,* 64118-64119.

12. *Ibid,* 64175-64176.

13. D J Weber, K K Hoffmann, A Rutala, "Management of the healthcare worker infected with human immunodeficiency virus: Lessons from nosocomial transmission of hepatitis B virus," *Infection Control and Hospital Epidemiology* 12 (October 1991) 628.

14. "AORN revised statement on the patient and health care workers with human immunodeficiency virus (HIV) and other bloodborne diseases," in *Standards, Recommended Practices, and Guidelines* (Denver: Association of Operating Room Nurses, Inc, 1999) 121.

15. Centers for Disease Control, "Recommendations for preventing transmission of human immunodeficiency virus and hepatitis B virus to patients during exposure-prone invasive procedures," *Morbidity and Mortality Weekly Report* 40 (July 12, 1991) 2.

16. "Occupational exposure to bloodborne pathogens; Final rule," 64156.

17. Garner, "Guideline for isolation precautions in hospitals," 65.

18. Centers for Disease Control, "Guidelines for preventing the transmission of *Mycobacterium tuberculosis* in health-care facilities," *Morbidity and Mortality Weekly Report* 43 (Oct 28, 1994) 54242, 54303.

19. Garner, "Guideline for isolation precautions in hospitals," 65-66.

20. Garner, "Guideline for isolation precautions in hospitals," 65-66; "New isolation guidelines written to ease confusion," *OR Manager* 11 (March 1995) 22.

21. Garner, "Guideline for isolation precautions in hospitals," 63, 68.

22. *Ibid,* 62.

23. *Ibid,* 64.

24. *Ibid,* 55.

25. "Occupational exposure to bloodborne pathogens; Final rule," 64175.

26. V Fox, "Passing surgical instruments, sharps without injury," (Clinical Issues) *AORN Journal* 55 (January 1992) 264-266; Garner, "Guideline for isolation precautions in hospitals," 69.

27. Centers for Disease Control, "Guidelines for preventing the transmission of *Mycobacterium tuberculosis* in health-care facilities," 9.

28. Garner, "Guideline for isolation precautions in hospitals," 55.

29. *Ibid.*

30. *Ibid.*

Originally published February 1993, *AORN Journal,* as "Recommended practices for universal precautions in the perioperative practice setting."
Revised November 1998 as "Recommended practices for standard and transmission-based precautions in the perioperative practice setting"; published February 1999, *AORN Journal.*
Reformatted July 2000.

The following recommended practices were developed by the AORN Recommended Practices Committee and have been approved by the AORN Board of Directors. They were presented as proposed recommended practices for comments by members and others. They are effective January 1, 2006.

These recommended practices are intended as achievable recommendations representing what is believed to be an optimal level of practice. Policies and procedures will reflect variations in practice settings and/or clinical situations that determine the degree to which the recommended practices can be implemented.

AORN recognizes the numerous settings in which perioperative nurses practice. These recommended practices are intended as guidelines adaptable to various practice settings. These practice settings include traditional operating rooms, ambulatory surgery centers, physicians' offices, cardiac catheterization suites, endoscopy suites, radiology departments, and all other areas where operative and other invasive procedures may be performed.

Purpose

These recommended practices provide guidance for establishing and maintaining a sterile field. The creation and maintenance of a sterile field can directly influence patient outcomes. Adherence to aseptic practices by all individuals involved in surgical interventions aids in fulfilling the professional responsibility to protect patients from injury. Aseptic practices are implemented preoperatively, intraoperatively, and postoperatively to minimize wound contamination and reduce patient risks for surgical site infections.

Recommended Practice I

Scrubbed persons should function within a sterile field.

1. Before donning sterile gowns and gloves, surgical hand antisepsis should be performed according to AORN's "Recommended practices for surgical hand antisepsis/hand scrubs"[1] and the manufacturer's written instructions for the antiseptic. Surgical hand antisepsis decreases the microbial counts on the skin and will reduce the transfer of microorganisms.

2. Personnel within the sterile field should be attired according to both AORN's "Recommended practices for surgical attire"[2] and "Recommended practices for standard and transmission-based precautions."[3] Personnel should wear scrub attire, caps, masks, eye protection, and sterile gowns and gloves to prevent microbial transference to the sterile field, surgical site, and patient during the surgical procedure and to reduce risk of occupational exposure to bloodborne pathogens and other potentially infectious materials.[4-7]

3. Scrubbed personnel should don sterile gowns and gloves from a sterile area away from the main instrument table to prevent contamination of the sterile field.[8-12]

4. Materials for gowns should be selected according to AORN's "Recommended practices for selection and use of surgical gowns and drapes"[13] and according to the required level of barrier protection as outlined in the Association for the Advancement of Medical Instrumentation (AAMI) guideline "Liquid barrier performance and classification of protective apparel and drapes intended for use in health care facilities."[14] Surgical gowns should be of sufficient size to adequately cover the scrubbed person. Surgical gowns should establish a barrier that minimizes the passage of microorganisms between nonsterile and sterile areas.[12,15]

5. The front of a sterile gown is considered sterile from the chest to the level of the sterile field. The sterile area of the gown front extends to the level of the sterile field because most scrubbed personnel work adjacent to a sterile bed and/or table. Gown sleeves are considered sterile from two inches above the elbow to the cuff, circumferentially.

   The neckline, shoulders, underarms, sleeve cuffs, and gown back are areas of friction and, therefore, are not considered effective microbial barriers. The gown back is considered nonsterile because it cannot be constantly monitored.

   Gowns of an adequate size to close completely in the back and a sleeve length adequate to prevent cuff exposure outside the glove should be selected.

6. Sleeve cuffs should be considered contaminated when the scrubbed person's hands pass beyond the cuff.[9,10,12]

   ♦ Cuffs of the gown should remain at or below the natural wrist area.
   ♦ Gown sleeves should not be pulled up, leaving cuffs exposed.
   ♦ Sleeves of the gown should be of sufficient length and should cover the back of the hand to avoid exposing the gown cuff when the gloves slide down.

7. Scrubbed personnel should inspect gloves for integrity after donning them. Intact gloves establish a barrier that minimizes the passage of microorganisms between nonsterile and sterile areas.[4,12,16] AORN's "Recommended practices for standard and transmission-based precautions"[3] should be followed. Policies and procedures in the practice setting should indicate when double-gloving is required to reduce the potential for hand contact with blood and body fluids.

8. Sterile gloves that become contaminated should be changed as soon as possible. The preferred method of changing gloves is assisted gloving, whereby one member of the sterile team assists another member. This technique allows a gowned and gloved team member to touch only the outside of the new glove when applying the glove to a team member's hand. If this method is not possible, the contaminated glove should be changed by the open-glove method. If it is not possible to change the glove at the moment the break in technique is noted, a new glove may be donned over the contaminated/damaged glove until it can be changed.[9,11,12]

Recommended Practice II

Sterile drapes should be used to establish a sterile field.

1. Surgical drapes should be selected according to AORN's "Recommended practices for selection and use of surgical gowns and drapes"[13] and the AAMI guideline "Liquid barrier performance and classification of protective apparel and drapes intended for use in health care facilities."[14] Surgical drapes should establish an aseptic barrier that minimizes the passage of microorganisms between nonsterile and sterile areas.[15,17,18]

2. To prevent transfer of microorganisms from nonsterile to sterile areas, sterile drapes should be placed on the patient, furniture, and equipment to be included in the sterile field.[19]

3. Sterile drapes should be handled as little as possible. Rapid movement of draping materials creates air currents on which dust, lint, and other particles can migrate.[20,21]

4. Draping material should be held in a compact manner, held higher than the OR bed, and placed from the surgical site to the periphery to minimize contamination of the surgical site. Some procedures may require modified draping techniques (eg, extremities).[9,10,12]

5. During draping, gloved hands should be protected by cuffing the drape material over the gloved hands to reduce the potential for contamination.[9,10,12]

6. The portion of the surgical drape that establishes the sterile field should not be moved after it is positioned. Shifting or moving the sterile drape can compromise the sterility of the field.[9,10,12]

Recommended Practice III

Items used within the sterile field should be sterile.

1. To ensure that only sterile items are presented to the sterile field, all items should be inspected immediately before presentation to the field for proper packaging, processing, seal, package container integrity, and inclusion of a sterilization indicator. The indicator should be inspected immediately to verify the appropriate color change for the sterilization process selected. If an expiration date is provided, the date should be checked before the package is opened and the contents are delivered to the field. Outdated items should not be used.[12,22]

   An event-related sterility system should be used. Event-related sterility is based on the concept that "sterility is not altered over time, but may be compromised by certain events or environmental conditions."[23] Shelf life refers to the time an item may remain on the shelf and still maintain its sterility. Shelf life is influenced by the type of packaging used, storage conditions (eg, open or closed shelves), humidity, temperature, transport conditions, use of dust covers, and the amount of handling the item receives.[12,22,23]

Spaulding's criteria are used to determine the potential for transmission of infectious agents.[24] Within this classification, items contacting the vascular system, the neurological system, and/or sterile tissues pose the greatest risk of infection and are classified as critical items. Using sterile items when contacting sterile tissues minimizes the risk of infection.[12,25-28]

2. Packaging materials should meet the criteria identified in AORN's "Recommended practices for selection and use of packaging systems."[29]

3. Methods of sterilization, event-related shelf life, and handling of sterile items should be in accordance with AORN's "Recommended practices for sterilization in the perioperative practice setting."[30] Sterilization provides the highest level of assurance that surgical items are free of viable microbes. High-level disinfection reduces the risk of microbial contamination, but it does not ensure the same margin of safety that sterilization provides.[25,26,28,31,32]

Recommended Practice IV

All items introduced to a sterile field should be opened, dispensed, and transferred by methods that maintain item sterility and integrity.

1. All invasive surgical procedures should be performed using sterile instruments and supplies, and the surgical team should practice aseptic technique for all surgical patients.

The mucous membranes of the mouth, urinary tract, and intestinal tract are effective bacterial barriers when intact. However, ear, nose, and throat procedures, hemorrhoidectomy, and other procedures are invasive and impair the integrity of the mucosal barrier. The normal flora found in these areas is not infectious to the individual in question, but it may be pathogenic when transferred to other tissues by contaminated surgical instruments.

Health care-acquired surgical infections are a leading cause of patient morbidity and mortality in the United States. Rigorous adherence to the principles of asepsis is the foundation of surgical site infection prevention and should never be circumvented to save time or money. A sterile field should be prepared and maintained for every surgical patient.[4,25,26]

2. Unscrubbed individuals should open wrapped sterile supplies by opening the wrapper flap farthest away from them first, to prevent contamination from passing an unsterile arm over a sterile item. Next, they should open each of the side flaps. The nearest wrapper flap should be opened last.[9-11]

3. All wrapper edges should be secured when supplies are presented to the sterile field. Securing the loose wrapper edges prevents them from contaminating the sterile field or a sterile item.[9,10]

4. Sterile items should be presented to the scrubbed person or placed securely on the sterile field. Items tossed onto a sterile field may roll off the edge, create a hole in the sterile drape, or cause other items to be displaced, leading to contamination of the sterile field.[9,10]

   ♦ Sharps and heavy objects should be presented to the scrubbed person or opened on a separate surface. These heavy items may penetrate the sterile barrier if dropped onto the sterile field.[9,10]

   ♦ Peel pouches should be presented to the scrubbed person to prevent contamination of the contents. The edges of the package may curl and the contents may slide over the unsterile edge, contaminating the contents of the package.

   ♦ Rigid container systems should be opened on a separate surface. The external indicator should be verified for appropriate color change. Locks should be inspected for security to verify there has not been a breach of the container seal prior to use. The lid should be lifted toward the person opening the container and away from the container. The filter should be checked and changed according to the manufacturer's written instructions.

5. All items should be delivered to the surgical field in a manner that prevents nonsterile objects or people from extending over the sterile field. Skin is a source of bacteria and scurf shedding; therefore, maintaining distance from

the sterile field can decrease the potential for contamination when items are passed from a nonsterile area to a sterile area.[9,10,19]

6. When solutions are dispensed, the labeled solution receptacle on the sterile field should be placed near the table's edge or held by the scrubbed person. The entire contents of the container should be poured slowly to avoid splashing. Splashing can cause strike-through and splash-back from nonsterile surfaces to the sterile field. Placing the solution receptacle near the edge of the sterile table allows the unscrubbed person to pour fluids without contaminating the sterile field. Any remaining fluids should be discarded. The edge of a container is considered contaminated after the contents have been poured; therefore, the sterility of the contents cannot be ensured if the cap is replaced. Reuse of open containers may contaminate solutions due to drops contacting unsterile areas and then running back over container openings.[9,10]

7. Medications should be delivered to the sterile field in an aseptic manner. Stoppers should not be removed from vials for the purpose of pouring medications. Sterile transfer devices (eg, sterile vial spike, filter straw, plastic catheter) should be used to dispense medications to the sterile field. Medications should be delivered to the sterile field according to AORN's "Recommended practices for safe care through identification of hazards in the surgical environment,"[33] AORN's "Guidance statement: Safe medication practices in perioperative practice settings,"[34] the "AORN latex guideline,"[35] and the policies and procedures of the practice setting.

Recommended Practice V

A sterile field should be maintained and monitored constantly.

1. The sterile field should be prepared in the location in which it will be used. Moving tables stirs air currents that can contaminate the sterile field.[36]

2. Sterile supplies should be opened for only one patient at a time. Opening several cases in a room at one time increases the risk of cross-infection.

3. One patient at a time should occupy the OR. Concurrent cases performed on two patients in the same room at the same time may expose patients to a variety of hazards and increase the risk of contamination and infection. The transmission of infectious diseases can occur by airborne, contact, and droplet methods. The risk of cross-contamination may be increased significantly when two sterile fields, two surgical teams, and two open surgical wounds are confined to one OR. Operating rooms in the United States are not designed to accommodate the additional personnel and equipment necessary to care for two patients simultaneously. In the United States, general ORs built to the standards of the American Institute of Architects (AIA) are 400 sq ft.[37] Some ORs may be as small as 360 sq ft. This square footage minimum is intended to accommodate the equipment and personnel necessary for one surgical field. To move around the sterile field without contaminating it, nonsterile personnel (eg, the circulating nurse) should maintain a distance of at least 12 inches from the sterile field. When two patients and two sterile fields occupy an area designed to accommodate one patient and one sterile field, contamination of the sterile field is likely.

4. Sterile fields should be prepared as close as possible to the time of use. The potential for contamination increases with time because dust and other particles present in the ambient environment settle on horizontal surfaces over time. Particulate matter can be stirred up by movement of personnel when opening the room and can settle on opened sterile supplies.[4,12,21,36,38,39] The OR environment can be breached by other vectors, such as insects, that potentially could come into contact with open sterile fields, unobserved, unless the sterile field is monitored.

There is no specified amount of designated time that a room can remain open and not used and still be considered sterile. The sterility of an open sterile field is event-related. An open sterile field requires continuous visual observation. Direct observation increases the likelihood of detecting a breach in sterility.[12,39-41]

5. Sterile fields should not be covered. Although there are no research studies to support or

discount the practice, removing a table cover may result in a part of the cover that was below the table level being drawn above the table level or air currents drawing microorganisms from a nonsterile area to the sterile field. It is important to continuously monitor all sterile areas for possible contamination.[12,21]

6. Conversations in the presence of a sterile field should be kept to a minimum to reduce the spread of droplets. Air contains microorganisms on airborne particles, such as respiratory droplets. The primary source of airborne bacteria is health care personnel.[7,12,21,31]

7. Surgical equipment (eg, cables, tubing) should be secured to the sterile field with nonperforating devices. Perforations in a barrier provide portals of entry and exit for microorganisms, blood, and other potentially infectious body fluids.

8. Nonsterile equipment (eg, Mayo stands, microscopes, C-arms) should be covered with sterile barrier material(s) before being introduced to or brought over a sterile field. Only sterile items should touch sterile surfaces. The equipment should be covered with a barrier material on the top, bottom, and all sides. Sterile barrier material also should be applied to the portion of the Mayo stand or other equipment that will be positioned immediately adjacent to the sterile field.[11]

Recommended Practice VI

All personnel moving within or around a sterile field should do so in a manner that maintains the sterile field.

1. Scrubbed personnel should remain close to the sterile field.[9,10] Walking outside the sterile field's periphery or leaving the OR in sterile attire increases the potential for contamination. Using a closed container system for flash sterilization and transport of items eliminates the need for the scrubbed person to leave the sterile field to retrieve instruments from a sterilizer. Scrubbed personnel should avoid leaving the sterile field when x-rays are taken. Protective devices for reducing radiological exposure should be provided to personnel who cannot leave the room or who cannot stand approximately 6 ft away from the source of radiation.[42]

2. Scrubbed personnel should move from sterile areas to sterile areas to prevent contamination. If they must change position, they should turn back to back or face to face while maintaining safe distances from each other and the sterile field.

3. Unscrubbed personnel should face sterile fields on approach, should not walk between two sterile fields, and should be aware of the need for distance from the sterile field. By establishing patterns of movement around the sterile field and keeping sterile areas in view, accidental contamination can be reduced.

4. Scrubbed personnel should keep their arms and hands above the level of their waists at all times. Hands should remain in front of the body above waist level so the hands remain visible. Contamination may occur when arms and hands are moved below waist level. Arms should not be folded with the hands in the axilla. This area has the potential to become contaminated by perspiration, allowing for strike-through of the gown and, ultimately, contamination of the gloved hands. The gown at the axilla also is an area of friction and, therefore, is not considered an effective microbial barrier.

5. Scrubbed personnel should avoid changing levels and should be seated only when the entire surgical procedure will be performed at that level. When changing levels, exposure of the nonsterile portion of the surgical gown is likely.

6. The number and movement of individuals involved in a surgical procedure should be kept to a minimum per AORN's "Recommended practices for traffic patterns in the perioperative practice setting."[36] Bacterial shedding increases with activity. Air currents can pick up contaminated particles shed from patients, personnel, and drapes and distribute them to sterile areas.[12,21,31,43]

7. When a break in sterile technique occurs, corrective action should be taken immediately unless the patient's safety is at risk. If the patient's safety is at risk, correct the break in technique as soon as it is safe to do so.

8. When a break in sterile technique occurs and cannot be corrected immediately, the organization should determine how it should be reported and recorded, and the wound classification

should be adjusted accordingly and documented on the operative record.

Recommended Practice VII

Policies and procedures for maintaining a sterile field should be developed, reviewed periodically, revised as necessary, and readily available in the practice setting.

1. Policies and procedures for maintaining a sterile field should be developed by each facility and should include, but not be limited to,
   ◆ aseptic technique, including handling sterile supplies and monitoring a sterile field;
   ◆ surgical hand antisepsis;
   ◆ gowning and gloving with sterile gown and gloves;
   ◆ masks, head coverings, and scrub attire;
   ◆ draping;
   ◆ event-related sterility;
   ◆ traffic patterns; and
   ◆ monitoring of environmental conditions, including OR air exchange rate and pressure, temperature, and humidity.

2. These recommended practices should be used as a guideline for developing policies and procedures in the perioperative practice setting. Policies and procedures serve as operational guidelines and establish authority, responsibility, and accountability within the facility.

3. Personnel and observers should be knowledgeable about the procedures involved in developing and maintaining a sterile field. An introduction and review of policies and procedures for maintaining the sterile field should be included in orientation to the perioperative setting for personnel and observers. Continuing education should be provided when new technologies (eg, sterilization containers, barrier materials) are introduced. Ongoing education of perioperative personnel facilitates the development of knowledge, skills, and attitudes that affect surgical patient outcomes. Policies and procedures also assist in the development of quality assessment and improvement activities.

4. The Perioperative Nursing Data Set (PNDS) should be used in the development of policies and procedures and documentation of nursing interventions related to maintenance of the sterile field. The expected outcome of primary importance to this recommended practice is outcome O10, "The patient is free from signs and symptoms of infection." This outcome falls within the domain of Physiological Responses (D2). The associated nursing diagnosis is X28, "Risk for infection." The associated interventions that may lead to the desired outcome may be I21, "Assesses susceptibility for infection"; I70, "Implements aseptic technique"; and I98, "Protects from cross-contamination."[44]

Glossary

Asepsis: Process for keeping away disease-producing microorganisms.

Aseptic technique: Methods by which contamination with microorganisms is prevented.

Assisted gloving: Method by which a gowned and gloved person assists another gowned person to don sterile gloves.

Closed gloving method: Used when wearing a sterile gown to prevent exposure of bare skin during gowning and donning of sterile gloves, thereby lessening the chance of contamination.

Critical item: An item that contacts the vascular system or enters sterile tissue, posing the highest risk of transmission of infection.

Event-related sterility: Shelf life of a packaged sterile item depends on the quality of the wrapper material, the storage conditions, the conditions during transport, and the amount of handling.

Noncritical item: An item that comes in contact with intact skin but not with mucous membranes, sterile tissue, or the vascular system.

Open-gloving method: Used when changing a glove during a surgical procedure. A method of donning sterile gloves in which the everted cuff of each glove allows the gowned person to touch the inner side of the glove with ungloved fingers and the outer side of the glove with gloved fingers.

Scurf: A bran-like desquamation of the epidermis.

Semicritical item: An item that comes in contact with mucous membranes or with skin that is not intact.

Sterile: The absence of all living microorganisms.

Sterile field: Area around the site of the incision into tissue or the site of introduction of an instrument into a body orifice that has been prepared for the use of sterile supplies and equipment. This area includes all furniture covered with sterile drapes and all personnel who are in sterile attire.

Sterile technique: Methods by which contamination with microorganisms is prevented to maintain sterility throughout the surgical procedure.

Sterilization: Processes by which all pathogenic and nonpathogenic microorganisms, including spores, are killed.

Strike-through: Contamination of a sterile surface by moisture that has originated from a nonsterile surface and penetrated the protective covering of the sterile item.

Time-related sterility: Expiration dates are established to indicate the maximum duration of time within which a sterile item is considered sterile and safe to use.

NOTES

1. "Recommended practices for surgical hand antisepsis/hand scrubs," in *Standards, Recommended Practices, and Guidelines* (Denver: AORN, Inc, 2005) 377-385.

2. "Recommended practices for surgical attire," in *Standards, Recommended Practices, and Guidelines* (Denver: AORN, Inc, 2005) 299-305.

3. "Recommended practices for standard and transmission-based precautions in the perioperative practice setting," in *Standards, Recommended Practices, and Guidelines* (Denver: AORN, Inc, 2005) 447-451.

4. A J Mangram et al, "Guideline for prevention of surgical site infection," *American Journal of Infection Control* 27 (April 1999) 97-134.

5. W A Rutala, D J Weber, "A review of single-use and reusable gowns and drapes in health care," *Infection Control and Hospital Epidemiology* 22 (April 2001) 248-257.

6. H Laufman, N L Belkin, K K Meyer, "A critical review of a century's progress in surgical apparel: How far have we come?" *Journal of the American College of Surgeons* 191 (November 2000) 554-568.

7. Association for Professionals in Infection Control and Epidemiology, *APIC Text of Infection Control and Epidemiology* (Washington, DC: Association for Professionals in Infection Control and Epidemiology, 2002) 27-1 to 27-4.

8. J S Heal et al, "Bacterial contamination of surgical gloves by water droplets spilt after scrubbing," *Journal of Hospital Infection* 53 (February 2003) 136-139.

9. D M Fogg, "Infection prevention and control," in *Alexander's Care of the Patient in Surgery,* 12th ed, J C Rothrock, ed (St Louis: Mosby, 2003) 97-158.

10. N F Phillips, *Berry & Kohn's Operating Room Technique,* 10th ed (St Louis: Mosby, 2004) 247-323.

11. P A Mews, "Establishing and maintaining a sterile field," in *Patient Care During Operative and Invasive Procedures,* second ed, M Phippen, M Wells, eds (Philadelphia: W B Saunders Co, 2000) 61-93.

12. B Gruendemann, S Mangum, *Infection Prevention in Surgical Settings* (Philadelphia: W B Saunders Co, 2001) 47-49, 88-97, 119-219, 250-257, 266-281, 365-371.

13. "Recommended practices for selection and use of surgical gowns and drapes," in *Standards, Recommended Practices, and Guidelines* (Denver: AORN, Inc, 2005) 371-375.

14. Association for the Advancement of Medical Instrumentation, *Liquid Barrier Performance and Classification of Protective Apparel and Drapes Intended for Use in Health Care Facilities,* ANSI/ AAMI PB70 (Arlington, Va: Association for the Advancement of Medical Instrumentation, 2003).

15. Association for the Advancement of Medical Instrumentation, *Selection of Surgical Gowns and Drapes in Health Care Facilities,* AAMI TIR no 11:1994 (Arlington, Va: Association for the Advancement of Medical Instrumentation, 2000.)

16. J Tanner, H Parkinson, "Double gloving to reduce surgical cross-infection," (Cochrane Review) in *The Cochrane Library,* issue 2 (Chichester, UK: John J Wiley & Sons, 2004). Abstract available at *http://www.cochrane.org/cochrane/revabstr/AB003087.htm* (accessed 26 Aug 2005).

17. A Lipp, "An assessment of the clinical effectiveness of surgical drapes," *Nursing Times* 99 (Dec 9, 2003) 28-31.

18. N Belkin, "Selecting surgical gowns and drapes for today's surgery," *SSM* 9 (December 2003) 41-44.

19. J Pournoor, "New scientific tools to expand the understanding of aseptic practices," *Surgical Services Management* 6 (April 2000) 28-32.

20. F Memarzadah, A P Manning "Comparison of operating room ventilation systems in the protection of the surgical site," session 4549, *ASHRAE Transactions,* proceedings of the 2002 annual meeting (Atlanta: American Society of Heating, Refrigerating, and Air-Conditioning Engineers, 2002). Abstract available at *http://resourcecenter.ashrae.org/store/ashrae* (accessed 26 Aug 2005).

21. C Edmiston et al, "Airborne particulates in the OR environment," *AORN Journal* 69 (June 1999) 1169-1183.

22. N Japp, "Packaging: Shelf life," in *Sterilization Technology for the Health Care Facility,* second ed, M Reichert, J Young, eds (Gaithersburg, Md: Aspen Publishers, 1997) 99-103.

23. L O'Connor, "Event-related sterility assurance: An opportunity for continuous quality improvement," *The Surgical Technologist* (January 1994) 8-12.

24. E H Spaulding, "Chemical disinfection of medical and surgical materials," in *Disinfection, Sterilization, and Preservation,* C A Lawrence, S S Block, eds (Philadelphia: Lea & Febiger, 1968) 517-531.

25. W Rutala, D Weber, "Modern advances in disinfection, sterilization, and medical waste management," in *Prevention and Control of Nosocomial Infections,* fourth ed, R P Wenzel, ed (Philadelphia: Lippincott Williams & Wilkins, 2003) 542-574.

26. M C Roy, "Modern approaches to preventing surgical site infections," in *Prevention and Control of Nosocomial Infections,* fourth ed, R P Wenzel, ed (Philadelphia: Lippincott Williams & Wilkins, 2003) 369-384.

27. "Medical devices; semicritical reprocessed single-use devices; termination of exemptions from premarket notification; requirement for submission of validation data," *Federal Register* 69 (April 13, 2004) 19433-19435.

28. W Rutala, "APIC guideline for selection and use of disinfectants," *American Journal of Infection Control* 24 (August 1996) 313-342.

29. "Recommended practices for selection and use of packaging systems," in *Standards, Recommended Practices, and Guidelines* (Denver: AORN, Inc, 2005) 415-420.

30. "Recommended practices for sterilization in perioperative practice settings," in *Standards, Recommended Practices, and Guidelines* (Denver: AORN, Inc, 2005) 459-469.

31. L Sehulster, R Y Chinn, "Guidelines for environmental infection control in health care facilities," *Morbidity and Mortality Weekly Report* 52 RR-10 (June 6, 2003) 1-42.

32. "Recommended practices for high-level disinfection," in *Standards, Recommended Practices, and Guidelines* (Denver: AORN, Inc, 2005) 313-319.

33. "Recommended practices for safe care through identification of potential hazards in the surgical environment," in *Standards, Recommended Practices, and Guidelines* (Denver: AORN, Inc, 2005) 387-393.

34. "Guidance statement: Safe medication practices in perioperative practice settings," in S*tandards, Recommended Practices, and Guidelines* (Denver: AORN, Inc, 2005) 196-198.

35. "AORN latex guideline" in *Standards, Recommended Practices, and Guidelines* (Denver: AORN, Inc, 2005) 117-132.

36. "Recommended practices for traffic patterns in the perioperative practice setting," in *Standards, Recommended Practices, and Guidelines* (Denver: AORN, Inc, 2005) 483-485.

37. American Institute of Architects Academy of Architecture for Health, *Guidelines for Design and Construction of Hospital and Health Care Facilities* (Washington, DC: American Institute of Architects, 2001).

38. A Tammelin et al, "Dispersal of methicillin-resistant *Staphylococcus epidermis* by staff in an operating room suite for thoracic and cardiovascular surgery: Relation to skin carriage and clothing," *Journal of Hospital Infection* 44 (February 2000) 119-126.

39. R Conner, "Washing and restringing instruments; bone debris; preparing setups; patient restraints; Group A *Streptococcus*," (Clinical Issues) *AORN Journal* 73 (April 2001) 835-838.

40. C Petersen, "Time for unused sterile setups; maintaining instrument count sheets; gowning off back tables; plants in the OR; count discrepancies," (Clinical Issues) *AORN Journal* 80 (August 2004) 321-324.

41. "Surgical site infections," in *APIC Handbook of Infection Control and Epidemiology,* third ed, J Jennings, J Wideman, eds (Washington, DC: Association for Professionals in Infection Control and Epidemiology) 312-321.

42. "Recommended practices for reducing radiological exposure in the practice setting," in *Standards, Recommended Practices, and Guidelines* (Denver: AORN, Inc, 2005) 437-442.

43. F Pryor, P Messmer, "The effect of traffic patterns in the OR on surgical site infections," *AORN Journal* 68 (October 1998) 649-660.

44. S C Beyea, ed, *Perioperative Nursing Data Set: The Perioperative Nursing Vocabulary,* second ed (Denver: AORN, Inc, 2002).

RESOURCES

American Society for Healthcare Central Service Professionals. "Eliminating sterile outdates," (self-study series) *Healthcare Purchasing News* (March 2003) 42-44.

Barrett, R; Stevens, J; Taranter, J. "A shelf-life trial: Examining the efficacy of event related sterility principles and its implications for nursing practice," *Australian Journal of Advanced Nursing* 21 (2003–2004) 8-12.

Belkin, N. "Barrier drapes and their impact on surgical site infections," *Infection Control Today* (May 2002).

Belkin, N. "Barrier materials: Their influence on surgical wound infections," *AORN Journal* 55 (June 1992) 1521-1528.

Bell, M. "Hospital uses team approach to improve processes, reduce costs," *AORN Journal* 68 (July 1998) 68-72.

Donovan, A; Turner, D W; Smith, A. "Successful, documented studies favoring indefinite shelf life," *Journal of Healthcare Materiel Management* 9 (March 1991) 34-40.

Garibaldi, R A, et al. "Comparison of nonwoven and woven gown and drape fabric to prevent intraoperative wound contamination and postoperative infection," *The American Journal of Surgery* 152 (November 1986) 505-509.

Groah, L, ed. "Limiting contamination sources in the operating room," in *Perioperative Nursing,* third ed (Stamford, Conn: Appleton & Lange, 1996) 137-162.

Gruendemann, B; Fernsebner, B. "Asepsis," in *Comprehensive Perioperative Nursing, Volume 1: Principles* (Boston: Jones and Bartlett Publishers, 1995) 180-288.

Hinchliff, S. "Innate defenses," in *Physiology for Nursing Practice,* S Hinchliff, S Montague, eds (London: Baillière Tindall, 1988) 549-578.

Mayworm, D. "Probably sterile," *Infection Control and Sterilization Technology* (March 1995) 7.

Nicolette, L. "Sterilization and disinfection," in *Perioperative Nursing,* third ed, L Groah, ed (Stamford, Conn: Appleton & Lange, 1996) 163-195.

Parker, L. "Rituals versus risks in the contemporary operating theatre environment," *British Journal of Theatre Nursing* 9 (August 1999) 341-345.

Roark, J. "Guidelines for maintaining the sterile field," *Infection Control Today* 7 (August 2003) 14-16.

Saunders, S. "Practical measures to ensure health and safety in theatres," *Nursing Times* 100 (March 16, 2004) 32-35.

Taylor, M; Campbell, C. "The multidisciplinary team in the operating department," *British Journal of Theatre Nursing* 9 (April 1999) 178-183.

Xavier, G. "Asepsis," *Nursing Standard* 13 (May 26, 1999) 49-53.

Originally published March 1978, *AORN Journal,* as "Recommended practices for aseptic technique." Format revision July 1982.

Revised March 1987, October 1991.

Revised June 1996; published November 1996, *AORN Journal.*

Revised and reformatted; published February 2001, *AORN Journal.*

Revised November 2005; published February 2006, *AORN Journal.*

Recommended Practices for Sterilization in the Perioperative Practice Setting

The following recommended practices were developed by the AORN Recommended Practices Committee and have been approved by the AORN Board of Directors. They were presented as proposed recommended practices for comments by members and others. They are effective January 1, 2006.

These recommended practices are intended as achievable recommendations representing what is believed to be an optimal level of practice. Policies and procedures will reflect variations in practice settings or clinical situations that determine the degree to which the recommended practices can be implemented.

AORN recognizes the numerous types of settings in which perioperative nurses practice. These recommended practices are intended as guidelines adaptable to various practice environments. These practice settings include traditional ORs, ambulatory surgery units, physicians' offices, cardiac catheterization suites, endoscopy suites, radiology departments, and all other areas where operative and other invasive or minimally invasive procedures may be performed.

Purpose

These recommended practices provide guidance for sterilizing items (eg, instruments, supplies, equipment, medical devices) to be used in the surgical environment. The creation and maintenance of an aseptic environment has a direct influence on patient outcomes. A major responsibility of the perioperative registered nurse is to minimize patient risk for surgical wound infection. The expected outcome of primary importance to this recommended practice is outcome O10, "The patient is free from signs and symptoms of infection."[1] One of the measures for preventing surgical wound infections is to provide surgical items that are free of contamination at the time of use. This can be accomplished by subjecting them to a sterilization process. Steam, ethylene oxide (EO), low temperature gas plasma, peracetic acid, ozone, and dry heat are sterilization methods that are used in the health care environment. Sterilization of each item to be processed must be validated by the product manufacturer. Directions for sterilizing items should be reviewed in consultation with the manufacturers of the sterilizer and the item to be sterilized. Each sterilization method, and some

instrumentation, has limitations; these limitations should be identified before purchasing and using any sterilizer. Sterilization provides the highest level of assurance that surgical items are free of viable microbes.

Recommended Practice I

Items to be sterilized should be cleaned and decontaminated in a controlled environment and in accordance with the device manufacturer's written instructions.

1. Factors to be controlled in the environment include room temperature, humidity, and ventilation. To aid in environmental control, there should be a physical separation between the decontamination and sterilization areas. Health care personnel should use standard precautions when performing decontamination activities. Appropriate personal protective attire must be worn, and cleaning procedures should minimize the possibility of spreading contamination.[2-4]

2. Items should be cleaned and dried thoroughly in accordance with AORN's "Recommended practices for cleaning and caring for surgical instruments and powered equipment," "Recommended practices for cleaning and processing endoscopes and endoscope accessories," and the "Multi-society guideline for reprocessing flexible gastrointestinal endoscopes."[5-7] The reliability of sterilization is affected negatively by the number, type, and inherent resistance of microorganisms, including biofilms, on the items to be sterilized. Soils, oils, and other materials may shield items from contact with the sterilant or combine with and inactivate the sterilant.[2,3,8]

Recommended Practice II

Items to be sterilized should be packaged according to guidelines established in AORN's "Recommended practices for selection and use of packaging systems."[9]

1. Items should be prepared and packaged so sterility can be achieved and maintained to the point of use. The Association for the Advancement of Medical Instrumentation (AAMI) provides guidance for the density of wrapped

Table 1

TYPICAL MINIMUM CYCLE TIMES FOR GRAVITY-DISPLACEMENT STEAM STERILIZATION[1]						
Item	Exposure time at 250° F (121° C)	Minimum drying time	Exposure time at 270° F (132° C)	Minimum drying time	Exposure time at 275° F (135° C)	Minimum drying time
Wrapped instruments	30 min	45 min	15 min	45 min	10 min	30 min
Textile packs	30 min	30 min	25 min	30 min	10 min	30 min
Wrapped utensils	30 min	30 min	15 min	30 min	10 min	30 min

1. Association for the Advancement of Medical Instrumentation, ANSI/AAMI ST8, Hospital Steam Sterilizers (2001); ANSI/AAMI ST46, Steam Sterilization and Sterility Assurance in Health Care Facilities (2002). Arlington, Va: Association for the Advancement of Medical Instrumentation.

packages. Manufacturers of packaging systems should be consulted for package preparation, configuration, and sterilization recommendations and the ability of the packaging to allow for presentation of the package contents to the sterile field in an aseptic manner.[3,9,10]

2. Instruments should be held in an open and unlocked position. Preparation and assembly procedures should consider the type of surgical instruments in the set and total set weight, configuration, and density. Paper/plastic peel pouches should not be placed in a container or wrapped set. Container or instrument manufacturers do not validate this configuration. Additional packaging materials inside a set can interfere with sterilization efficacy and drying.[3]

3. Instrument sets and container systems should be of a weight specified by the manufacturers of the surgical instruments, sterilizers, and container systems. If instrument sterilization/container systems are used, the manufacturer's written instructions for maximum weight, set preparation, sterilizer loading procedures, exposure times, and drying cycles should be followed. Sets weighing more than approximately 20 lbs are known to be difficult to dry without lengthy drying times. The manufacturer of the instrument sterilization/container system being used should provide written data to support its recommendations.[11] The National Institute for Occupational Safety and Health (NIOSH) has published a lifting equation for calculating a recommended weight for speci-

fied, two-handed lifting tasks. This document and the accompanying Applications Manual for the Revised NIOSH Lifting Equation should be consulted.[12-14]

Recommended Practice III

Saturated steam under pressure is the preferred sterilization method and should be used to sterilize heat- and moisture-stable items unless otherwise indicated by the device manufacturer.

1. Manufacturers' written instructions for operating steam sterilizers should be followed. Steam under pressure is inexpensive and sterilizes both porous and nonporous materials relatively rapidly.[15] Steam sterilizers vary in design and performance characteristics; therefore, cycle parameters recommended by the device manufacturer should be reconciled with the sterilizer manufacturer's written instructions for the specific sterilization cycle and load configuration.[3,11,16]

2. A variety of steam sterilization cycles are used in health care facilities. Some examples are gravity-displacement cycles, prevacuum cycles, and abbreviated steam sterilization (ie, flash) cycles. Tables 1 and 2 provide typical minimum sterilization times for gravity displacement and dynamic air-removal steam sterilizers.

3. If a sterilizer container system is used, the container manufacturer's written recommendations for exposure and drying times should be reconciled with those of the sterilizer's manufacturer. Certain types of equipment and implants

Table 2

TYPICAL MINIMUM CYCLE TIMES FOR DYNAMIC AIR-REMOVAL STEAM STERILIZATION[1]				
Item	Exposure time at 270° F (132° C)	Minimum drying time	Exposure time at 275° F (135° C)	Minimum drying time
Wrapped instruments	4 min	30 min	3 min	16 min
Textile packs	4 min	5 min	3 min	3 min
Wrapped utensils	4 min	20 min	3 min	16 min

1. *Association for the Advancement of Medical Instrumentation, ANSI/AAMI ST8, Hospital Steam Sterilizers (2001); ANSI/AAMI ST46, Steam Sterilization and Sterility Assurance in Health Care Facilities (2002). Arlington, Va: Association for the Advancement of Medical Instrumentation.*

(eg, some pneumatically powered instruments; specialty orthopedic, neurosurgery, trauma instruments) may require prolonged exposure times or drying times.[3,11] Current manufacturers' written instructions should be reviewed and followed.

4. Packages should be thoroughly dried and cooled before they are handled or removed from the sterilizer. At the end of the steam sterilization cycle and after an appropriate drying time, items still may contain some steam vapor. Touching packages at this vulnerable stage could compromise the barrier properties of the packaging material by causing moisture to wick through the wrapper. Warm or hot items should not be placed on cool or cold surfaces. When hot and cold surfaces are brought together, moisture condenses from both inside and outside the package. If this liquid breaches the packaging material, items inside the package are considered unsterile. When impermeable materials of any type (eg, closed containers, plastic-reinforced wrappers, woven or nonwoven wrappers, peel or other pouches) are used and condensate is observed within the package, the device should be considered unsterile and should not be used.[3,11]

5. For instruments or devices used on high-risk tissue (eg, brain, spinal cord, eyes), known or suspect Creutzfeldt-Jakob disease (CJD), or variant CJD patients, refer to AORN's "Recommended practices for cleaning and caring for surgical instruments and powered equipment."[5]

6. User manuals for all sterilization equipment should be readily available to the sterilizer operators. The manuals should be retained for the life of the sterilizers.

Recommended Practice IV

Flash sterilization should be used only in selected clinical situations and in a controlled manner. Use of flash sterilization should be kept to minimum.

1. Flash sterilization should be considered only if all of the following conditions are met.[17]
   - The device manufacturer's written instructions are available and followed.
   - Items are disassembled and thoroughly cleaned with detergent and water to remove soil, blood, body fats, and other substances.
   - Lumens are flushed with the cleaning solution and rinsed thoroughly
   - Items are placed in a sterilization container or tray in a manner that allows steam to contact all instrument parts.
   - Measures are taken to prevent contamination during transfer to the sterile field.
   - Documentation of cycle information and monitoring results is maintained to provide for tracking of the flashed item(s) to the individual patient.[3,17]

   Flash sterilization should be used only when there is insufficient time to process by the preferred wrapped or container method. Flash sterilization should not be used as a substitute for sufficient instrument inventory.

2. Flash sterilization may be associated with increased risk of infection to patients because of pressure on personnel to eliminate one or more steps in the cleaning and sterilization process. It is essential that all steps in the sterilization process be performed in a conscientious manner.[17]

3. Before sterilization, instruments should be thoroughly cleaned and dried in a manner consistent with AORN's "Recommended practices for cleaning and caring for surgical instruments and powered equipment"[5] and AAMI's standards for decontamination, steam sterilization, and EO sterilization.[2,3,5,18] Proper decontamination is essential in removing bioburden and preparing an item for sterilization by any method. Cleaning is the first step in decontamination. To remove debris from all parts of the instrument, the instrument should be disassembled (if possible) before cleaning.[2] Failures in instrument cleaning have resulted in transmission of infectious agents.

4. Packaging and wrapping (eg, textiles, paper/plastic pouches, nonwoven wrappers) should not be used in flash sterilization cycles unless the sterilizer specifically is designed and labeled for this use. Special handling of unwrapped packages during transport to the point of use is necessary. This includes the use of sterile gloves and the avoidance of contact with unsterile surfaces. Specialized flash sterilization containers are commercially available and may reduce the risk of contamination during transport. These containers should be used and cleaned according to the manufacturers' written instructions. Items with lumens should be prepared according to AORN's "Recommended practices for cleaning and caring for surgical instruments and powered equipment."[5]

5. Flash sterilization exposure times, temperature settings, and drying times, if recommended, should be according to the device and sterilizer manufacturers' written instructions.[17] Table 3 provides examples of typical flash sterilization cycle parameters.

6. Flash sterilization should not be used for implantable devices.[17,19,20] Implants are foreign bodies, and they increase the risk of surgical site infection. Careful planning, appropriate packaging, and inventory management in cooperation with suppliers can minimize the need to flash sterilize implantable medical devices. When an implantable device is sterilized at a health care facility, a biological indicator should be run with the load and the implant should be quarantined until the results of the biological indicator are known.[3,19,20] If an emergency situation makes flash sterilization unavoidable, a rapid-action biological monitoring device should be used along with a class V chemical integrator. The implant should not be released until the rapid-action indicator provides a negative result. After the rapid-action negative result is obtained, the implant can be released for use in the immediate situation. If the implant is not used, it cannot be saved as sterile for future use. Resterilization of the device is required. If the biological indicator is later determined to have a positive result, the surgeon should be notified as soon as the results are known.

7. Each sterilization cycle should be monitored to verify that parameters required for sterilization have been met. The physical parameters of time and temperature should be recorded for each cycle and verified by the sterilizer operator before transferring the item(s) to the point of use. Sterilizer function should be monitored with mechanical, chemical, and biological indicators to meet all of the monitoring standards established for gravity displacement and prevacuum sterilizers.[3,17] Sterilization process monitoring devices intended for flash sterilization cycles should be used according to manufacturers' written instructions. A sterilization process-monitoring device should be used with each load that is flash sterilized. The routine use of monitoring devices, including biological indicators or integrators, provides information to demonstrate that conditions for sterilization have been met.[3,17]

8. Documentation should be maintained to allow for traceability of every load to the patient for whom the instruments were used. A sterilization log or database should include information on each load, including the device(s) processed, the patient receiving the item(s), and the reason for flash sterilization.[3]

Table 3

EXAMPLES OF TYPICAL FLASH STEAM STERILIZATION PARAMETERS[1]		
Type of sterilizer	**Load configuration**	**Time**
High-speed gravity displacement*	Metal or nonporous items only (ie, no lumens)	3 minutes
	Metal items with lumens and porous items (eg, rubber, plastic) sterilized together	10 minutes
Pulsing gravity	Nonporous, nonlumened instruments only	See manufacturers' written instructions for time and temperature
Dynamic air-removal (prevacuum)*	Metal or nonporous items only (ie, no lumens)	3 minutes
	Metal items with lumens and porous items sterilized together	4 minutes
Abbreviated prevacuum	Nonporous, nonlumened instruments	See manufacturers' written instructions for time and temperature

* Temperature settings for both the high-speed gravity displacement and dynamic air-removal (prevacuum) flash sterilizers should be 270°–272° F (132°–135° C).

Note: The sterilizer manufacturer's instructions for use of express cycles should be followed. One sterilizer manufacturer provides an express flash cycle that permits flash sterilization with a single-ply wrapper to help contain the device to the point of use. This cycle is not recommended for devices with lumens. Express cycles should be used only if the sterilizer is designed with this feature.

1. *Association for the Advancement of Medical Instrumentation, ANSI/AAMI ST37,* Flash Sterilization: Steam Sterilization of Patient Care Items for Immediate Use *(Arlington, Va: Association for the Advancement of Medical Instrumentation, 1996).*

Recommended Practice V

Ethylene oxide sterilization is a low-temperature process that may be used for heat- and moisture-sensitive surgical items.

1. The manufacturer's written instructions should be reviewed to determine if a heat- or moisture-sensitive item is compatible with EO sterilization. Ethylene oxide is an alkylating agent that results in microbial death under controlled parameters.

2. Manufacturers' written instructions should be followed for EO sterilization parameters and placement of items within the sterilizer. Ethylene oxide sterilizers differ in design and operating characteristics. Items should be placed in EO sterilizers in baskets or on loading carts in a manner that allows free circulation and penetration of the EO.[18]

3. Items, including all lumens, should be clean and dry before being packaged for EO sterilization. Soil inhibits sterilization, and moisture may produce toxic by-products.

4. Compatibility of materials with the EO sterilization process should be established before attempting sterilization by this method.

5. Mechanical monitors of EO sterilizers should record the essential parameters for sterilization, including
   - temperature,
   - exposure time,
   - relative humidity, and
   - sterilant concentration.[18]

6. Documentation for EO processed items should include
   - the assigned lot number;
   - contents of each load; and
   - results of mechanical, chemical, and biological monitors.

Recommended Practice VI

Items sterilized in EO sterilizers should be properly aerated in a mechanical aerator to remove EO.

1. All EO-sterilized items must be completely aerated before they can be used safely. Manufacturers' written instructions should be followed for specific aeration requirements. Ethylene oxide residues can be harmful to patients and personnel. Ethylene oxide is a known human carcinogen and a chemical that has the potential to cause adverse reproductive effects in humans. The Occupational Safety and Health Administration (OSHA) has established exposure limits for EO in the workplace.[21-23]

2. Health care facilities use 100% concentrations of EO or EO in mixtures with inert diluent gases (eg, carbon dioxide, hydrochlorofluorocarbons [HCFC]) for EO sterilization procedures. Until the 1990s, chlorofluorocarbons (CFCs) were used as diluents for EO. Chlorofluorocarbons cause depletion of the ozone layer and are no longer produced in the United States. Hydrochlorofluorocarbons also deplete the ozone layer but to a lesser degree than CFCs. Users of HCFCs should be aware of and comply with federal, state, and local regulations regarding HCFC use in EO sterilizers.[18,21,24]

3. The EO absorbed into EO-sterilized items represents a hazard to patients and health care personnel if it is not removed. The EO vapors and residues diffuse from sterilized items over time. This aeration or degassing process can be expedited by raising the temperature and by increasing the flow of air around the item. Whenever possible, EO-sterilized items should be processed in sterilizers that have an integrated aeration cycle. When using a separate mechanical aerator, health care personnel should be protected from EO vapors and residue. To prevent health care personnel from breathing EO gas or coming in contact with EO residues, sterilized items should be handled as little as possible before aeration. Pulling, rather than pushing, sterilizer carts during transfer to aerators directs the flow of EO vapors and residues away from health care personnel. Butyl rubber or neoprene gloves provide protection to the skin of health care personnel handling EO-sterilized items. Specific aeration times necessary for surgical items depend on many variables that include, but are not limited to,

   ◆ item composition and size,
   ◆ item preparation and packaging,
   ◆ density of the load,
   ◆ type of EO sterilizer used,
   ◆ type of aerator used, and
   ◆ temperature penetration pattern of the aerator's chamber.[18]

4. Items should remain in aerators until the aeration time has been completed. Manufacturers of medical device and packaging systems should provide written instructions on the necessary aeration time and temperature for their products. Adequate aeration time reduces EO to a level safe for exposure of both patients and health care personnel. Aeration requirements for the most difficult-to-aerate products may require increased time frames.

5. Aeration cycles should never be interrupted to remove items for use. Items not sufficiently aerated may cause patient or personnel injury (eg, chemical burns). Aeration is the only safe and effective way to remove EO.[18,21]

6. All aeration cycle parameters should be documented and verified as to the accuracy of the correct aeration time and temperature.

Recommended Practice VII

A program for monitoring occupational exposure to EO must be established.

1. To protect personnel from excessive exposure, OSHA has determined maximum limits for EO exposure. The EO monitoring program in each facility must comply with OSHA regulations.[21-23] Compliance with regulations promotes a safe work environment that is within federally mandated limits.

2. Specific OSHA regulations should be consulted to accurately determine the airborne concentrations of EO permissible within the health care setting. Employee breathing zone monitoring and sampling provide a means to determine that environmental EO concentrations in an

employee's breathing zone have not exceeded the OSHA action level of 0.5 parts per million as an eight-hour, time-weighted average. Personnel who have the potential for exposure should wear EO-monitoring badges that meet NIOSH standards for accuracy.[3,25] Monitoring of short-term excursion levels (STEL) over a 15-minute period also is required while specific activities are being performed. The OSHA permissible STEL is 5 ppm over a 15-minute sampling period. The action level and STEL test cannot be combined. General environmental monitoring is not required, although it does provide an indicator of problems with the ventilation or EO system.[18]

3. Documentation of EO employee breathing zone monitoring should be maintained in employees' health records. These records must be retained for the duration of employment plus 30 years after termination of employment.[18,26] Documentation establishes a continuous history of the work environment.

4. Health and safety procedures should be developed for health care personnel. Personnel should be informed about the health effects and potential hazards associated with exposure to EO. This information should be provided at the time of assignment to an area where EO is used and at least annually thereafter. Periodic physical assessment and testing should be carried out and documented according to current OSHA regulations.[18,26] Personnel should be familiar with the facility's emergency spill plan.[22] People who have inhaled concentrated EO gas should seek fresh air immediately. Administration of oxygen may be necessary. Cardiopulmonary resuscitation may be necessary if respiratory or cardiac collapse occurs.[18] Refer to the material data safety sheet for the type of EO used for specific first-aid measures.

Recommended Practice VIII

Low-temperature gas plasma sterilization methods may be used for moisture-stable, moisture-sensitive, and heat-sensitive items.

1. Only one gas plasma sterilization system cleared by the US Food and Drug Administration (FDA) currently is marketed in the United States. This system uses a combination of hydrogen peroxide

vapor and low-temperature gas plasma.[27] In this process, microbial life is disrupted when free radicals created from hydrogen peroxide gas plasma interact with microbial cell membranes, enzymes, or nucleic acids.[21,28]

2. When using a low-temperature gas plasma sterilization system, the manufacturer's written instructions for use, monitoring, and maintenance should be followed. Hydrogen peroxide is considered nonmutagenic, and the hydrogen peroxide residuals/by-products formed in the currently available hydrogen peroxide system are nontoxic and noncarcinogenic.[21,29] Items processed in this system require no aeration because the residuals and by-products are nontoxic.[21,30]

3. Documentation of items that can and cannot be processed in hydrogen peroxide gas plasma should be obtained from the device and sterilizer manufacturers. Cellulosic (eg, paper-based) packaging materials, products, and liquids are not suitable for hydrogen peroxide gas plasma sterilization. Items to be gas plasma sterilized should be packaged in nonwoven polypropylene wraps or in high-density polyethylene (ie, Tyvek) or biaxially oriented polyethylene terephthalate polyester film (ie, Mylar) pouches. Trays designed and validated for use with low-temperature gas plasma sterilization should be used.

4. Sterilization of devices to be processed in hydrogen peroxide gas plasma should be validated by the device manufacturer. Devices to be sterilized should comply with the sterilizer manufacturer's lumen claims relating to diameter and length of the device.[31-33]

Recommended Practice IX

Sterilization systems using peracetic acid as a low-temperature liquid sterilant may be used for heat-sensitive surgical items that can be immersed.

1. One FDA-cleared liquid peracetic acid sterilization system is currently marketed in the United States. This system uses a chemical formulation of 35% peracetic acid, hydrogen, and water. Peracetic acid is a strong oxidizing agent. An anticorrosive additive prevents harm to instruments and items being sterilized. Liquid peracetic acid sterilization should be considered a

just-in-time sterilization process and should not be used for items to be stored and used at a later time without additional processing.

2. Sterilization systems using liquid peracetic acid should be used, monitored, and maintained according to the manufacturer's written instructions. Peracetic acid is an effective sterilizing agent that does not leave toxic residues on sterilized items when items are rinsed properly. Serious injuries (eg, burns) may result if the chemical is not handled, neutralized, and rinsed properly. Peracetic acid is corrosive to the skin at concentrations of 3.4% or higher and corrosive to eyes at concentrations of 0.35% or higher.[32,33]

3. When using peracetic acid, as with other sterilization/disinfection processes, health care personnel should clean and process endoscopes and their accessories according to AORN's "Recommended practices for cleaning and processing endoscopes and endoscope accessories" and the manufacturer's specific instructions.[6]

4. When use of adapters is recommended by the sterilizer manufacturer, health care personnel should verify proper selection and connection of the adapter to the device. Failure to do so may result in failure to sterilize the lumen of the item.

5. Items sterilized in an automated system using peracetic acid should be transported and used immediately. Items sterilized with peracetic acid are wet, and the cassette or container is not sealed to prevent contamination.

6. The ability to successfully process devices intended for use with a peracetic acid system should be validated by the device manufacturer and comply with the sterilizer manufacturer's written instructions.

7. Documentation of items that can and cannot be processed in liquid peracetic acid should be obtained from the device and sterilizer manufacturers.

Recommended Practice X

Sterilization systems using ozone may be used for moisture-stable, moisture-sensitive, heat-sensitive items.

1. Only one FDA-cleared ozone sterilization system is currently marketed in the United States. Ozone is a strong oxidizer, which makes ozone sterilization an effective low-temperature sterilization process. Manufacturers' written instruction for operating, monitoring, and maintaining ozone sterilizers should be followed. Ozone is generated within the sterilizer using only oxygen and water. On completion of the sterilization cycle, ozone is exhausted through a catalytic converter where it is converted back into the raw materials of oxygen and water. No aeration of sterilized items is necessary because these by-products are nontoxic.

2. Ozone has been cleared by the FDA for use in the sterilization of metal and plastic surgical instruments, including some lumened instruments. Manufacturers' written instructions should be consulted for specific use limitations. All devices should comply with the sterilizer manufacturer's claims for lumen length and diameter.

3. Cellulose-based packaging materials and products are not suitable for ozone processes. Items to be processed in ozone should be packaged in nonwoven pouches or reusable rigid sterilization containers.[34]

Recommended Practice XI

Dry-heat sterilization should be used to sterilize anhydrous (ie, waterless) items that can withstand high temperatures.

1. Dry-heat sterilizers should be used, monitored, and maintained according to the manufacturer's written instructions. Dry heat is an oxidation or slow burning process that coagulates protein in the microbial cells. There is no moisture present in a dry-heat process, so microorganisms are destroyed by a very slow process of heat absorption. Dry-heat sterilizers vary in design and performance characteristics.

2. Sharp instruments that would be damaged by the moisture of steam may be sterilized by dry heat.[15] Dental instruments, burrs, reusable needles, glassware, and heat-stable powders and oils are examples of items that can withstand the high temperatures generated by dry-heat sterilization.

3. When possible, small containers should be used for items to be dry-heat sterilized, and package density should be as low as possible.[35] Packaging materials designed for dry-heat sterilization processing should allow for easy heat penetration, provide an adequate barrier to microorganisms, resist tearing or puncture, have a proven seal integrity, and be free of toxic ingredients and non-fast dyes. Only materials designed to withstand the high temperature of the dry-heat sterilization process should be used. If they are not formulated for dry-heat sterilization, pouches may char, compromising the aseptic presentation of sterilized items. Before packaging materials are selected for dry-heat sterilization, the manufacturer should be consulted to confirm the compatibility of the packaging material with sterilizer temperatures.[35] Closed containers or cassettes may extend the time needed to achieve sterilization; therefore, the use of such containers should be based on manufacturers' instructions and biological monitoring results. Most types of tape are not designed to withstand the high temperatures. Tape adhesive melts and may leave a sticky residue on sterilized packages or compromise the packaging.

4. Packages should be cooled before being handled or removed from the dry-heat sterilizer. Burns are the most common safety hazard associated with dry-heat sterilization. On completion of the sterilization cycle, both the sterilizer chamber and the items in the chamber are very hot and should not be touched. The operator should be aware of the hazards associated with dry-heat sterilization and use the appropriate protective equipment (eg, insulated gloves, handles).[35]

5. Dry-heat sterilizers are not commonly available in ORs or central processing departments. When used, their main purpose is to sterilize talcum powder for surgical procedures. Presterilized oils and powders are commercially available and should be considered before purchasing a dry-heat sterilizer.

Recommended Practice XII

The shelf life of a packaged sterile item is event related.

1. An event must occur to compromise package content sterility. Events that may compromise the sterility of a package include, but are not limited to,
   ◆ multiple handling that leads to seal breakage or loss of package integrity,
   ◆ moisture penetration, and
   ◆ exposure to airborne contaminants.[3,18,35,36]

2. These conditions should be evaluated before policies and procedures on event-related sterility are written for perioperative practice settings.

3. Sterile packages should be stored under environmentally controlled conditions.

Recommended Practice XIII

Transportation of sterile items should be controlled.

1. Sterile items should be transported in covered or enclosed carts with solid-bottom shelves. Sterile items placed in covered or enclosed carts will be protected from exposure to environmental contaminants along the transportation route. Loss of sterility is event related and depends on the amount of handling, conditions during transportation and storage, and the quality of the packaging material. An evaluation of these conditions should occur before policies and procedures on the transportation of sterile items are written for perioperative practice settings.[3,11,18,35,36]

2. Written policies and procedures should address prevention of physical damage and maintenance of package sterility during transport. Procedures for transporting sterile items can help preserve the quality of sterile packages and maintain the integrity of processed items until the time of use.[3,18]

Recommended Practice XIV

A quality control program should be established and maintained.

1. Quality control programs that enhance personnel performance and monitor sterilization efficacy should be established to promote patient and employee safety. These programs should include, but not be limited to,

♦ orientation programs,

♦ continuing education,

♦ documented competency, and

♦ tracking of unusual occurrences.

Operator and processing errors are minimized with regularly scheduled education, training, and competency demonstration.[3,17,18] Analysis of unusual occurrences helps identify systems failures that may lead to erroneous practice.

2. Continuous attention to all aspects of the sterilization process and sterilizer performance will help achieve and maintain the sterility of processed items.[3,11,17,18,35,36] Quality control parameters for the sterilization process should include, but not be limited to,

♦ sterilizer maintenance and repair history;

♦ sterilization process monitoring by mechanical, chemical, or biological indicators (chemical and biological indicators should be used in a process challenge device where appropriate);

♦ dynamic air-removal testing (ie, Bowie-Dick test) of prevacuum steam sterilizers;

♦ visual inspection of packaging materials; and

♦ lot control and traceability of load contents. Lot control numbers should identify the sterilizer used, the cycle or load number, and the date of sterilization. Lot control numbers allow items to be identified or retrieved in the event of a sterilizer failure or malfunction.[3,18,35,36]

3. Information should be recorded from each sterilization cycle and should include, but not be limited to,

♦ identification of sterilizer (eg, sterilizer #1)

♦ type of sterilizer and cycle used;

♦ lot control number;

♦ load contents (eg, major set, three Kelly clamps)

♦ critical parameters for the specific sterilization methodology (eg, exposure time and temperature for steam sterilization)

♦ operator's name; and

♦ results of sterilization process monitoring (ie, biological, chemical, mechanical).

4. Documentation establishes accountability. Documentation is necessary for every sterilization cycle, including steam (eg, wrapped, unwrapped), EO, hydrogen peroxide gas plasma, liquid peracetic acid, ozone, and dry heat.

5. All records should be maintained for a time period specified by the health care facility's risk manager and in compliance with local, state, and federal regulations. Accurate and complete records are required for process verification and used in sterilizer malfunction analyses.[3,11,17,18,35]

6. Mechanical monitors should be used to verify time, temperature, and pressure recordings for steam sterilization cycles. The printout should be reviewed at the end of each cycle and signed by the sterilizer operator verifying that all sterilization parameters were met. Recordings of mechanical data should be used, when available, for all sterilization methodologies to ascertain that sterilization systems function within manufacturers' specifications.[3,11,17,18]

7. A sterilization process indicator should be used in each package to be sterilized and included with all items being flash sterilized. When the process indicator is not visible from the outside of the package, a separate process indicator should be used on the exterior of the package. The purpose of the external process indicator is to differentiate between processed and unprocessed items. Although external sterilization process indicators do not verify sterility, they help detect procedural errors and equipment malfunctions; therefore, the color change should be verified before opening.

8. Internal process monitors do not establish whether the item is sterile, but they show that the sterilant was able to penetrate the package, exposing the package contents to conditions of sterilization. The internal chemical indicator should be reviewed for acceptance in color change before placing on the sterile field. If the interpretation of the external or internal process monitors suggests inadequate processing, the item should not be used.[3,17,18,37]

9. For wrapped cycles, sterilizer efficacy should be monitored routinely at regular intervals with a biological indicator placed in an appropriate process challenge device (ie, test pack). The AAMI standards for quality assurance testing of rigid containers should be followed.[11] For flash cycles (ie, unwrapped high-speed gravity or dynamic air removal), biological testing should be performed in an open mesh pan and/or in a

flash container to simulate in-use conditions. Additional monitoring of three consecutive sterilization cycles should be performed after installation, major repair, redesign, or relocation of sterilizers. This testing is performed in an otherwise empty sterilizer. Packs should be placed in the area(s) of the sterilizer least favorable to sterilization, as identified by the sterilizer manufacturer.[3,17,18] If a steam sterilizer is intended to be used for multiple types of cycles (eg, gravity displacement, dynamic air removal, flash), each sterilization mode should be tested.[3] The following provides guidance for sterilizer testing.[3,17,18,35-37]

Steam sterilizers—*Geobacillus stearothermophilus* (formerly *Bacillus stearothermophilus*) spore testing should be performed at least weekly and preferably daily.

Prevacuum sterilizers—An air-removal test (ie, Bowie-Dick test) should be performed daily in an empty chamber. The air-removal test is designed to detect residual air in the sterilizer chamber. Whenever a prevacuum sterilizer is newly installed, relocated, or undergoes a major repair, three consecutive air-removal tests should be performed before the biological testing.

Ethylene oxide sterilizers—*Bacillus atropheus* (formerly *Bacillus subtilis*) spore testing should be performed with every load.

Low-temperature hydrogen peroxide gas plasma sterilizers—*Geobacillus stearothermophilus* spore testing should be performed at the same interval as testing of other sterilizers in the facility. Consult the sterilizer manufacturer for specific product(s) to be used and location of the biological test pack.

Ozone sterilizers—*Geobacillus stearothermophilus* spore testing should be performed at the same interval as testing of other sterilizers in the facility. Consult the sterilizer manufacturer for specific product(s) to be used.

Low-temperature liquid peracetic acid sterilizers—*Geobacillus stearothermophilus* spore testing should be performed daily. The product used should be designed specifically for use with liquid peracetic acid processes. The sterilizer manufacturer's written instructions for use should be followed.

Dry-heat sterilizers—*Bacillus atropheus* indicators should be used upon unit installation and after any major repairs. For tabletop gravity convection units, sterilization loads should be monitored biologically at least once per week. Mechanical convection (ie, forced air) dry-heat sterilizers should be monitored according to the manufacturer's recommendations.

Sterilization process monitoring devices ascertain whether items have been subjected to sterilization conditions. Sterility of the sterilizer load is evidenced by the killing of all spores on the biological test indicator.

10. A biological indicator (preferably a process challenge device) should be included in all loads containing an implant(s), and the implant(s) should be quarantined until the results of the biological indicator are known.[3,19,20]

11. All biological indicator test results, including results from controls, should be interpreted by qualified personnel in the time frame specified by the biological test manufacturer and should be included in the sterilization records. All control vials must be from the same lot number as the biological test vial for the test to be considered valid.[3] Positive biological indicator test results should be reported immediately so that appropriate action can be taken. Accurate interpretation and reporting of positive results promotes safe patient care.[3]

12. In the event of a positive biological indicator test, the sterilizer printout should first be checked to determine if the cycle parameters were met. Chemical indicators should be reviewed for proper color or other change. The positive biological indicator vial should be sent to the laboratory for subculturing for bacillus. If retrievable, items processed in the suspect sterilizer (ie, back to the last known negative biological indicator test) should be retrieved and reprocessed before use.[3] All actions taken in response to a positive biological indicator test should be documented.[3]

Recommended Practice XV

Preventive maintenance on sterilizers should be performed by qualified personnel on a scheduled basis.

1. Inspection and cleaning should be performed as outlined in the manufacturer's written

instructions.[3,16-18] Proper inspection and cleaning minimizes sterilizer downtime and helps prevent sterilizer malfunctions. Preventive maintenance should be performed as specified in the manufacturer's written instructions. Periodic inspections, maintenance, and replacement of components subject to wear (eg, recording devices, steam traps, filters, valves, drain pipes, gaskets) help maintain proper functioning of sterilizers.

2. Maintenance records should be kept for each sterilizer. Accurate and complete records are required for sterilization process verification. Information should include, but not be limited to,
   ♦ date of service;
   ♦ sterilizer model and serial number;
   ♦ sterilizer location;
   ♦ description of malfunctions;
   ♦ name of person and company performing maintenance;
   ♦ description of service and parts replaced;
   ♦ results of biological validation and testing, if performed;
   ♦ results of air-removal test results and, where appropriate, the name of the person requesting the service; and
   ♦ the signature and title of the person acknowledging the completed work.

Recommended Practice XVI

Policies and procedures for sterilization processes should be developed, reviewed periodically, and readily available in the practice setting.

1. These recommended practices for sterilization should be used to guide the development of policies and procedures within individual perioperative practice settings. Policies and procedures establish authority, responsibility, and accountability and serve as operational guidelines. An introduction and review of policies and procedures should be included in the orientation and ongoing education of health care personnel to assist in the development of knowledge, skills, and attitudes that affect patient outcomes. Policies and procedures also assist in the development of continuous quality improvement activities.

2. The uniform perioperative nursing vocabulary should be used in the development of policies and procedures and documentation of nursing interventions related to sterilization. The perioperative nursing vocabulary is a clinically relevant and empirically validated standardized nursing language. This standardized language consists of the Perioperative Nursing Data Set (PNDS) and includes perioperative nursing diagnoses, interventions, and outcomes.[1] The expected outcome of primary importance to this recommended practice is outcome O10, "The patient is free from signs and symptoms of infection." This outcome falls within the domain of Safety (D1). Interventions that might lead to the desired outcome include I98, "Protects from cross-contamination"; I121, "Assesses susceptibility for infection"; and I188, "Monitors for signs and symptoms of infection."

3. As new technologies are introduced for use in perioperative practice settings, it is imperative that health care personnel strictly follow manufacturers' written instructions for the operation and maintenance of sterilization equipment and are aware of the occupational hazards that different sterilants may pose to patients, health care personnel, and the environment. Compliance with the Safe Medical Device Act of 1990, which was amended in 2000, is required and will contribute to patient safety.[38] When selecting a new sterilization technology, perioperative nurses and nurse managers should follow AORN's "Recommended practices for product selection in perioperative practice settings."[39]

4. Policies and procedures for routine cleaning of sterilizer chambers, carts, and exterior surfaces should be developed and implemented. The sterilizer manufacturer's written instructions for cleaning should be followed.

Glossary

Aeration: Method by which absorbed EO is removed from EO-sterilized items by circulating warm air in an enclosed cabinet specifically designed for this purpose.

Anhydrous: Items that are free of water.

Bioburden: Population of viable microorganisms on raw material, components, finished products, or packaging.

Biofilms: Microscopic organisms that have the ability, when growing in water, water solutions, or in vivo (eg, the bloodstream), to adhere to a surface and then exude over themselves a protective polysaccharide matrix. This matrix prevents antimicrobial agents from reaching the microbial cells.

Biological indicator: A sterilization process-monitoring device commercially prepared with a known population of highly resistant spores that tests the effectiveness of the method of sterilization being used. The indicator is used to demonstrate that conditions necessary to achieve sterilization were met during the sterilizer cycle being monitored.

Chemical indicator: A sterilization process-monitoring device used to monitor the attainment of one or more critical parameters required for sterilization. A characteristic color or other visual change indicates a defined level of exposure based on the classification of the chemical indicator used (eg, chemically treated paper, pellet sealed in a glass tube, pressure-sensitive tape).

Chemical integrator: A Class V indicator that parallels a biological indicator without containing spores. Used to monitor all the critical parameters of the sterilization cycle and provide a result immediately at the end of the cycle. Cannot be used as a substitute for a biological indicator.

Decontamination: The use of physical or chemical means to remove, inactivate, or destroy bloodborne or other pathogens on a surface or item to the point where they no longer are capable of transmitting infectious particles and the surface or item is rendered safe for handling or disposal.

Dynamic air removal: Mechanically assisted air removal from the sterilization chamber.

Dynamic air-removal test (ie, Bowie-Dick test): A diagnostic test to determine the adequacy of air removal from the chamber of a prevacuum steam sterilizer. The air-removal test is not a test for sterilization.

Downtime: A period of time when an item or device is not operational.

Emergency spill plan: A plan of action for any unanticipated release of ethylene oxide into the workplace.

Flash sterilization (ie, abbreviated/express cycle): A process designed for the steam sterilization of patient care items for immediate use.

Mechanical indicator: Automated devices (eg, graphs, gauges, printouts) that monitor sterilization parameters for the sterilization method in use.

Process challenge device (PCD): A predetermined item/package (ie, test pack) designed to simulate the product to be sterilized and that is used to assess the efficacy of the sterilization process.

Shelf life: The length of time an item is considered sterile and safe to use.

Sterilization process monitoring device: A device used to monitor sterilization processes. Sterilization monitoring devices can be biological, chemical, or mechanical.

NOTES

1. S C Beyea, ed, *Perioperative Nursing Data Set: The Perioperative Nursing Vocabulary,* second ed (Denver: AORN, Inc, 2002).

2. Association for the Advancement of Medical Instrumentation, ANSI/AAMI ST35, *Safe Handling and Biological Decontamination of Reusable Medical Devices in Health Care Facilities and in Nonclinical Settings* (Arlington, Va: Association for the Advancement of Medical Instrumentation, 2003).

3. Association for the Advancement of Medical Instrumentation, ANSI/AAMI ST46, *Steam Sterilization and Sterility Assurance in Health Care Facilities* (Arlington, Va: Association for the Advancement of Medical Instrumentation, 2002).

4. Occupational Safety and Health Administration, "Final rule on occupational exposure to bloodborne pathogens," *Federal Register* 56 (6 Dec 1991) 64004. Also available at *http://www.osha.gov/pls/oshaweb /owadisp.show_document?p_table=STANDARDS&p_id= 10051* (accessed 13 Sept 2005).

5. "Recommended practices for cleaning and caring for surgical instruments and powered equipment," in *Standards, Recommended Practices, and Guidelines* (Denver: AORN, Inc, 2005) 395-403.

6. "Recommended practices for cleaning and processing endoscopes and endoscope accessories," in *Standards, Recommended Practices, and Guidelines* (Denver: AORN, Inc, 2005) 341-346.

7. American Society for Gastrointestinal Endoscopy, "Multi-society guideline for reprocessing flexible gastrointestinal endoscopes," *Gastrointestinal Endoscopy* 58 (July 2003) 1-8.

8. C J Alvarado, M Reichelderfer, 1997-1999 APIC Guidelines Committee, "APIC guideline for infection prevention and control in flexible endoscopy," *American Journal of Infection Control* 28 (April, 2000) 138-155.

9. "Recommended practices for selection and use of packaging systems," in *Standards, Recommended Practices, and Guidelines* (Denver: AORN, Inc, 2005) 415-420.

10. Association for the Advancement of Medical Instrumentation, ANSI/AAMI/ISO 11607, *Packaging for Terminally Sterilized Medical Devices* (Arlington, Va: Association for the Advancement of Medical Instrumentation, 2000).

11. Association for the Advancement of Medical Instrumentation, ANSI/AAMI ST33 *Guidelines for the*

Selection and Use of Reusable Rigid Container Systems for Ethylene Oxide Sterilization and Steam Sterilization in Health Care Facilities (Arlington, Va: Association for the Advancement of Medical Instrumentation, 2000).

12. "Revised NIOSH equation for the design and evaluation of manual lifting tasks," *Ergonomics* 36 (July 1993) 749-776.

13. H G Wickes, Jr, G S Nelson, "Manual lifting: The revised NIOSH lifting equation (1993) for evaluations acceptable weights for manual lifting," National Institute for Occupational Safety and Health, *http://www.hazard control.com/ml-niosh93.html* (accessed 13 Sept 2005).

14. "Applications manual for the revised NIOSH lifting equation," US Department of Health and Human Services (NIOSH) Publication 94-110 (January 1994). Also available at *http://www.cdc.gov/niosh/94-110.html* (accessed 13 Sept 2005).

15. L J Joslyn, "Sterilization by heat," in *Disinfection, Sterilization, and Preservation,* fifth ed, S S Block, ed (Philadelphia: Lippincott Williams & Wilkins, 2001) 695-728.

16. Association for the Advancement of Medical Instrumentation, ANSI/AAMI ST8, *Hospital Steam Sterilizers* (Arlington, Va: Association for the Advancement of Medical Instrumentation, 2001).

17. Association for the Advancement of Medical Instrumentation, ANSI/AAMI ST37, *Flash Sterilization: Steam Sterilization of Patient Care Items for Immediate Use* (Arlington, Va: Association for the Advancement of Medical Instrumentation, 1996).

18. Association for the Advancement of Medical Instrumentation, ANSI/AAMI ST41, *Ethylene Oxide Sterilization in Health Care Facilities: Safety and Effectiveness* (Arlington, Va: Association for the Advancement of Medical Instrumentation, 2000).

19. J S Garner, *Guideline for Prevention of Surgical Wound Infections, 1985* (Atlanta: Centers for Disease Control and Prevention, 1985).

20. A J Mangram et al, "Guideline for prevention of surgical site infection, 1999," *Infection Control and Hospital Epidemiology* 20 (April 1999) 247-280.

21. L J Joslyn, "Gaseous chemical sterilization," in *Disinfection, Sterilization, and Preservation,* fifth ed, S S Block, ed (Philadelphia: Lippincott Williams & Wilkins, 2001) 337-359.

22. Occupational Safety and Health Administration, "Occupational exposure to ethylene oxide, final standard," *Federal Register* 53 (April 6, 1988) 11414-11438. Also available at *http://www.osha.gov/pls/oshaweb /owadisp.show_document?p_table=STANDARDS&p_ id=10070* (accessed 13 Sept 2005).

23. "Ethylene oxide," 29 CFR 1910.1047, Occupational Safety and Health Administration, *http://www.osha.gov /pls/oshaweb/owadisp.show_document?p_table= STANDARDS&p_id=10070* (accessed 13 Sept 2005).

24. T Crane, R Prezoptto, "Hospital sterilization after the CFC phaseout," *Surgical Services Management* 2 (July 1996) 10-11.

25. P M Schneider, "Ethylene oxide sterilization: Employee monitoring," in *Sterilization Technology for the Heath Care Facility,* second ed, M Reichert, J H Young, eds (Gaithersburg, Md: Aspen Publishers, 1997) 220-227.

26. "Access to employee exposure and medical records," 29 CFR 1910.1020, Occupational Safety and Health Administration, *http://www.osha.gov/pls/oshaweb /owadisp.show_document?p_table=STANDARDS &p_id=10027* (accessed 13 Sept 2005).

27. D F Smith, *STERRAD 200 Sterilization System* (Irvine, Calif: Advanced Sterilization Products, 2000).

28. American Society for Healthcare Central Service Professionals, "Sterilization," in *Training Manual for Health Care Central Service Technicians,* fourth ed (San Francisco: American Hospital Association Press/Jossey-Bass, 2001) 140-173.

29. "Material safety data sheet: Hydrogen peroxide solution" (Irvine, Calif: Advanced Sterilization Products, Aug 7, 2003).

30. W A Rutala, M F Gergen, D J Weber, "Comparative evaluation of the sporicidal activity of new low-temperature sterilization technologies: Ethylene oxide, two plasma sterilization systems, and liquid peracetic acid," *American Journal of Infection Control* 26 (August 1998) 393-398.

31. P T Jacobs, S M Lin, "Sterilization processes utilizing low-temperature plasma," in *Disinfection, Sterilization, and Preservation,* fifth ed, S S Block, ed (Philadelphia: Lippincott Williams & Wilkins, 2001) 751-758.

32. Association for the Advancement of Medical Instrumentation, AAMI TIR 7, *Chemical Sterilants and High-Level Disinfectants: A Guide to Selection and Use* (Arlington, Va: Association for the Advancement of Medical Instrumentation, 2000).

33. P S Machesky, "Medical applications of peracetic acid," in *Disinfection, Sterilization, and Preservation,* fifth ed, S S Block, ed (Philadelphia: Lippincott Williams & Wilkins, 2001) 979-996.

34. L K Weavers, G B Wickramanayake, "Disinfection and sterilization using ozone," in *Disinfection, Sterilization, and Preservation,* fifth ed, S S Block, ed (Philadelphia: Lippincott Williams, & Wilkins, 2001) 205-214.

35. Association for the Advancement of Medical Instrumentation, ANSI/AAMI ST40, *Table-Top Dry Heat (Heated Air) Sterilization and Sterility Assurance in Dental and Medical Facilities* (Arlington, Va: Association for the Advancement of Medical Instrumentation, 2000).

36. Association for the Advancement of Medical Instrumentation, ANSI/AAMI ST42, *Steam Sterilization and Sterility Assurance Using Table-Top Sterilizers in Office-Based, Ambulatory-Care, Medical, Surgical, and Dental Facilities* (Arlington, Va: Association for the Advancement of Medical Instrumentation, 1998).

37. Association for the Advancement of Medical Instrumentation, AAMI TIR 25, *Chemical Indicators— Guidance for the Selection, Use, and Interpretation of Results* (Arlington, Va: Association for the Advancement of Medical Instrumentation, 2000).

38. "Medical device reporting: Manufacturer reporting, importer reporting user facility reporting, distributor reporting; final rule," *Federal Register* 65 (26 Jan 2000) 4112-4121. Also available at *http://www.fda.gov/OHRMS /DOCKETS/98fr/012600c.pdf* (accessed 13 Sept 2005).

39. "Recommended practices for product selection in perioperative practice settings," in *Standards, Recommended Practices, and Guidelines* (Denver: AORN, Inc, 2005) 433-436.

RESOURCES

Bailey, A. "Updating sterilization technology," *Infection Control and Sterilization Technology* 2 (June 1995) 31-33.

Bastedo, G. "Ethylene oxide sterilization," (Viewpoint) *Surgical Services Management* 1 (July 1995) 9-10.

Bronowicki, J P et al. "Patient-to-patient transmission of hepatitis C virus during colonoscopy," *The New England Journal of Medicine* 337 (July 1997) 237-240.

Centers for Disease Control and Prevention, "Bronchosopy-related infections and pseudoinfections—New York, 1996 and 1998," *Morbidity and Mortality Weekly Report* 48 (July 9, 1999) 557-560. Also available at *http://www.cdc.gov/mmwr/preview/mmwrhtml/mm4826a1.htm* (accessed 9 Sept 2005).

Chobin, N. "Cost analysis of three low-temperature sterilization systems at Saint Barnabas Medical Center," *Journal of Healthcare Materials Management* 12 (August 1994) 29-32.

DesCoteaux, J G, et al. "Residual organic debris on process surgical instruments," *AORN Journal* 62 (July 1995) 23-30.

Gross, D. "Ethylene oxide sterilization and alternative methods," (Viewpoint) *Surgical Services Management* 1 (July 1995) 11-12.

"Hazard communication in the 21st century workplace," March 2004, Occupational Safety and Health Administration, *http://www.osha.gov/dsg/hazcom/finalmsdsreport.html* (accessed 9 Sept 2005).

Lagergren, E. "Gas plasma sterilization," (Viewpoint) *Surgical Services Management* 1 (July 1995) 18-20.

Rutala, W A; Weber, D J. "Creutzfeldt-Jakob disease: Recommendations for disinfection and sterilization." *Clinical Infectious Diseases* 32 (May 2001) 1348-1356.

Spry, C. "Sterilization regulations—Who's in charge here?" (Focus on Quality) *Surgical Services Management* 1 (July 1995) 56-59.

Steelman, V. " Creutzfeldt-Jacob disease: Recommendations for infection control," *American Journal of Infection Control* 22 (October 1994) 312-318.

Tablan, O C, et al. "Guidelines for preventing health care-associated pneumonia, 2003: Recommendations of the CDC and the Healthcare Infection Control Practices Advisory Committee," *Morbidity and Mortality Weekly Report* 53 (RR03) (March 26, 2004) 1-36. Also available at *http:// www.cdc.gov/mmwr/preview/mmwrhtml/rr5303a1.htm* (accessed 4 Feb 2006).

US Environmental Protection Agency. "Identification and listing of hazardous waste," in *Code of Federal Regulations* 40: Protection of Environment, Part 261. Available at *http://www.epa.gov/epacfr40/chapt-I.info/chi-toc.htm* (accessed 4 Feb 2006).

Ward, S. "Today's new sterilization technology presents new decision variables," (Editorial) *Surgical Services Management* 1 (July 1995) 4-5.

Originally published August 1980, *AORN Journal*.

Format revision July 1982.

Revised February 1987, October 1992.

Published as proposed recommended practices in July 1994.

Revised; published August 1999, *AORN Journal*.

Reformatted July 2000.

Revised November 2005; scheduled for publication in the *AORN Journal* in 2006.

Recommended Practices for Surgical Tissue Banking

The following recommended practices were developed by the AORN Recommended Practices Committee and have been approved by the AORN Board of Directors. They were presented as proposed recommended practices for comments by members and others. They are effective January 1, 2006.

These recommended practices are intended as achievable recommendations representing what is believed to be an optimal level of practice. Policies and procedures will reflect variations in practice settings and/or clinical situations that determine the degree to which the recommended practices can be implemented.

AORN recognizes the numerous settings in which perioperative nurses practice. These recommended practices are intended as guidelines adaptable to various practice settings. These practice settings include traditional operating rooms, ambulatory surgery centers, physicians' offices, cardiac catheterization suites, endoscopy suites, radiology departments, and all other areas where operative and other invasive procedures may be performed.

Purpose

Surgical tissue banking encompasses procuring, processing, preserving, and/or storing selected human cells and tissue. Human tissue includes, but is not limited to, bone, cartilage, ligaments, tendons, fascia, dura mater, sclera, corneas, heart valves/conduits, bone marrow, vessels, and skin. It is beyond the scope of these recommended practices to address all areas of tissue banking, solid organ transplantation, or nonhuman tissue. These recommended practices provide guidance for developing organizational policies and procedures that are specific to the needs of surgical patients and address the perioperative practice setting and expertise required of personnel.

A tissue bank should be established only where a need exists. Before the decision is made to establish a tissue bank, consideration should be given to personnel, equipment, and practical operational requirements for providing safe, reliable, and biologically useful products.

In 1997, the US Food and Drug Administration (FDA) announced a program for comprehensive regulatory oversight of tissue banking.[1] In support of this program, the FDA has published proposed guidance documents that were later clarified as final rules.[2-6] The agency intends to propose more regulations in the future in the form of guidance documents. Adherence to these regulations is required during the development and ongoing operation of a human tissue bank. In addition, the standards published by the American Association of Tissue Banks (AATB)[7] should be referred to for additional direction.

Effective July 1, 2005, the Joint Commission on Accreditation of Healthcare Organizations (JCAHO) standards for tissue banking have been updated in the laboratory accreditation program and additionally applied to ambulatory care, critical access hospital and hospital accreditation programs, and office-based surgery practices. The standards apply to organizations that store or issue human, nonhuman, and synthetic tissue, including surgery and outpatient centers.[8]

Recommended Practice I

Facilities procuring, processing, and/or preserving tissue, and facilities storing tissue for potential transfer to a different facility, must register as tissue banks with the FDA.[4]

1. A list of types of human cells, tissue, and cellular and tissue-based products must be submitted with the application to the FDA.[4] Facilities that recover, screen, test, process, label, package, and/or distribute human cells or tissue for implantation, transplantation, or infusion must register with the FDA. The registration form includes a list of tissues and cells to be used in this process.[4] Facilities must register within five days after beginning operations, notify the FDA within six months of changes in products, and update the registration annually in December. Facilities storing only purchased tissue for use within the same facility, or those who recover autologous skin or skull bone flaps for later reimplantation into the same patient, are not required to register as tissue banks. Additional clarification is available from the FDA.

2. Facilities should verify that tissue and cells acquired from outside sources have been procured, processed, stored, and distributed by tissue banks registered with the FDA and licensed by state agencies.[8] Depending on the type of

tissue being acquired, outside sources of cells or tissues also should be accredited by the AATB, the Eye Bank Association of America (EBAA), or the AABB (formerly known as the American Association of Blood Banks). Accreditation by any of these agencies demonstrates that these sources periodically pass inspections by the accrediting agency and provides minimum assurance of quality control for the recovery, screening, testing, processing, storage, and distribution of the tissue. Some tissue banks purchase tissue procured or processed by other tissue banks and have limited registration or accreditation. All tissue banks involved in handling the tissue must be registered and should be accredited. Copies of current certificates should be requested annually and kept on file.

Recommended Practice II

Facilities procuring, processing, preserving, storing, or distributing tissue to other facilities should have defined oversight with authority and accountability for all activities performed.[8]

1. A facility performing any tissue-banking activities should appoint an administrator or oversight group accountable for these activities. The administrator of a tissue bank is accountable for all aspects of the tissue bank's activities, including compliance with regulations. This role requires a broad understanding of the processes and responsibilities involved.

2. Administrative personnel should be knowledgeable about
   ◆ all applicable federal, state, and local regulations;
   ◆ applicable standards of the AATB, EBAA, and AABB;
   ◆ accrediting agency requirements;
   ◆ screening and testing criteria;
   ◆ the grieving process;
   ◆ aspects of informed consent;
   ◆ donor and recipient rights;
   ◆ quality control;
   ◆ documentation and record-keeping requirements;
   ◆ confidentiality and release of information;
   ◆ requirements for release of tissue;
   ◆ adverse event reporting; and
   ◆ ethical considerations.

3. A physician or medical advisory committee should be available to provide direction for medical decisions. The AATB recommends that a medical director be appointed.[7]

4. Tissue ordering and receiving, procuring, processing, preserving, storing, and distributing should be coordinated throughout the health care facility.[8] Centralized oversight of all aspects of tissue banking is necessary to ensure that all tissue received and stored is safe for implantation, that processes are validated and monitored on an ongoing basis, and that all tissue can be traced back to the source or easily recalled if necessary.

Recommended Practice III

Surgical tissue bank personnel must be knowledgeable about the aspects of tissue banking in which they participate.[6]

1. Personnel should be knowledgeable about the importance of the tissue bank products and services. An understanding of the importance of tissue bank activities instills an attitude of attention to detail, and may minimize errors.

2. Personnel soliciting tissue donations must be knowledgeable about
   ◆ federal and state regulations,
   ◆ screening and testing criteria,
   ◆ the grieving process,
   ◆ aspects of informed consent,
   ◆ donor and recipient rights, and
   ◆ ethical considerations.

   Requesting authorization for donation of tissue requires unique interpersonal communication skills to ensure that donations are legally and ethically solicited and accepted.

3. Personnel screening potential donors must be knowledgeable about
   ◆ the grieving process;
   ◆ screening and testing criteria;
   ◆ sources of information for screening (eg, relevant medical records, knowledgeable historian);
   ◆ techniques to obtain accurate and complete information; and
   ◆ resources and options available when screening results are ambiguous or unclear.

Screening requires specific training to learn the best sources of medical history and behavioral risk assessment information. This source may be friends rather than family members. Obtaining the most accurate information requires strategies for interviewing. At times, the results of screening may not be clear. The screening individual needs to know what resources are available to assist with the determination of suitability.

4. Personnel processing and/or packaging tissue must be knowledgeable about
   - environmental conditions required,
   - steps in the processing procedures,
   - labeling requirements,
   - packaging,
   - documentation,
   - appropriate measures to be taken when tissue is compromised, and
   - disposal of unsuitable tissue.

   Understanding the steps of tissue processing is essential to preventing errors that may alter the integrity and/or function of the tissue, contaminate it, or negatively affect the outcomes of transplantation. Disposal of human tissue must be done in compliance with federal and state regulations. Complete and accurate documentation for tracing tissue disposition is required by the FDA.

5. Administrators should ensure that initial and ongoing educational opportunities are provided to meet the needs of personnel who perform tasks within the surgical tissue bank. Regulations and standards affecting tissue bank activities are evolving. Initial education provides a baseline to support a beginning level of job performance. Ongoing education offers personnel an opportunity to enhance skills and learn about changes in regulations and standards. An introduction and review of tissue banking policies and procedures should be included in the orientation and ongoing education of personnel to assist in the development of knowledge, skills, and attitudes that positively affect patient outcomes.

6. Administrators should ensure that the employees performing tasks within the surgical tissue bank are competent to perform these tasks.

Competency assurance is essential because errors may cause breaches in regulations, compromise the integrity or function of the tissue, contaminate it, and/or lead to negative outcomes of transplantation.

Recommended Practice IV

Potential donors, their families, and recipients of tissue should be treated with respect, dignity, and sensitivity, and their rights should be protected.

1. Personnel approaching living donors or families of potential deceased donors to request consent for donation should be sensitive to the level of distress the situation may cause and respect the individual's rights. Tissue donation is frequently requested at the time of an unexpected death. This event creates distress in the survivors and is emotionally charged. Sensitivity to the needs of the survivors is essential to a successful donation. Perioperative personnel also should recognize that the deceased donor is an individual with the same rights that would be afforded to any other patient. At times, donation is requested of a living relative. This situation also may trigger strong emotions and ethical dilemmas. The person's rights should be honored.

2. Personnel should obtain informed consent from the donor or donor's responsible party before tissue recovery. Permission to retrieve tissue from nonliving donors should be sought from next of kin in order of legal precedence. If the next of kin is unavailable, local, state, and federal regulations should be followed. The Uniform Anatomical Gift Act (UAGA) of 1968, passed in all 50 states, provides guidelines within which consent may be obtained upon death of the donor, including an order of priority for the potential donor's next of kin. Additional guidelines concerning donations appear in the 1987 amendments to the UAGA and were clarified in 2001 by the US Department of Health and Human Services.[9] Individual state laws may vary. Some states expressly honor the donor's documented wishes (eg, donor registry, driver's license, donor card or directive) as legal consent in lieu of obtaining additional authorization from the next of kin.

Key elements of an informed consent include
- identification of tissues to be recovered;
- explanation of the potential uses of the tissue (eg, transplantation, research, education);
- a general description of the recovery process; and
- explanations that the family may limit or restrict the use of the tissue.[9]

3. Personnel should provide the family with written materials disclosing the intended uses of the tissue and the nature of the donation, including
- a copy of the signed consent form,
- instructions on how to follow up with the tissue bank should concerns arise,
- a description of the uses for which donated tissue may be applied, and
- a list and description of other companies and entities with which the tissue bank has relationships for processing and distributing tissue.

The tissue bank is responsible for ensuring that accurate, sensitive, and appropriate information is shared with the person giving consent. Using written materials ensures consistency and allows the person providing consent an opportunity to review the material again.[2]

4. Allograft donations from living donors should be accepted only if the medical, legal, and ethical conditions surrounding the donations meet approved criteria. Questionable conditions include undue medical risk to the donor, coercion, promises of monetary gain, and the diminished capacity of the donor to evaluate the medical or surgical risks.[7]

5. Informed consent should be obtained from patients receiving tissue transplants, following a discussion of the risks, benefits, and alternatives.

Recommended Practice V

Tissue for transplantation must be recovered only from suitable donors.

1. A responsible individual(s) must determine allograft donor suitability based on results of required screening and testing for risk factors or the presence of relevant communicable disease agents and diseases.[5,7] Individuals making the determination of donor suitability must be knowledgeable about the legal requirements and medical risks involved and must have the formal authority to make this determination. This responsibility may rest with a medical director or a medical advisory committee.

2. A responsible individual should screen donors of allografts for risk factors and clinical evidence of relevant infectious agents and diseases before recovery of tissues. Screening includes documenting the review of relevant medical records, performing a strict physical assessment, and conducting detailed interviews with a knowledgeable historian. Donor screening minimizes the risk of transmission of infectious agents and diseases to the recipient and minimizes the risk of retrieving tissue that is not suitable for transplantation.

3. Allograft donor exclusion criteria include the following:
- active systemic viral, bacterial, or fungal infection;
- disease history of unknown etiology;
- risk associated with human transmissible spongiform encephalopathy (eg, Creutzfeldt-Jakob disease [CJD], a blood relative with noniatrogenic CJD, rapidly progressive dementia, receipt of human pituitary-derived hormones, receipt of human dura mater grafts, travel/residency risks associated with variant CJD);
- certain autoimmune diseases;
- fever associated with a possible infectious etiology; and
- meeting any of the high-risk criteria for relevant communicable disease agents identified by the FDA, including
  - physical evidence for risk of sexually transmitted diseases such as genital ulcerative disease, herpes simplex, syphilis, chancroid;
  - for a male donor, physical evidence of anal intercourse, including perianal condyloma;
  - physical evidence of nonmedical percutaneous drug use, such as needle tracks, (note any tattoos that may be covering needle tracks);
  - physical evidence of recent tattooing, ear piercing, or body piercing;
  - disseminated lymphadenopathy;

– oral thrush;

– blue or purple spots consistent with Kaposi's sarcoma;

– unexplained jaundice, hepatomegaly, or icterus (note that hepatomegaly may not be apparent in a physical assessment unless an autopsy is performed);

– physical evidence of sepsis, such as unexplained generalized rash;

– large scab consistent with recent small-pox immunization;

– eczema vaccinatum;

– generalized vesicular rash (ie, generalized vaccinia);

– severely necrotic lesion consistent with vaccinia necrosum; and/or

– corneal scarring consistent with vaccinial keratitis.[10]

The medical director or medical advisory committee should evaluate potential donors with metabolic or bone disease, malignancy or malignant neoplasm, or disease of unknown etiology on a case-by-case basis. Some diseases have a range of severity that may cause the tissue to be appropriate or inappropriate for donation. A physician with knowledge and oversight responsibilities should evaluate these potential donors and make this determination. Potential donors are screened to minimize the risk of transmission of infection or disease. Recipients of pituitary-derived human growth hormone, human dura mater, or gonadotropin, as well as those who meet the travel/residency parameters associated with an increased exposure risk to the human form of bovine spongiform encephalopathy (BSE), may be at risk of carrying the agent causing CJD or variant CJD and should be excluded from consideration for tissue procurement.[5,10] Xenotransplantation recipients and their intimate contacts should be excluded from potential transplantation because xenotransplants may harbor infectious agents from the donor animal. These infectious agents also may have been transmitted to intimate contacts of the xenotransplant recipient. The FDA considers these individuals not to be suitable donors.[5,10]

Donor screening minimizes the risk of transmitting infectious agents and diseases to tissue recipients through transplantation.[10] Contraindications and exclusion criteria are evolving as new knowledge is gained and infectious disease threats are identified. Tissue bank administrations should remain informed of changes in the recommendations of the Centers for Disease Control and Prevention (CDC), FDA, and AATB and incorporate these changes into screening criteria.

4. Donors of allografts must be tested with FDA-approved, cleared, or licensed tests by laboratories compliant with the Clinical Laboratory Improvement Amendments of 1988 and found negative for relevant infectious agents and diseases, including, but not limited to

   ◆ HIV type 1 and type 2 (anti-HIV-1 and anti-HIV-2);

   ◆ hepatitis B virus (HBV) surface antigen (HBsAg);

   ◆ total antibody to hepatitis B core antigen (antiHBc)—(IgG+IgM);

   ◆ hepatitis C virus (HCV) (anti-HCV);

   ◆ *Treponema pallidum* (syphilis) confirmatory test;

   ◆ human T-lymphotropic virus (Types I and II); and

   ◆ cytomegalovirus.[5]

Living donors should be tested for hepatitis HBc core antibody (anti-HBc) and should be retested 180 days after recovery before tissues are released for allogenic use. Testing for these infectious agents minimizes the risk of transmission and is required by the FDA final rule.[3] Donors of dura mater grafts also must be tested for the infectious agent that causes CJD; this includes a recommendation that a qualified pathologist perform an examination of the donor's entire brain.[5]

Recommended Practice VI

Tissue must be recovered, processed, and transplanted in clean, controlled environments appropriate for sterile surgical procedures.

1. Traffic patterns should be established and maintained in accordance with AORN's "Recommended practices for traffic patterns in the perioperative practice setting."[11] Traffic control in the OR minimizes the potential for contamination of the tissue retrieved. Eyes usually are procured with intact corneas in less controlled

environments; however, the corneas should be removed from the eyes, processed, and transplanted in an OR-type environment.

2. The environment should be cleaned in accordance with AORN's "Recommended practices for environmental cleaning in the surgical practice setting."[12] Cleaning should be performed on a routine basis and as needed to reduce the amount of organic and inorganic debris and microbial load that can potentially contaminate the tissue. The FDA requires that the facility for tissue recovery be controlled to minimize the risk for contamination or cross-contamination through the introduction or transmission of communicable disease.[6(p68683)]

3. Surgical attire should be worn during recovery and transplantation of tissue in accordance with AORN's "Recommended practices for surgical attire."[13] Clean surgical attire minimizes contamination of the tissue.

4. Only powder-free gloves should be used. Glove powder is aerosolized when powdered gloves are used.[14] Powder can contaminate recovered tissue and may lead to adverse reactions or rejections of the tissue by the recipient.[15-23]

5. When it is known that the potential tissue recipient has antibodies to natural rubber proteins, the tissue should be recovered with latex-free supplies in accordance with the "AORN latex guideline."[24] Transplanting tissue with an antigen to which the recipient is allergic can lead to adverse outcomes, including tissue rejection, impaired healing, and allergic reaction.

Recommended Practice VII

Tissue must be recovered and processed in a manner that minimizes microbial growth, contamination, and cross-contamination.[6(p68681)]

1. Postmortem donors should be placed in refrigeration within 12 hours of asystole, and tissue should be procured within 24 hours of asystole. Refrigeration minimizes cell oxygen consumption and microbial growth. Prolonged times between cell ischemia and tissue recovery provides an opportunity for microbial proliferation. Recommendations for maximum duration of time between recovery and transplantation have been established by the AATB.[7]

2. A sterile field should be established and maintained in accordance with AORN's "Recommended practices for maintaining a sterile field."[25] Aseptic practices are used to prevent contamination of the tissue and minimize the risk of subsequent infection. Sterile surgical drapes provide a barrier to minimize contamination of the recovered tissue.

3. The donor site and operative site should be prepared in accordance with AORN's "Recommended practices for skin preparation of patients."[26] Adequate skin preparation reduces the microbial count of the skin that can lead to contamination of recovered tissue.

4. The surgical team should perform surgical hand antisepsis and wear sterile gowns and gloves during recovery of tissue, in accordance with AORN's "Recommended practices for surgical hand antisepsis/hand scrubs."[27] Surgical hand antisepsis reduces microbial flora and may reduce the contamination of the tissue. Gowns and gloves provide a barrier to microbial contamination. When corneas are recovered, the sterile field is very small, and gowns may not be necessary.

5. Transplantation of tissue has resulted in transmission of viral, bacterial, and fungal infections. Inadequate tissue processing and quality controls have resulted in postoperative infections and graft failures.[6(p68651)] In 2002, the CDC published an investigation of 26 reported cases of allograft-associated infections.[28] During an investigation of voluntary reports, the FDA identified failure to validate procedures to prevent contamination and cross-contamination during processing in more than half of reported adverse events.[6(p68652)] Proper processing and quality controls minimize the risk of adverse events associated with transplanted tissue.

Recommended Practice VIII

Tissue must be prepared, processed, and preserved in a manner that minimizes microbial growth and optimizes the condition of the tissue for transplantation.[6(p68681)]

1. Aerobic and anaerobic tissue cultures should be collected when tissue is retrieved. Culture results may identify tissue that is inappropriate for transplantation and also provide a baseline for evaluation of processing and storage.

2. Tissue that will not undergo a sterilization process should be aseptically prepared and transferred to a sterile storage container. Aseptic technique is used to prevent contamination of tissue.

3. The package or container selected should provide an adequate barrier to microbial contamination and should be compatible with the type of sterilization, preservation, and storage conditions. Packages of refrigerated and frozen tissue become wet during storage and form condensation upon removal from storage. Containers should be impervious to moisture.

4. For sterilization of tissue, FDA-approved technology should be used in accordance with the FDA current good tissue practices[6] and AATB standards for guidance. The FDA regulations and recommendations are evolving as new knowledge is gained. The AATB periodically reviews and revises the standards for tissue banking. It is important to review information from these sources to minimize risks of tissue processing.

5. Pooling (ie, commingling) of tissue from two or more donors must not occur.[6(p68684)]

6. When processing dura mater, a validated procedure must be used to minimize the risk of transmitting human transmissible spongiform encephalopathy (eg, prion disease, CJD).[6(p68683)] Transplantation of contaminated tissue has resulted in transmission of viral, bacterial, and fungal infections.[6] Proper processing and quality controls minimize the risk of adverse events associated with transplanted tissue.

Recommended Practice IX

Tissue must be labeled in a manner that provides direction for preparation and implantation and minimizes the risk of errors.[6,7]

1. Proper labeling of tissue minimizes the risk of errors. The allograft package/storage container should be labeled with the following information:

 - tissue identification number (this may include a bar code);
 - description of the tissue;
 - name, address, and telephone number of the tissue bank responsible for determining donor suitability, processing, storage, and distribution of the allograft;
 - recovery or distribution center that is responsible for determining donor suitability, processing, and distribution;
 - recovery date and time;
 - expiration date, if applicable, including the month and year;
 - acceptable storage conditions, including recommended storage temperature and acceptable storage temperature range;
 - the disinfection or sterilization method used, if applicable;
 - if not sterilized, whether the tissue was procured and prepared under aseptic conditions;
 - quantity of tissue expressed as volume, weight, dimensions, or a combination of these units of measure, if applicable;
 - potential residues of processing agents and solutions (eg, antibiotics, ethanol, ethylene oxide, dimethyl sulfoxide); and
 - package inserts containing instructions for use, indications and contraindications, preparation of tissue for use, expiration dates, and specific tests performed on tissues, warnings and potential adverse reactions, and instructions for opening packages or containers.[6,7]

2. The autograft package/storage container should be labeled with the following information:
 - name, address, and telephone number of the tissue bank responsible for processing, storing, and distributing the autograft;
 - the statements "For Autologous Use Only" and "Autologous Donation";[7(p86)]
 - disinfection/sterilization method, if used;
 - if not sterilized, whether the tissue was recovered and prepared under aseptic conditions;
 - the warning "Not Evaluated For Infectious Substances" if infectious disease testing has not been performed;
 - the warning "Biohazard" if infectious disease tests were performed and found to be positive;
 - two unique identifiers of the donor/recipient (eg, name, medical records number), including bar code;

- description of the tissue;
- recovery date and time;
- expiration date, if applicable, including the month and year;
- acceptable storage conditions, including recommended storage temperature and acceptable storage temperature range;
- method of preservation, if applicable; and
- potential residues of processing agents and solutions (eg, antibiotics, ethanol, ethylene oxide, dimethyl sulfoxide).[6,7] This information is necessary for release of the autograft for reimplantation only into the same donor/patient, quality control, and appropriate tissue preparation for implantation.

This documentation is required for certification by the AATB. Some of the information also is required by the FDA. Autografts have not undergone testing for infectious agents and diseases and must be released only to the donor. Release to another recipient may cause serious injury. Using two unique donor/recipient identifiers is consistent with JCAHO's safety goal of patient identification.[29] The application of bar code labeling facilitates matching of tissue to the desired recipient and accurate record keeping. These strategies minimize the potential for errors. The FDA requires that a procedure be maintained to verify the accuracy of labels when labeling human tissue.[6(p68684)]

Recommended Practice X

Allograft tissue obtained from an outside tissue bank should be handled in a manner consistent with the source facility's or manufacturer's written instructions.

1. Incoming tissue should be recorded, including the unique identifiers of the tissue and expiration date, the identification of the person accepting the tissue, and the date and time of receipt.

2. The packaging and transport conditions of incoming tissue should be examined to verify that the tissue integrity and temperature are acceptable and have been maintained during transport.

3. The tissue should be transferred to storage in manner consistent with the source facility's and manufacturer's written instructions.

Recommended Practice XI

Tissue is transported and stored in a manner that minimizes the risk of compromise or contamination.[6]

1. Containers for transporting and/or temporarily storing tissue must protect the tissue from contamination and maintain tissue at appropriate temperatures during transport.[6(p68660), 8(PC.17.10.C)]

2. Tissue for transplantation at a later date should be contained and frozen as soon as possible after recovery. Warm tissue is a medium for microbial growth. Tissue contamination may be multifactorial, and no finite time frame has been established. Institutions should determine this time frame with consideration of the type of tissue and recovery conditions.

3. Tissue must be stored in a secure area, with access restricted to authorized personnel, to minimize the risk of mix-ups, contamination, or improper distribution of tissue.[6(p68685)]

4. Temperatures selected for storage should be consistent with the AATB standards.[7]
   - Lyophilized or dehydrated musculoskeletal tissue should be stored at ambient temperature or cooler (but not be frozen).
   - Refrigerated musculoskeletal and osteoarticular tissue should be aseptically recovered, stored in an isotonic solution containing suitable antibiotics, and stored at 33.8° F (1° C) to 50° F (10° C).
   - Refrigerated skin should be stored at 33.8° F (1° C) to 50° F (10° C).
   - Frozen musculoskeletal and osteoarticular tissue should be processed and stored at –40° F (–40° C) or colder for long-term storage; and between –4° F (–20° C) to –40° F (–40° C) for short-term storage (fewer than six months).
   - Frozen or cryopreserved skin should be stored at –40° F (–40° C) or colder.
   - Frozen, cryopreserved cardiovascular tissue should be stored at –148° F (–100° C) or colder.
   - Reproductive cells should be frozen and cryopreserved in a liquid nitrogen freezer. Storage may be in either the liquid or vapor phase.

◆ Refrigeration minimizes oxygen consumption of cells and prolongs their life. Dead cells provide a medium for microbial growth. Refrigeration minimizes microbial growth.

5. Autologous tissue should be segregated from allografts.[7] Autologous tissue usually has not undergone testing for infectious diseases or suitability screening for use for other patients, and its use is restricted to the donor only. Segregation minimizes the risk of error that may result in a negative outcome to a tissue recipient.

6. An expiration date for each tissue must be assigned. This expiration date must be based on tissue type, processing, preservation, storage, and packaging.[6(p68683)] The expiration time of tissue should not exceed the following recommendations of the AATB:[7]
   ◆ refrigerated musculoskeletal tissue: five days;
   ◆ refrigerated skin: 14 days;
   ◆ frozen and cryopreserved cells and tissue (–40° F [–40° C] or colder): five years; and
   ◆ lyophilized or dehydrated tissue: five years.

   Safe duration of storage of autografts may be influenced by processing and packaging methods and should be defined by the facility, not to exceed the recommendations of the AATB listed above. A process should be in place to minimize the number of autografts in storage to those that will be reimplanted. This is facilitated by periodic communication with surgeons or review of medical records to determine whether patients have survived.

7. Refrigerator and freezer units used for storing tissue should
   ◆ be monitored and daily temperature checks recorded,
   ◆ have annual calibration checks, and
   ◆ have an alarm system that is continuously monitored and that sounds when the temperature is not within the acceptable range.

   Restricted access is required to verify the safety and security of tissues. Maintenance of temperatures within the refrigerator or freezer unit ensures tissue integrity. Acceptable temperature range limits for the storage of tissue at each phase of the operation should be set in accordance with established standards and federal and state regulations. Temperature fluc-

tuations outside the recommended temperature range may render tissue unsafe for patient use. The source facility should be consulted if this occurs. The alarm should sound in an area where an individual is present at all times to initiate immediate corrective action.

8. Personnel should have a specific contingency plan for refrigerator or freezer malfunction. Storage freezers and refrigerators should be attached to an emergency power system. In the event of failure of a refrigerator or freezer, the temperature of tissue should be monitored and maintained to prevent compromise of the tissue. All events should be properly documented.

Recommended Practice XII

Tissue should be quarantined until all steps of the tissue banking process have been reviewed and found acceptable.

1. Allografts should be segregated and not released until all screening, testing, processing, labeling, and storage criteria have been reviewed and determined to be satisfactory. The tissue should remain in an area segregated from available tissue until this review has been completed and the tissue is available for implantation. Segregation minimizes the risk of implanting unsuitable tissue. A checklist of criteria for release provides a standardized method of verifying release criteria and minimizes the potential for errors.

2. Autografts should be segregated and not released until all processing, labeling, and storage criteria have been reviewed and determined to be satisfactory. Segregation minimizes the risk of implanting unsuitable tissue. A checklist of criteria for release provides a standardized method of verifying release criteria and minimizes the potential for errors.

3. Autografts meeting all criteria for release should be released only for reimplantation in the autologous donor. Two unique identifiers (eg, donor name, medical record number) should be used for release of autografts. Autografts usually have not undergone testing for infectious agents and diseases and must be released only for reimplantation in the donor. Release to another recipient may cause serious

injury. Using two unique donor identifiers is in accordance with the Joint Commission's safety goal of patient identification.[29] This strategy minimizes the potential for errors.

4. Tissue not meeting the release criteria should be considered compromised and should be destroyed in accordance with state and federal regulations. Regulations addressing human tissue disposal vary from state to state. Tissue that has not undergone sterilization is considered biohazardous.

5. Before dispensing tissue from the tissue bank, the processes used should be reviewed, and the suitability of the tissue for implantation should be determined. A standardized process should be in place to verify the donor tissue and recipient match, when applicable.

6. Verification of tissue availability should be incorporated into the verification process used to ensure the correct patient, procedure, site, position, and implants.[30]

7. The contents of the package, expiration date, and other pertinent information should be read back and verified before the tissue is dispensed onto the sterile field. Use of bar coding technology facilitates matching tissue to the desired recipient and keeping accurate records.

Recommended Practice XIII

Each tissue bank must maintain donor, tissue, and recipient records to ensure that pertinent data are retrievable.

1. The surgical tissue bank should have a tissue identification system that allows for tracking of tissues from the donor source to the recipient patient or institution, and vice versa.[6] Quality control issues and infections from implanted tissue have been reported. An identification system provides a means to determine what tissue is affected, rapidly quarantine the tissue, and follow up with affected recipients to ensure timely intervention to minimize morbidity.

2. Surgical tissue banks procuring, processing, distributing, and storing tissues should keep accurate records of the distribution of each tissue according to donor identification number,

tissue type and identifying number, and identifying information for the receiving center, along with the dates of recovery and distribution.[6] This information provides a means to recall tissue that may be compromised.

3. Records should be developed and maintained according to the recommendations of AATB and in compliance with FDA rules. Records should include the following information:
   ♦ FDA registration, if applicable;
   ♦ copies of FDA registration and AATB accreditation of outside vendors from whom tissue is obtained (EBAA for ocular tissue, AABB for stem cells);
   ♦ listing of all tissue products ordered, stored, and used;
   ♦ informed consent documents;
   ♦ donor suitability assessment criteria;
   ♦ recovery;
   ♦ processing;
   ♦ preservation;
   ♦ labeling;
   ♦ storage;
   ♦ quarantining;
   ♦ testing record review;
   ♦ releasing;
   ♦ distribution;
   ♦ ordering and receipt of tissue acquired from other sources:
      − package integrity upon receipt,
      − transport temperature-controlled and acceptable, and
      − source facility and unique identifier of the tissue;
   ♦ instructions/procedures for reconstitution;
   ♦ identity of personnel preparing, accepting, and issuing tissue;
   ♦ dates and times of preparing, accepting, and issuing tissue;
   ♦ documentation in the recipient's health record of the unique identifier of the tissue;
   ♦ quality management records;
   ♦ recall criteria and procedures; and
   ♦ disposal of tissue.

   For tissue obtained from outside tissue banks, copies of pertinent records should be forwarded to the source facility. Documentation assists in clinical evaluation and in tracking recipients if an adverse event is identified.[6]

4. Records must be maintained for 10 years after tissue is dispensed or the tissue expiration date is reached, whichever is longer.[6] Tissue may be used years after recovery. For that reason, the FDA requires that records must be maintained for 10 years.

Recommended Practice XIV

A quality management program must be in place to evaluate the structure, processes, and outcomes of tissue bank services.[6(p68682)]

1. An initial program review should be performed by a multidisciplinary committee, comparing procedures with regulations and standards. Program review should be done annually to ensure ongoing compliance with regulations and ensure safe tissue banking practices.

2. Quality indicators should include, but not be limited to,
   - donor screening and testing;
   - tissue processing procedures;
   - labeling procedures;
   - storage requirements;
   - criteria for release of tissue;
   - the use of two unique donor identifiers for release of autografts; and
   - adverse events (including posttransplantation infections), corrective action, and evaluation.

   Tissue bank services involve significant risks to recipients if errors are made. The FDA requires any facility performing tissue banking to maintain a quality management program intended to prevent the introduction, transmission, or spread of communicable disease for every step of tissue banking performed.[6(p68682)] Ongoing quality management involves verifying that these steps are done in a safe, efficacious manner. These quality indicators address specific issues that may compromise the tissue. Specific quality indicators will depend on the services provided.

3. The FDA final rule for current good tissue practices requires the following aspects of quality management:[6]
   - ensuring that required procedures are established and maintained;
   - ensuring the appropriate analysis and sharing of information that could affect the potential contamination of the product or the potential transmission of communicable disease by the product;
   - ensuring that appropriate corrective actions are taken and documented;
   - ensuring proper training and education of personnel;
   - establishing and maintaining appropriate monitoring systems;
   - establishing and maintaining a system of records;
   - investigating and documenting product deviations and making certain required reports; and
   - conducting evaluations, investigations, audits, and other actions necessary to ensure compliance with the regulations.[6]

   This quality framework is required by the FDA. Administrative personnel should be familiar with this requirement and its application to the components of tissue banking performed.

4. Facilities should report adverse events, including infections for which there is a reasonable possibility that the transplanted tissue caused the event. The tissue bank manufacturing the tissue is required to report adverse events to the FDA.[6] These reports are submitted through MedWatch at *http://www.fda.gov/medwatch/report/instruc.htm*. For events that result from tissue acquired from an outside tissue vendor, the report should be sent to the vendor and also may be submitted to the FDA.

Recommended Practice XV

Policies and procedures for preserving, storing, and maintaining tissue should be established, reviewed annually, and readily available in the practice setting.

1. Policies establishing authority, responsibility, and accountability for tissue handling and appropriate donor testing within the practice setting must be established and maintained for all steps performed by the facility.[6(p68683)] These policies may include, but are not limited to,
   - authority and accountability for processes;
   - screening and testing criteria;
   - obtaining informed consent from the donor;

♦ providing information and obtaining informed consent from the allograft recipient;

♦ evaluating culture and serology tests with appropriate interventions for positive results;

♦ processing and preserving tissue;

♦ packaging and labeling tissue;

♦ sterilizing processes, if applicable;

♦ monitoring temperature during storage;

♦ maximum storage duration;

♦ handling frozen tissue if there is a freezer malfunction or power outage;

♦ warming or reconstituting preserved tissue;

♦ rinsing solutions from tissues;

♦ criteria for return of unused tissue into inventory;

♦ disposal of tissue;

♦ documenting implanted and discarded tissue in a retrievable format, and notifying recipients or recalling released tissues;

♦ responses to adverse events; and

♦ responses to recalls of tissue from tissue vendors.

2. Before implementation, procedures must be approved by the responsible authority within the health care organization.[6(p68683)] Institutional policies and procedures may seriously affect patient safety and should be reviewed by designated authorities within the facility (eg, infection control committee, pathology department). Tissue may be used years after recovery. For that reason, the FDA final rule for good tissue practices requires that policies and procedures be reviewed periodically, be readily available in the practice setting, and be archived for 10 years after recovery or the expiration date of the tissue, whichever is longer.[6(p68685)] These recommended practices should be used as guidelines, along with the standards of the AATB and regulations and recommendations of the FDA, for the development of policies and procedures for surgical tissue banking in the practice setting. Policies and procedures establish authority, responsibility, and accountability and serve as operational guidelines.

3. The uniform perioperative nursing vocabulary should be used to document perioperative nursing care of the transplant donor and recipient on the intraoperative patient record. The perioperative nursing vocabulary is a clinically relevant and empirically validated standardized nursing language. This standardized language consists of the Perioperative Nursing Data Set (PNDS) and includes perioperative nursing diagnoses, interventions, and outcomes. The expected outcome of primary importance to these recommended practices is outcome O10, "The patient is free from signs and symptoms of infection." This outcome falls within the domain of Safety (D1). Interventions that might lead to the desired outcome include I98, "Protects from cross-contamination"; I121, "Assesses susceptibility for infection"; and I188, "Monitors for signs and symptoms of infection."[31]

Editor's note: The American Association of Tissue Banks can be reached at 1320 Old Chain Bridge Road, Suite 450, McLean, VA 22101; telephone (703) 827-9582.

Glossary

Allografts: Grafts taken from a living or nonliving donor for transplantation to a different individual.

American Association of Tissue Banks (AATB): A nonprofit organization that defines the standards for tissue banking.

Autografts: Tissue derived from an individual for implantation exclusively on or in the same individual.

Donor screening: Review of the donor's relevant medical records and physical assessment for evidence of past or present risk factors for relevant infectious agents or disease.

Donor testing: Laboratory tests on blood specimens collected from a potential donor.

Prion diseases: A classification of infectious diseases, including Creutzfeldt-Jakob disease (CJD), caused by a unique proteinaceous agent.

Tissue bank: A facility that participates in procuring, processing, preserving, and/or storing human cells and tissue for transplantation.

Xenotransplant: Cells or tissue from a nonhuman animal source that are transplanted, implanted, or infused into a human.

Xenotransplantation: Any procedure that involves the transplantation, implantation, or infusion into a human recipient of either (a) live cells, tissues, or organs from a nonhuman animal source (eg, bovine heart valves); or (b) human body fluids, cells, tissues, or organs that have had ex vivo contact with live nonhuman animal cells, tissues, or organs.

Notes

1. US Food and Drug Administration, *Proposed Approach to Regulation of Cellular and Tissue-Based Products* (Rockville, Md: US Food and Drug Administration, Feb 28, 1997) 1-37.

2. US Food and Drug Administration, "Current good tissue practice for manufacturers of human cellular and tissue-based products; inspection and enforcement; proposed rule," *Federal Register* 66 (January 8, 2001) 1507-1559. Also available at *http://www.fda.gov/OHRMS /DOCKETS/98fr/010801c.pdf* (accessed 13 Sept 2005).

3. US Food and Drug Administration, "Suitability determination for donors of human cellular and tissue-based products; proposed rule," *Federal Register* 64 (Sept 30, 1999) 52696-52718. Also available at *http:// www.fda.gov/OHRMS/DOCKETS/98fr/093099a.pdf* (accessed 13 Sept 2005).

4. US Food and Drug Administration, "Human cells, tissues, and cellular and tissue-based products; establishment registration and listing; final rule," *Federal Register* 66 (Jan 19, 2001) 5447-5469. Also available at *http:// www.fda.gov/OHRMS/DOCKETS /98fr/011901a.pdf* (accessed 13 Sept 2005).

5. US Food and Drug Administration, "Eligibility determination for donors of human cells, tissues, and cellular and tissue-based products; final rule and notice," *Federal Register* 69 (May 25, 2004) 29785-29834. Also available at *http://www.fda.gov/OHRMS/DOCKETS /98fr/04-11245.pdf* (accessed 13 Sept 2005).

6. US Food and Drug Administration, "Current good tissue practice for human cell, tissue, and cellular and tissue-based product establishments; inspection and enforcement; final rule," *Federal Register* 69 (Nov 24, 2004) 68612-68688.

7. American Association of Tissue Banks, *Standards for Tissue Banking*, 10th ed (McLean, Va: American Association of Tissue Banks, 2002).

8. Joint Commission on Accreditation of Healthcare Organizations, "Standards approved for transplant and implant tissue storage and issuance," *Joint Commission Perspectives* (February 2005) 8-11.

9. Office of Inspector General, *Informed Consent in Tissue Donation: Expectations and Realities*, publ OEI-01-00-00440 (Boston: US Department of Health and Human Services, January 2001).

10. US Food and Drug Administration, *Guidance for Industry: Eligibility Determination for Donors of Human Cells, Tissues, and Cellular and Tissue-Based Products (HCT/Ps): Draft Guidance* (Rockville, Md: US Food and Drug Administration, May 2004) 1-52.

11. "Recommended practices for traffic patterns in the perioperative practice setting," in *Standards, Recommended Practices, and Guidelines* (Denver: AORN, Inc, 2005) 483-485.

12. "Recommended practices for environmental cleaning in the surgical practice setting," in *Standards, Recommended Practices, and Guidelines* (Denver: AORN, Inc, 2005) 361-366.

13. "Recommended practices for surgical attire," in *Standards, Recommended Practices, and Guidelines* (Denver: AORN, Inc, 2005) 299-305.

14. D Beezhold, D Kostyal, J Wiseman, "The transfer of protein allergens from latex gloves: A study of influencing factors," *AORN Journal* 59 (March 1994) 605-613.

15. D Abeck et al, "Latex allergy and repeated graft rejections," *The Lancet* 339 (June 27, 1992) 1609.

16. D Beezhold, W Beck, "The absorbability and immunology of starch glove powders," *Complications in Surgery* (July/August 1992) 36-40.

17. C Bene, G Kranias, "Possible intraocular lens contamination by surgical glove powder," *Ophthalmic Surgery* 17 (May 1986) 290-291.

18. I Singh, W L Chow, L V Chablani, "Synovial reaction to glove powder," *Clinical Orthopaedics and Related Research* 99 (March/April 1974) 285-292.

19. P H McKee, E F McKeown, "Starch granulomata of the endocardium," *Journal of Pathology* 126 (October 1978) 103-105.

20. S Moriber-Katz et al, "Contamination of perfused donor kidneys by starch from surgical gloves," *American Journal of Clinical Pathology* 90 (July 1988) 81-84.

21. D I Vâge et al, "Elutable factors from latex-containing materials activate complement and inhibit cell proliferation: An in vitro biocompatibility study of medical devices," *Complement Inflammation* 7 (January-February 1990) 63-70.

22. C M Ruhl et al, "A new hazard of cornstarch, an absorbable dusting powder," *The Journal of Emergency Medicine* 12 (January/February 1994)11-14.

23. D A A Verkuyl, "Glove powder introduced in the circulation by autotransfusion and severe cardiac failure," *The Lancet* 340 (Aug 29, 1992) 550.

24. "AORN latex guideline," in *Standards, Recommended Practices, and Guidelines* (Denver: AORN, Inc, 2005) 117-132.

25. "Recommended practices for maintaining a sterile field," in *Standards, Recommended Practices, and Guidelines* (Denver: AORN, Inc, 2005) 453-457.

26. "Recommended practices for skin preparation of patients," in *Standards, Recommended Practices, and Guidelines* (Denver: AORN, Inc, 2005) 443-446.

27. "Recommended practices for surgical hand antisepsis/hand scrubs," in *Standards, Recommended Practices, and Guidelines* (Denver: AORN, Inc, 2005) 377-385.

28. Centers for Disease Control and Prevention, "Update: Allograft-associated bacterial infections—United States," *Morbidity and Mortality Weekly Report* 51 (March 15, 2002) 207-210. Also available at *http://www.cdc.gov /mmwr/preview/mmwrhtml/mm5110a2.htm* (accessed 13 Sept 2005).

29. "2005 Hospitals' National Patient Safety Goals," Joint Commission on Accreditation of Health Care Organizations, *http://www.jcaho.org /accredited+organizations /patient+safety/05+npsg/05_npsg _hap.htm* (accessed 13 Sept 2005).

30. "Universal protocol for preventing wrong site, wrong procedure, wrong person surgery," Joint Commission on Accreditation of Health Care Organizations, *http://www.jcaho.org/accredited+organizations/patient+safety/universal+protocol/universal_protocol.pdf* (accessed 13 Sept 2005).

31. S C Beyea, ed, *Perioperative Nursing Data Set: The Perioperative Nursing Vocabulary,* second ed (Denver: AORN, Inc, 2002).

RESOURCES

Bren, L. "Keeping human tissue transplants safe," *FDA Consumer Magazine* 39 (May/June 2005) 30-36.

Verble, M; Worth, J. "Cultural sensitivity in the donation discussion," *Progress in Transplantation* 13 (March 2003) 33-37.

Verble, M; Worth, J. "Fears and concerns expressed by families in the donation discussion," *Progress in Transplantation* 10 (March 2000) 48-55.

Originally published September 1984, *AORN Journal.* Revised April 1991.

Published as proposed recommended practices, February 1994.

Revised November 1998; published March 1999, *AORN Journal.* Reformatted July 2000.

Revised November 2003; published February 2004, *AORN Journal.*

Revised November 2005; published February 2006, *AORN Journal.*

Recommended Practices for Traffic Patterns in the Perioperative Practice Setting

The following recommended practices were developed by the AORN Recommended Practices Committee and have been approved by the AORN Board of Directors. They were presented as proposed recommended practices for comments by members and others. They are effective January 1, 2006.

These recommended practices are intended as achievable recommendations representing what is believed to be an optimal level of practice. Policies and procedures will reflect variations in practice settings and/or clinical situations that determine the degree to which the recommended practices can be implemented.

AORN recognizes the numerous settings in which perioperative nurses practice. These recommended practices are intended as guidelines adaptable to various practice settings. These practice settings include traditional ORs, ambulatory surgery centers, physicians' offices, cardiac catheterization suites, endoscopy suites, radiology departments, emergency departments, labor and delivery units that have OR suites, and all other areas where operative and other invasive procedures may be performed.

Purpose

These recommended practices provide guidance for establishing traffic patterns in perioperative practice areas. Traffic control patterns suggest movement into and out of the surgical suite as well as movement within the suite. Clearly defined and enforced traffic control practices protect personnel, patients, supplies, and equipment from potential sources of cross-contamination; safeguard the privacy of patients; and provide security.

The building design of the surgical suite often predetermines traffic patterns. Implementation of all elements of these recommended practices may not be feasible within every facility because of the physical limitations of the setting.

Recommended Practice I

Traffic patterns should be designed to facilitate movement of patients and personnel into, through, and out of defined areas within the surgical suite. Signs should clearly indicate the appropriate environmental controls and surgical attire required.

1. The surgical suite should be divided into three designated areas that are defined by the physical activities performed in each area. Increasing environmental controls and surgical attire as progression is made from unrestricted to restricted areas decreases the potential for cross-contamination.

   The **unrestricted** area includes a central control point that is established to monitor the entrance of patients, personnel, and materials. Street clothes are permitted in this area, and traffic is not limited. The entrance to the surgical suite should be restricted to authorized personnel based on organizational policies.

   The **semirestricted** area includes the peripheral support areas of the surgical suite. It has storage areas for clean and sterile supplies, work areas for storage and processing of instruments, scrub sink areas, and corridors leading to the restricted areas of the surgical suite. Traffic in this area is limited to authorized personnel and patients. Personnel are required to wear surgical attire and cover all head and facial hair.[1]

   The **restricted** area includes ORs, procedure rooms, and the clean core area. Surgical attire and hair coverings are required. Masks are required where open sterile supplies or scrubbed persons are located. All persons entering the restricted area should follow the AORN "Recommended practices for surgical attire."[1]

   Persons entering the semirestricted or restricted areas of the surgical suite for a brief time for a specific purpose (eg, law enforcement officers, parents, biomedical engineers) should cover all head and facial hair and may don either freshly laundered surgical attire or a single-use coverall suit (eg, jumpsuit) designed to totally cover outside apparel.

2. Movement of personnel from unrestricted areas to either semirestricted or restricted areas should be through a transition zone. A transition zone exists where one can enter the area in street clothing and exit into the semirestricted or restricted zone in surgical attire. Locker rooms serve as transition zones between the outside and inside of a surgical suite and may serve as a security point to monitor people admitted to the suite.

3. Patients entering the surgical suite should wear clean gowns, be covered with clean linens, and have their hair covered. Clean gowns, linens, and hair coverings are worn by patients to minimize particulate shedding during surgical procedures.

Patients are not required to wear masks while in the surgical suite unless they are under airborne precautions (eg, a patient with active pulmonary tuberculosis or other airborne respiratory disease).[2] While in the restricted area, the mask could hinder access to the face and airway and might increase the patient's anxiety.

Personal undergarments may be worn when they will not interfere with the surgical site. Consideration should be given for management of potential incontinence. Many health care organizations now allow specific patients to wear clean personal clothing, including socks and underwear, into the surgical suite to promote the patient's comfort and sense of dignity. The most common surgical procedures that incorporate this new patient care practice are cataract extractions and carpal tunnel releases. Access to patients below the waist usually is not necessary for these surgical procedures. In addition, sterile fields can be maintained easily without the risk of contamination from patient clothing.

Recommended Practice II

Operating room suites should be secure.

1. The design of perioperative areas and traffic patterns should include the following.
   ♦ Patient privacy must be provided for as required by the Health Insurance Portability and Accountability Act of 1996 (HIPAA).[3]
   ♦ Patient, personnel, and visitor safety should be ensured.
   ♦ Supplies and equipment should be protected from tampering and theft.

2. Identification badges should be worn at all times according to organizational policy.

Recommended Practice III

Movement of personnel should be kept to a minimum while invasive and noninvasive procedures are in progress.

1. Careful assessment of the patient and planning for patient care needs should reduce the need for excessive movement and activity during the procedure. Air is a potential source of microorganisms that can contaminate surgical wounds. Because microbial shedding increases with activity, greater amounts of airborne contamination can be expected with increased movement of surgical team members.[4]

2. Doors to the operating or procedure rooms should be closed except during movement of patients, personnel, supplies, and equipment. The air pressure within each operating or procedure room should be greater than in the semirestricted area. The air in the OR should be maintained under positive pressure with a minimum of 15 total room air exchanges per hour.[5] When the doors are left open, the heating, ventilation, and air conditioning system is unable to maintain these critical environmental parameters. Leaving the door open can disrupt pressurization and cause turbulent airflow that could increase airborne contamination. Traffic in and out of the OR should be minimized by preplanning so that turbulence from this activity is minimized during the procedure or when sterile supplies are opened.

3. Talking and the number of people present should be minimized during procedures. An increase in airborne microorganisms can occur with an increased number of people present. Movement, talking, and uncovered skin areas can contribute to airborne contamination.[4]

Recommended Practice IV

The movement of clean and sterile supplies and equipment should be separated from contaminated supplies, equipment, and waste by space, time, or traffic patterns.

1. Surgical supplies prepared for surgical procedures outside the surgical suite (eg, in central processing) should be transported to the surgical suite to maintain cleanliness and sterility and to prevent physical damage. Protecting items from contamination, physical damage, and loss during transportation facilitates their safe use. Use of correct procedures for transporting items preserves the qualities of the sterile and clean environment.[6]

2. Supplies and equipment should be removed from external shipping containers and web-edged or corrugated cardboard boxes in the unrestricted area before transfer into the surgical suite. External shipping containers and web-edged cardboard boxes may collect dust, debris, and insects during shipment and may carry contaminants into the surgical suite.[6]

3. When there is a clean core, the movement of supplies should be from the clean core through the operating or procedure room to the peripheral corridor.

   ♦ Soiled supplies, instruments, and equipment should not reenter the clean core area. They should be contained in closed or covered carts or containers for transport to a designated decontamination area.

   ♦ The decontamination area and soiled linen and trash collection areas should be separated from personnel and patient traffic areas. Separation of clean and sterile supplies and equipment from soiled materials by space, time, and traffic patterns decreases the risk of infection.[6]

Recommended Practice V

During construction and renovation, specific traffic patterns should be established and maintained in accordance with applicable state regulations.

1. Specific traffic plans for construction personnel and movement of supplies, equipment, and debris should be developed and implemented following applicable guidelines for construction in health care facilities, with infection control personnel monitoring the process.[7,8] Infections have been transmitted through the dissemination of microorganisms from disruptions of environmental reservoirs (eg, drywall, ceiling tiles, flooring, casework).[9]

2. Surgical personnel should be able to move from place to place without contaminating their surgical scrubs. Clean or sterile supplies and equipment must be transported to storage areas by a route that minimizes contamination from the construction site and prevents contact with soiled or contaminated trash and linen. Since traffic patterns may not be easily altered to meet these requirements, the construction

personnel may need to work during off hours. If infection control requirements still cannot be met, some areas may need to be relocated or closed temporarily.[9]

3. A multidisciplinary assessment should be completed to determine the infection control and safety risks involved in a construction, renovation, or maintenance project. A multidisciplinary team performing the assessment should include infection control, safety, and project personnel. An infection control risk assessment (ICRA) matrix may facilitate the process. The ICRA matrix helps the team identify important preventive strategies that may include, but are not limited to,

   ♦ types of barriers necessary,
   ♦ maintenance of barrier integrity,
   ♦ attire for workers,
   ♦ special entrances and exits,
   ♦ negative pressure and high-efficiency particulate air filters, and
   ♦ other infection control prevention and surveillance measures (eg, particulate counts).[9]

   Thorough planning and coordination is necessary to minimize the risk for airborne infection both during projects and after their completion.[10]

4. Compliance with barrier precautions and traffic patterns should be monitored on an ongoing basis throughout and until the completion of the construction, renovation, or repair project. Monitoring provides an opportunity to rapidly correct any barrier or traffic restriction breach.

Recommended Practice VI

Policies and procedures for traffic patterns for patients, personnel, supplies, and equipment should be developed, reviewed periodically, revised as necessary, and kept readily available in the practice setting.

1. These recommended practices should be used as guidelines for developing written policies and procedures in the practice setting. Policies and procedures establish authority, responsibility, and accountability and serve as operational guidelines. Policies and procedures establish guidelines for performance improvement activities to be used when monitoring and evaluating traffic patterns in the surgical practice setting.

2. Information on traffic patterns and methods of handling supplies and equipment should be included in the orientation and continuing education of personnel to assist in the development of knowledge, skills, and attitudes that affect surgical patient outcomes. This education should include ancillary support or delivery personnel whose work activities require them to be within the semirestricted or restricted areas.

3. Policies and procedures should assist in the development of patient safety and quality assessment and improvement activities.

4. The uniform perioperative nursing vocabulary should be used in the development of policies and procedures related to traffic patterns. The perioperative nursing vocabulary is a clinically relevant and empirically validated standardized language. This standardized language consists of the Perioperative Nursing Data Set (PNDS) and includes perioperative nursing diagnoses, interventions, and outcomes. The expected outcome of primary importance to these recommended practices is outcome O10, "The patient is free from signs and symptoms of infection." This outcome falls within the domain of Physiological Responses (D2). The associated nursing diagnosis is X28, "Risk for infection." The associated interventions that may lead to the desired outcome may be I121, "Initiates traffic control"; I109, "Protects from cross-contamination"; I117, "Maintains continuous surveillance"; and I111, "Minimizes the length of invasive procedure by planning care."[11]

Glossary

Corrugated cardboard box: Web-edged box used for the purpose of containing items to be shipped for use in the OR.

Jumpsuit: One-piece suit that completely covers street clothes and can be worn in the semi restricted areas of the OR. *Synonyms:* coveralls, bunnysuit.

NOTES

1. "Recommended practices for surgical attire," in *Standards, Recommended Practices, and Guidelines* (Denver: AORN, Inc, 2005) 299-305.

2. J S Garner, Centers for Disease Control and Prevention Hospital Infection Control Practices Advisory Committee, "Guideline for isolation precautions in hospitals," *Infection Control and Hospital Epidemiology* 17 (January 1996) 53-80.

3. "The Health Insurance Portability and Accountability Act of 1996 (HIPAA)," Centers for Medicare and Medicaid Services, *http://www.cms.hhs.gov/hipaa* (accessed 13 Dec 2005).

4. A J Mangram et al, Centers for Disease Control and Prevention Hospital Infection Control Practices Advisory Committee, "Guideline for prevention of surgical site infection, 1999," *American Journal of Infection Control* 27 (April 1999) 97-134.

5. American Institute of Architects Academy of Architecture for Health, *Guidelines for Design and Construction of Hospital and Health Care Facilities* (Washington, DC: American Institute of Architects Press, 2001).

6. Association for the Advancement of Medical Instrumentation, *Steam Sterilization and Sterility Assurance in Health Care Facilities* (Arlington, Va: Association for the Advancement of Medical Instrumentation, 2002).

7. J M Bartley, "APIC state-of-the-art report: The role of infection control during construction in health care facilities," *American Journal of Infection Control* 28 (April 2000) 156-169.

8. J Bartley, "Construction and renovation," in *APIC Text of Infection Control and Epidemiology,* rev ed, J A Pfeiffer, ed (Washington, DC: Association for Professionals in Infection Control and Epidemiology, 2002) 72-1 to 72-11.

9. S A David, J A Fernandez, L A Herwaldt, "Infection control issues in construction and renovation," in *Practical Handbook for Healthcare Epidemiologists,* second ed, E Lautenbach, K F Woeltje, eds (Thorofare, NJ: Slack, 2004) 337-360.

10. Centers for Disease Control and Prevention, *Guidelines for Environmental Infection Control in Health-Care Facilities* (Atlanta: Centers for Disease Control and Prevention, 2003).

11. S C Beyea, ed, *Perioperative Nursing Data Set: The Perioperative Nursing Vocabulary,* second ed (Denver: AORN, Inc, 2002).

RESOURCE
"Infection control risk assessment matrix of precautions for construction and renovation," US Army Health Facility Planning Agency, *http://hfpa.otsg.amedd.army.mil/refs/docs/icra_assessment_form.pdf* (accessed 9 Dec 2005).

Originally published March 1982, *AORN Journal.*
Format revision July 1982.
Revised November 1988; May 1993.
Revised November 1995; published March 1996, *AORN Journal.*
Revised; published February 2000, *AORN Journal.*
Reformatted July 2000.
Revised November 2005; scheduled for publication in the *AORN Journal* in 2006.

ADDITIONAL RESOURCES

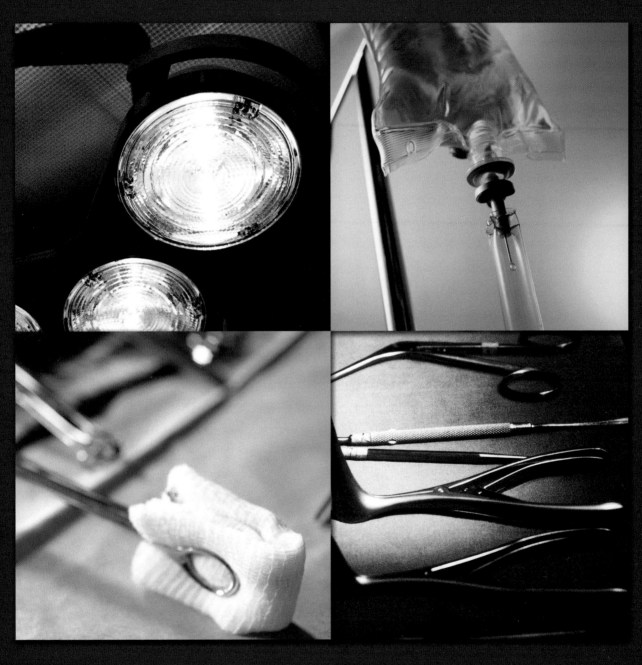

Section Four

Appendix A: Glossary of Times Used for Scheduling and Monitoring of Diagnostic and Therapeutic Procedures

The following glossary was developed by the Association of Anesthesia Clinical Directors (AACD) and was approved by their board of directors in October 1995. It has been endorsed by AORN, Inc, and the Society for Technology in Anesthesia and has been accepted without revision by the American Society of Anesthesiologists Committee on Quality Improvement and Practice Management. It is reprinted here with permission of the AACD.

Background

Elevated concerns regarding the economics of health care are dramatically intensifying the pressure for health care providers to establish critical pathways and/or total quality management programs. In addition, negotiating fiscally sound managed care contracts with health maintenance organizations and health insurance carriers, as well as meeting state and federal government documentation requirements, requires justification for each aspect of patient care as well as improved techniques in cost factor analysis and accounting. Few hospital administrators would deny that operating rooms/procedure rooms (OR/PR) are expensive to run, and all would concur that economic analyses of running OR/PRs are not readily available.

During the planning for multicenter studies of OR/PR scheduling, utilization, and efficiency, members of the Association of Anesthesia Clinical Directors (AACD) felt semantics were introducing a major impediment to data comparison and economic analysis. To provide a universal lexicon for the acquisition of data, the AACD has developed a glossary which inclusively, yet restrictively, defines the procedural times that permit comprehensive analyses of OR/PR scheduling, utilization, and efficiency. The AACD proposes adopting this lexicon as a standardized "Glossary of Times Used for Scheduling and Monitoring of Diagnostic and Therapeutic Procedures."

The glossary is divided into four sections: 1) Procedural Times, 2) Procedural and Scheduling Definitions and Time Periods, 3) Utilization and Efficiency Indices, and 4) Patient Categories. The terms defined under Procedural Times are listed in what is the usual chronological order, while terms defined in the other sections are presented in alphabetical order.

Glossary

1. Procedural Times

(For purposes of analyzing efficiency, each of the times defined below may be further classified by the subscripts S and A, for "Scheduled" and "Actual," respectively.)

1.1 Patient in Facility (PIF) = Time patient arrives at health care facility (applicable to outpatient or same day admission patients).

1.2 Patient Ready for Transport (PRT) = Time when all preparations required prior to transport (eg, labs, consent, gowning) have been completed.

1.3 Patient Sent-for (PS) = Time when transporting service is notified to deliver patient to the OR/PR.

1.4 Patient Available (PA) = Time the patient arrives in the OR/PR preprocedure area.

1.5 Room Set-up Start (RSS) = Time when personnel begin setting up, in the OR/PR, the supplies and equipment for the next case.

1.6 Anesthesia Start (AS) = Time when a member of the anesthesia team begins preparing the patient for an anesthetic.

1.7 Room Ready (RR) = Time when room is cleaned and supplies and equipment necessary for beginning of next case are present (see Discussion).

1.8 Patient In Room (PIR) = Time when patient enters the OR/PR.

1.9 Anesthesiologist, First Available (AFA) = Time of arrival in OR/PR of first anesthesiologist who is qualified to induce anesthesia in patient (see Discussion).

1.10 Procedure Physician, First Available (PPFA) = Time of arrival in OR/PR of first physician/surgeon qualified to position and prep the patient (see Discussion).

1.11 Anesthesiologist of Record In (ARI) = Time of arrival in OR/PR of anesthesiologist of record (see Discussion).

1.12 Anesthesia Induction (AI) = Time when the anesthesiologist begins the administration of agents intended to provide the level of anesthesia required for the scheduled procedure.

1.13 Anesthesia Ready (AR) = Time at which the patient has a sufficient level of anesthesia established to begin surgical preparation of the patient, and remaining anesthetic chores do not preclude positioning and prepping the patient (see Discussion).

1.14 Position/Prep Start (PS) = Time at which the nursing or surgical team begins positioning or prepping the patient for the procedure.

1.15 Prep-Completed (PC) = Time at which prepping and draping have been completed and patient is ready for the procedure or surgery to start.

1.16 Procedure Physician of Record In (PPRI) = Arrival time of physician/surgeon of record (see Discussion).

1.17 Procedure/Surgery Start Time (PST) = Time the procedure is begun (eg, incision for a surgical procedure, insertion of scope for a diagnostic procedure, beginning of exam under anesthesia [EUA], shooting of x-ray for radiological procedure).

1.18 Procedure/Surgery Conclusion Begun (PCB) = Time when diagnostic or therapeutic maneuvers are completed and attempts are made by the physician or surgical team to end any noxious stimuli (eg, beginning of wound closure, removal of bronchoscope).

1.19 Procedure Physician of Record Out (PPRO) = Time when physician/surgeon of record leaves the OR/PR (see Discussion).

1.20 Procedure/Surgery Finish (PF) = Time when all instrument and sponge counts are completed and verified as correct; all postoperative radiological studies to be done in the OR/PR are completed; all dressings and drains are secured; and the physician/surgeons have completed all procedure-related activities on the patient.

1.21 Patient Out of Room (POR) = Time at which patient leaves OR/PR.

1.22 Room Clean-up Start (RCS) = Time housekeeping or room personnel begin clean-up of OR/PR.

1.23 Arrival in PACU/ICU (APACU) = Time of patient arrival in PACU or ICU.

1.24 Anesthesia Finish (AF) = Time at which anesthesiologist turns over care of the patient to a postanesthesia care team (either PACU or ICU).

1.25 Room Clean-up Finish (RCF) = Time OR/PR is clean and ready for set-up of supplies and equipment for the next case.

1.26 Ready-for-Discharge from Postanesthesia Care Unit (RDPACU) = Time that patient is assessed to be ready for discharge from the PACU.

1.27 Discharge from Postanesthesia Care Unit (DPACU) = Time patient is transported out of PACU.

1.28 Arrival in Same Day Surgery Recovery Unit = Time of patient arrival in same day surgery recovery unit.

1.29 Ready-for-Discharge from Same Day Surgery Recovery Unit (RDSDSR) = Time that patient is assessed to be ready for discharge from the same day surgery recovery unit.

1.30 Discharge from Same Day Surgery Recovery Unit (DSDSR) = Time patient leaves SDSR unit (either to home or other facility).

2. Procedural and Scheduling Definitions and Time Periods

(For purposes of analyzing efficiency, each of the time periods defined below may be further classified by the subscripts E and A for "Estimated" and "Actual," respectively.)

2.1 Anesthesia Preparation Time (APT) = Time from Anesthesia Start to Anesthesia Ready Time.

2.2 Average Case Length (ACL) = Total hours divided by total number of cases performed within those hours.

2.3 Block Time (BT) = Hours of OR/PR time reserved for a given service or physician/surgeon. Within a defined cutoff period (eg, 72 hours prior to day of surgery), this is time into which only the given service may schedule. (NB: In some institutions, this is known as available or allocated time.)

2.4 Case Time (CT) = Time from Room Set-up Start to Room Clean-up Finished (see Discussion).

2.5 Early Start Hours (ESH) = Hours of Case Time performed prior to the normal day's start time when it is not expected that the Patient Out of Room Time will be before the normal start time for that day.

2.6 Evening/Weekend/Holiday Hours (EWHH) = Hours of Case Time performed outside of Resource Hours.

2.7 In-own Block Hours (IBH) = Hours of Case Time performed during a service's own Block Time. (NB: For a case to be counted in IBH, it must begin during that given service's Block Time.)

2.8 Open Time (OT) = Hours of OR/PR time not reserved for any particular service, into which any service or physician/surgeon may schedule according to the rules established by the given institution. (NB: In some institutions, this is known as discretionary time).

2.9 Outside-own Block Hours (OBH) = Hours of Case Time performed during Resource Hours but outside of the service's Block Time.

2.10 Overrun Hours (OVRH) = Hours of Case Time completed after the scheduled closure time of the OR/PR (ie, after the end of that day's Resource Hours).

2.11 Released Time (RT) = Hours of OR/PR time that are released from a service's Block Time and converted to Open Time (typically done when a service anticipates that it will be unable to use the Block Time due to meetings or vacation).

2.12 Resource Hours (RH) = Total number of hours scheduled to be available for performance of procedures (ie, the sum of all available Block Time and Open Time). This is typically provided for on a weekly recurring basis, but may be analyzed on a daily, weekly, monthly, or annual basis (see Discussion).

2.13 Room Clean-up Time (RCT) = Time from Patient Out of Room to Room Clean-up Finished.

2.14 Room Close (RC) = Time at which the room should be empty and the assigned personnel free to be discharged.

2.15 Room Open (RO) = Time when appropriate staff are scheduled to be present and are expected to have the OR/PR available for patient occupancy.

2.16 Room Set-up Time (RST) = Time from Room Set-up Start to Room Ready.

2.17 Service = A group of physicians or surgeons that together perform a circumscribed set of operative or diagnostic procedures (eg, cardiothoracic surgery, interventional radiology). Generally, any member of a service may schedule into that service's block time. Similarly, OR/PR time used by a given physician or surgeon is credited to his/her service's Total Hours.

2.18 Surgical Preparation Time (SPT) = Time from Position/Prep Start to Procedure/Surgery Start Time.

2.19 Start Time (ST) = Patient In Room Time (see Discussion).

2.20 Total Cases (TC) = Cumulative total of all cases done in a given time period. May be subdivided by service or physician/surgeon.

2.21 Total Hours (TH) = Sum of all Case Times for a given period of time. TH = IBH + OBH + EWHH. May be subdivided by service or individual physician/surgeon.

2.22 Turnover Time (TOT) = Time from prior Patient Out of Room to succeeding Patient In Room Time for sequentially scheduled cases (see Discussion).

3. Utilization and Efficiency Indices

3.1 Adjusted-Percent Service Utilization (ASU) = (IBH + OBH) x 100 ÷ BT. This measures the percentage of time a service utilizes their Block Time during Resource Hours. It is adjusted, compared to Raw Utilization, in that it gives a service "credit" for the time necessary to set up and clean up a room, during which time a patient cannot be in the room. It may exceed 100% because of the inclusion of cases performed during Resource Hours that are Outside-own Block Hours (see Discussion).

3.2 Adjusted-Percent Utilized Resource Hours (AURH) = (Total Hours-Evening/Weekend/Holiday Hours) ÷ Resource Hours x 100. This calculation provides the percentage of time that the OR/PRs are being prepared for a patient, are occupied by a patient, or are being cleaned after taking care of a patient during Resource Hours. It is adjusted, compared to Raw Utilization, in that it includes the time necessary to set up and clean up a room, during which time a patient cannot be in the room (see Discussion).

3.3 Delays may be due to:

    3.3.1 Patient issues
        Insurance problems
        Patient arrived late
        Patient ate/drank
        Abnormal lab values
        Surgery issues
        Complications arose

    3.3.2 System issues
        Test results unavailable
        Blood unavailable
        Patient not ready on floor
        Transport delay
        Elevator delay
        Previous case ran late
        Case bumped for emergency case
        Equipment unavailable
        Equipment malfunction
        X-rays unavailable
        X-ray technician unavailable
        Delay in receiving floor bed
        Insufficient post procedure care beds
        ICU delay
        Instrument problem

    3.3.3 Practitioner issues
        Needs more workup (eg, labs, consults)
        No consent
        Physician/surgeon arrived late
        Anesthesiologist arrived late
        Physician/surgeon unavailable
        Anesthesiologist unavailable
        Inaccurate posting
        Prolonged set-up time

3.4 Early Start = When Patient In Room, Actual, is prior to Patient In Room, Scheduled.

3.4.1 With overlap—When a case starts early but prior to the Room Clean-up Finished, Actual, of the case originally scheduled to precede it (this occurs when either the preceding or following case is moved to a different OR/PR than originally scheduled).

3.4.2 Without overlap—When a case starts early but after the Room Clean-up Finished, Actual, of the case originally scheduled to precede it (this may occur because there is no preceding case or because the preceding case finishes earlier than scheduled).

3.5 Late Start = When Patient In Room, Actual, is after Patient In Room, Scheduled.

3.5.1 With no interference—when the Room Clean-up Finished, Actual, of the preceding case occurs before the Room Set-up Start, Scheduled, of the following case (ie, the OR/PR is available prior to or at the time that preparation for the next case is supposed to begin).

3.5.2 With interference—When Room Clean-up Finished, Actual, of the preceding case occurs after the Room Set-up Start, Scheduled, of the following case (ie, the OR/PR is not available at the time that preparation for the next case is supposed to begin, either because it is still occupied or because it has not been cleaned).

3.6 Overrun = When Room Clean-up Finished, Actual, for the last scheduled case of the day is later than Room Close. This may be caused by a late start; a Case Time, Actual, greater than Case Time, Scheduled; or a combination of late start and longer than scheduled Case Time.

3.7 Productivity Index (PI) = Percent of time per hour that a patient is in the OR/PR during the prime shift time (eg, first 8 hours).

3.8 Raw Utilization (RU) = For the system as a whole, this is the percent of time that patients are in the room during Resource Hours (see Adjusted-Percent Utilized Resource Hours). For an individual service, this is the percent of its Block Time during which a service has a patient in the OR/PR (see Adjusted-Percent Service Utilization).

3.9 Room Gap = Time OR/PRs are vacant during Resource Hours.

3.9.1 Empty Room (or Late Start) Gap (LSG)
Planned—When Patient In Room, Scheduled, is later than Room Open.

Unplanned—When Patient In Room, Actual, is later than Room Open.

3.9.2 Between Case Gaps (BCG)
Planned—When Patient In Room, Scheduled, is later than the Room Clean-up Finished, Actual, of the preceding case.
Unplanned—When Patient In Room, Actual, is later than the Room Clean-up Finished, Actual, of the preceding case.

3.9.3 End of Schedule Gaps (ESG)
Planned—When Room Clean-up Finished, Scheduled, occurs before Room Close.
Unplanned—When Room Clean-up Finished, Actual, occurs before Room Close.

3.9.4 Total Gap Hours (TGH) = LSG + BCG + ESG.

4. Patient Categories

4.1 In-house (IH) = Patient admitted to and residing in the hospital prior to scheduled surgery/procedure.

4.2 Outpatient (OP) = Patient who is coming in on the day of surgery/procedure and is expected to return home following the procedure.

4.3 Same Day Admit (SDA) = Patient who is coming in on the day of surgery/procedure and will be admitted to the hospital following the procedure.

4.4 Overnight-Recovery (ONR) = Patient who comes in on the day of surgery/procedure but requires overnight recovery prior to returning home. These patients are never admitted to the hospital as inpatients, but may remain in the recovery facility for 12 to 23 hours post surgery/procedure.

Discussion

The foregoing list of the procedural times was intentionally made exhaustive in order to be all inclusive. This by no means suggests that all of the data points defined need to be collected by all institutions. Where problems with OR/PR efficiency exist, whether they are real or perceptual, collecting the appropriate times listed above, and calculating the pertinent time periods, will permit objective evaluation of where the real problems lie. Use of common definitions across the country will also permit inter-institutional comparisons that have been previously impossible.

Several terms listed in the "Procedural Times Glossary" have not had heretofore universally accepted definitions. For several of these, the authors, the board of directors of the Association of Anesthesia Clinical Directors, and the Society for Technology in Anesthesia National Database Committee felt that there existed significant controversy over which definition should be chosen. Although for each of these a consensus was generated which led to the definition chosen, general acceptance of these choices may be improved if the logic behind the decision is known. For those terms which created serious debate, the following discussion of terms is provided.

Adjusted-Percent Service Utilization (ASU) = (IBH + OBH) x 100 ÷ BT. This measures the percentage of time a service utilizes its Block Time during Resource Hours. It is adjusted, compared to raw utilization, in that it gives a service "credit" for the time necessary to set up and clean up a room, during which time a patient cannot be in the room. It may exceed 100% because of the inclusion of cases performed during Resource Hours that are Outside-own Block Hours.

Adjusted-Percent Utilized Resource Hours (AURH) = (Total Hours-Evening/Weekend/Holiday Hours) ÷ Resource Hours x 100. This calculation provides the percentage of time that the OR/PRs are being prepared for a patient, are occupied by a patient, or are being cleaned after taking care of a patient during Resource Hours. It is adjusted, compared to raw utilization, in that it includes the time necessary to set up and clean up a room, during which time a patient cannot be in the room.

Raw Utilization (RU) = For the system as a whole, this is the percent of time that patients are in the room during Resource Hours (see Adjusted Percent Utilization Resource Hours). For an individual service, this is the percent of its Block Time during which a service has a patient in the OR/PR (see Adjusted-Percent Utilization).

Frequently, institutions attempt to assess the extent to which a service uses its allotted Block Time by calculating a utilization percentage. Such a calculation should be performed for the system as a whole to measure the extent to which the "normal" hours of operation are actually used for patient care. If one considers only the time that a patient is in the OR/PR (raw utilization), then the percent of time that a service uses its Block Time is

artificially lowered because the time necessary to set up and clean up a room, during which time a patient cannot be in the room, is not accounted for. Similarly, the calculation of percentage utilization of Resource Hours is artificially reduced if only Patient In Room time is used. The larger the number of procedures done in a given room during Resource Hours, the greater the error.

Cost-effective utilization requires highly effective scheduling and optimum utilization of the Resource Hours, with minimal overtime and/or uses of more highly paid on-call personnel. For proper assessment of the extent to which a service or system utilizes its Block or Resource Hours, respectively, the utilization calculations should be adjusted as defined above. For the individual service, this provides a fairer determination of how much of its Block Time is truly used. For the system as a whole, it provides the actual percentage of time that the OR/PRs are being used for patient care. Perhaps as important, it provides an accurate percentage of time that is not used and therefore available for efficiency improvements.

Anesthesiologist, First Available (AFA) = Time of arrival in OR/PR of first anesthesiologist who is qualified to induce anesthesia in patient.

Procedure Physician, First Available (PPFA) = Time of arrival in OR/PR of first physician/surgeon qualified to position and prep the patient.

If delays in starting cases are thought to be due to the late arrival of either a qualified anesthesiologist or surgeon, recording of these times will allow documentation of the extent of that cause of delay.

Anesthesia Ready (AR) = Time at which the patient has a sufficient level of anesthesia established to begin surgical preparation of the patient, and remaining anesthetic chores do not preclude positioning and prepping the patient.

To maximize efficiency, surgical preparation of the patient should begin as soon as an adequate level of anesthesia has been obtained. In some instances however, the anesthesiologist may need to continue anesthetic preparation of the patient (eg, insertion of Swan-Ganz catheter) that precludes moving or prepping the patient. Anesthesia Ready is thus defined as that time when the anesthesiologist may allow surgical preparation to begin.

Anesthesiologist of Record In (ARI) = Time of arrival in OR/PR of anesthesiologist of record.

Procedure Physician of Record In (PPRI) = Arrival time of physician/surgeon of record.

In academic settings, delays may be due to the late arrival of either the attending anesthesiologist or surgeon. Recording of these times will allow one to determine if tardiness of either attending contributes to delays. Further, in the future, accrediting bodies and insurance carriers may require documentation of the time of presence of the physicians of record.

Case Time (CT) = Time from Room Set-up Start to Room Clean-up Finished.

This definition includes all of the time for which a given procedure requires an OR/PR. It allows for the different duration of Room Set-up and Room Clean-up Times that occur because of the varying supply and equipment needs for a particular procedure. For purposes of scheduling and efficiency analysis, this definition is ideal because it includes all of the time that an OR/PR must be reserved for a given procedure.

Procedure Physician of Record Out (PPRO) = Time when physician/surgeon of record leaves the OR/PR.

Because perceptual differences of turnover times abound, it is important to note when the physician of record leaves the OR/PR, as this may be significantly earlier than when the patient leaves the OR/PR. In those situations when an anesthesiologist is supervising another anesthesia care provider (resident or CRNA), the anesthesiologist of record may be in and out of the OR/PR multiple times, and thus no analogous definition has been provided for.

Resource Hours = Total number of hours scheduled to be available for performance of procedures (ie, the sum of all available Block Time and Open Time). This is typically provided for on a weekly recurring basis, but may be analyzed on a daily, weekly, monthly, or annual basis.

For a given institution, this is the time during which an optimum number of appropriate personnel are available to do cases. This may include more than one shift of personnel, or personnel working extended shifts (ie, greater than 8 hours), in order to gain vertical expansion of OR/PR hours. It may also include electively scheduled time on weekends to gain horizontal expansion of OR/PR hours. Resource hours do not include time gained through overtime or use of on-call personnel, even though this time may be routinely accrued at a given institution.

Room Ready (RR) = Time when room is cleaned and supplies and equipment necessary for beginning of next case are present. To maximize efficiency, the patient should be brought into the OR/PR as early as possible. Although some wish to have all the supplies and equipment necessary for the entire case present and open before the patient is brought in, institutions that have minimized turnover times move patients into the OR/PR as soon as it is clean and only the minimum supplies and equipment (ie, those needed to start the case) are present, but not necessarily open. In those institutions, room preparation continues as anesthesia in induced, allowing an overlap of processes (anesthesia induction and room preparation) that saves time.

Start Time (ST) = Patient in Room Time. Significant debate, indeed, even argument, exists over the proper definition of Start Time. Operating and procedural room nurses generally feel that they have properly accomplished their preparatory tasks if the room is ready at the scheduled start time (Room Ready = Start Time, Estimated), regardless of where the patient is at that time. Anesthesiologists often feel that they are "on time" if anesthesia induction has been completed by the scheduled start time (Anesthesia Ready = Start Time, Estimated). Surgeons generally believe start time should be the time at which the procedure is begun (Procedure/Surgery Start Time = Start Time, Estimated). Since Room Set-up Time is procedure specific and therefore generally known at the time of scheduling, one can reasonably predict Room Ready Time. Anesthesia Preparation Time, however, depends on both the procedure and patient needs. It is thus more variable and not known at the time a procedure is scheduled, making accurate prediction of Anesthesia Ready Time impossible.

This variability in Anesthesia Preparation Time also makes prediction of Procedure/Surgery Start Time inaccurate. Variability in Case Times, due to varying length of surgery, makes prediction of Start Times after the first scheduled case of the day even more inaccurate.

Much of the concern over Start Time is for the first case of the day, particularly when a service or surgeon follows herself/himself in the same OR/PR throughout the day. Prediction, then, of accurate Start Times for the first case of the day appears to be most critical. Once the procedure is known, it is almost always possible to have the Room Ready at any time that is desired for the start of the day. It should also be possible, and desirable for maximizing efficiency, to have the patient in the room for the first case of the day as soon as the room is ready. For maximizing scheduling accuracy and attempting to encourage the most efficient patient flow, the authors have elected to define Start Time as Patient In Room Time.

Turnover Time (TOT) = Time from prior Patient Out of Room to succeeding Patient In Room Time. Strong perceptual differences exist over the definition of Turnover Time. Anesthesiologists and OR/PR nurses usually consider turnover time to be the time between cases when the room is not occupied by a patient. Surgeons consider any time when they are unable to operate as "down time," and thus more often consider turnover time to be the time between the end of surgery on one case and the beginning of surgery on the next case. The latter may appear to be particularly long to an academic surgeon who leaves an OR before the wound is closed (allowing the residents to close and dress the incision) and does not re-enter the OR until the next patient is ready for incision.

As with Start Time, the variability of Anesthesia Preparation Time (APT) makes prediction of turnover times inaccurate if APT were to be included. Thus, to maximize scheduling accuracy and to encourage distinction of time spent preparing the OR/PR from time spent preparing the patient, the authors have elected to define Turnover Time as time from prior Patient Out of Room to succeeding Patient In Room Time for sequentially scheduled cases. As this definition attempts to include the time spent cleaning and preparing the OR/PR for the next case, it should only be calculated if a subsequent case is scheduled to immediately follow. With nonsequential cases, idle time between Room Clean-up Finished for the prior case to Room Set-up Start for the subsequent case should be identified and recorded under the appropriate room-gap category.

Copyright © Association of Anesthesia Clinical Directors, 1997. Reprinted with permission.

Index to 2006 Edition

A

AABB (American Association of Blood Banks) 646

Administrative practice standards 393-396

Advanced cardiac life support 434

Advanced practice nurse
APN, definition 427
definition, position statement 352
in RNFA programs 425

Air exchanges per hour, OR 660

Air pressure, OR 660

Airborne precautions 617, 660; *See also* Standard and transmission-based precautions

Ambulatory surgery guidelines
application of PNDS 295-302, 303-308
postoperative patient care 295-302
preoperative patient care 303-308

American Association of Nurse Anesthetists (AANA) 442

American Association of Tissue Banks (AATB) 656

American Conference of Governmental Industrial Hygienists (ACGIH) 473

American Society for Gastrointestinal Endoscopy 469

American Society of Anesthesiologists (ASA) 435, 442

American Society of Bariatric Surgeons (ASBS) 140

American Society of PeriAnesthesia Nurses 295

ANA Code of Ethics, perioperative explications for 167-198; *See also* Explications for perioperative nursing

Analgesia and moderate sedation 433-440
advanced cardiac life support (ACLS) 434
adverse reactions 436
assessment 435
clinical competency 434
complications of 436
continuum of depth of sedation 434
discharge instructions 437
documentation 437
equipment selection and use 435-436
monitoring the patient 434
objectives of sedation 433
physical status classification 435, 436
policies and procedures for 438

Anesthesia equipment, cleaning, handling, and processing 441-450
aseptic technique in 441
bacterial filters, use of 445
CDC recommendations for 441, 442, 443
competency of personnel 442
critical items 441

exterior surfaces, cleaning 443
guidelines for processing 446
hazards, potential 446
humidifiers, use of 445
internal components, cleaning 445
malignant hyperthermia (MH) risk 444
medication administration 441
noncritical items 443
performance and safety criteria 444
personal protective equipment (PPE) for 446
policies and procedures for 447
reprocessing single-use devices 444
reusable equipment 443
semicritical items 442
sharps handling 446
single-use items 443-444
storage of items 442
waste disposal 445

Anesthesia, local 571-574; *See also* Local anesthesia

Antisepsis, surgical hand scrub 537-546; *See also* Hand antisepsis, surgical

Antiseptic agent for skin prep 604

AORN explications for perioperative nursing 167-198; *See also* Explications for perioperative nursing

Archived position statements 344

Artificial nails 538

Aseptic practices 621-628; *See also* Sterile field, maintaining

Association for Professionals in Infection Control and Epidemiology, Inc (APIC) 442

Association for the Advancement of Medical Instrumentation (AAMI) 262, 621, 629

Association of Anesthesia Clinical Directors (AACD) glossary 665-672; *See also* Glossary of procedural times

Attire, surgical 451-458
cover apparel, use of 452
disposal of 451
fabric selection 451
gloves, selection and use 454
hair, head and facial 453
head covers, use of 453
home laundering of 451-452
in restricted and semirestricted areas 451-452
jewelry 453
laundering 451-452
masks, when to wear 453, 454
nonscrubbed personnel 452
personal protective equipment (PPE) for 452
policies and procedures for 455

knowledge of wound healing 422
participation in plan of care 422
participation in rehabilitation process 421
right to privacy 423
value system, lifestyle, ethnicity, culture 423
perioperative safety 416-418
chemical injury 416
electrical injury 416
laser injury 417
medication safety 417
positioning injury 417
radiation injury 417
transfer/transport injury 417
physiologic responses 418-420
cardiovascular function 419
fluid, electrolyte, and acid-base balances 419
infection 418
neurological function 420
normothermia 418
pain control 420
respiratory function 419
wound/tissue perfusion 418

P

Packaging systems 575-580
aseptic presentation 576-577
evaluation of 575
event related sterility 578
for ethylene oxide (EO) 575-576
for hydrogen peroxide plasma sterilization 576
for steam sterilization 575
labeling 578
manufacturers' instructions 575, 576
packaging materials 576
peel packages 576, 577
rigid container systems 577
sequential wrapping 576
shelf life 578
sterilization compatibility 575-576
Pain management 64-66, 420
PASS (acronym) 256
Patient attire 660
body piercing 486
jewelry 486
masks 660
personal undergarments 660
Patient focused model, perioperative; See Perioperative patient focused model
Patient positioning, See Positioning the patient

Patient safety culture, guidance statement on 289-294
accountability model 291, 292
accountable, definition 293
adverse event, definition 293
culture, definition 289
disciplinary system theory approach 290
failure mode and effects analysis (FMEA) 289, 293
flexible culture 290
just culture 290, 293
learning culture 290
medical error, definition 293
near miss 293
negligence, definition 293
nonpunitive environment vs individual accountability 290
patient-centric safety culture 289, 290, 293
relationship between discipline and patient safety 291
reporting culture 289
root cause analysis (RCA) 289, 293
wary culture 290
Patient skin prep 603-606; See also Skin preparation, surgical
Patient's right to privacy 89
Patients with IEDs, perioperative care of 265-288
application of PNDS 279-278
cardiac IEDs 267-270, 284
gastric electronic stimulation 279
gastric stimulation devices 287
general patient management 266-267
general safety issues 266
implantable hearing devices 272-275, 286
implantable infusion pumps 275-276, 286
neurological IEDs 285
neurostimulators 270-272
osteogenic stimulators 276-279, 287
sacral nerve stimulators 276, 287
Peel pouches 576, 577, 623
Perioperative care coordinator nurse competency statements 125-136
Perioperative nurse, definition 7, 15
Perioperative nursing
administrative practice standards 393-396
clinical practice standards 397-400
patient care quality 389-390
patient outcomes standards 415-424
position statements 345-386
quality and performance improvement standards 405-414
standards of 391-392

S